Perspectives in Exercise Science
and Sports Medicine: Volume 8

Exercise in Older Adults

Edited by

Carl V. Gisolfi, Ph.D.
University of Iowa

David R. Lamb, Ph.D.
The Ohio State University

Ethan Nadel, Ph.D.
Yale University School of Medicine

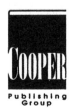

COOPER
Publishing
Group

Library of Congress Cataloging in Publication Data:
LAMB, DAVID R., 1939–
PERSPECTIVES IN EXERCISE SCIENCE AND SPORTS MEDICINE
VOLUME 8: EXERCISE IN OLDER ADULTS

Cover Design: Gary Schmitt

Library of Congress Catalog Card number: 88-70343

ISBN: 1-884125-20-4

Printed in the United States of America by Cooper Publishing Group, 1048 Summit Drive, Carmel, IN 46032
10 9 8 7 6 5 4 3 2

Contents

Contributors

Kenneth M. Baldwin, Ph.D.
Department of Physiology and
Biophysics
University of California
Irvine, CA 92717

Oded Bar-Or, M.D.
McMaster University
Chedoke Hospital
Hamilton, ON L8N 3Zs
CANADA

Susan A. Bloomfield, Ph.D.
Dept. of Health & Kinesiology
Texas A&M University
College Station, TX 77843

Jeffery B. Blumberg, Ph.D.
USDA Human Nutrition Research
Center on Aging
Tufts University
Boston, MA 02111

Claude Bouchard, Ph.D.
Physical Activity Science
Laboratory
Laval University
Ste. Foy, Quebec G1K 7P4
CANADA

Priscilla M. Clarkson, Ph.D.
University of Massachusetts
Boyden Building—Exercise Science
Amherst, MA 01003

Edward T. Coyle, Ph.D.
Human Performance Laboratory
The University of Texas at Austin
Austin, TX 78712

J. Mark Davis, Ph.D.
University of South Carolina
Department of Exercise Science
Columbia, SC 29208

Jerome A. Dempsey, Ph.D.
Preventive Medicine
University of Wisconsin
Center for Health Science
Madison, WI 53706

Loretta DiPietro, Ph.D.
John B. Pierce Foundation Laboratory
Yale University School of Medicine
New Haven, CT 06519

Dennis Eddy, Ph.D.
Gatorade Exercise Physiology
Laboratory
The Gatorade Company
Barrington, IL 60010

V. Reggie Edgerton, Ph.D.
Department of Kinesiology
University of California
Los Angeles, CA 90024

E. Randy Eichner, M.D.
University of Oklahoma
Health Sciences Center
Hematology Laboratory
Oklahoma City, OK 73190

William Evans, Ph.D.
Noll Laboratory
The Pennsylvania State University
University Park, PA 16802

Carl V. Gisolfi, Ph.D.
Department of Exercise Science
University of Iowa
Iowa City, IA 52242

Steven Gregg, Ph.D.
Gatorade Exercise Physiology
Gatorade Europe, Inc.
1200 Brussels
BELGIUM

William J. Haskell, Ph.D.
Stanford Center for Research
in Disease Prevention
Stanford University
Palo Alto, CA 94304-1583

Walter Hempenius, Ph.D.
The Gatorade Company
Barrington, IL 60010

Mitch Kanter, Ph.D.
Gatorade Exercise Physiology
Laboratory
The Gatorade Company
Barrington, IL 60010

W. Larry Kenney, Ph.D.
Noll Laboratory
Pennsylvania State University
University Park, PA 16802

Howard G. Knuttgen, Ph.D.
Pennsylvania State University
Center for Sports Medicine
University Park, PA 16802

Ricardo Javornik, M.D.
Productos Quaker, C.A.
Caracas
VENEZUELA

Edward G. Lakatta, M.D.
Gerontology Research Center
National Institute on Aging
Baltimore, MD 21224

David R. Lamb, Ph.D.
Sport and Exercise Science Faculty
The Ohio State University
Columbus, OH 43210

Ronald Maughan, Ph.D.
University Medical School
Department of Environmental
and Occupational Medicine
Foresterhill, Aberdeen A39 2ZD
SCOTLAND

Mohsen Meydani, Ph.D.
USDA Human Nutrition Research
Center on Aging
Tufts University
Boston, MA 02111

Francisco Mora, Ph.D.
Department of Physiology
Faculty of Medicine
Central University
28040 Madrid
SPAIN

Robert Murray, Ph.D.
Gatorade Exercise Physiology
Laboratory
The Gatorade Company
Barrington, IL 60010

Ethan Nadel, Ph.D.
John B. Pierce Foundation Laboratory
Yale University School of Medicine
New Haven, CT 06519

Mark S. Nash, Ph.D.
University of Miami
School of Medicine
Miami, FL 33136

David C. Nieman, Ph.D.
Appalachian State University
Dept. of Health, Leisure
and Exercise Science
Boone, NC 28608

Wayne T. Phillips, Ph.D.
Stanford Center for Research
in Disease Prevention
Stanford University
Palo Alto, CA 94304-1583

Gerald M. Reaven, M.D.
GRECC-182B
VA Medical Center
Palo Alto, CA 94304

Ronald Rogowski, Ph.D.
The Gatorade Company
Barrington, IL 60010

Douglas R. Seals, Ph.D.
University of Colorado
Dept. of Kinesiology
Boulder, CO 80309

Waneen W. Spirduso, Ed.D.
University of Texas at Austin
Dept. of Kinesiology and Health
Education
Austin, TX 78712

Lawrence L. Spriet, Ph.D.
University of Guelph
School of Human Biology
Guelph, ON N1G 2W1
CANADA

John R. Sutton, M.D.
Cumberland College of Health Sciences
New South Wales 2141
AUSTRALIA

Ronald L. Terjung, Ph.D.
Department of Physiology
SUNY Health Science Center
Syracuse, NY 13210

Charles M. Tipton, Ph.D.
Department of Exercise and Sport
Sciences
University of Arizona
Tucson, AZ 84721

Timothy P. White, Ph.D.
Dept. of Human Biodynamics
University of California
Berkeley, CA 94720

Clyde Williams, Ph.D.
Loughborough University
Department of Physical Education,
Sport Studies and Recreation
Loughborough, Leicestershire LB11
3TU
ENGLAND

Acknowledgement

As part of our continuing commitment to research and education in sports science and sports nutrition, Gatorade is proud to sponsor the series, *Perspectives in Exercise Science and Sports Medicine.* As with the previous seven volumes of the series, this book resulted from our annual Gatorade Sports Science Institute *Perspectives* Conference at which invited scientists of international repute discuss a variety of scientific issues related to an annual theme; in this case, the participants enthusiastically debated the effects and potential benefits of habitual physical activity in older adults.

We hope that you will find this volume to be a valuable addition to your professional library. Congratulations to the authors, reviewers, and editors for a job extremely well done.

James F. Doyle
President
Quaker Oats Beverages

Foreword

The **Perspectives in Exercise Science and Sports Medicine** series reflects an enduring commitment by The Gatorade Company, and the Gatorade Sports Science Institute to enhance the field of exercise science and sports medicine. This volume joins seven others that are widely recognized as essential holdings in our personal and institutional libraries, as they provide a scholarly treatment to selected topics of central importance to our field.

On behalf of the members, fellows, officers, and trustees of the American College of Sports Medicine (ACSM), I extend a hearty thank you to The Gatorade Company a thoughtful supporter of ACSM, which is a not-for-profit scientific and medical society dedicated to improving health through physical activity. The generosity of Gatorade for over a decade has enriched many of ACSM's programs, including the Annual Meeting and Research Roundtables. Indeed, all of the royalties from the sale of the **Perspectives** series are donated to the ACSM Foundation, where they are used to support our research and educational initiatives.

I congratulate the editors, authors, and organizers of the Gatorade Sports Science Institute conference that led to the publication of this volume focused on exercise in older adults. It is apparent that impairments in human performance are inevitable consequences of longevity and that they affect the very fabric of life. Declines with age in strength, mobility, balance, and endurance result in large measure from the alterations in molecules, cells, organs, and systems that comprise the human organism. The impairments can negatively affect fundamental levels of human performance, such as the accomplishment of life's daily activities. In turn, these fundamental abilities provide the basis for independence, which is of profound importance for the quality of life of older persons. Obviously, age-associated declines in the ability to generate and sustain muscular power also affect the performance of recreational and elite participants in sports and dance.

There are rich opportunities for scientific and medical discoveries in aging and for exercise interventions that can improve the quality of life of older persons. This volume holds high promise to stimulate further work in physical activity and aging.

Timothy P. White, Ph.D.
President
American College of Sports Medicine

Preface

The primary goal of this volume was to evaluate the hypothesis that increased physical activity preserves function during the aging process. In addressing this hypothesis, the chapters of this volume are intended to provide insight into i) the mechanisms associated with the decrements in functional status with aging, ii) the mechanisms underlying any improvements in function that may be induced by increased activity, and iii) issues related to exercise and aging that require further study.

The traditional view of the aging process has been that of a progressive decline in health and in the ability to function independently. The emerging view of the aging process distinguishes the decline in function due to biological aging from that caused by the reduced participation in physical activity that is so common in older people. Any decline in function caused by inactivity could theoretically be attenuated or even reversed by adopting a more active lifestyle.

In this volume, leaders in the field address the mechanisms by which physiological deficits occur with aging and the extent to which the rates of decline are altered by increasing physical activity. Chapter topics range from the relationships among aging, fitness, health, and longevity to the influences of physical activity on insulin resistance and immune function in older adults. The timeliness and importance of the topics in this volume are clear. More than 30 million persons living in the United States—12% of the population—are 65 years of age or older. Accompanying these demographics of aging is the increasing prevalence of functional impairment and chronic disease in the older population. Americans over 65 years account for approximately 30% of U.S. health care expenditures, and most of these costs are incurred in the last five years of life. Clearly, the benefits to society, not to mention to those afflicted, would be enormous if the onset of functional limitations could be postponed or eliminated altogether.

We gratefully acknowledge the support of the Gatorade Company, which since 1987 has sponsored free and open scientific exchanges by experts invited to the discussion table at outstanding scientific conferences, has facilitated the publication of the proceedings of these conferences in *Perspectives in Exercise Science and Sports Medicine*, and has generously donated the proceeds from the book sales to the American College of Sports Medicine. We are particularly grateful for the continuing support of Jim Doyle, President of Gatorade Worldwide, Ron Rogowski, Ph.D., Vice President of Gatorade Worldwide Research and Development, and Bob Murray, Ph.D., Director of the Gatorade Exercise Physiology Laboratory. We are also indebted to Cozette Lamb, whose extensive editorial contributions have markedly enhanced the quality of this volume, and to Joan Seye and Betty Dye, who did a marvelous job of rapidly transcribing the chapter discussions for editing by the scientist participants before the conference was concluded. We also appreciate the efforts of Butch and Joanne Cooper and their colleagues at the Cooper Publishing Group, especially Kendal Gladish, the superb copy editor, for insuring that the book was produced in a first-rate manner. Finally, we thank Kathryn Bowling and her associates at McCord Travel Management; they excelled at arranging international travel to the conference, at coordinating the conference functions, and at organizing various social functions.

Carl V. Gisolfi
David R. Lamb
Ethan R. Nadel

1

Introduction to Exercise in Older Adults

LORETTA DIPIETRO, Ph.D., M.P.H.

DOUGLAS R. SEALS, Ph.D.

INTRODUCTION

The aging process has traditionally been viewed as a progressive decline in health, leading to infirmity and death. Although many physiological functions are known to decline with age, the emerging view of the aging process distinguishes the decline in function due to biological aging from the decline in function associated with the reduced physical activity so common in older people. Bortz (1982) was an early proponent of the hypothesis that inactivity causes many of the functional losses attributed to aging, at every level from cellular and molecular to tissue and organ systems. He noted that many of the physiological changes ascribed to aging are similar to those induced by enforced inactivity, such as during bedrest or during prolonged space flight. He proposed that the decline in function due to inactivity could be attenuated, or even reversed, by exercise and stated that this prospect holds much promise for sustained lifetime health. Numerous studies (e.g., Fiatarone & Evans, 1990) and reviews (e.g., Evans, 1986; Holloszy, 1983) have provided data in support of this notion. However, the mechanisms by which the deficits occur with aging

1

and the extent to which and the means by which these are reversible by increasing physical activity are not yet known.

A primary goal of this volume is to discuss and evaluate the hypothesis that increased physical activity preserves function during the aging process. In addressing this hypothesis, the chapters and discussions will provide insight into the mechanisms associated with the reductions in functional status with aging, how some improvements in function can be induced by increased activity, and some of the issues that require further study.

DEMOGRAPHICS OF AGING IN THE UNITED STATES

As those born in the baby boom of the 1940s and 1950s in the United States move through their life spans, and as the mortality rates in these age cohorts continue to decline, the size of the population of older adults shows a rapid and continuing rise (Figure 1-1). In 1990, women born in the United States had a life expectancy of 78.8 y and men 71.8 y, approximately a 4 y increase from just 20 y earlier, when life expectancy was 74.7 y and 67.1 y for women and men, respectively (National Center for Health Statistics, 1993). The population aged 65 y and older currently numbers about 31 million and represents 12% of the total U.S. population but is projected to approach 60 million and become 20% of the population by 2025 (Figure 1-1). Perhaps of even greater concern in terms of health care is the increase in the "oldest old" segment of the population, i.e., those 85 and older. Since 1930, these oldest old have more than doubled in number every 30 y and are projected to be the fastest growing group in the older population well into the next century (United States Bureau of Census, 1989). For example, in 1990 there were approximately 3 million persons aged 85 y or older living in the U.S., and this number is projected to increase to between 10 and 18 million by 2040 (Figure 1-1). The impact of this change in age structure has enormous implications for the entire population, but especially for those persons involved in planning for the various components of health care.

SOCIETAL COSTS OF CHRONIC DISEASE IN OLDER ADULTS

Accompanying the demographics of aging is the increasing prevalence of functional impairment and chronic disease in this population. Approximately 80% of older adults have at least one chronic health problem, such as cardiovascular disease, cancer, diabetes, and auditory and/or visual impairment (Guralnik et al., 1989; U.S. Dept. of Health and Human Services, 1984). Nearly a third of those over 85 y suffer some degree of dementia (Skoog et al., 1993). The extent to which these are the conse-

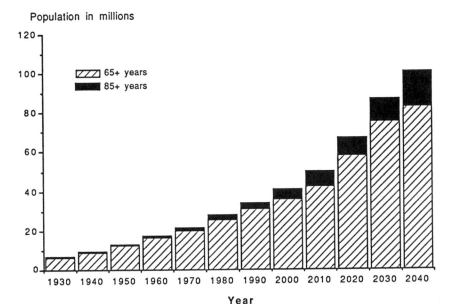

Population in millions

FIGURE 1-1. *Population estimates and projections for persons aged 65 y and older and those aged 85 y and older who live(d) in the United States between the years 1930 and 2040.* Data from Taeuber and Rosenwaike (1992).

quences of aging or the cumulative effects of physical inactivity or nutritional deficits that accompany aging is of concern to biologists and economists alike.

Chronic health problems among older Americans exact a considerable toll on the economy. Americans over 65 y account for approximately 30% of U.S. health care expenditures, or more than $50 billion annually (U.S. Dept. of Health and Human Services, 1984), despite accounting for only 12% of the population. Aside from the costs incurred to the individual and to society, functional impairment has negative consequences for autonomy and quality of life (King, 1991). Approximately 42% of older adults suffer some functional limitations, with about 10% likely to be so severely restricted in mobility that they require institutionalization (Katz, 1983; World Health Organization, 1987). The use of long-term care services and the associated costs increase exponentially with age (Schneider & Guralnik, 1990). Clearly, the benefits to society, not to mention to those afflicted, would be enormous if the onset of functional limitations could be postponed or if they could be eliminated altogether.

There is encouraging evidence that the rates of disease and disability among older Americans have begun to decline, particularly among those age 85 and older. With recent emphasis shifting from tertiary care toward preventing or delaying the onset of chronic disease, the maintenance of functional well-being may be extended to a time closer to the life expectancy (Bortz, 1982). This "compression of morbidity" (Fries et al., 1989) will inevitably improve the quality of life and preserve autonomy among older people, as well as reduce health costs to the individual and society (Bladeck & Firman, 1983; King, 1991; Manton & Soldo, 1985). To further accelerate this compression of morbidity, we need to improve our ability to distinguish mandatory from facultative aging; if we can better make this distinction, we can more effectively learn to manipulate variables, i.e., those related to facultative aging, over which we have some control.

MECHANISMS UNDERLYING MANDATORY CELLULAR AGING

Mandatory aging is that over which we have no control. In the absence of disease or injury, biological cells, tissues, systems, and organs undergo a process of irreversible aging. The basis for mandatory aging has been discussed and debated for decades. This volume does not address this issue directly, so a very brief review follows.

There are two general classes of hypotheses that attempt to define the cellular basis of aging (Dice, 1993). The first of these proposes that aging is the consequence of a progressive accumulation of errors in the makeup of the cell because the cell's repair processes do not keep up. The consequence of the error buildup is that the genetic foundation of the cell becomes altered and the expression of essential protein is either limited or cannot proceed at all. The second of these classes of hypotheses proposes that the aging process is actively programmed by the cell's genetic machinery.

In the first case, random environmental events such as oxygen free radical damage (Starke-Reed, 1989), somatic cell gene mutation (Hayflick, 1975), or cross linkage among macromolecules, particularly proteins (Zs.-Nagy & Nagy, 1980), render the cell incapable of functioning normally. Normal function is defined as the ability to transfer information from DNA to RNA to the synthesis of protein. Synthesis of aberrant protein or a failure to express essential protein when required eventually leads to the cell's inability to contribute to tissue homeostasis. Individual cell loss is not catastrophic to tissue or organ function until a significant complement of cells in the tissue or organ fails.

In the second case, proponents of the programmed cell-death hypothesis cite examples such as the death of certain cell lines during development and maturation to support their case. While the examples cited are real enough, indicating that programmed cell death does occur in very specific cases, the relevance of this process to the aging of the organism has not been established.

PHYSICAL INACTIVITY—A MECHANISM UNDERLYING FACULTATIVE CELLULAR AGING

Lean body mass (Fleg & Lakatta, 1988), basal metabolic rate (Poehlman & Horton, 1990), aerobic capacity (Seals et al., 1984b; Seals, 1993), and insulin sensitivity (Laws & Reaven, 1991) all have been reported to decline with both increasing age and decreasing level of physical activity (Fiatarone & Evans, 1990). Is this mandatory, or can some of the decline be attributed to the relative inactivity associated with growing older? Older people become increasingly limited in their abilities to perform activities of daily living because of poor balance, reduced endurance, generalized weakness, or repeated falls. Again, it is unclear how these limitations are related to the aging process.

Of increasing interest is the extent to which physical activity influences these aging-related changes in physiological function. In population studies, physical activity has been shown to be inversely associated with several chronic conditions, including coronary heart disease (Blair et al., 1989; Leon et al., 1987; Paffenbarger et al., 1993; Powell et al., 1987), hypertension (Hagberg et al., 1987; Seals et al., 1984a, 1994), diabetes (Helmrich et al., 1991; Manson et al., 1991, 1992), osteoporotic fractures (Paganini-Hill et al., 1991; Farmer et al., 1989), and cancer (Albanes et al., 1989; Gerhardsson et al., 1988; Lee et al., 1991), as well as cognitive decline (Chodzko-Zajko & Moore, 1994; Hultsch et al., 1993). Therefore, physical activity may be particularly beneficial for older adults, in whom the prevalence of these conditions is disproportionally high. There is also evidence that increased levels of physical activity may provide additional benefits to older people by attenuating functional impairment, even when chronic disease is present (Fiatarone et al., 1990, 1994; Frontera et al., 1988; Tinetti et al., 1988). Thus, regular physical activity and improved physical fitness have the potential to enhance the functional well-being of older people and consequently to reduce the aging-related increases in chronic disease morbidity and mortality.

The prevalence of depression-like symptoms is considerable among older populations. Such symptoms may be secondary to health status in general (Chodzko-Zajko, 1990) and to psychosocial factors, such as isolation, bereavement, spousal illness, or limited financial resources (Lebowitz & Niederehe, 1992). There is a lack of empirical research establishing the causal mechanisms by which physical activity or exercise may attenuate, or possibly prevent, the occurrence of depression (O'Connor et al., 1993). Specific hypotheses have addressed the potential for exercise to reregulate monoaminergic brain systems and the hypothalamic-pituitary axis because these physiological systems have been reported to be altered in depressed individuals (Dunn & Dishman, 1991). Plausible mediating factors to explain a beneficial association between exercise and improved psychological function in older people include increased opportunity for social interaction (North et al., 1990) and improvements in feelings of self-efficacy, confidence, and mastery over physical tasks (Hughes, 1984; Sonstroem & Morgan, 1989).

METHODOLOGICAL ISSUES IN RESEARCH ON AGING AND EXERCISE

Both cross-sectional and longitudinal experimental approaches have been used to study the influence of aging on human physiology at rest and in response to acute and chronic exercise (Hagberg, 1994; Lakatta, 1993; Saltin, 1986; Seals, 1993). Most studies of aging effects have employed the cross-sectional approach, in which subjects are studied either over one broad continuous age range, e.g., from age 20 y through age 85 y, or in two or more distinct groups representing young, e.g., 20–25 y, and older, e.g., 65–75 y, age ranges. Only a limited amount of longitudinal information on the effects of aging on physiology has been obtained from making serial measurements in the same subjects over time, typically, periods of 10–20 y. In general, these two approaches to studying the effects of aging on the physiological responses to acute and chronic exercise have yielded qualitatively (i.e., directionally) consistent findings (Hagberg, 1994; Lakatta, 1993; Saltin, 1986; Seals, 1993).

Cross-sectional and longitudinal approaches have been used not only to study the influence of aging on physiology, but also to study the influence of regular physical activity (physical training) on the physiology and the risk of disease in older adults (Hagberg, 1994; Heath, 1981; Lakatta, 1993; Saltin, 1986; Seals, 1993). The cross-sectional approach in this case has typically consisted of comparisons of groups of middle-aged and older "masters" athletes with groups of untrained controls who are matched on age and gender. Longitudinal studies have examined the adaptations to a period of physical training in sedentary middle-aged and older adults. Generally speaking, previously sedentary older subjects (and young adults, for that matter) who undergo physical training are unable to attain the same high levels of physiological adaptations demonstrated by their athletic peers. This is probably due to the athletes' genetic advantages as well as to their abilities to exercise regularly at much greater intensities and durations than is possible for non-athletic older adults, who have much lower physical work capacities and, therefore, reduced tolerance for vigorous exercise.

Limitations of Existing Data on Aging and Exercise

Many methodological limitations of the research on aging and exercise make it difficult to interpret the available experimental data, especially when attempting to distinguish the *primary* versus the *secondary* effects of the aging process on a particular function. For example, many factors associated with increasing age can independently influence the physiological responses to exercise. These factors include disease, physical inactivity (deconditioning), loss of muscle mass, increased body fatness (Folkow & Svanborg, 1993; Hagberg, 1994; Lakatta, 1993; Seals, 1993), and a variety of psychosocial factors (Rowe & Kahn, 1987). In general, these potentially confounding factors were poorly controlled in earlier investigations. Over the last decade or so, attempts have been made in both cross-sectional and longitudinal investigations to account for or control such influences, thereby better isolating the direct effects of the aging process *per se* (Hagberg, 1994; Lakatta, 1993). These newer approaches, however, have their own inherent limitations (Seals, 1993).

A related problem is the failure in many studies to determine true maximal exercise capacities in older subjects (Lakatta, 1993). This would confound interpretation of, for example, not only the effects of aging on maximal oxygen consumption but also the responses to submaximal exercise that typically are based on a certain percentage of the individual's peak work capacity. Collectively, this factor along with those mentioned above would cause the physiological changes due to the direct effects of the aging process to be *over*estimated. In fact, it has been proposed by Rowe and Kahn (1987) that in some cases physiological differences between young and older populations may be due only in small part to aging *per se*.

Other limitations of much of the research in this field include: 1) the arbitrary nature of the criteria used to define young and older subject groups, and 2) the relative lack of data on resistance exercise compared to endurance exercise, on women, and on subjects of both genders who are greater than 80 years of age. The gender issue is important in light of the marked effects of menopause, as well as the influence of estrogen therapy on the physiology and risk of disease in the aging woman (Eaker et al., 1993; Manolio et al., 1993).

It is also important to appreciate that almost all of the emphasis to date in describing the influence of aging on physiological function at rest and during exercise has been on *average* (i.e., group) responses. In reality, the effects of advancing age are highly specific, with substantial variability among individuals. Rowe and Kahn (1987) have described a qualitative spectrum of aging from "successful" (least functional changes) to "usual" to "diseased" to "impaired" (greatest functional changes). These different types of physiological aging among individuals will have significant effects on the rate of decline in many bodily functions. More research is needed to identify the physiological, as well as any behavioral, mechanisms associated with the observed heterogeneity between older and younger populations in response to exercise.

Finally, selective survival may influence the variability of adaptations to exercise training both within older populations and between younger and older adults. The individuals most susceptible to putative risk factors, and who might benefit most from training, die at earlier ages. Thus, research results may be biased because they are derived from studies of the effects of exercise training on the more robust surviving cohort. This is especially true when investigators fail to directly assess physical activity in their subjects and instead rely on maximal oxygen uptake and other markers of fitness as indices of training status. Such fitness markers are known to be heavily influenced by genetic predisposition so that research results based on these fitness characteristics may be more indicative of the effects of heredity rather than the effects of exercise training.

SUMMARY

The chapters in this volume document the latest information concerning the effects of physical activity on physiological processes in older adults. In certain cases, e.g., from studies of older athletes, it is clear that increased activity aids in the maintenance of function in older people. In other cases, it is not so clear. Fascinating recent studies (Fiatarone et al., 1994) demonstrate that people even in their tenth decade of life retain the plasticity of their skeletal muscle systems to respond favorably to a strength training stimulus. While increased activity may not elevate these people to the status of Olympic caliber athletes, the increased strength may be just enough to enable them to rise from chairs or to climb flights of stairs without faltering.

Equally important to documenting the improvements in function is the understanding of the biological basis for the changes. This allows a better understanding of the aging process itself, allows the partitioning of the aging process into mandatory and facultative categories more readily, and thus provides clues as to what can and what cannot be expected to change with increased activity. We need to know more about the aging process to plan effectively for the future, both on an individual and on a societal basis. Understanding the role of physical activity in retarding the facultative component of the aging process has important implications for meeting the needs of the world's increasing population of older people.

BIBLIOGRAPHY

Albanes, D., A. Blair, and P.R. Taylor (1989). Physical activity and the risk of cancer in the NHANES I population. *Am. J. Public Health* 79:744–750.
Bladeck, B., and J. Firman (1983). The aging of the population and health services. *Annals* 468:132–148.
Blair, S.N., H.W. Kohl, III, R.S. Paffenbarger, D.G. Clark, K.H. Cooper, and L.W. Gibbons (1989). Physical fitness and all-cause mortality:a prospective study of healthy men and women. *J. Am. Med. Assoc.* 262:2395–2401.

Bortz, W.M. (1982). Disuse and aging. *J. Am. Med. Assoc.* 248:1203–1208.

Chodzko-Zajko, W.J. (1990). The influence of general health status on the relationship between chronological age and depressed mood state. *J. Geriatr. Psychiatr.* 23:13–22.

Chodzko-Zajko, W.J., and K.A. Moore (1994). Physical fitness and cognitive function in aging. In: J.O. Holloszy (ed.) *Exercise and Sport Sciences Reviews*, Vol. 22. Baltimore, MD: Williams & Wilkins, pp. 195–220.

Day, J.C (1993). Bureau of the Census. Current population reports, P-25, no 1104. Population projections of the United States, by age, sex, race, and Hispanic origin: 1993 to 2050 (middle series). Washington, D.C.: U.S. Government Printing Office.

Dice, J.F. (1993). Cellular and molecular mechanisms of aging. *Physiol. Rev.* 73:149–159.

Dunn, A.L., and R.K. Dishman (1991). Exercise and the neurobiology of depression. In: J.O. Holloszy (ed.) *Exercise and Sport Sciences Reviews*, Vol. 19. Baltimore, MD: Williams & Wilkins, pp. 41–98.

Eaker, E.D., J.H. Chesebro, F.M. Sacks, N.K. Wenger, J.P. Whisnant, and M. Winston (1993). Cardiovascular disease in women. *Circulation* 88:1999–2009.

Evans, W.J. (1986). Exercise and muscle metabolism in the elderly. In: H.N. Munroe and M.L. Hutchenson (eds.) *Nutrition and Aging.* New York: Academic Press, pp. 179–191.

Farmer, M.E., T. Harris, J.H. Madans, R.B. Wallace, J. Cornoni-Huntley, et al. (1989). Anthropometric indicators and hip fracture. The NHANES I Epidemiologic Follow-up Study. *J. Am. Geriatr. Soc.* 37:9–16.

Fiatarone, M.A., E.F. O'Neill, N.D. Ryan, K.M. Clements, G.R. Solares, et al. (1994). Exercise training and nutritional supplementation for physical frailty in very elderly people. *N. Engl. J. Med.* 330:1769–1775.

Fiatarone, M.A., and W.J. Evans (1990). Exercise in the oldest old. *Topics Geriatr. Rehab.* 5:63–77.

Fiatarone, M.A., E.C. Marks, N.D. Ryan, C.N. Merideth, L.A. Lipsitz, and W.J. Evans (1990). High-intensity strength training in nonagenarians:effects on skeletal muscle. *J.Am. Med. Assoc.* 263:3029–3034.

Fleg, J.L., and E.G. Lakatta (1988). Role of muscle loss in the age-reduction in maximal oxygen consumption. *J. Appl. Physiol.* 65:1147–1151.

Folkow, B., and A. Svanborg (1993). Physiology of cardiovascular aging. *Physiol. Rev.* 73:725–764.

Fries, J.F., L.W. Green, and S. Levine (1989). Health promotion and the compression of morbidity. *Lancet* 1:481–484.

Frontera, W.R., C.A. Meredith, K.P O'Reilly, and W.J. Evans (1988). Strength conditioning in older men: skeletal muscle hypertrophy and improved function. *J. Appl. Physiol.* 64:1038–1044.

Gerhardsson, M., B. Floderus, and S.E. Norell (1988). Physical activity and colon cancer risk. *Int. J. Epidemiol.* 17:743–746.

Guralnik, J.M., A.Z. LaCroix, D.F. Everitt, and M.G. Kovar (1989). Aging in the eighties: the prevalence of comorbidity and its association with disability. *Advance Data from Vital and Health Statistics.* No 170. Hyattsville, M.D.: National Center for Health Statistics.

Hagberg, J.M. (1987). Effect of training on the decline of $\dot{V}O_2$max with aging. *Fed. Proc.* 46:1830–1837.

Hagberg, J. M. (1994). Physical Activity, Fitness, Health, and Aging. In: C. Bouchard, R. Shephard, and T. Stephens (eds.) *Physical Activity, Fitness, and Health.* Champaign, IL: Human Kinetics, pp. 993–1005.

Hayflick, L. (1975). Current theories of biological aging. *Fed. Proc.* 34:9–13.

Heath G.W., J.M. Hagberg, A.A. Ehsani, and J.O. Holloszy (1981). A physiological comparison of young and older endurance athletes. *J. Appl. Physiol.* 51:634–640.

Helmrich, S.P., D.R. Ragland, R.W. Leving, and R.S. Paffenbarger, Jr. (1991). Physical activity and reduced occurrence of non-insulin-dependent diabetes mellitus. *N. Engl. J. Med.* 325:147–152.

Holloszy, J.O. (1983). Exercise, health and aging: a need for more information. *Med. Sci. Sports Exerc.* 15:1–5.

Hughes, J.R. (1984). Psychological effects of habitual aerobic exercise. A critical review. *Prev. Med.* 13:66–78.

Hultsch, D.F., M. Hammer, and B.J. Small (1993). Age differences in cognitive performance in later life: relationships to self-reported health and activity lifestyle. *J. Gerontol.* 48:1–11.

Katz, S. (1983). Assessing self-maintenance. *J. Am. Geriatr. Soc.*2 31:721–727.

King, A.C. (1991). Physical activity and health enhancement in older adults: current status and future prospects. *Ann. Behav. Med.* 13:87–90.

Lakatta, E.G. (1993). Cardiovascular regulatory mechanisms in advanced age. *Physiol. Rev.* 73:413–467.

Laws, A., and G.M. Reaven (1991). Physical activity, glucose tolerance, and diabetes in older adults. *Ann. Behav. Med.* 13:125–132.

Lebowitz, B.D., and G. Niederehe (1992). Concepts and issues in mental health and aging. In: J.E. Birren, R.B. Sloan, and G.D. Cohen (eds.) *Handbook of Mental Health and Aging.* San Diego: Academic Press, pp. 3–27.

Lee, I-M., R.S. Paffenbarger, Jr., and C.C. Hsieh (1991). Physical activity and risk of developing colorectal cancer among college alumni. *J. Nat. Cancer Inst.* 83:1324–1329.

Leon A.S., J. Connett, D.R. Jacobs, and R. Raauramaa (1987). Leisure time physical activity and risk of coronary heart disease and death: the Multiple Risk Factor Intervention Trial. *J. Am. Med. Assoc.* 258:2388–2395.

Manolio, T.A., C.D. Furberg, L. Shemanski, B.M. Psaty, D.H. O'Leary, R.P. Tracy, and T.L. Bush (1993). Associations of postmenopausal estrogen use with cardiovascular disease and its risk factors in older women. *Circulation* 88:2163–2171.

Manson, J.E., D.M. Nathan, A.S. Krolewski, M.J. Stampfer, W.C. Willett, and C.H. Hennkins (1992). A prospective study of exercise and incidence of diabetes among US male physicians. *J. Am. Med. Assoc.* 268:63–67.

Manson, J.E., E.B. Rimm, M.J. Stampfer, G.A. Golditz, W.C. Willett, et al. (1991). Physical activity and incidence of non-insulin-dependent diabetes mellitus in women. *Lancet* 338:774–778.

Manton, K.G., and B.J. Soldo (1985). Dynamics of health changes in the oldest old: new perspectives and evidence. *Milbank Mem. Fund Quart., Health Soc.* 63:206–285.

National Center for Health Statistics (1993). Monthly vital statistics report. *Advance Report of Final Mortality Statistics, 1990,* 41 (7). Washington, D.C.: U.S. Government Printing Office.

North, T.C., P. McCullagh, and Z.V. Tran (1990). Effects of exercise on depression. In: K.B. Pandolf and J.O. Holloszy (eds.) *Exercise and Sport Sciences Reviews,* Vol. 18. Baltimore, MD: Williams & Wilkins, pp. 379–415.

O'Connor, P.J., L.E. Aenchbacher, and R.K. Dishman (1993). Physical activity and depression in the elderly. *J. Aging Phys. Act.* 1:34–58.

Paffenbarger R.S., Jr., R.T. Hyde, A.L. Wing, I-M. Lee, D.L. Jung, and J.B. Kampert (1993). The association of changes in physical activity level and other lifestyle characteristics with mortality among men. *N. Eng. J. Med.* 328:538–545.

Paganini-Hill, A., A. Chao, R.K. Ross, and B.E. Hendersen (1991). Exercise and other factors in the prevention of hip fracture: the Leisure World Study. *Epidemiology* 2:16–25.

Poehlman, E.T., and E.S. Horton (1990). Regulation of energy expenditure in aging humans. *Ann. Rev. Nutr.* 10:255–275.

Powell, K.E., P.D. Thompson, C.J. Caspersen, and J.S. Kendrick (1987). Physical activity and incidence of coronary heart disease. *Ann. Rev. Public Health* 8:253–287.

Rowe, J.W., and R.L. Kahn (1987). Human aging: usual and successful. *Science* 237:143–149.

Saltin, B. (1986). The aging endurance athlete. In: J.R. Sutton and R.M. Brock (eds.) *Sports Medicine for the Mature Athlete.* Carmel, IN: Cooper Publishing Group, pp. 59–80.

Schneider, E.L., and J.M. Guralnik (1990). The aging of America: Impact of health care costs. *J. Am. Med. Assoc.* 263:2335–2340.

Seals, D.R. (1993). Influence of aging on autonomic-circulatory control in humans at rest and during exercise. In: D.R. Lamb and C.V. Gisolfi (eds.) *Perspectives in Exercise Science & Sports Medicine, Vol. 6: Exercise, Heat, and Thermoregulation.* Indianapolis, IN: Brown & Benchmark, pp.257–304.

Seals, D.R., J.M. Hagberg (1984a). The effect of exercise training on human hypertension: a review. *Med. Sci. Sports Exerc.* 16:207–215.

Seals, D.R., J.M. Hagberg, B.F. Hurley, A.A. Ehsani, and J.O. Holloszy (1984b). Endurance training in older men and women: I. cardiovascular responses to exercise. *J. Appl. Physiol.* 57:1024–1031.

Seals, D.R., J.A. Taylor, A.V. Ng, and M.D. Esler (1994). Exercise and aging: autonomic control of the circulation. *Med. Sci. Sports Exerc.* 26:568–576.

Skoog, I., L. Nilsson, B. Palmertz, L-A. Andreasson, A. Svanborg (1993). A population-based study of dementia in 85-year-olds. *N. Engl. J. Med.* 328:153–158.

Sonstroem, R.J., and W.P. Morgan (1989). Exercise and self-esteem rationale and model. *Med. Sci. Sports Exerc.* 21:329–337.

Starke-Reed, P.E. (1989). The role of oxidative modification in cellular protein turnover and aging. *Prog. Clin. Biol. Res.* 287:269–276.

Taeuber, C.M., and I. Rosenwaike (1993). A demographic portrait of America's oldest old. In: R.M. Suzman, D.P. Willis, and K.G. Manton (eds.) *The Oldest Old.* Oxford, England: Oxford Unversity Press, pp. 17–49.

Tinetti, M.E., M. Speechley, and S.F. Ginter (1988). Risk factors for falls among elderly persons living in the community. *N. Engl. J. Med.* 319:1701–1707.

United States Bureau of the Census (1989). Projections of the Population of the United States by Age, Sex, and Race; 1988–2080. Current Population Reports, series, CPH-L-74, no. 1018. Washington, DC: U.S. Government Printing Office.

U.S. Department of Health and Human Services (1984). *Executive summary: aging and health promotion: market research for public education.* Washington, DC: U.S. Government Printing Office.

World Health Organization (1987). *Prevention of Cardiovascular Disease Among the Elderly: Report of a WHO Meeting.* Geneva, Switzerland: March 26–27.

Zs.-Nagy, I. and K. Nagy (1980). On the role of cross-linking of cellular proteins in ageing. *Mech. Age. Dev.* 14:245–281.

2

Exercise Training, Fitness, Health, and Longevity

WILLIAM L. HASKELL, Ph.D.

WAYNE T. PHILLIPS, Ph.D.

INTRODUCTION

The advancing age structure of the population in the United States over the next 30–50 y will influence all aspects of our social structure, including the characteristics of the work force, the nature and magnitude of retirement programs, the design and support of the educational system, and the demands on the delivery of health care services. Health care is of particular concern because older persons experience more disability days requiring greater medical care and related services. Thus, a major objective in providing comprehensive health care for the aging population is to include strategies that will not only promote longevity, but will decrease disability days and enhance overall quality of life. A wide variety of procedures and services is being considered for achieving these goals, with programs for maintaining or increasing physical activity among the more attractive options.

There is no doubt that appropriate exercise training regimens favorably influence the functioning of various bodily systems in older as well as younger individuals. This fact is documented in substantial detail in the other chapters of this volume. The primary purpose of this chapter is to review research that addresses the issue of how exercise training and/or general increases in physical activity by older adults may influence longevity, health status as evaluated by indices of morbidity and risk factors for disease, functional status for daily living, and physical disability. The final section provides an overview of the research needed to better define these issues.

Definitions

For the purposes of this chapter, the term *older adults* refers to men and women over 65 y of age, even though organizations such as the American Association of Retired Persons consider individuals over age 50 as "seniors." *Exercise* will be used according to the definition presented by Caspersen et al. (1985): "Physical activity that is planned, structured, repetitive, and purposeful in the sense that one or more components of physical fitness is an objective." *Physical activity* is defined in the same report as "any bodily movement produced by skeletal muscles that results in energy expenditure." Exercise or exercise training is considered a subset of physical activity. *Physical fitness* is defined "as the ability to carry out daily tasks with vigor and alertness, without undue fatigue and with ample energy to enjoy leisure-time pursuits and to meet unforeseen emergencies" (President's Council on Physical Fitness and Sports, 1971). The definition of *health* is that provided in the 1988 International Consensus Conference on Physical Activity, Physical Fitness, and Health (Bouchard et al., 1990): "a human condition with physical, social, and psychological dimensions, each characterized on a continuum with positive and negative poles. Positive health is associated with a capacity to enjoy life and to withstand challenges; it is not merely the absence of disease. Negative health is associated with morbidity and, in the extreme, with premature mortality."

PHYSICAL ACTIVITY, PHYSICAL FITNESS, AND LONGEVITY

Substantial evidence demonstrates that higher levels of physical activity (Berlin & Colditz, 1990; Leon et al., 1987; Morris et al., 1990; Paffenbarger et al., 1984; Powell et al., 1987; Shaper & Wannamethee, 1991) and endurance fitness (Blair et al., 1989; Ekelund et al., 1988; Sandvik et al., 1993) in men living in technologically advanced countries are significantly associated with reduced all-cause and selected cause-specific mortality rates, and with some increase in life expectancy (Paffenbarger et al., 1986; Pekkanen et al., 1987). Unfortunately, no randomized clinical trial of adequate size or duration has been conducted to test the causality of this hypothesis, but features of the designs and results of many observational studies are consistent with the interpretation that a more physically active lifestyle independently contributes to reduced mortality and increased longevity (Blair, 1993; Powell et al., 1987). Such features include a proper sequence of events (physical activity precedes the clinical event), a reasonable dose-response relationship between activity level and benefit, associations observed in relevant populations, independence of association from other established risk factors, and biological plausibility of a causal relationship.

In observational prospective studies in which physical activity has been assessed for both younger (<65 y) and older men and women, follow-up for the next 8–20 y usually demonstrates that the risk ratio between sedentary and active persons for either coronary heart disease or all-cause mortality is at least as great or greater for the older as for the younger persons (Morris et al., 1980; Salonen et al., 1982). It may be that this greater risk ratio is due to the higher overall mortality rate in the elderly, but it does indicate that the more favorable outcomes observed in physically active younger persons are not lost with advancing age.

It appears that if middle-aged men have been habitually active or become active, they are more likely to reach old age than if they remain sedentary (Paffenbarger et al., 1993; Pekkanen et al., 1987). Men aged 35–39 y who are assumed to have sedentary jobs but who expend more than 2,000 kcal/wk during leisure time have a life expectancy 2.51 y longer than similar men who expend less than 500 kcal/wk (Paffenbarger et al., 1986). At ages 55–59 this difference decreased to 2.02 y, and at ages 65–69 the difference was only 1.35 y. Given that the average life expectancy of American men at age 65 was approximately 15.1 y in 1990, the more physically active man at age 65 would appear to have increased his life expectancy by approximately 9% over his sedentary counterpart. The data from Paffenbarger and colleagues (1986) are similar to those reported by Pekkanen et al. (1987) for Finnish men living in rural areas. The adjusted gain in life expectancy for middle-aged men with high levels of physical activity was 2.1 y.

Other studies of men tend to support these results of increased longevity for more active persons; they report significantly lower age-specific or age-adjusted all-cause mortality rates for more active versus sedentary men (Leon et al., 1987; Morris et al., 1980; Shaper & Wannamethee, 1991). This increased longevity attributed to a more physically active lifestyle is likely caused by the effects of activity on reducing mortality due to coronary artery disease (Berlin & Colditz, 1990; Lakka et al., 1994; Powell, et al., 1987) and type-II diabetes mellitus (Manson et al., 1992). Other possible contributors to a lower mortality rate in older physically active persons include a reduced incidence of stroke (Wannamethee & Shaper, 1992), other complications due to hypertension (Reaven et al., 1991), site-specific cancers (Kohl et al., 1988), and osteoporotic fractures (Nevitt et al., 1989). Very few data are available on sufficiently large samples of women to address the issue of increased longevity as a result of increased physical activity or physical fitness, but the evidence shows lower all-cause and cause-specific mortality rates for more physically active and fit younger and older women and is consistent with data reported for men (Blair et al., 1989; Salonen et al., 1982).

While earlier published studies comparing the life expectancy of athletes versus non-athletes or the general population demonstrated some differences in cause-specific mortality rates, overall longevity was unaffected (Hartley & Llewellyn, 1939; Rook, 1954). Also, more recent reports have not observed any increases in life expectancy of college athletes versus non-athletes, even when following these men to their seventh or eighth decades (Quinn et al., 1990). It appears that the major reason that little or no difference in longevity has been observed in studies comparing college-age athletes and non-athletes is that habitual activity throughout one's lifetime, or at least performing activity in the recent past, is what provides protection, not activity performed only during youth or early adulthood (Kahn, 1963; Paffenbarger et al., 1986). Thus, as the population ages, it appears that it will be important for most people to continue a physically active lifestyle to well beyond age 65.

The data demonstrating a reduced mortality for persons with higher levels of physical activity or fitness in older as well as younger persons are consistent with the results of studies evaluating the effects of exercise training on various health-related biological variables. These studies have documented that older persons generally respond in a similar manner and magnitude as younger persons when exposed to a similar relative exercise stress (Adams & de Vries, 1973; Schwartz et al., 1992). Also, many of the exercise training and detraining studies typically show that most exercise-induced, health-related, biological changes are quite transient and require that activity be maintained on a reasonably regular basis to improve long-term health and longevity (Hickson et al., 1985). Thus, if these physiological changes are the mechanisms by which exercise alters mortality, then the cited studies provide "biological plausibility" to the inverse association between physical activity and mortality observed in older persons.

PHYSICAL ACTIVITY, PHYSICAL FITNESS, AND CLINICAL STATUS

Coronary Heart Disease

There are substantially more data linking physical activity or physical fitness to reductions in all-cause and CHD-related mortality than to the prevalence of morbidity due to most diseases in younger or older persons. For example, in the past there has not been good documentation that a high level of physical activity reduces the incidence of non-fatal manifestations of CHD, including non-fatal myocardial infarction and angina pectoris. In several studies where higher levels of activity are associated with lower CHD mortality, there was no association between activity status and non-fatal manifestations of CHD (Morris et al., 1953; Shapiro et al., 1969). Recently, Lakka and colleagues (1994) from Finland reported an inverse relationship between the incidence of acute myocardial infarction and both the level of physical activity and maximal oxygen uptake. Data were not reported separately for non-fatal and fatal events, probably because there were only 42 myocardial infarctions over 4.9 y of follow-up in 1166 men free of cardiovascular disease at baseline. The apparent difference in the association between physical activity and CHD mortality versus morbidity could be due to true biological differences in acquiring the disease compared to dying from it, or to the known difficulty of collecting accurate morbidity data for many chronic diseases, including CHD, in population-based studies.

Data from secondary prevention or cardiac rehabilitation studies support the possibility that physical inactivity may be more associated with dying from CHD than with non-fatal clinical manifestations. In a meta-analysis of the effects of exercise-based cardiac rehabilitation programs on cardiac morbidity and mortality there was a 25% lower CHD mortality rate in the rehabilitation program participants but a nonsignificant slightly greater prevalence of non-fatal myocardial infarction and angina pectoris (Oldridge et al., 1988). Similar results evaluating a larger number of exercise-based rehabilitation programs were reported by O'Conner and colleagues (O'Conner et al., 1989). Also, autopsy studies have observed no difference in the magnitude of coronary atherosclerosis in men who were classified as inactive or active by their major occupations, but there was less myocardial damage in the more active men (Morris & Crawford, 1958).

Physical activity could reduce CHD mortality without affecting morbidity by favorably altering the "triggering event" for acute myocardial infarction or cardiac arrest. Recent data indicate that the primary triggering event for many myocardial infarctions is the acute rupture of atherosclerotic lesions and the rapid closure of the arterial lumen due to platelet aggregation and cell proliferation (Fuster et al., 1992). It could be that physical activity reduces either the risk of lesion rupture, platelet aggregation, or cell proliferation, thus reducing CHD mortality but not the development of atherosclerosis, which may be more related to the development of non-fatal clinical manifestations of myocardial ischemia.

Hypertension

There are observational data demonstrating that a more physically active lifestyle or a greater endurance exercise capacity is associated with a lower mean arterial blood pressure and a lower prevalence of hypertension in older men and women (Paffenbarger et al., 1983; Reaven et al., 1991). Lower blood pressure in the more physically active older adults may be due to the effects of lifelong activity helping to prevent the age-related rise in pressure observed in most Western countries, or to a more recent effect in older persons who initiated exercise later in life (American College of Sports Medicine, 1993). Because low-intensity activity has at least as much, if not more, of an effect on lowering blood pressure as does higher intensity exercise (Jennings et al., 1986), this benefit appears to be well within the capacity of most ambulatory older adults. A comprehensive review of the effects of endurance exercise training on blood pressure found that hypertensive patients participating in endurance exercise training experienced a reduction in systolic and diastolic blood pressure of approximately 9 mm Hg, whereas borderline hypertensive patients and normotensive persons experienced a 6 and 3 mm Hg reduction in systolic and diastolic pressures, respectively (Fagard & Tipton, 1994). This magnitude of blood pressure reduction in response to endurance exercise training has been reported for men and women age 60 y and older (Cononie et al., 1991; Hagberg et al., 1989).

Non-Insulin Dependent Diabetes Mellitus (NIDDM)

Prospective observational studies have reported an inverse relationship between the level of reported habitual physical activity and the incidence of NIDDM in men (Helmrich et al., 1991; Manson et al., 1992) and women (Manson et al., 1991). While the incidence of NIDDM increased with age in these studies, no analyses were presented to determine if the inverse association between activity and incidence of NIDDM was similar for older as for younger persons. The type and amount of activity associated with the decreased incidence of NIDDM was well within the capacity of many older persons. For example, in the University of Pennsylvania alumni study (Helmrich et al., 1991), every increase of 500 kcal of energy expenditure per week was associated with a 6% lower incidence of NIDDM, and this association existed for moderate intensity activity as well as for vigorous sports play. Prior retrospective studies of athletes versus non-athletes and of active versus inactive cultures have reported similar associations, but it is impossible to determine if the activity preceded the onset of NIDDM.

Osteoporotic Fractures

Peak bone mass occurs in both men and women around the age of 30 and subsequently declines by approximately 0.5% per year in men and 1% per year in women (Riggs & Melton, 1986). Although some authors have argued that older persons with hip fractures are no more osteoporotic than non-injured persons (Cummings, 1985; Cummings & Black, 1986), most experts agree that the decline in bone mass observed throughout the life cycle does contribute to an increased incidence of osteoporotic fractures, which rises exponentially with age and is a major contributing factor to disability in the elderly (Drinkwater, 1994; Smith & Gilligan, 1991). The increased risk of osteoporosis associated with inactivity has long been recognized (Buchner et al., 1992), and since exercise was identified as a potential mediator for bone decrement more than 20 y ago (Chalmers & Ho, 1970), a large body of research has developed to clarify mechanisms and optimize training protocols that may allow exercise to increase bone integrity, maintain it, or slow its loss.

Weight-bearing physical activity is an essential requirement for bone health (Drinkwater, 1994), and it is therefore logical to assume not only that habitual physical activity is instrumental in preventing osteoporosis, but that becoming more active may increase bone mass in previously sedentary people. While some authors support this hypothesis and feel that physical activity is underutilized as a preventive measure for osteoporosis (Smith & Gilligan, 1991), others are more cautious (Drinkwater, 1994), citing the lack of randomized trials in this area (Buchner et al., 1992) and/or the lack of adequate methodological control (Block et al., 1989). Nevertheless, recent reviews of this topic that incorporated some 50 cross-sectional and longitudinal studies show a positive trend (Block et al., 1989; Buchner et al., 1992; Drinkwater, 1994; Smith & Gilligan, 1991). The majority of these studies, using different populations, age groups, exercise interventions, and measuring technologies, produced fairly consistent, if relatively small, positive results.

In reviewing studies involving post-menopausal females, Drinkwater (1994) noted that the apparent effectiveness of physical activity for increasing bone mass depended on both the type of study (cross-sectional or longitudinal) and the type of activity (load bearing or non-load bearing).

Attribution of causality also becomes more tenuous in this older population because there are few well-controlled randomized trials, and the results in those that are reported are inconsistent (Block et al., 1989; Buchner et al., 1992). Although positive effects of exercise on calcium bone index (Chow et al., 1987) and lumbar bone mineral density (Notelovitz et al., 1991) have been reported, other randomized studies have found negative results (Sandler et al., 1987; Sinaki & Offord, 1988). A closer look at the methodologies of these studies reveals factors that could well disguise the true effects of the intervention. For example, the impact of exercise on bone mineral density is reported as being site specific (Drinkwater, 1994), but Sandler et al. (1987) measured bone mineral density at the radius when the major focus of their exercise intervention was predominantly on the lower body. Similarly, Prince et al. (1991) reported a slower rate of bone loss at the radius in a group receiving calcium supplements compared to an exercise only group, but the exercise intervention consisted of low-impact aerobics plus walking, which would be expected to stress the upper body only minimally.

Improved specificity in both measurement techniques and exercise interventions as well as a more careful focus on methodology in future studies (Block et al., 1989), may well help to confirm the potential for exercise to elicit small but positive changes in bone mineral content. Even relatively small increases may well be beneficial in reducing the incidence of fractures in the elderly (Drinkwater, 1994).

Bone mineral content, however, is only one factor to be considered in this respect, because incidence of fractures will obviously also be affected by incidence of falls. It may be that the greatest effect on alleviating the increasing rate of osteoporotic fractures in this population is not derived from the direct effect of exercise on strengthening bones but, rather, on its potential to improve muscular strength and perhaps balance and/or gait, thus reducing the actual incidence of falls. These aspects are reviewed below.

PHYSICAL ACTIVITY, PHYSICAL FITNESS, FUNCTIONAL STATUS, AND DISABILITY

Effects of Exercise on Selected Components of Physical Fitness in Older Adults

The decline in physical fitness with aging was, until recently, considered to be not only inevitable, but also very resistant to change. Hollman (1964), for example, stated that "commencement of physical training in a person unaccustomed to sport caused slight effects of adaptation after forty, while after the age of sixty there is practically no observable effect."

Other studies reported a similar lack of response to endurance exercise (Benestad, 1965; Katsuki & Masuda, 1969; Wilmore et al., 1970). However, differentiation of chronological age from physiological age led to the concept of disuse atrophy (DeVries, 1975) and to the suggestion that such disuse may account for as much as 50% of the functional decline commonly associated with aging (Smith, 1980). In support of this concept was the apparent paradox of an elderly population being viewed as frail and in a state of constant decline (Suzman et al., 1993), while masters athletes in their 60s and 70s performed exceptionally well in athletic events such as the marathon (Cunningham & Paterson, 1990). A potential for exercise as an intervention for maintaining functional capacity in the elderly was established, as was a need expressed for information to separate "wishful thinking" from actuality (Holloszy, 1983).

Aerobic Capacity. Studies over the past decade examining the links between age and fitness have consistently reported lower rates of decline in maximal oxygen uptake ($\dot{V}O_2$max) in older adults who are physically active (Paterson et al., 1988) and trained (Kasch et al., 1988; Pollock et al., 1987), compared to older sedentary individuals (Buskirk & Hodgson, 1987; Paterson et al., 1988). Early studies that showed a lower capability for adaptation to dynamic endurance training in individuals over 65 y compared to younger subjects (Hagberg, 1987; Raven & Mitchell, 1980) have also been superseded by more recent evidence. Programs of endurance training have shown increases of 22–30% in $\dot{V}O_2$max for 60–70 y old men and women (Hagberg et al., 1989; Kohrt et al., 1991), proportionally as great as those of younger populations when the change is expressed as a percentage of baseline (Hickson et al., 1981). In addition, although recommendations to increase $\dot{V}O_2$max are usually based on a training intensity of approximately 65% $\dot{V}O_2$max (American College of Sports Medicine, 1993), older populations, perhaps due to their lower initial fitness status, may benefit from lower intensities. Seals et al. (1984) and Seals and Reiling (1991), for example, have reported $\dot{V}O_2$max increases of 12% and 9%, respectively, for older men and women following a six-month training program at 40–45% of heart rate reserve.

Although the effects of lifelong training in older male athletes on fitness variables have been well documented (Hagberg, 1994), fewer longitudinal studies of exercise training programs on sedentary or previously inactive elderly have been published. In one such study of a 13-y follow-up involving men aged 40–59 y who had CHD risk factors, MacKeen et al. (1985) found that those who persevered with their exercise programs reduced the loss of fitness over time compared to those who had not. Other studies (Buskirk & Hodgson, 1987; Kasch et al., 1988; Paterson et al., 1988; Pollock et al., 1987) reported similar effects and lend continuing support to the hypothesis that the decline in aerobic fitness with aging may be slowed by regular endurance exercise of low to moderate intensity.

Muscle Strength. Strength, until recently, has been little explored and an underrated aspect of fitness in the elderly. Early studies (Rodriguez et al., 1965) reported that strength training was ineffective in the elderly, with Muller (1957) stating that "the gift . . . to increase strength by training is lost in the course of aging." When training effects did result, a "widely held view" (Fiaterone et al., 1990) attributed such improvements to learning effects rather than to actual increases in strength (Moritani & DeVries, 1979).

Such lack of response to strength training programs may have had more to do with social attitudes towards older persons than to exercise theory. As little as 20 y ago, strength training in this population was regarded as an activity that needed to be approached with great caution, and guidelines were biased very much towards low-resistance training. Shephard (1978), in a review of studies generally categorized as strength training, detailed exercise protocols more correctly categorized as endurance training, including programs that incorporated cycle ergometry and calisthenics. Meusel (1986) counseled against static and dynamic strength exercises and excluded movements such as push-ups and pulls-ups for all but the most active elders. Other studies (Harris, 1984) and reviews (Stamford, 1988) revealed similar biases towards low-intensity exercise.

Research in recent years has produced well-controlled studies utilizing state-of-the-art measuring protocols to convincingly demonstrate that high-intensity resistance training can safely produce significant strength increases as well as muscular hypertrophy in older men and women. Frontera et al. (1988) used a dynamic weight training program of 3 sets of 8 repetitions, 3 times per week, for 12 weeks in a group of 12 men aged 62–70 y. The initial training resistance was set at 80% of a subject's one repetition maximum (1 RM) and maintained at this level throughout the program. Significant increases in the strength of knee flexors and extensors were found, as well as increases in total thigh and quadriceps cross-sectional areas measured by computer-assisted tomography. In an even older population, Fiaterone et al. (1990) reported strength gains following a similar but shorter duration (8-wk) protocol. This group of 6 women and 4 men, average age 90 ± 1 y (range 86–96), showed strength increases of 174 ± 31% and increases in mid-thigh area of 9 ± 4.5%.

These two landmark studies heralded a focus of attention on strength increases with high-intensity training, whether utilizing lower body exercises only (Meredith et al., 1992), upper body exercises only (Roman et al., 1993), whole body dynamic exercise (Dupler & Cortes, 1993, Nichols et al., 1993), or whole body static exercise (Rantanen et al., 1994). With the exception of the static exercise study, significant muscle hypertrophy was also produced. In addition, Hamdy et al. (1994) reported a small (1%) but significant increase in lean muscle mass and a significant increase in the performance of strength-related calisthenics exercises in subjects over 55 y, following a training program of aerobic (60–85% of predicted maximal heart rate) and strength (50–65% of 1 RM) exercise. Häkkinen (1994) incorporated explosive leg training with heavy resistance strength training in two groups of men and women, each of which consisted of subgroups that were about 50 y and 70 y old. Following 12 wk of training, significant increases were reported in strength and cross-sectional areas of the quadriceps for all four groups. This same laboratory (Häkkinen et al., 1994), using a graduated low- to high-intensity strength training program extended over a period of 6 mo, reported strength improvements for a group of middle-aged patients afflicted with recent-onset rheumatoid arthritis. Thus, as was the history with aerobic training, early negative and/ or cautious reports on strength training for older adults have been superseded by a growing body of research that demonstrates the capacity of the elderly not only to cope safely with high-intensity training but to adapt and improve at rates similar to those for younger cohorts.

Flexibility. Defined as the maximum ability to move a joint through a range of movement (American College of Sports Medicine, 1993), flexibility has been measured at all major joint complexes using a variety of different assessment techniques and protocols (Alter, 1988; Corbin, 1984; Holland, 1968). The majority of measures, however, have focused on aspects of spinal range of movement and/or trunk mobility (Skinner & Oja, 1994) because restricted spinal movement is considered to be a risk factor for low back pain (Corbin & Lindsey, 1993; Frymoyer & Cats-Baril, 1987; Riihimaki 1991). The muscles of the low back and the hamstrings are considered to be particularly relevant to trunk mobility and to healthy back functioning (Plowman, 1992), especially in the elderly (Raab et al., 1988). Although the modified Schober test represents a clinical measure of spinal range of motion (Battie et al., 1987), the sit-and-reach test has been the field measure of choice in assessing and comparing flexibility for standardized test batteries (AAHPERD, 1986; American Health and Fitness Foundation, 1986; Canadian Standardized Test of Fitness, 1986; Golding et al., 1989) as well as for many observational and interventional studies. Although some authors consider this test to assess both low back and hip flexibility (AAPHERD, 1986; Howley & Franks, 1986), others report very low correlations with criterion measures of low back flexibility and consider the test to be predominantly a measure of hamstring flexibility (Jackson & Baker, 1986; Jackson & Langford, 1988).

A decline of flexibility with age is reported by a number of authors (Allender et al., 1974; Germain & Blair, 1983; Raab et al., 1988; Shephard, 1990), and this is reflected in tables of normative values for the standardized test batteries referred to above. Shephard (1990) has reported that sit-and-reach performance deteriorates by 20–30% between 20 and 70 y, with further reductions occurring by the age of 80 (Figure 2-1). Although sit-and-reach is often the only measure of flexibility status reported in

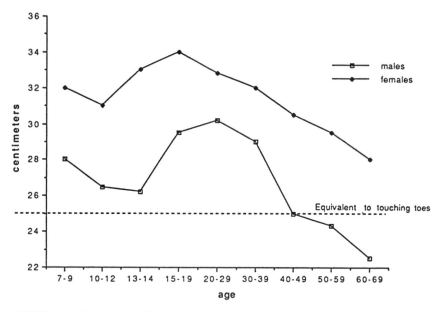

FIGURE 2-1. *Changes in flexibility with aging as measured by the sit-and-reach test.* Data from Shephard (1990).

standardized test batteries, this belies the fact that flexibility is joint specific (Harris, 1969; Skinner & Oja, 1994) and that low correlations are found between range of movement measures at different joint complexes (Shephard, 1990).

Exercise generally is recommended for improving all aspects of flexibility in the elderly (Barry et al., 1966; Lampman & Savage, 1987; Shephard, 1990), and cross-sectional studies report higher levels of flexibility in active compared to inactive older persons (Germain & Blair, 1983; Rikli & Busch, 1986). Studies have examined the effects of both general and specific exercise. In a 7-mo controlled trial of exercise at two residential homes, McMurdo and Rennie (1993) reported a significant increase in spine flexibility following a randomized controlled program of seated exercise versus conversational sessions with 49 subjects who were 64–91 years old. In a randomized controlled trial of persons living in a community, McMurdo and Burnett (1992) found that exercise significantly improved knee flexibility by 5% and spine flexibility by 44% in 87 healthy 60–81-year-old volunteers randomly assigned for 32 wk to either an aerobic exercise program or to a health education class. Significant improvements were retained for spine flexibility in an 8-mo follow-up test. Improvements in range of movement for other joint complexes have also been reported when the training program utilized specific stretching programs. In 46 women aged 65–89 y, Raab et al. (1988) found that shoulder flexion and abduction, ankle dorsiflexion, and cervical rotation all significantly improved following a program of light resistance and flexibility exercises three times weekly for 25 wk when compared to a non-exercise control group. In this program that utilized both active and passive stretching techniques, the addition of ankle and wrist weights, during stretching improved joint flexibility more than in the control group, but with the exception of shoulder abduction flexibility improved more in subjects who stretched without weights. Hip flexion, as a measure of hamstring flexibility, improved nonsignificantly for all groups. Interpretation of results in this study is limited because the assignment of subjects to either exercise or control conditions was not random.

Most flexibility studies have used healthy subjects, whether institutionalized or community-based, but Morey et al. (1989), in a randomized, prospective, longitudinal study, examined the effects of exercise on a geriatric population suffering from a variety of chronic diseases. This study involved 69 men over 64 y of age in a program of exercise that included stationary cycling and walking, as well as 20-min strength and flexibility sessions focusing on lower back and abdominal musculature. Hamstring range of motion increased 15.7% from baseline following a 90-min program of supervised exercise 3 times per week for 12 wk. Figure 2-2 summarizes the results of intervention studies that have reported small but significant range of motion increases in people aged 60–85+ y; results were measured in degrees (Figure 2-2a) or in inches (Figure 2-2b). Such increases in flexibility have been achieved with a variety of exercise and testing protocols, in both community and institutional settings, and in debilitated geriatric patients.

Balance, Gait, and Falls. A fall has been defined as "an event which results in a person coming to rest inadvertently on the ground or other lower level and other than as a consequence of the following: sustaining a violent blow; loss of consciousness; sudden onset of paralysis, as in a stroke; or an epileptic seizure" (Kellogg International Work Group, 1987). Falls are the most common of all accident events in the elderly (Cwikel & Fried, 1992) and are the leading cause of death from injury in this population (National Safety Council, 1990; Nevitt, 1990). In 1986 there were 58.9 million days of restricted activity and 18.8 million bed days reported for persons aged 65 and over (National Center for Health Statistics, 1987), the majority of which were probably the result of a fall (Nevitt, 1990). The ramifications of this number of "disability days" in terms of health care costs has been variously estimated at $7–10 billion per year (Rice & Mackenzie, 1989).

Nevitt (1990) has described a fall in terms of three phases: (a) an initiating event that displaces the body's center of gravity beyond its base of support, (b) a failure to detect this displacement and correct it in time to prevent a fall, and (c) impact of the body with environmental surfaces,

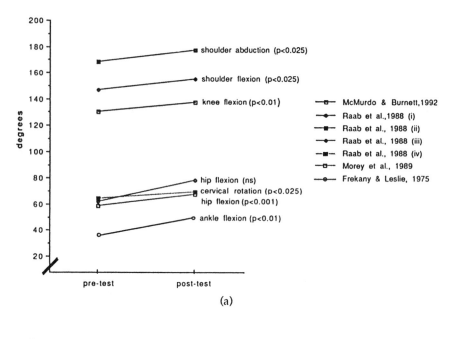

(a)

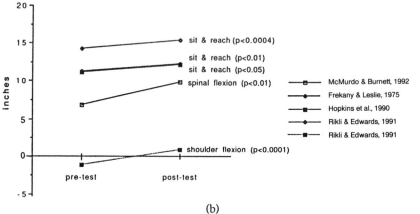

(b)

FIGURE 2-2. *Flexibility improvements following various exercise programs in elderly populations.*

resulting in the transmission of forces to body tissue and organs. For the purposes of this chapter, it is of importance to note that gait, balance, and muscular weakness are causally implicated in the first two phases (Nevitt, 1990). Additionally, an active musculature depending mostly on muscle strength serves as "the body's most effective energy absorber" (Sattin, 1992). Thus, relative muscular strength may also be implicated in the third phase of falling by potentially reducing the severity of the impact.

Other authors have reported strong associations between falls and reduced lower body strength (Whipple et al., 1987), including strength measured by the ability to rise from a chair (Tinetti et al., 1986); by gait abnormalities (Costa, 1991); by poor postural control and/or instability (Tinetti et al., 1986); and by reduced walking speed (Hindmarsh & Estes, 1989). Although there is general agreement in the literature on these associations (Cwikel & Fried, 1992; Nevitt, 1990; Nevitt et al., 1989, 1991; Sattin, 1992), studies using exercise as an intervention for these factors report more equivocal results, and these are discussed below.

Disability in Older Adults

Definitions. Disability has been defined by The International Classification of Impairments, Disabilities and Handicaps as "a restriction or lack . . . of ability to perform an activity in the manner or within the range considered normal for a human being" (Chamie, 1990). The Committee on a National Agenda for the Prevention of Disabilities (Pope & Tarlov, 1991), using data from the National Health Interview survey (LaPlante, 1988), classified the causes of disability for all ages into four main categories (Figure 2-3). In the elderly, chronic disease is considered to be a

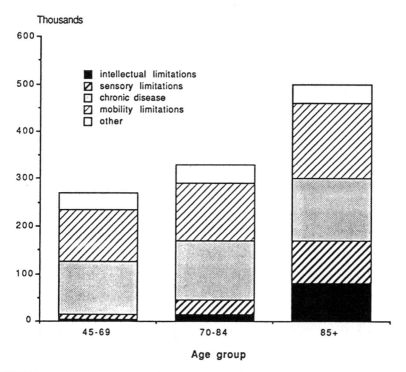

FIGURE 2-3. *Main causes of activity limitation for persons living in the United States between 1983 and 1985.* Data adapted from: Pope and Tarlov (1991).

major contributor to activity limitation (Pope & Tarlov, 1991), and La-
Plante (1988), using data from the National Health Interview Survey,
cites arthritis, heart disease, blindness/visual impairments, lower extremity impairments, and cerebrovascular disease as the five most common
causes of disability in persons aged 70–84. The situation is also complicated by the fact that many of these conditions in the elderly exist simultaneously. Guralnik et al.(1989b), using data from the Supplement on
Aging (Fitti & Kovar, 1987), considered nine common chronic conditions
and their effects, both singly and in combination, on the ability to perform
six common daily activities (bathing/showering, dressing, eating, getting
in and out of a bed or chair, walking, and using the toilet). There was a
very clear and significant association between the number of chronic conditions and the proportion of people unable to perform these activities.

Although disability in the elderly involves a variety of interrelated
domains, including cognitive, social, emotional, and sensory functions
(Buchner et al., 1992; Guralnick & Simonsick, 1993; Ory et al., 1993; Pope
& Tarlov, 1991), at least 50% of the functional decline in the elderly has
been attributed to a lack of activity (DeVries, 1975; Pope & Tarlov, 1991;
Smith, 1980). The remainder of this section will focus predominantly on
disability related to physical functioning and on the potential of exercise
to prevent or ameliorate disabling conditions.

Assessment of disability. A wide variety of different measures has
been used to assess limitations in physical functioning, all of which may
be categorized under three general dimensions of daily functioning: basic
self-care, physical task performance, and components of health related
fitness.

Basic self-care. The most commonly assessed indicators of physical disability are referred to as activities of daily living (ADL) and include such
basic self-care activities as bathing, dressing, transferring from bed to
chair, using the toilet, eating, and walking a short distance (Branch &
Jette, 1984; Guralnick & Simonsick, 1993; Katz et al., 1983; World Health
Organization, 1980).

Physical tasks performance. More difficult and/or complex aspects of daily
functioning have been referred to as instrumental activities of daily living
(IADL) and include necessary aspects of independent living such as shopping, food preparation, housekeeping, doing laundry, using transportation, and using the telephone (Fulton et al., 1989; Lawton & Brody, 1969;
World Health Organization, 1980).

Components of fitness. Aspects of daily functioning relating directly or indirectly to the components of fitness such as mobility, strength, endurance, and range of movement, have also been utilized as indicators of disability in the elderly (Nagi, 1976; Rosow & Breslau, 1966). Such aspects
are referred to as complementary activities of daily living (CADL) and
have included performance tests such as $\dot{V}O_2$max, 1 RM, and sit-and-

reach; tests simulating commonly performed daily activities such as the ability to lift arms above shoulders, walking flights of stairs, and stooping (Guralnik et al., 1989a); as well as measures of gait, balance, and coordination that are linked to the incidence of falls in the elderly (Clark et al., 1993).

Effects of Exercise on the Activities of Daily Living and On Disability in Older Adults

The conventional image of older persons has been one of disability and frailty, and projections of increasing numbers of disabled persons with increasing age tend to reinforce this impression (Figure 2-4). In reality, although the absolute number of people who are disabled increases with age, this number represents a relatively small proportion of all older people (Figure 2-4). Most older persons are able to live quite independent lives without personal assistance, and efforts should be made to minimize the increase in the percentage of the elderly who lose their independence and consume a disproportionately large fraction of the heath care budget (Manton & Soldo, 1993). One approach to this problem is to investigate those who suffer little or no decline in function over a period of time in an

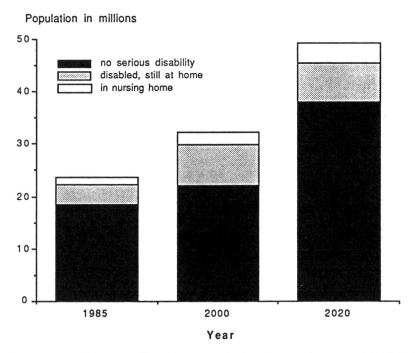

FIGURE 2-4. *Disability among older people: projections for the population aged 65 years and older living in the United States between 1985 and 2020.* Data from: Manton et al. (1993b).

attempt to identify factors that suggest therapeutic interventions in those members of this population who are disabled or likely to become disabled.

Some 77% of the those aged 65+ y and 51% of those 85 years of age and older experience little difficulty in independently performing everyday activities (NCHS, 1987); 43% of the oldest old remain in the community with some help from another person (Suzman et al., 1993). In addition, significant numbers of older persons can maintain or even regain mobility/independence over time. The National Long Term Care Survey reported a significant decline in chronic disability and institutional prevalence in the U.S. older population in the period 1982–1989 (Manton et al., 1993a).

Such results demonstrate the heterogeneity of the elderly population and suggest capacities that may be regarded as the opposite of disability. The Longitudinal Study on Aging defined such capacity as "robustness," which was characterized by the authors as the absence of difficulty in performing four tasks utilizing basic gross motor skills considered to underlie many ADL and IADL (Harris et al., 1989). Tasks consisted of walking ¼ mile; stooping, crouching, or kneeling; lifting 10 lbs; and walking up 10 steps without resting. Two years later, 50% of the women and 40% of the men who were categorized as robust at baseline continued to meet the criteria for robustness at follow-up. In addition, 11% of the women and 7% of the men in the disabled group at baseline were able to achieve the criteria for robustness at follow-up. Factors such as cardiovascular disease, hypertension, arthritis, body weight, and less education were associated with the onset of a new disability during this period (Harris et al., 1989). This gives rise to some optimism for restoration of function because some of these factors are amenable to exercise intervention.

More direct links between exercise and improved daily functioning have been suggested by a few surveys that report inverse correlations between activity and disability, although in certain of these studies methodological problems may compromise the determination of inactivity (Simonsick et al., 1993). However, a prospective multi-center study of four community-based populations, the Established Populations for Epidemiological Studies of the Elderly (EPESE), found that over a 3-y period persons who participated in moderate to high levels of recreational activity were less likely to develop impairments in their abilities to walk ½ mile, climb stairs, and do heavy housework (Simonsick et al., 1993). Other studies (Branch & Jette, 1984; Kaplan et al., 1987) that controlled for baseline health or that excluded physically impaired persons from their analysis (Mor et al., 1989) have reported similar findings. The projections for the decrease in ADL performance (Figure 2-5) highlights the importance of developing a body of research aimed at clarifying the contribution of particular components of fitness to the disability process.

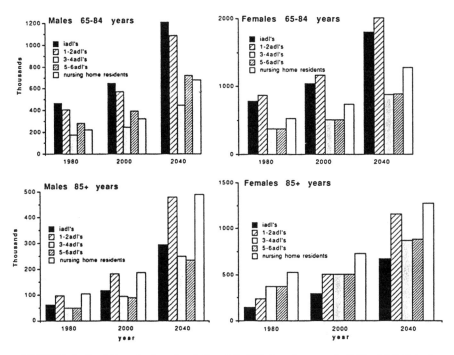

FIGURE 2-5. *Population estimates and projections of disability by performance of activities of daily living for older males and females in the United States between 1980 and 2040.* Data from Manton & Soldo (1993).

Effect of Selected Components of Fitness on Activities of Daily Living and On Diability in Older Adults

Aerobic/Cardiovascular Fitness. As evidenced earlier in this chapter, exercise of a predominantly aerobic nature and of varying intensities is associated with improvements in clinical health status and may ameliorate the effect of certain chronic diseases in older adults. While the consequences of increased activity appear to be beneficial in terms of improved mortality and life expectancy, in practical terms such improvements will be of most benefit only if accompanied by an increase in what has variously been termed "active life expectancy" (Katz et al., 1983), "successful aging" (Rowe & Kahn, 1987), or "compression of morbidity" (Fries, 1989). This potential for dying young as late as possible will be enhanced less by a reduction of diagnosed risk factors or diseases than by a capacity in the elderly to remain functionally independent (Guralnik et al., 1989a) and is likely to involve components of fitness in addition to cardiovascular fitness, traditionally the major focus of health-related research.

Muscle Strength: Observational Studies. The decline of strength with aging is detailed in Chapter 4 of this volume. For the elderly, such a decline potentially has more severe consequences for activities of daily living than does a decline in cardiovascular fitness (Frontera et al., 1988; Fiaterone et al., 1990). Musculoskeletal conditions have been cited as the most common cause of disability in older adults (Manton et al., 1993a). Lower limb muscular weakness appears to predispose the elderly to falls (Lord et al., 1993; Whipple et al., 1987), and strength, whether absolute or relative, is an obvious component of many ADL and IADL. Pendergast et al. (1993), in a cross-sectional study (n = 20 men and 20 women per decade), reported a hierarchical decrement of physical function preceded by significant decreases in activity occurring as early as the fourth decade. Decreases in peak and sustained power did not occur until the fifth decade, followed by declines in muscular endurance in the sixth decade and muscular strength in the seventh decade. The authors proposed that cardiopulmonary function, as determined by $\dot{V}O_2max$, was not a limitation for ADL performance in the frail elderly, whereas muscle function interfered both with ADL and $\dot{V}O_2max$. The authors' findings argue for exercise, and particularly strength training, as an early intervention in the maintenance of daily functioning with aging. They reported that a rehabilitation program based on these results (commencing with strength training and proceeding to endurance training) "shows promise for improving not only physiological function but functional performance as well."

In support of these findings, Bassey et al. (1992) have reported significant associations between leg extensor power and a range of functional performances (chair-rising speed, stair-climbing speed, walking speed, and stair-climbing power) in a group of 26 very old institutionalized men and women with multiple pathologies. In this study, those who needed a walking frame had less than half the leg extensor power of those who were able to walk freely, and this was interpreted by the authors to indicate that the lack of balance for which a walking frame is generally prescribed may be due to inadequate musculature rather than to a deficiency in balance mechanisms *per se*. In addition, the authors reported that more than 86% of the variance in walking speed in women was explained by leg extensor power, a factor that is not linked to balance.

Muscle strength may also be linked to feelings of physical competence because Konczak et al. (1992), in a study involving 24 older subjects (mean age 71.1 ± 5.9 y), reported significant associations ($r = 0.7$, $p < 0.05$) between leg strength (peak torque to body weight ratio) and *perception* of maximal stair-climbing ability, as well as between leg strength and *actual* maximal stair-climbing ability ($r = 0.8$, $p < 0.05$).

Muscle Strength: Intervention Studies. A strong case is evolving for the validity of using strength training as an intervention for an ADL endpoint, the available evidence indicating that the improvement of strength may provide a springboard to increased independence in the elderly. Despite this, clinical investigations of ADL performance, in terms of the extent of its relationship to or dependence on strength measures, have to date been fairly narrowly focused, with most studies generally confined to measures involving factors associated with gait and balance. Significant improvements in single-leg balance have been reported in randomized controlled trials of both endurance exercise (Hopkins et al., 1990; Stones & Kozma, 1987), strength exercise (Judge et al., 1993), and various "combined" exercise programs. Judge et al. (1993) reported significant differences in measures of single-leg balance between subjects who participated in a "combined" exercise program consisting of leg strengthening (knee extension and seated leg press), walking, and simple tai chi movements and subjects in a control group who performed flexibility exercises.

Sauvage et al. (1992) implemented randomly assigned programs of inactivity or strength and endurance exercise of moderate to high intensity in elderly nursing home residents. Quadriceps muscle strength and lower limb muscle endurance improved in the exercise group versus the control. Significant improvements were also found in the exercise group for mobility scores, stride length, and gait velocity, but stance time and gait duration were not significantly affected. This study also found no significant differences in postural sway, which was not in agreement with the findings of Era (1988), who found training-associated improvements in force platform measures of both lateral and antero-posteral sway.

Lichtenstein et al. (1989), in a randomized controlled pilot study, found inconsistent results in force platform postural sway measures following a 16-wk program of balance, flexibility, and reaction time practice exercises. The program was performed twice daily, 4 d/wk, for 16 wk, and the authors reported a subgroup analysis showing that compliance with this exercise program was a determinant of degree of change in the outcome measures.

As indicated above, the case for improved strength as an ameliorative factor in gait abnormalities is promising, though still equivocal. The results of several of the randomized studies cited above have been criticized from a methodological perspective (Buchner et al., 1992), and a number of other non-randomized studies (Barry et al., 1966; Brown & Holloszy, 1991; Gutman et al., 1977) have reported non-significant effects of exercise on gait and balance measures.

Few studies have investigated the effects of strength gains on other aspects of functional performance. Fisher et al. (1991) conducted a pilot study on the effects of a 6-wk muscle strengthening program in 18 functionally impaired, nursing-home residents (age range 60–90 y). The authors reported that 75% of patients demonstrated improved muscle function, with the female subjects (n = 10) showing significant improvements in maximal isometric force and isometric endurance of the knee extensors at hip angles of 90°, 135°, and 180°. These improvements were maintained in the nine subjects retested at 4-mo follow-up. In terms of ADL improvements, the authors reported that 75% of the participants felt the program was beneficial and enjoyable. A subjective survey of the nursing staff conducted by the authors indicated that participants in the study were observed to be more independent and active. In their discussion, the authors stated that such results imply an improvement in functional performance, which "when sustained, served to maintain muscle function, thus creating a positive feedback loop". McMurdo and Rennie (1993), in a more quantitative evaluation, utilized a 7-mo program of seated exercise in a group of 49 institutionalized patients aged 64–91 y. They reported significant improvements for the exercise group, compared to those of a discussion group, in chair-to-stand time and in self-reported ADL performance.

The strongest evidence to date for strength-induced ADL benefits comes from Fiaterone et al. (1994) who, as part of a larger study (Ory et al., 1993), investigated the effect of a high-intensity strength-training program, both with and without nutritional supplementation, on 100 elderly men and women (mean age 87.1 ± 0.6 y, range 72–98 y). The training protocol consisted of a 10-wk, 3 times weekly program of leg presses and leg extensions at a constantly maintained 80% of each subject's 1 RM. The emphasis in this protocol also seemed to be on movements producing high degrees of tension, because each repetition lasted 6–9 s. Three measures of ADL were used as outcome variables: gait speed, stair-climbing power (Bassey et al., 1992), and physical activity as measured by a large-scale, integrated activity monitor (LaPorte et al., 1979). Following the exercise intervention, significant increases were reported in all strength measures and in muscle cross-sectional area. For the ADL measures, gait speed increased by 9%, stair-climbing power by 34%, and physical activity by 51%. This randomized, placebo-controlled, clinical trial provides powerful initial evidence of the important role strength may play in ameliorating the debilitating effects of frailty in the elderly.

Flexibility: Observational Studies. Lack of flexibility is associated with poor performance in a variety of activities of daily living (Table 2-1) and can be a major cause of discomfort and disability in the elderly (Jette & Bottomley, 1987; Vandervoort et al., 1992; Wood & Turner, 1985). The criteria against which such limitations are assessed are those established by The American Association of Orthopaedic Surgeons (AAOS) (Heck et al., 1965). Despite the fact that range of motion decreases with age (Figure 2-1), no definitive values for the geriatric population have yet been established (Fiebert et al., 1992), although the need for such norms has been documented by a number of authors (Chakravarty & Webley 1993; Fiebert et al. 1992; Smith & Walker, 1983; Walker et al., 1984). In support of this contention is the fact that some authors have reported age-attributable deviations from mean AAOS values for range of motion for the shoulder (Bassey et al., 1989), hip (Walker et al., 1984), knee (Smith &

TABLE 2-1. *Studies relating flexibility measures with performance of activities of daily living.*

Component of ADL	Authors	Joint motion	Correlations (All sig.)	Criterion measure
Mobility	*Badley et al., 1984	Knee flex	0.56	WHO Classification
Bending, Stooping	*Badley et al., 1984	Hip flex	0.53	WHO Classification
Reaching up	*Badley et al., 1984	Shoulder abd	0.78	WHO Classification
Dexterity	*Badley et al., 1984	Thumb ext	0.65	WHO Classification
Boarding public transport	†Bergstrom et al., 1985	Knee ROM	N/A	N/A
Stairclimbing ability	†Konczak et al., 1992	Hip flex (Standing Trunk–Thigh angle)	0.42 (Achieved) 0.43 (Perceived)	Self estimated maximum capability
Self care activities	†Chakravaty & Webley, 1993	Shoulder ROM	$p < 0.001$	Katz ADL scale
Falls	¥Gehlsen & Whaley, 1990	Hip Flex	$p < 0.01$	vs non fallers
Falls	¥Gehlsen & Whaley, 1990	Ankle flex	$p < 0.01$	vs non fallers
Falls	¥Patla et al., 1990	Ankle ROM	N/A	vs non fallers
Falls	¥Studenski et al., 1991	Ankle flex	$p < 0.02$	vs non fallers
Gait speed	§Bowes et al., 1992	Hip flex	$p < 0.0001$	vs non-Parkinson Disease suffers

Note: ¥ = Fallers vs Non Fallers
　† = Healthy
　* = With Arthritis
　§ = With Parkinson's Disease
　N/A = Not available

Walker, 1983), wrist (Svanberg, 1988), cervical vertebrae, and bilateral sidebending (Lind et al., 1989), whereas others (Fiebert et al., 1992; Roach & Miles, 1991) have reported no age-related differences in range of motion for these joints. Clarification on this issue is important from a disability perspective, because not only is adequate flexibility considered to be necessary for normal daily physical functioning, but accurate normative values for range of motion are essential to support predictions of rehabilitation potential and to serve as "an indication of final functional capacity" (Fiebert et al., 1992).

Task specific ranges of motion for particular joints have been reported by some authors. For example, Perry (1978) suggested an optimal range of 120–140° of flexion at the elbow, whereas Brumfield and Champoux (1984), using an electrogoniometer, recorded the active range of wrist movement required to accomplish a variety of ADL and IADL. In this latter study, activities such as grooming and washing required between 10° of flexion to 15° of extension, whereas activities such as eating, reading a newspaper, and using a telephone required between 5° of flexion to 35° of extension. The authors suggested that these results may be used as the basis for disability evaluations. No age effect was reported in this study, despite the wide age range (25–60 y) of their subjects.

While flexibility has been referred to as a component of "muscular fitness" (ACSM, 1993), particularly in the elderly, it may be more accurately termed "connective tissue fitness." As one of the major limitations to range of motion (Alter, 1988; Threlkeld, 1992), connective tissue tends to increase with age in proportion to muscle mass (Fitts, 1980; Menard & Standish, 1989), to become less hydrated (Alter, 1988), and to change its relative composition of collagen and elastin (Shephard, 1978), all of which contribute to its increased density and rigidity (Beyer, 1983). The result of this change is an increase in passive mechanical resistive torque (PRT) in response to stretching of the connective tissues in and around the involved joint complex, a condition which contributes to a phenomenon referred to as "joint stiffness" (Wright, 1973), and thus to a decrease in range of motion. Passive resistive torque has been measured on the finger (Barnett & Cobbold, 1968, Wright & Johns, 1961), knee (Such et al., 1975), and elbow (Wiegner & Watts, 1986), with only the latter showing no significant age-related increase in PRT.

The contribution of muscle stiffness to disability in older persons is illustrated in a recent study by Vandervoort et al. (1992). In a randomized controlled study, they examined the ankle joint complex because of its significant role in gait, posture control, and many activities of daily living. They found a significant increase of PRT with age for both men and women, as well as significant decreases in the range of motion for active dorsiflexion and in voluntary isometric dorsiflexion strength. The authors suggested that this combination of greater PRT with decreasing dorsiflexor strength would increase the difficulty of turning up the foot during walking. This, in turn, could potentially result in inadequate foot clearance, a factor that has been implicated in accidental stumbles and falls (Patla et al., 1990). Vandervoort et al. (1992) interpreted their results as indicating a need to increase the strength of the dosiflexors so as to overcome the high resistive torque of the antagonist muscles. Equally effective, however, may be a flexibility program designed to increase the range of motion and/or decrease the "stiffness" of the muscles opposing dorsiflexion. This approach is validated by the studies cited above.

Other authors have also acknowledged the involvement of joint flexibility in gait regulation (Bowes et al., 1992; Koch et al., 1994; Schultz, 1992) and have recognized impaired range of motion as a risk factor for falls and mobility problems (Koch et al., 1994; Studenski et al., 1991; Tinetti et al., 1993a). Accordingly, a slowing of the inevitable decline in flexibility may help reduce either the incidence or the severity of such falls and difficulties in maintaining mobility. This is graphically illustrated in Figure 2-6, in which each of the three plotted training studies of women used the sit-and-reach test as its outcome measure. All three studies reported remarkably similar improvements in flexibility (2.4–2.5 cm), and when these results are superimposed on the comparable curve of Figure 2-1 (Shephard, 1990) the "zone" thus formed indicates the gains in flexibility potentially achievable by women who undergo appropriate exercise programs. Such gains may help to slow the deterioration in performance of daily living activities that generally accompanies aging.

Flexibility: Intervention Studies. Although flexibility has been shown to be amenable to improvement with exercise in the elderly (Figure 2-2), very few studies have examined this in terms of its potential to improve performance in activities of daily living. Koch et al. (1994) included measurements of both upper and lower body range of motion and strength in the development of a protocol for assessing and treating impairment and disability. In terms of flexibility, a criterion for intervention ("If range of motion is less than considered necessary for activities of daily living") was set for various movement planes of the shoulder, elbow, hip, and ankle joints, and a criterion value in degrees of range of motion was established for each of these joints. This newly developed protocol has been used in recent multicenter trials (Tinetti et al., 1993a), and preliminary results at 12 mo of follow-up show a reduced number of falls (30% vs 46%) in the intervention group compared to a "usual care" group (Tinetti et al., 1993b). With the exception of this one study, much of the literature describing the benefits of adequate flexibility and range of motion has been found in the field of physical therapy, where the abilities of patients to perform activities of daily living are crucial (DiFabio, 1992; Farrell & Jensen, 1992).

Flexibility exercises to improve range of motion have probably been more utilized in rehabilitation than in exercise training settings. Much may

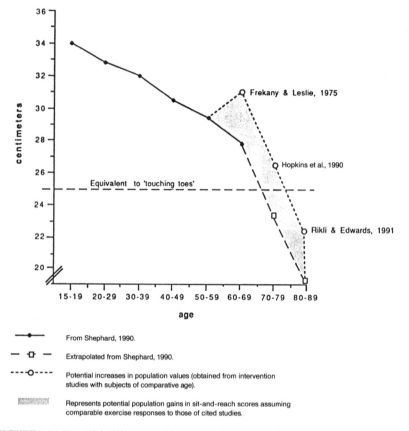

FIGURE 2-6. *Potential flexibility gains with exercise in the female population age 60–90 y.*

be gained from encouraging the inclusion of flexibility training in preventive exercise/activity programs. However, caution is still needed in attributing causality for improvements in activities of daily living to increases in flexibility because even in the more narrowly focused field of physical therapy, there is still a lack of scientifically validated treatment outcomes (DiFabio, 1992; Farrell & Jensen, 1992; Kane, 1994). There remains a need for randomized, controlled trials to directly address causality.

Multidisciplinary Approaches to Disability in Older Adults

Disability is a multifactorial phenomenon (Buchner et al., 1992; Guralnik & Simonsick, 1993; Ory et al., 1993; Pope & Tarlov, 1991), and one explanation for many of the inconsistent results found in the exercise training literature may be that most investigations were unidimensional. Multidisciplinary interventions such as those recently carried out in geriatric assessment units show promise for combinations of exercise, cognitive, and environmental/social treatments in the alleviation of disability in institutionalized populations (Applegate et al., 1990; Epstein et al., 1987), although the effects of such interventions vary with the setting and type of service (McVey et al., 1989; Rubenstein, 1987) and appear to be most effective for at-risk patients when assessment is combined with intensive treatment (National Institutes of Health, 1988).

Multidisciplinary approaches have also been used in community settings. For example, Svanborg (1993) reported the favorable progress of an ongoing community intervention in Gothenburg, Sweden, that utilized a team approach, including medical, social, nutritional, economic, architectural, and physical interventions. In the United States, the recently completed study entitled Frailty and Injuries: Cooperative Studies of Intervention Techniques (FICSIT) (Ory et al., 1993) is the largest investigation to date designed to assess optimal approaches to the amelioration of frailty and injuries in later life. FICSIT is a multi-center, randomized trial funded by the National Institute on Aging and by The Centers for Disease Control that is structured to maximize the amount of information from each of the eight centers by providing mechanisms for developing shared measures of subject characteristics, interventions, and outcomes (Ory et al., 1993). Several different intervention strategies are being tested in both community and institutionalized populations, with the aim of improving physical capacities, optimizing health behaviors, and/or improving the safety of environmental conditions (Ory et al., 1993). For example, the Seattle FICSIT trial (Buchner et al., 1993) is investigating the effect of exercise on gait and balance, utilizing either whole-body strength training (10 repetitions at 50–80% of 1 RM) or endurance training (walking, cycling or aerobic dance, generally at 50–70% of maximum heart rate reserve), or a both strength and endurance training. All the training was designed to simulate typical community exercise programs in terms of frequency and duration, and all exercise sessions were conducted 3 d/wk for approximately 1 h. The Atlanta FICSIT group (Wolf et al., 1993) utilize two exercise protocols involving center-of-mass feedback and tai chi training as interventions to reduce frailty in community-dwelling elders older than 70 y. Outcome measures in this study include both balance and environmental factors. Data analysis for the FICSIT trials should contribute much to the task of identifying the most effective techniques for systematically reducing the debilitating effects of frailty in our growing population of older adults.

DIRECTIONS FOR FUTURE RESEARCH

There are sufficient data indicating that adults of all ages benefit clinically from a program of moderate-intensity physical activity performed on most days to justify the widespread promotion of such a program, but there is still a substantial amount of information that needs to be scientifically documented. In terms of the effects of physical activity on longevity or mortality in older adults, all of the data demonstrating a favorable association are observational. Randomized clinical trials with mortality or longevity as the primary outcome are needed to demonstrate a causal relationship. Such studies are highly unlikely given their high costs and difficult logistics. Thus, additional prospective observational studies relating physical activity to all-cause and cause-specific mortality need to be conducted, especially in older women. However, these studies should include the measurement of known potential confounders so that they can be accounted for in the analysis. Additional data are needed on the "profile of activity" required to achieve specific health outcomes. For example, the type and intensity of activity required to optimize bone strength are likely to be different from what is needed to enhance insulin-mediated glucose uptake.

There is greater likelihood that randomized clinical trials can be conducted to determine if an increase in physical activity in older persons reduces the morbidity caused by specific chronic degenerative diseases, including hypertension, NIDDM, CHD, stroke, and osteoporotic fractures. For each of these disorders, research is needed on the role of physical activity in primary disease prevention (which may need to be conducted in persons at younger ages) and in secondary prevention, as well as on the use of activity in disease management or rehabilitation. Exercise training as part of rehabilitation following myocardial infarction has been shown to reduce mortality in meta analysis studies of existing data (O'Conner et al., 1989; Oldridge et al., 1988) and to be associated with modest reductions in blood pressure in hypertensive patients (Fagard & Tipton, 1994), but there are few data from randomized studies on the effects of specific exercise regimens on the clinical outcomes of patients with other disorders. A high priority for research in this area is randomized trials to determine the role of physical activity in the prevention of NIDDM and the contribution of physical activity to the management of NIDDM patients; clinical complications should be the major outcome variables. This research is especially important in older women, given their higher incidence of NIDDM and the increased risk for CHD conferred by NIDDM in these women.

As for the components of physical fitness, it is well established that there is sufficient plasticity in the tissues of sedentary older persons so that appropriate exercise regimens will produce increases in aerobic capacity, muscle strength, muscle endurance, flexibility, and gait speed. Less is understood regarding the improvement in balance, and little is known about how much and at what level of attainment (e.g., at what functional threshold) these components of fitness causally influence the various activities of daily living that lead to independent living and enhanced quality of life in the elderly. Studies are needed that link laboratory-based, exercise-induced improvements in aerobic capacity, muscular strength, endurance, flexibility, and balance with measures of daily functioning. Prime target populations for this research are older frail persons and those at high risk of clinical frailty in the near future, living both in community and institutional settings.

A major goal of this research also should be to determine which exercise regimens lead to significant reduction in the number of disability days as well as to ensure that the exercises can be performed in the community (senior centers, schools, homes, etc.) or in long-term care facilities. This requires a translation of methods suitable for programs based in the laboratory or clinic that use expensive and bulky equipment to methods suitable for programs that can be conducted in the community and used by a large percentage of older persons.

Better performance outcome measures are also needed that are relevant to the maintenance of independent living by the elderly. Traditional laboratory-based tests such as 1 RM and $\dot{V}O_2$max need to be superseded, or at least complemented, by tests that more accurately reflect the requirements for activities of daily living. Simulated tasks that aim to duplicate commonly performed activities such as rising from a chair, stooping, lifting, and carrying need to be used to develop validated instruments that can more accurately assess outcome measures related to independence. Both self-report and performance protocols need to be developed.

Finally, to successfully conduct research that better defines the relationship between physical activity and various clinical and performance outcomes in older persons, better physical activity measurement methodology needs to developed. Physical activity questionnaires that accurately and reliably define the physical activity profile (type, intensity, duration, frequency) of older adults are still lacking, especially for determining the activities of daily living in persons who perform only light and moderate intensity activity. Movement or/and physiologic monitoring systems need to be developed that can quantify levels of activity throughout the day, thus providing measures that are objective and do not depend on the limited short-term recall of many older persons.

SUMMARY

Performance of moderate-intensity physical activity on a regular basis appears to be an important ingredient in the recipe for growing older successfully. Men who remain physically active during middle and older age appear to live longer than their sedentary counterparts. Older men and women who self-select a physically active lifestyle experience a lower incidence of some chronic degenerative diseases and a lower age-specific mortality rate. However, these associations are based on observational studies and are potentially confounded by the self-selection of healthy people who choose to be more active. In addition to the possibility of increasing longevity, being more active may increase disability-free days in the elderly and help promote independent living. These projections are made from observational studies and preliminary randomized trials that demonstrate an enhanced capacity for performing activities of daily living following exercise training. Studies evaluating the effects of exercise training on aerobic capacity and muscle strength document improvements in the elderly similar to those observed in younger persons. Additional data are needed on the influence of various exercise regimens on dynamic balance and risk of falling in the oldest old and the relationship of each of the components of physical fitness to maintenance of independence and quality of life.

BIBLIOGRAPHY

Adams, G.H., and H.A. de Vries (1973). Physiological effects of exercise training regimen upon women age 52 to 79 years. *J. Gerontol.* 28:50–55.
Allender, E., O.J. Björnsson, O. Olsafsson, N. Sigfusson, and J. Thornsteinsson (1974). Normal range of joint movements in shoulder, hip, wrist, and thumb with special reference to side: comparison between two populations. *Int. J. Epidemiol.* 3:253–261.
Alter, M.J. (1988). *The Science of Stretching.* Champaign, IL: Human Kinetics Publishers.
American Alliance for Health, Physical Education, Recreation and Dance. (1986). *Physical Best Manual.* Reston, VA: American Alliance for Health, Physical Education, Recreation and Dance.
American College of Sports Medicine (1993). Physical activity, physical fitness, and hypertension. *Med. Sci. Sports Exerc.* 25:i–x.
American Health and Fitness Foundation (1986). *Fit Youth Today.* Austin, TX: American Health and Fitness Foundation.
Applegate, W.B., S.T. Miller, M.J. Graney, J.T. Elam, R. Burns, and D.E. Akins (1990). A randomized, controlled trial of a geriatric assessment unit in a community rehabilitation hospital. *New Engl. J. Med.* 322:1572–1578.
Badley, E.M., S. Wagstaff, and P.H.N. Wood (1984). Measures of functional ability (disability) in arthritis in relation to impairment of range of joint movement. *Ann. Rheumat. Dis.* 43:563–569.
Barnett, C.H., and A.F. Cobbold (1968). Effects of age on the mobility of human finger joints. *Ann. Rheumat. Dis.* 20:36–45.
Barry, A.J., J.R. Steinmetz, H. Page, and K. Rodahl (1966). The effects of physical conditioning on older individuals. II. Motor performance and cognitive function. *J. Gerontol.* 21:192–199.
Bassey, E.J., M.A. Fiatarone, E.F. O'Neill, M. Kelly, W.J. Evans, and L.A. Lipsitz (1992). Leg extensor power and functional performance in very old men and women. *Clin. Sci.* 82:321–327.
Bassey, E.J., K. Morgan, H.M. Dallasso, and S.B.J. Ebrahim (1989). Flexibility of the shoulder joint measured as range of abduction in a large representative sample of men and women over 65 years of age. *Eur. J. Appl. Physiol.* 58:353–360.
Battie, M.C., S.J. Bigos, A. Sheehy, and M.J. Wortley (1987). Spinal flexibility and individual factors that influence it. *Phys. Ther.* 67:653–658.
Benestad, A.M. (1965). The trainability of old men. *Acta Medica Scand.* 178:321–327.
Bergstrom, G., A. Aniansson, A. Bjelle, G. Grimby, B. Lungren-Lindquist, and A. Svanborg. (1985). Functional consequences of joint impairment at age 79. *Scand. J. Rehab. Med.* 17:183–190.
Berlin, J.A., and G.A. Colditz (1990). A meta-analysis of physical activity in the prevention of coronary heart disease. *Am. J. Epidemiol.* 132:612–628.
Beyer, R.E. (1983). Regulation of connective tissue metabolism in aging and exercise: A review. In: K.T. Borer, D.W. Edington, and T.P. White (eds.) *Frontiers in Exercise Biology.* Champaign, IL: Human Kinetics Publishers, pp. 85–99.
Blair, S.N., H.W. Kohl, R.S. Paffenbarger, D.G. Clark, K.H. Cooper, and L.W. Gibbons (1989). Physical fitness and all-cause mortality: A prospective study in healthy men and women. *J. Am. Med. Assoc.* 262:2395–2401.

Blair, S.N. (1993). C.H. McCloy research lecture: Physical activity, physical fitness, and health. *Res. Quart. Exerc. Sport* 54:365–376.

Block, J.E., R. Smith, A. Friedlander, and H.K. Grant (1989). Preventing osteoporosis with exercise: A review with emphasis on methodology. *Med. Hypoth.* 30:9–19.

Bouchard, C., R.J. Shephard, T. Stephens, J.R. Sutton, and B.D. McPherson (eds.) (1990). *Exercise, Fitness and Health. A Consensus of Current Knowledge.* Champaign, IL: Human Kinetics Publishers.

Bowes, S.G., A. Charlett, R.J. Dobbs, D.D. Lubel, R. Mehta, C.J.A. O'Neill, C. Weller, J. Hughes, and S.M. Dobbs (1992). Gait in relation to idiopathic Parkinsonism. *Scand. J. Rehab. Med.* 24:181–186.

Branch, L.G., and A.M. Jette (1984). Personal health practices and mortality among the elderly. *Am. J. Publ. Health* 74:1126–1129.

Brown, M., and J.O. Holloszy (1991). Effects of a low intensity exercise program on selected physical performance characteristics of 60- to 71-year-olds. *Aging* 3:129–139.

Brumfield, R.H., and J.A. Champoux (1984). A biomechanical study of normal functional wrist motion. *Clin. Orthopaed. Rel. Res.* 4:23–25.

Buchner, D.M., S.A. Beresford, E.B. Larson, A.Z. LaCroix, and E.H. Wagner (1992). Effects of physical activity on health status in older adults II: Intervention studies. *Ann. Rev. Publ. Health* 13:469–488.

Buchner, D.M., M.E. Cross, E.H. Wagner, B.J. deLateur, R. Price, and I.B. Abrass (1993). The Seattle FICSIT/Move It Study: The effect of exercise on gait and balance in older adults. *J. Amer. Geriatric Soc.* 41:321–325.

Buchner, D.M., and E.B. Larson (1987). Falls and fractures in patients with Alzheimer's type dementia. *J. Am. Med. Assoc.* 257:1492–1495.

Buskirk, E.R., and J.L. Hodgson (1987). Age and aerobic power: The rate of change in men and women. *Fed. Proc.* 46:1824–1829.

Canadian Standardized Test of Fitness (CSTF) Operations Manual, 3rd Ed. (1986). Ottawa, Canada: Fitness and Amateur Sport Canada.

Caspersen, C.J., K.E. Powell, and G.M. Christenson (1985). Physical activity, exercise, and physical fitness: Definitions and distinctions for health related research. *Publ. Health Rep.* 100:126–131.

Chakravarty, K., and M. Webley (1993). Shoulder joint movement and its relationship to disability in the elderly. *J. Rheumatol.* 20:1359–1361.

Chalmers, J., and K.C. Ho. (1970). Geographical variations in senile osteoporosis, *J. Bone Joint Surg.* 52:667–675.

Chamie, M. (1990). The status and use of the International Classification of Impairments, Disabilities, and Handicaps (ICIDH). *World Health Stat. Quart.* 43:273–280.

Chow, R., J.E. Harrison, and C. Notarius (1987). Effect of two randomised exercise progammes on bone mass of healthy postmenopausal women. *Br. Med. J.* 295:1441–1444.

Clark, R.D., S.R. Lord, and I.W. Webster (1993). Clinical parameters associated with falls in an elderly population. *Gerontology* 39:117–123.

Cononie, C.C., J.E. Graves, M.L. Pollock, M.I. Phillips, C. Summers, and J.M. Hagberg (1991). Effect of exercise training on blood pressure in 70- to 79-yr-old men and women. *Med. Sci. Sports Exerc.* 23:505–511.

Corbin, C.B. (1984). Flexibility. *Clin. Sports Med.* 3:101–117.

Corbin, C.B., and R. Lindsey (1993). *Fitness for Life.* Glenville, IL: Scott, Foresman, and Company.

Costa, A.J. (1991). Preventing falls in your elderly patient. *Postgrad. Med.* 89:139–142.

Cummings, S.R. (1985). Are patients with hip fractures osteoporotic? *Am. J. Med.* 78:487–494.

Cummings, S.R., and D. Black (1986). Should perimenopausal women be screened for osteoporosis? *Ann. Intern. Med.* 104:817–823.

Cunningham, D.A., and D.H. Paterson (1990). Discussion: Exercise, fitness and aging. In: C. Bouchard, R.J. Shephard, T. Stephens, J.R. Sutton, and B.D. McPherson (eds.) *Exercise, Fitness and Health. A Consensus of Current Knowledge.* Champaign, IL.: Human Kinetics Publishers, pp. 699–704.

Cwikel, J., and A.V. Fried (1992). The social epidemiology of falls among community-dwelling elderly: guidelines for prevention. *Disabil. Rehabil.* 14:113–121.

DeVries, H.A. (1975). The physiology of exercise and aging. In: D.S. Woodruff and J.R. Birren (eds.) *Aging: Scientific Perspectives and Social Issues.* New York: D. Van Nostrand Co., pp. 257–276.

DiFabio, R.P. (1992). Efficacy of manual therapy. *Phys. Ther.* 72:853–864.

Drinkwater, B.L. (1994). Physical activity, fitness and osteoporosis. In: C. Bouchard, R.J. Shephard, and T. Stephens (eds.) *Physical Activity, Fitness, and Health: International Proceedings and Consensus Statement.* Champaign, IL: Human Kinetics Publishers, pp. 724–736.

Dupler, T.L., and C. Cortes (1993). Effects of a whole body resistive training regimen in the elderly. *Gerontology* 39: 314–319.

Ekelund, L.G., W.L. Haskell, J.L. Johnson, F.S. Wholey, M.H. Criqui, and D.S. Sheps (1988). Physical fitness in the prevention of cardiovascular mortality in asymptomatic North American men. *New Engl. J. Med.* 319:1379–1384.

Epstein, A.M., J.A. Hall, and R. Besdine (1987). The emergence of geriatric assessment units: the "new technology of geriatrics." *Ann. Inter. Med.* 106: 299–303.

Era, P. (1988). Posture control in the elderly. *Intern. J. Tech. Aging* 1: 166–169.

Fagard, R.H., and C.M. Tipton (1994). Physical activity, fitness and hypertension. In: C. Bouchard, R.J. Shephard, and T. Stephens (eds.) *Physical Activity, Fitness, and Health: International Proceedings and Consensus Statement.* Champaign, IL: Human Kinetics Publishers, pp. 633–655.

Farrell, J.P., and G.M. Jensen (1992). Foreword: manual therapy. *Phys. Ther.* 72:842.

Fiatarone, M.A., E.C. Marks, N.D. Ryan, C.N. Meredith, L.A. Lipsitz, and W.J. Evans (1990). High intensity strength training in nonagenarians. *J. Am. Med. Assoc.* 263:3029–3034.

Fiatarone, M.A., E.F. O'Neill, N.D. Ryan, K.M. Clements, G.R. Solares, M.E. Nelson, S.B. Roberts, J.J. Kehayias, L.A. Lipsitz, and W.J. Evans (1994). Exercise training and nutritional supplementation for physical frailty in very elderly people. *New Engl. J. Med.* 330:1769–1775.

Fiebert, I., J.R. Fuhri, and M. Dahling (1992). Elbow, forearm and wrist passive range of motion in persons aged sixty and older. *Phys. Occupat. Ther. Geriatr.* 10:17–32.

Fisher, N.M., D.R. Pendergast, and E. Calkins (1991). Muscle rehabilitation in impaired elderly nursing home residents. *Arch. Phys. Med. Rehab.* 72:181–185.

Fitti, J.E., and M.G. Kovar (1987) The supplement on aging to the 1984 National Health Interview Survey. *Vital and Health Statistics, Series 1, No. 21. Dept. Health and Human Services pub. (PHS) 87–1323.* Hyattsville, MD: National Center for Health Statistics.

Fitts, R.H. (1980). Aging and skeletal muscle. In: E.L. Smith and R.C. Serfass (eds.) *Exercise and Aging: The Scientific Basis.* Hillside, NJ: Enslow Publishers, pp. 31–44.

Frekany, G.A., and D.K. Leslie (1975). Effects of an exercise program on selected flexibility measurements of senior citizens. *Gerontologist* 15:174–175.

Fries, J.F. (1989). The compression of morbidity: Near or far? *Millbank Quart.* 67:208–231.

Frontera, W.R., C.N. Meredith, K.P. O'Reilly, H.G. Knuttgen, and W.J. Evans (1988). Strength conditioning in older men: skeletal muscle hypertrophy and improved function. *J. App. Physiol.* 64:1038–1044.

Frymoyer, J.W., and W. Cats-Baril (1987). Predictors of low-back pain disability. *Clin. Orthop.* 221:89–98.

Fulton, J.P., S. Katz, S.S. Jack, and G.E. Hendershot (1989). Physical functioning of the aged: United States, 1984. *Vital and Health Statistics, Series 10, No. 167. Dept. Health and Human Services pub. (PHS) 89–1595.* Hyattsville, MD: National Center for Health Statistics.

Fuster, V., L. Badimon, J.J. Badimon, and J.H. Chesebro (1992). The pathogenesis of coronary artery disease and the acute coronary syndromes. *New Engl. J. Med.* 326:241–250.

Gehlsen, G.M., and M.H. Whaley (1990). Falls in the elderly: Part I, Gait. *Arch. Phys. Med. Rehab.* 71:735–738.

Germain, N.W., and S.N. Blair (1983). Variability of shoulder flexion with age, activity and sex. *Am. Correc. Ther. J.* 32:156–160.

Golding, L.A., C.R. Myers, and W.E. Sinning (eds.) (1989). *The Y's Way to Physical Fitness, 3rd Ed.* Champaign, IL: Human Kinetics Publishers

Guralnik, J.M., L.G. Branch, S.R. Cummings, and J.D. Curb (1989a). Physical performance measures in aging research. *J. Gerontol.: Med. Sci.* 44: M141–146.

Guralnik, J.M., A.Z. LaCroix, D.F. Everett, and M.G. Kovar (1989b). Aging in the eighties: the prevalence of comorbidity and its association with disability. *Advance Data from Vital and Health Statistics; Series 3, No. 170. Dept. Health and Human Services pub. (PHS) 89–1250.* Hyattsville, MD: National Center for Health Statistics.

Guralnik, J.M., and E.M. Simonsick (1993). Physical disability in older Americans. *J. Gerontol.* 48 (Special Issue):3–10.

Gutman, G.M., C.P. Herbert, and S.R. Brown (1977). Feldenkrais versus conventional exercises for elderly. *J. Gerontol.* 32:562–572.

Hagberg, J.M. (1987). Effect of training on the decline of $\dot{V}O_2$ max with aging. *Fed. Proc.* 46:1830–1837.

Hagberg, J.M. (1994). Physical activity, fitness, health and aging. In: C. Bouchard, R.J. Shephard, and T. Stephens (eds.) *Physical Acivity, Fitness, and Health. International Proceedings and Consensus Statement.* Champaign, IL: Human Kinetics Publishers, pp. 993–1005.

Hagberg, J.M., S.C. Montain, W. H. Martin, and A.A. Ehsani. (1989). Effect of exercise training in 60- to 69-year-old persons with essential hypertension. *Am. J. Cardiol.* 64:348–353.

Häkkinen, K. (1994). Neuromuscular adaptations during strength training and detraining in middle-aged and elderly people. Stairmaster Conference on Aging and Physical Activity, Virginia Beach, Virginia, October 21–23, 1993. In: *J. Aging Phys. Activ.* (Conference Abstracts) 1:100.

Häkkinen, A., K. Häkkinen, and P. Hannonen (1994). Effects of strength training on neuromuscular function in middle-aged patients with recent-onset rheumatoid arthritis. Stairmaster Conference on Aging and Physical Activity, Virginia Beach, Virginia, October 21–23, 1993. In: *J. Aging Phys. Activ.* (Conference Abstracts) 1:100–101.

Hamdy, R.C., J. Beamer, K. Whalen, M. Doman, S. Moore, H. Cancellaro, and J. Anderson (1994). Are aerobic exercises as beneficial on the musculoskeletal system as weight lifting exercises in subjects 55 years and older? Stairmaster Conference on Aging and Physical Activity, Virginia Beach, Virginia, October 21–23, 1993. In: *J. Aging Phys. Activ.* (Conference Abstracts) 1:101–102.

Harris, M.L. (1969). Flexibility: A review of the literature. *Phys. Ther.* 49:591–601.

Harris, R. (1984). Diagnostic and therapeutic aspects of physical exercise and sport in clinical health care of the aging. In: B.D. McPherson (ed.) *Sport and Aging.* Champaign, IL: Human Kinetics Publishers, pp. 159–160.

Harris, T., M.G. Kovar, R. Suzman, J.C. Kleinman, and J.J Feldman (1989). Longitudinal study of physical ability in the oldest old. *Am. J. Publ. Health.* 79:698–702.

Hartley, P., and G.F. Llewellyn (1939). The longevity of oarsmen: A study of those who rowed in the Oxford and Cambridge boat race from 1829 to 1928. *Brit. Med. J.* 1:657–662.

Heck, C.V., I.E. Hendryson, and C.R. Rowe (1965). *Joint motion: methods of measuring and recording.* Chicago, IL: American Academy of Orthopedic Surgeons, pp. 27–43

Helmrich, S.P., D.R. Ragland, R.W. Leung, and R.S. Paffenbarger (1991). Physical activity and reduced occurrence of non-insulin-dependent diabetes mellitus. *New Engl. J. Med.* 325:147–152.

Hickson, R.C., C. Foster, M.L. Pollock, T.M. Galassi, and S. Rich (1985). Reduced training intensities and loss of aerobic power, endurance and cardiac growth. *J. Appl. Physiol.* 58:492–499.

Hickson R.C., J.M. Hagberg, A.A. Ehani, and J.D. Hollozy (1981). Time course of the adaptive responses of aerobic power and heart rate. *Med. Sci. Sports Exerc.* 13:17–20.

Higgins, P.G. (1988). Biometric outcomes of a geriatric health promotion programme. *J. Adv. Nursing* 13:710–715.

Hindmarsh, J.J., and E.H. Estes Jr. (1989). Falls in older persons: causes and interventions. *Arch. Int. Med.* 149:2217–2222.

Holland, G. (1968). The physiology of flexibility: A review of the literature. *Kinesiol. Rev.* 1:49–62.

Hollman, W. (1964). Changes in the capacity for maximal and continuous effort in relation to age. In: E. Jokl and E. Simon (eds.) *International Research in Sport and Physical Education.* Springfield, IL: Charles C. Thomas, pp. 369–371.

Holloszy, J.O. (1983). Exercise, health and aging: A need for more information. *Med. Sci. Sports Exerc.* 15:1–5.

Hopkins, D.R., B. Murrah, W.W.K. Hoegar, and R.C. Rhodes (1990). Effect of low-impact aerobic dance on the functional fitness of elderly women. *Gerontologist* 30:189–192.

Howley, E.T., and B.D. Franks (1986). *Health/Fitness Instructors Handbook.* Champaign, IL: Human Kinetics Publishers.

Jackson, A.W., and A.A. Baker (1986) The relationship of the sit-and-reach test to criterion measures of hamstring and back flexibility in young females. *Res. Quart. Exerc. Sport* 57:183–186.

Jackson, A.W., and N.J. Langford (1988). The criterion-related validity of the sit-and-reach test: Replication and extension of previous findings. *Res. Quart. Exerc. Sport* 60:384–387.

Jennings, G., L. Nelson, P. Nestel, M. Esler, P. Korner, D. Burton, and J. Bazelmans. (1986). The effects of changes in physical activity on major cardiovascular risk factors, hemodynamics, sympathetic function, and glucose utilization in man: A controlled study of four levels of activity. *Circulation* 73:30–40.

Jette, A.M., and J.M. Bottomley (1987). The greying of America. Opportunities for physical therapy. *Phys. Ther.* 67:1537–1542.

Judge, J.O., C. Lindsey, M. Underwood, and D. Winsemius. (1993). Balance improvements in older women: Effects of exercise training. *Phys. Ther.* 73:254–265.

Kahn, H.A. (1963). The relationship of reported coronary heart disease mortality to physical activity of work. *Am. J. Publ. Health.* 53:1058–1067.

Kane, R.L. (1994). Looking for physical therapy outcomes. *Phys. Ther.* 74: 425–429.

Kaplan, G.A., T.E. Seeman, R.D. Cohen, L.P. Knudsen, and J. Guralnik (1987). Mortality among the elderly in the Alameda County Study: behavioral and demographic risk factors. *Am. J. Publ. Health.* 77:307–312.

Kasch, F.W., J.P. Wallace, S.P. Van Camp, and L. Verity (1988). A longitudinal study of cardiovascular stability in active men aged 45–65 years. *Phys. Sports Med.* 16:117–124.

Katsuki, S., and M. Masuda (1969). Physical exercise for persons of middle and older age in relation to their physical ability. *J. Sports Med.* 9:193–199.

Katz, S., L.G. Branch, M.H. Branson, J.A. Papsidero, J.C. Beck, and D.S. Greer (1983). Active life expectancy. *New Engl. J. Med.* 309:1218–1223.

Kellogg International Work Group on the Prevention of Falls in the Elderly (1987). The prevention of falls in later life. *Danish Med. Bull. Suppl.* 4:34.

Koch, M., M. Gottschalk, D.I. Baker, S. Palumbo, and M.E. Tinetti (1994). An impairment and disability assessment and treatment protocol for community-living ederly persons. *Phys. Ther.* 74:286–298.

Kohl, H.W., R.E. LaPorte, and S.N. Blair (1988). Physical activity and cancer: An epidemiological perspective. *Sports Med.* 6:222–237.

Kohrt, W.M., M.T. Malley, A.R. Coggan, R.J. Spina, T. Ogawa, J.O. Holloszy (1991). Effects of gender, age, and fitness level on response of $\dot{V}O_2$max to training in 60–71 yr. olds. *J. Appl. Physiol.* 71:2004–2011.

Konczak, J., H.J. Meeuwsen, and M.E. Cress (1992). Changing affordances in stair climbing: The perception of maximum climbability in young and older adults. *J. Exper. Psychol. Human Percep. Perform.* 18:691–697.

Lakka, T.A., J.M. Venalainen, R. Rauramaa, R. Salonen, J. Tuomilehto, and J.T. Salonen (1994). Relation of leisure-time physical activity and cardiorespiratory fitness to the risk of acute myocardial infarction in men. *New Engl. J. Med.* 330:1549–1554.

Lampman, R.M., and P.J. Savage (1987). Exercise and aging: A review of benefits and a plan for action. In: J.R. Sowers and J.V. Felicetta (eds.) *The Endocrinology of Aging.* New York: Raven Press, pp. 307–355.

LaPlante, M.P. (1988). Data on disability from the National Health Interview Survey 1983–1985. *An InfoUse Report.* Washington, DC: National Institute on Disability and Rehabilitation Research.

LaPorte, R.E., L.H. Kuller, D.J. Kupfer, R.J. McPartland, G. Matthews, and C. Casperson (1979). An objective measure of physical activity for epidemiologic research. *Am. J Epidemiol.* 109:158–168.

Lawton, M.P., and E.M. Brody (1969). Assessment of older people: self-maintaining and instrumental activities of daily living. *Gerontologist* 9:179–186.

Leon, A.S., J. Cornett, D.R. Jacobs, R. Rauramaa (1987). Leisure-time physical activity levels and risk of coronary heart disease and death: The Multiple Risk Factor Intervention Trial. *J. Am. Med. Assoc.* 258:2388–2395.

Lichtenstein, M.J., S.L. Shields, R.G. Shiavi, and C. Burger (1989). Exercise and balance in aged women: A pilot controlled clinical trial. *Arch. Phy. Med. Rehab.* 70:138–143.

Lind, B., H. Sihlbom, A. Nordwall, and H. Malchau (1989). Normal range of motion of the cervical spine. *Arch. Phys. Med. Rehab.* 70:692–695.

Lord, S.R., G.A. Caplan, and J.A. Ward (1993). Balance, reaction time, and muscle strength in exercising and nonexercising older women: A pilot study. *Arch. Phys. Med. Rehab.* 74:837–839.

MacKeen, P.C., J.L. Rosenberger, J.S. Slater, W.C. Nicholas, and E.R. Buskirk (1985). A 13 year follow-up of a coronary heart disease risk factor screening and exercise program for 40–59-year-old men: exercise habit maintenance and physiologic status. *J. Cardiopul. Rehab.* 5:510–523.

Manson, J.E., D.M. Nathan, A.S. Krolewski, M.J. Stampfer, W.C. Willett, and C.H. Hennkens (1992). A prospective study of exercise and incidence of diabetes among US male physicians. *J. Am. Med. Assoc.* 268:63–67.

Manson, J.E., E.B. Rimm, and M.J. Stampfer (1991). Physical activity and incidence of non-insulin-dependent diabetes mellitus in women. *Lancet* 3:774–778.

Manton, K.G., L.S. Corder, and E. Stallard (1993a). Estimates of change in chronic disability and institutional incidence and prevalence rates in the U.S. elderly population from the 1982, 1984, and 1989 National Long Term Care Survey. *J. Gerontol. Soc. Sci.* 48:S153–S166.

Manton, K.G., and B.J. Soldo (1993). Disability and mortality among the oldest old: Implications for current and future health and long-term care service needs. In: R.M. Suzman, D.P. Willis, and K.G. Manton (eds.) *The Oldest Old.* Oxford, England: Oxford University Press.

Manton, K.G., E. Stallard, and M.A. Woodbury (1993b). A multivariate event history model based upon fuzzy states: Estimation from longitudinal surveys with informative non-response. In: R.M. Suzman, D.P. Willis, and K.G. Manton (eds.) *The Oldest Old.* Oxford, England: Oxford University Press, p. 10.

McMurdo, M.E., and L. Burnett (1992). Randomized controlled trial of exercise in the elderly. *Gerontology* 38:292–298.

McMurdo, M.E., and L. Rennie (1993). A controlled trial of exercise by residents of old people's homes. *Age Aging* 22:11–15.

McVey, L.J., P.M. Becker, C.C. Saltz, J.R. Feussner, and H.J. Cohen (1989). Effect of a geriatric consultation team on functional status of elderly hospitalized patients. *Ann. Internal Med.* 110:79–84.

Menard, D., and W.D. Standish (1989). The aging athlete. *Am. J. Sports Med.* 17:187–196.

Meredith, C.N., W.R. Frontera, K.P. O'Reilly, and W.J. Evans (1992). Body composition in elderly men: effect of dietary modification during strength training. *J. Am. Geriatr. Soc.* 40:155–162.

Meusel, H. (1986). Health and well-being for older adults through physcal exercises and sport—outline of the Giessen Model. In: B.D.McPherson (ed.) *Sport and Aging.* Champaign, IL: Human Kinetics Publishers, pp. 107–115.

Mor, V., J. Murphy, and S. Masterson-Allen (1989). Risk of functional decline among well elders. *J. Clin. Epidemiol.* 42:895–904.

Morey, M.C., P.A. Cowper, J.R. Feussner, R.C. DiPasquale, G.M. Crowley, D.W. Kitzman, and R.J. Sullivan (1989). Evaluation of a supervised exercise program in a geriatric population. *J. Am. Geriatr. Soc.* 37:348–354.

Moritani, T., and H.A. deVries (1979). Neural factors versus hypertrophy in the time course of muscle strength gain. *Am. J. Phys. Med.* 58:115–131.

Morris, J.N., D.G. Clayton, M.G. Everitt, A.M. Semmence, and E.H. Burgess. (1990). Exercise in leisure time: Coronary attack and death rates. *Brit. Heart J.* 63:325–334.

Morris, J.N., and M.D. Crawford (1958). Coronary heart disease and physical activity of work: Evidence of a national necropsy survey. *Brit. Med. J.* 5111:1485–1496.

Morris, J.N., J.A. Heady, and P.A.B. Raffle (1953). Coronary heart disease and physical activity of work. *Lancet* 1053:1111–1119.

Morris, J.N., R. Pollard, M.G. Everitt, and S.P.W. Chave (1980). Vigorous exercise in leisure time: Protection against coronary heart disease. *Lancet* 8206:1207–1214.

Muller, E.A. (1957). The regulation of muscular strength. *J. Assoc. Phys. Mental Rehab.* 11:41–47.

Nagi, S.Z. (1976). An epidemiology of disability among adults in the United States. *Millbank Mem. Fund Quart./Health Soc.* 54:439–468.

National Center for Health Statistics (1987). Current estimates from the national health interview survey, United States. *Vital and Health Statistics, Series 10, No. 166. Dept. Health and Human Services Pub. No. 1 (PHS) 88-1594.* Washington, D.C.: U.S. Government Printing Office.

National Center for Health Statistics (1993). Monthly Vital Statistics Report. *Advance Report of Final Mortality Statistics, 1990.* 41 (7).

National Institutes of Health (1988). National Institutes of Health Consensus Development Conference Statement: Geriatric Assessment Methods for Clinical Decision-Making. *J. Am. Geriatr. Soc.* 36:342–347.

National Safety Council (1990). *Accident Facts.* Chicago, IL: National Safety Council.

Nevitt, M.C. (1990). Falls in older persons: risk factors and prevention. In: R.L. Berg and J.S. Cassello (eds.) *The Second Fifty Years, Promoting Health and Preventing Disability.* Washington, D.C.: Institute of Medicine, National Academy Press, pp. 263–290.

Nevitt, M.C., S.R. Cummings, and E.S. Hudes (1991). Risk factors for injurious falls: A prosective study. *J. Gerontol.* 46:M164–170.

Nevitt, M.C., S.R. Cummings, S.R. Kidd, and D. Black (1989). Risk factors for recurrent nonsyncopal falls: A prospective study. *J. Am. Med. Assoc.* 261: 2663–2668.

Nichols, J.F., D.K. Omizo, K.K. Peterson, and K.P. Nelson (1993). Efficacy of heavy-resistance training for active women over sixty: muscular strength, body composition, and program adherence. *J. Am. Geriatr. Soc.* 41:205–210.

Notelovitz, M., D. Martin, R. Tesar, L. McKenzie, and C. Field (1991). Estrogen therapy and variable resistance weight training increases bone mineral in surgically menopausal women. *J. Bone Min. Res.* 6:583–590.

O'Conner, G.T., J.E. Boving, and S. Yusuf (1989). An overview of randomized trials of rehabilitation with exercise after myocardial infarction. *Circulation* 80:234–245.

Oldridge, N.B., G.H. Guyatt, M.E. Fisher, and A.A. Rimm (1988). Cardiac rehabilitation after myocardial infarction: Combined exercise of randomized clinical trials. *J. Am. Med. Assoc.* 260:945–950.

Ory, M.G., K.B. Schechtman, J.P. Miller, E.C. Hadley, M.A. Fiatarone, M.A. Province, C.L. Arfken, D. Morgan, S. Wiess, M. Kaplan, and The FICSIT Group (1993). Frailty and injuries in late life: The FICSIT Trials. *J. Am. Geriatr. Soc.* 41:283–296.

Paffenbarger, R.S., R.T. Hyde, A.L. Wing, and C-C. Hsieh (1986). Physical activity, all-cause mortality and longevity of college athletes. *New Engl. J. Med.* 314:605–613.

Paffenbarger R.S., R.T. Hyde, A.L. Wing, I-M. Lee, D.L. Jung, and J.B. Kampert (1993). The association of changes in physical activity level and other lifestyle characteristics with mortality among men. *New Engl. J. Med.* 328:538–545.

Paffenbarger, R.S., R.T. Hyde, A.L. Wing, and C.H. Steinmetz (1984). A natural history of athleticism and cardiovascular health. *J. Am. Med. Assoc.* 252:491–495.

Paffenbarger, R.S., A.L. Wing, R.T. Hyde, and C. Hsieh (1983). Physical activity and incidence of hypertension in college alumni. *Am. J. Epidemiol.* 117:245–257.

Paterson, D.H., D.A. Cunningham, J.E. Himann, and P.A. Rechnitzer (1988). Long term effects of exercise training on $\dot{V}O_2$max in older men. *Canad. J. Sports Sci.* 13:124P–125P.

Patla, A., J. Frank, and D. Winter (1990). Assessment of balance control in the elderly: Major issues. *Physiother. Canada* 42:89–97.

Pekkanen, J., B. Marti, A. Nissinen, J. Tuomilehto, S. Punsar, and M. Karvonen (1987). Reduction of premature mortality by high physical activity: 20-year follow-up of middle-aged Finnish men. *Lancet* 1136:1473–1477.

Pendergast, D.R., N.M. Fisher, and E. Calkins (1993). Cardiovascular, neuromuscular and metabolic alterations with age leading to frailty. *J. Gerontol.* 48 (Special Issue): 61–67.

Perry, J. (1978). Normal upper extremity kinesiology. *Phys. Ther.* 58:265–278.

Plowman, S.A. (1992). Physical activity, physical fitness, and low back pain. *Exerc. Sport Sci. Rev.* 20:221–242.

Pollock, M.L., C. Foster, D. Knapp, J.L. Rod, and D.H. Schmidt (1987). Effect of age and training on aerobic capacity and body composition of master athletes. *J. Appl. Physiol.* 62:725–731.

Pope, A.M., and A.R. Tarlov (eds.) (1991). *Disability in America: Towards a National Agenda for Prevention.* Washington, D.C.: Institute of Medicine, National Academy Press.

Powell, K.E., P.D. Thompson, C.J. Caspersen, and J.S. Kendrick (1987). Physical activity and the incidence of coronary heart disease. *Ann. Rev. Publ. Health* 8:253–287.

President's Council on Physical Fitness and Sports (1971). *Phys. Fit. Res. Digest,* Series I, No. 1. Washington, D.C.

Prince, R., M. Smith, I.M. Dick, R.I. Price, P.G. Webb, K. Henderson, and M. Harris (1991). Prevention of osteoporosis: A comparative study of exercise, calcium supplementation, and hormone-replacement therapy. *New Engl. J. Med.* 325:1189–1195.

Quinn, T.J., H.A. Sprague, W.D. Van Huss, and H.W. Olson (1990). Caloric expenditure, life status, and disease in former male athletes and non-athletes. *Med. Sci. Sports Exerc.* 22:742–750.

Raab, D.M., J.C. Agre, M. McAdam, and E.L. Smith (1988). Light resistance and stretching exercise in elderly women: effect upon flexibility. *Arch. Phys. Med. Rehab.* 69: 268–272.

Rantanen, R., P. Era, and E. Heikkinen (1994). Maximal isometric strength and mobility among 75-year-old men and women. *Age Ageing.* 23:132–137.

Raven, P.B., and J.H. Mitchell (1980). Effect of aging on the cardiovascular response to dynamic and static exercise in the aging heart: Its function and response to stress. In: M.L. Weisfeldt (ed.) *Aging*, Vol. 12. New York: Raven Press.

Reaven, P.D., E. Barrett-Conner, and S. Edelstein (1991). Relation between leisure-time physical activity and blood pressure in older women. *Circulation* 83:559–565.

Rice, D.P., and E.J. Mackenzie (1989). *Cost of injury in the United States: A report to Congress.* San Francisco CA: Institute for Health and Aging, University of California; and Baltimore, MD: Injury Prevention Center, The Johns Hopkins University, pp. 37–86.

Riggs, B.L., and L.J. Melton (1986). Involutional osteoporosis. *New Engl. J. Med.* 311:1601–1606.

Riihimaki, H. (1991). Low-back pain, its origin and risk indicators. *Scand. J. Work Environ. Health.* 17:81–90.

Rikli, R., and S. Busch (1986). Motor performance of women as a function of age and physical activity level. *J. Gerontol.* 41:654–659.

Rikli, R.E., and D.J. Edwards (1991). Effects of a three-year exercise program on motor function and cognitive processing speed in older women. *Res. Quart. Exerc. Sport* 62:61–67.

Roach, K.E., and T.P Miles (1991). Normal hip and knee active ranges of motion; The relationship of age. *Phys. Ther.* 71:656–665.

Rodriguez, M.J., J.J. Depalma, and H.D. Daykin (1965). Isometric exercise in general practice. *J. Assoc. Phys. Mental Rehab.* 19:197–200.

Roman, W.J., J. Fleckenstein, J. Stray-Gundersen, S.E. Alway, R. Pechock, and W.J. Gonyea (1993). Adaptations in the elbow flexors of elderly males after heavy resistance training. *J. Appl. Physiol.* 74:750–754.

Rook, A. (1954). An investigation into the longevity of Cambridge sportsmen. *Br. Med. J.* 1:773–777.

Rosow, I., and N. Breslau (1966). A Guttman health scale for the aged. *J. Gerontol.* 21:556–559.

Rowe, J., and R. Kahn (1987) Human aging: usual and successful. *Science* 237:143–149.

Rubenstein, L.Z. (1987). Geriatric assessment: An overview of its impacts. *Clin. Geriatr. Med.* 3:1–15.

Salonen, J.T., P. Puska, and J. Tuomilehto (1982). Physical activity and risk of myocardial infarction, cerebral stroke and death: A longitudinal study in Eastern Finland. *Am. J. Epidemiol.* 115:526–537.

Sandvik L., J. Erikssen, E. Thaulow, G. Erikssen, R. Mundal, and K. Rodhal (1993). Physical fitness as a predictor of mortality among healthy, middle-aged Norweigan men. *New Engl. J. Med.* 328:553–557.

Sandler, R.B., J.A. Cauley, D.L. Hom, D. Sashin, and A.M. Kriska (1987). The effects of walking on the cross-sectional dimensions of the radius in postmenopausal women. *Calcif. Tiss. Internat.* 41:65–69.

Sattin, R.W. (1992). Falls among older persons: A public health perspective. *Ann. Rev. Publ. Health* 13:489–508.

Sauvage, L.R., B.M. Myklehurst, J. Crow-Pan, S. Novak, P. Millington, M.D. Hoffman, A.J. Hartz, and D. Rudman (1992). A clinical trial of strengthening and aerobic exercise to improve gait and balance in elderly male nursing home residents. *Am. J. Phys. Med. Rehab.* 71:333–342.

Schultz, A.B. (1992). Mobility impairment in the elderly: challenges for biomechanics research. *J. Biomech.* 25:519–528.

Schwartz, R.S., K.C. Cain, W.P. Shuman, V. Larson, J.R. Stratton, J.C. Beard, S.E. Kahn, M.D. Cerqueira, and I.B. Abrass (1992). Effect of intensive endurance training on lipoprotein profiles in young and older men. *Metabolism* 41:649–654.

Seals, D.R., and M.J. Reiling (1991). Effect of regular exercise on 24-hour arterial blood pressure in older hypertensive humans. *Hypertension* 18:583–592.

Seals, D.R., J.M. Hagberg, B.F. Hurley, A.A. Ehsani, and J.O. Hollozy (1984). Endurance training in older men and women: I. Cardiovascular responses to exercise. *J. Appl. Physiol.* 57:1024–1029.

Shaper, A.G., and G. Wannamethee (1991). Physical activity and ischaemic heart disease in middle-aged British men. *Brit. Heart J.* 66:384–394.

Shapiro, S., E. Weinblatt, C.W. Frank, and R.V. Sager (1969). Incidence of coronary heart disease in a population insured for medical care (HIP). *Am. J. Publ. Health* (Suppl.) 59:1–76.

Shephard, R.J. (1978). *Physical activity and aging.* London: Croom Helm.

Shephard, R.J. (1990). The scientific basis of exercise prescribing for the very old. *J. Am. Geriatr. Soc.* 38:62–70.

Simonsick, E.M., M.E. Lafferty, C.L. Phillips, C.F. Mendes de Leon, S.V. Kasl, T.E. Seeman, G. Fillenbaum, P. Hebert, and J.H. Lemke (1993). *Am. J. Publ. Health* 83:1443–1450.

Sinaki, M., and K.P. Offord (1988). Physical activity in postmenopausal women: Effect on back muscle strength and bone mineral density of the spine. *Arch. Phys. Med. Rehab.* 69:277–280.

Skinner, J.S., and P. Oja. (1994). Laboratory and field tests for assessing health related fitness. In: C. Bouchard, R.J. Shephard, and T. Stephens (eds.) *Physical Activity, Fitness, and Health: International Proceedings and Consensus Statement.* Champaign, IL: Human Kinetics Publishers, pp. 160–179.

Smith, E.L. (1980). Age: The interaction of nature and nurture. In: E.L. Smith and R.C. Serfass (eds.) *Exercise and Aging. The Scientific Basis.* Englewood Cliffs, NJ: Enslow Publishers, p. 11–17.

Smith, E.L., and C. Gilligan (1991). Physical activity effects on bone metabolism. *Calcif. Tiss. Internat.* (Suppl.) 49:S50-S54.

Smith, J.R., and J.M. Walker (1983). Knee and elbow range of motion in healthy older individuals. *Phys. Occupat. Ther. Geriatr.* 2:31-38.

Stamford, B.A. (1988). Exercise and the elderly. *Exerc. Sport Sci. Rev.* 9:341-379.

Stones, M.J., and A. Kozma (1987). Balance and age in the sighted and blind. *Arch. Phys. Med. Rehab.* 68:85-89.

Studenski, S., P.W. Duncan, and J. Chandler (1991). Postural responses and effector factors in persons with unexplained falls: Results and methodological issues. *J. Am. Geriatr. Soc.* 39:229-234.

Such, C.H., A. Unsworth, V. Wright, and D. Dowson (1975). Quantitative study of stiffness in the knee joint. *Ann. Rheum. Dis.* 34:286-291.

Suzman, R.M., T. Harris, E.C. Hadley, M.G. Kovar, and R. Weindruch (1993). The robust oldest old: optimistic perspectives for increasing healthy life expectancy. In: R.M. Suzman, D.P. Willis, and K.G. Manton (eds.) *The Oldest Old.* Oxford, England: Oxford University Press, pp. 341-358.

Svanborg, A. (1988). Practical and functional consequences of aging. *Gerontology* 34:11-15.

Svanborg, A. (1993). A medical-social intervention in a 70-year-old Swedish population: Is it possible to postpone functional decline in aging? *J. Gerontol.* 48(Spec. No.):84-88.

Threlkeld, A.J. (1992). The effects of manual therapy on connective tissue. *Phys. Ther.* 72:893-902.

Tinetti, M.E., D.I. Baker, and P.A. Garrett (1993a). Yale FICSIT: Risk factor abatement strategy of fall prevention. *J. Am. Geriatr. Soc.* 41:315-320.

Tinetti, M.E., D.I. Baker, and M.C. Koch (1993b). Multiple risk factor fall prevention trial: one-year results. *Clin. Res.* 41:190A.

Tinetti, M.E., F.T. Williams, and R. Mayewski (1986). A fall risk index for elderly patients based on number of chronic disabilities. *Am. J. Med.* 80:429-434.

Vandervoort, A.A., B.M. Chesworth, D.A. Cunningham, D.H. Paterson, P.A. Rechnitzer, and J.J. Koval (1992). Age and sex effects on mobility of the human ankle. *J. Gerontol.* 47:M17-21.

Walker, J.M., S.D. Miles-Elkousy, N. Ford, and G. Trevelyan (1984). Active mobility in the extremities of older subjects. *Phys. Ther.* 64:919-923.

Wannamethee, G., and A. G. Shaper (1992). Physical activity and stroke in British middle-aged men. *Brit. Med. J.* 304:597-601.

Whipple, R.H., L.I. Wolfson, and P.M. Amerman (1987). The relationship of knee and ankle weakness to falls in nursing home residents: An isokinetic study. *J. Am. geriatr. Soc.* 35:13-20.

Wiegner, A.W., and R.L. Watts (1986). Elastic properties of muscles measured at the elbow in man: I. Normal controls. *J. Neurol. Neurosurg. Psych.* 49:1171-1176.

Wilmore, J.H., J. Royce, R.N. Girandola, F.I. Katch, and V.I. Katch (1970). Physiological alterations resulting from a 10 week program of jogging. *Med. Sci. Sports Exerc.* 2:7-14.

Wolf, S.L., N.G. Kutner, R.C. Green, and E. McNeely (1993), The Atlanta FICSIT study: Two exercise interventions to reduce frailty in elders. *J. Am. Geriatr. Soc.* 41:329-332.

Wood, D.W., and R.J. Turner (1985). The prevalence of physical disability in southwestern Ontario. *Canad. J. Publ. Health* 76:262-265.

World Health Organization (1980). *International Classification of Impairments, Disabiliies, and Handicaps—A Manual* of Classification Relating to the Consequences of Disease. Geneva: World Health Organization.

Wright, J., and R.J. Johns. (1961). Quantitative and qualitative analysis of joint stiffness in normal subjects and in patients with connective tissue diseases. *Ann. Rheu. Dis.* 20:36-45.

Wright, J. (1973). Stiffness: A review of its measurement and physiological importance. *Physiotherapy* 59:107-111.

DISCUSSION

KNUTTGEN: The times required for recovery from and adaptation to aerobic and strength conditioning programs in the elderly must be very different from those for younger people. Is there any information about the efficacy of multiple short bouts of exercise instead of one long bout, or training every other day versus every day or every third day?

HASKELL: When training is expressed as a percentage of $\dot{V}O_2$max, older individuals can get significant increases in aerobic capacity at a somewhat lower training intensity than is true for younger people. There are probably four or five studies showing that in men and women over age 60, endurance exercise three times a week, 30–40 min/session, at intensities of about 40–50% $\dot{V}O_2$max, particularly in the first three to six months of training, will evoke improvements in $\dot{V}O_2$max on the order of 10–15%. To my knowledge, there have been few studies of the elderly that have examined other components of the exercise prescription. My overall impression is that if elderly people are detrained not because of a chronic disorder, but simply due to inactivity, moderate durations of moderate intensity exercise over the first six months or so will produce significant improvements in $\dot{V}O_2$max. These improvements are accompanied by improvements in the abilities of these elderly people to perform their normal daily activities.

I have been impressed with recent work with older subjects suggesting that some of the intensity guidelines for strength training may be higher than needed for older sedentary persons. To produce significant improvements in strength, we typically think of a minimal intensity somewhere above 75% of one repetition maximum (RM) being required for improvements in strength. There are three or four studies that have recently reported improvements of 15–30% in strength with regimens that required no more than about 50% of 1 RM as the stimulus. Also, investigators have moved from three sets/session down to two sets/session or even one set/session (at 80% of 1 RM with eight repetitions per set) and have observed significant strength improvements.

A major problem related to exercise prescription is determining how to successfully implement an exercise program on a very broad scale for older persons. It is apparent that exercise programs can be implemented in a much broader way if they are done at a lower intensity. Also, the lower the intensity, the less medical supervision is required.

KNUTTGEN: Can you comment on the interactions among exercise, fitness, and the psychological aspects of health?

HASKELL: In older individuals, quality of life, e.g., being able to get out of bed, out of a chair, or out of the bathtub, is very important; it has a profound effect on one's psychological status. I think there is a strong interaction between physical and psychological functioning at this very low level.

WILLIAMS: It seems that those people studying the fitness of older people are using indices of fitness that are combinations of traditional measurements and measures of what is best described as "beneficial capacity." This latter term describes the ability of older people to undertake activities that allow them to have an independent lifestyle. There are two problems that present themselves when interpreting traditional forms of fitness assessment. First, the improvements in $\dot{V}O_2$max are small compared with the increases in functional capacity. For example, a 10–15% increase in $\dot{V}O_2$max as a result of endurance training is often accompanied by a 400–500% improvement in submaximal endurance capacity. Secondly, improvement in $\dot{V}O_2$max and strength do not translate easily into a prediction of the capacity of an older individual to successfully complete his or her daily domestic and social activities. We should reexamine the concept of a battery of functional fitness tests for the elderly and try to develop tests that are more meaningful in the context of daily living.

HASKELL: This is a very important issue. We know a great deal about the effects of standard exercise regimens conducted in the laboratory or clinic, but we still know very little about how to translate these programs into activities of daily living.

LAKATTA: As long as we are on the topic of sacrificing the "holy cow," i.e., $\dot{V}O_2$max, and emphasizing functional capacity and better definitions of fitness, could we also expand our future definition of fitness to include preventive measures? A fit person ought to be not only capable of independent daily living at older age, but also able to do things at a younger age to prevent the occurrence or clinical manifestations of those degenerative diseases that occur later in life. It is widely recognized that exponential increases in coronary heart disease, hypertension, and heart failure occur with aging. Thus, these are essentially diseases of older people. The burden of these diseases on our society might be tremendously reduced if we had a definition of fitness that included preventive lifestyles for all young people in our society that could be followed because it was natural for them to do that. We need to establish by studies just how much exercise is required to prevent specific disease endpoints.

HASKELL: I fully agree. One of the difficulties is that we have different exercise recommendations from the bone experts, from the cardiovascular authorities, and the psychological experts. I think it is very important to think about the whole person in coming up with one set of recommendations. I would rather focus on the simple tests of fitness behaviors that individuals can accomplish in or near their places of residence, rather than on a complicated set of tests that require people to go some place to have the tests administered.

BALDWIN: Energy intake seems to be a key variable in fitness, life extension, and the quality of life. There is a great deal of evidence in laboratory animals that longevity can be extended, oxygen pulse can be lowered, and blood pressure reduced by curtailing daily energy intake. I would like you to comment on this issue.

HASKELL: There appears to be a great deal of synergy between increased physical activity and reduced calorie intake that is related to a reduction in adiposity. As you point out, similar effects on adiposity result from restricting energy intake or from increasing physical activity, particularly in the existing U.S. population that tends to be over-fat. My colleague, Peter Wood, has shown a similar equivalence of effects of energy restriction and activity enhancement on changes in lipid metabolism; in either case, triglycerides go down and HDLC goes up. The same phenomenon seems to occur when considering insulin metabolism. So reducing adiposity, whether by decreasing energy intake or increasing energy expenditure seems to have widespread beneficial effects. Also, synergistic effects result when one combines both energy restriction and increased energy expenditure. Extreme restriction of energy intake as done with rats would require, if applied to humans, the equivalent of reducing energy intake to less than 1000 kcal/d. We have too little evidence to say what happens under these conditions. It surely seems to me that decreased overall mortality is best achieved by a reasonable energy intake that provides access to needed micronutrients as well as adequate physical activity to get a synergistic effect on reducing body fat.

REAVEN: In-vivo insulin action will vary 6–8 fold in healthy, normal, non-diabetic subjects. If you try to define the mechanisms responsible for this variability, you can account for about half of the variability by differences in $\dot{V}O_2$max and body mass index, which are both equally powerful. This is true of individuals of European descent and of Pima Indians. Energy expenditure and energy intake also seem to be equally powerful in explaining variability in various metabolic factors.

EVANS: In one of our studies, we observed a significant decrease in depressive symptoms in those people who exercised. Because this was a randomized, placebo-controlled trial, we concluded that those subjects who received as much attention in the nursing home but did not exercise did not manifest any changes in depressive symptoms.

Also, we need to be careful about the intensity of the exercise intervention. In the nursing home, or in the frail elderly, it may well be that a 25–35% increase in strength doesn't translate into real changes in functions related to daily activities. We do know that high-intensity resistance training can cause a 200–300% increase in strength. Such training doesn't present much of a cardiovascular challenge to this population; they can tolerate it easily and perform the exercises very effectively. In addition, it is now clear that quantity of training needed by the elderly to maintain strength is far less than that needed to gain it. Many of the nursing home patients in our study have been strength training for one day a week, and they have been able to maintain the strength that they initially achieved in our three-month training intervention for 2–4 y.

WHITE: Dr. Knuttgen, in your opening question, the premise was that the time course for recovery from and adaptation to exercise must differ with age. The premise is not necessarily correct in all aging models. For example, in rodents if one induces a change in the contractile activity pattern of a muscle by surgical means, the adaptive response in the old is the same or even greater than that in younger rats.

KNUTTGEN: My intention was, indeed, to call attention to differences among age groups. According to the information presented by Bill Evans, the adaptations might be faster in the older individual. It is definitely my assumption that the recovery from tissue disruption and/or injury would be slower in the older individual.

WHITE: There is good evidence that the regenerative response of skeletal muscle to ischemic and exercise-induced injury in the old is slow compared to adults or young.

HASKELL: I would agree that the recovery period is very important in older versus younger persons. We don't have much data in humans to justify any conclusive statement concerning the rate of the recovery response. Frequently, measurements are taken only at baseline and again after 8–12 wk of training. In a study reported by Frontera et al., in which 1 RM was tested weekly for 16 wk, there was a nearly linear increase in both knee extensor and flexor strength. My impression is that in extremely detrained persons, particularly older persons who have been bed-ridden, the early rapid increase in strength upon initiation of resistance training may be related as much to neuroactivation as to changes in muscle morphology and occurs very rapidly.

WHITE: Digby Sale and others have shown in young adults that strength and power improvements occurring at the onset of training are the consequences of optimization of neural recruitment patterns. Dr. Evans, you might know if this phenomenon is more profound in the old human.

EVANS: We see increases in muscle strength on the order of 10–15% per week in the first 8 wk of training. The improvement is quite dramatic.

BAR-OR: When children expend energy during a structured physical activity intervention lasting 30 min, they often reduce their spontaneous activity during the remaining 23.5 h so that there is no net increase in total energy expenditure in the 24 h period. Are there similar data regarding adults or the elderly? On another issue, one reason for the scant information available on muscle endurance and peak power in older adults is that we don't have accepted methods of measuring these variables. We recently modified the Wingate test for use with the elderly. People with advanced chronic obstructive lung disease (mean age approximately 65 y) performed a 15-s abbreviated Wingate test in duplicate. We found this protocol to be safe and to have a high test-retest reliability.

HASKELL: We have some data on individuals over the age of 50 where we used our Vitalog activity monitors and measured heart rate and motion continuously for 3 d after we prescribed activity. The subjects did indeed reduce normal daily activity when they engaged in the structured activity program. This is a critical issue if variables under investigation are presumably affected by total energy expenditure. More work needs to be done in this area, too.

MORA: If we are going to understand exercise, fitness, health, and longevity in relation to aging, we should consider the physiological mechanisms underlying motivation. We know some of the neurochemical systems in the brain that are the basis of motivation, and these systems should be investigated in the exercise context, given the obvious importance of motivation in the scheme of physical training.

HASKELL: I didn't address this important issue because I don't know anything about it.

NASH: Other important factors influencing fitness and longevity include life satisfaction or dissatisfaction, social and psychobiological challenges, psychic and physiologic stresses, marital status, support mechanisms, coping strategies, and familial dependencies.

HASKELL: I agree; those are certainly important factors.

EICHNER: I agree with your suggestion that rheology and blood viscosity play a role in risk of heart attack. Fibrinogen seems to be a new discovered independent coronary risk factor that may be associated with hematocrit, which all along has been a weak coronary risk factor. I think the simplest hypothesis is that exercise dilutes down both fibrinogen and hematocrit by lieu of expanding the baseline plasma volume. This reduces the risk of heart attack.

HASKELL: This is an intriguing area in relation to our understanding of the altered etiology of acute cardiac events over the last 3–5 years. We are no longer talking about just the atherosclerotic process, but an atherosclerotic-thrombotic process in which the triggering event is probably an interaction between plaque rupture and thrombolysis associated with local growth factors released during the plaque rupture. In people who exercise regularly, there may be less platelet aggregation upon plaque rupture. Perhaps this is a mechanism whereby exercise influences clinical outcomes of heart disease but not the underlying disease process that leads to angina. In secondary prevention studies over the last several years, there has been a 25% reduction in fatal events in active people, but there has been little change in angina or other symptoms. It may be that exercise is moderating the effects of the triggering event, i.e., plaque rupture and platelet aggregation, rather than the underlying disease.

3

Aging and Motor Control

Waneen W. Spirduso, Ed.D.

INTRODUCTION

The coordination of movements is necessary to accomplish almost everything that people do. Without neuromuscular control, it is impossible to breathe, eat, dress, walk, drive a car, sew, or dial a telephone. In the absence of the ability to control movement, it is impossible to communicate ideas to another person. Motor control as a topical area of study includes how the central nervous system (CNS) processes sensory information, integrates reflex and postural neurosynergistic adjustments, and coordinates voluntary movements to accomplish goals. The control of movements can be developed relatively early in life to exceptionally high levels of sophistication, as is evident in child prodigy pianists, violinists, gymnasts, and skaters.

As is true of other physiological systems, aging exacts a toll on the function of the CNS. For example, the speed with which adults react to environmental stimuli and the speed with which they can move the trunk, head, and limbs inevitably slows with aging. The ability to coordinate complex movements, particularly two or more movements at once, gradually declines. With passage of enough time, motor skills such as driving an automobile and even functional activities such as dressing and toileting become eroded to a point at which independent living is impossible. These losses are so threatening to self-image, self-esteem, and quality of life that most individuals fear the consequences of an aging motor system.

Because all human movement is based upon at least some minimal level of muscular strength, endurance, and flexibility, it is reasonable to question whether exercise and muscular training can contribute to the maintenance of motor control, thus slowing age-related declines in motor skill. This question seems even more appropriate in light of the observation that the CNS is more vulnerable to oxygen inadequacy than other physiological systems. Cortical tissue, for example, cannot survive without oxygen for more than 5–10 min, whereas it takes 20–30 min of oxygen deprivation in other systems to make damage irreversible (McFarland, 1963). Thus, the maintenance of the oxygen delivery system seems a highly appropriate preventive behavior to postpone premature aging. Surprisingly little attention has been paid to the role of exercise in the *control* of motor behavior. Although the effects of aerobic training and strength training on muscular strength and endurance, locomotion, and basic activities of daily living among aged populations have enjoyed considerable research attention in the last decade, the role that exercise plays in the integration of basic and neurosynergistic reflexes with the voluntary control of complex movements of aging adults has been virtually ignored.

After a brief section in which the medical, clinical, and health implications of an aging motor system are discussed, the focus of this chapter will be on the effects of aging and exercise on sensory functions related to motor control, basic mechanisms of motor control, reflexes and motor synergies, static and dynamic postural control, and reactive and planned coordinated movements. In cases in which little or no research information on the effects of exercise is available, some conjectures are made with regard to the general benefits exercise might provide. The chapter will conclude with a short discussion of nutritional contributions to motor control and with suggested directions for future research.

AGE-RELATED CHANGES IN MOTOR CONTROL: MEDICAL, CLINICAL, AND HEALTH CONCERNS

Losses of motor control evoke at least two major medical, clinical, and health concerns: the loss of mobility, along with the concomitant increased risk for falling and subsequent injury, and the loss of independence, which inevitably leads to high costs of health and caregiving. For most elderly adults independent living, or at least independent decision making, is a necessity to maintain a reasonable quality of life (Figure 3-1). In fact, among the greatest fears of the elderly are the fears of being a burden and/or of losing one's liberty (Moss & Halamandaris, 1977). One of the greatest threats to liberty is the loss of the physical ability required to carry out the activities of daily living and thus live independently. Losses of muscular strength threaten mobility, in that minimal levels of leg strength and flexibility are necessary to sweep or clean a floor, make a bed, or rise out of a chair.

Impaired balance, slow and inadequate postural adjustments to perturbations in the environment, poor leg strength, and compromised locomotor patterns escalate the risk for falling, and the consequences of falling for old adults are, more often than not, catastrophic. Falls account for 87% of all fractures in the elderly, and more than 65% of accidental deaths in the elderly are caused by falling (Azar & Lawton, 1964). More

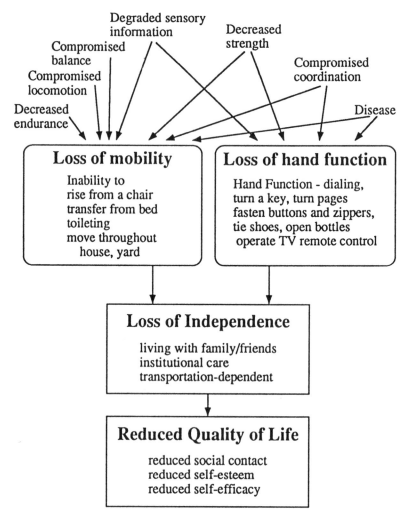

FIGURE 3-1. *Pictorial diagram of proposed relationships among losses of sensory and physical function, disease, and quality of life.*

than 50% of old adults who fracture hips from falls do not live more than one year after the falls (Rubenstein et al., 1983). In the United States by the end of the 1980s, the national health care cost related to hip fractures was $37.3 billion per year (Russell, 1989).

Degraded locomotion has other negative consequences for quality of life. The inability to move around the house and neighborhood not only limits the social contacts outside the home that an older adult has, but it also has the potential to decrease the individual's independence and reduce his or her sense of control (Spirduso, 1995). Having a sense of control over their lives is important to the well-being of the elderly and thus to their quality of life (Kozma & Stones, 1978).

Also of great significance for independent living is the maintenance of hand function. The loss of hand function is most predictive of the need for assistance in living either by family support or by an institution (Jette et al., 1990). For example, motor tasks such as dialing a telephone, turning a key in a lock, picking up small objects, fastening buttons and zippers, tying shoes, opening pharmacy bottles and vials, using scissors, and cutting food are necessary for independent living.

Impairments of balance, locomotion, and hand function associated with human frailty and dependence are often accompanied by losses of the perceptual and motor-coordination skills required for driving an automobile. Driving a car is a learned psychomotor skill, requiring perceptual acuity, attention, memory, rapid information processing, higher-order cognitive functions, and motor programming. Driving, for many millions of adults in American society, is the only means of transportation and mobility within the community. Driving, therefore, is almost tantamount to freedom and independence. Most adults passionately resist the notion of relinquishing their driving privileges in the face of advancing age. Yet all of the perceptual and physical attributes necessary to drive are negatively affected by aging, and the costs of failure in this motor task are great, from both a personal and societal perspective. Although the safest driving records are reported for adults between the ages of 40 and 65, the accident rate climbs precipitously after the age of 70, and adults over this age are 4 times more likely to be injured or killed than are younger adults (Reuben et al., 1988). These statistics have great significance for society in terms of health care costs, property damages, and other economic costs. The impact of these costs should be considered in light of the prediction that by the year 2000, more than 25% of the American driving population will be older than 55 (Transportation Research Board, 1988).

The medical and health concerns that accumulate from age-related changes in perceptual-motor processing, anticipatory and reactive postural reflexes, and coordinated movements are considerable. Exercise, working in concert with good dietary and other health habits, has the potential to modify sensory and neurophysiological processes and to enhance their integration so that complex tasks can be executed. It is, therefore, important to understand the relationships among aging, exercise, and motor control, and it is to these issues that we now turn.

BASIC PHYSIOLOGICAL MECHANISMS OF MOTOR CONTROL

At the most basic level, the control of movement is an elaborate, complex, and ongoing integration of sensory information, motor effector properties, and descending influences from higher CNS centers. The function of sensory receptors, which provide information from the periphery and the external environment, is critical to effective movement.

Sensory Function Related to Motor Control

Information from the environment (sight, sound, smell) and sensations from the body (touch, proprioception, pain, and temperature) are integral inputs for controlling movements, including those required in daily living. The receptors in these sensory systems provide information regarding the type of modality activated (sight, sound, smell) and the intensity, duration, and location of the stimulus. The sensory systems most closely related to motor control are the visual, vestibular (inner ear/balance), and proprioceptive systems (vibration, touch, limb and body position, detection of force). Constant and accurate information from these systems is required to initiate, modify, and terminate movement. However, these systems age at different rates, so that an elderly person may have deficient tactile sensation but unimpaired mechanical sensitivity at the same site (Kenshalo, 1986).

The effect of aging on the processing of sensory information, particularly on those systems involved in the sensation of movement, has attracted relatively less attention than motor control issues perhaps because these sensations are extremely difficult to measure accurately. It is, however, important to distinguish among the contributions of various sensory and motor systems to the control of a sensory motor task. Some tests of sensory capacity require motor output for responses. For example, one test of a blindfolded subject's ability to detect the position of the right elbow joint would be for the subject to mimic the right arm position with the left elbow. It might be assumed that a failure to place the left elbow in the same position is a failure in joint position sense. It may, however, be due to a failure in motor programming skill. The sensory system may be maintained, but the motor expression of the sensory recognition is impaired. In this case, an interpretation that the sensory system has deteriorated might be incorrect. Conversely, some motor output depends on sensory information. It would be an error to assume that motor processes had deteriorated if impaired sensory systems were limiting behavior.

Vision. Vision provides information not only about the environment but also about the location, direction, and speed of movement of the organism within the environment. Visual input, as well as vestibular input, trigger postural reflexes that maintain balance and prepare the body for subsequent movement. Consequently, losses in vision affect balance and locomotion as well as coordination. Age-related losses in visual acuity frequently occur as early in life as the fourth decade and can have profound effects upon motor control. Associated with increased aging are losses in visual processing speed, dynamic vision, visual search, size of visual field, estimation of velocity, acuity in low illumination, accommodation reserve, and resistance to glare (Ball & Owsley, 1991; Kline et al., 1992). Other changes occur in the ability to detect the spatial relationships of objects (Sekuler & Hutman, 1980), in depth perception, and in peripheral vision, all of which contribute substantially to balance (Manchester et al., 1989). An example of how vision can affect even simple motor function was provided by Woollacott et al. (1988). In their study, the dynamic balance of older adults was compared to that of young adults as both age groups wore special goggles that limited their access to: a) central vision only, b) peripheral vision only, or c) visual feedback unrelated to body sway (translucent goggles were worn). The older adults lost their balance 38% of the time when only central vision was available, whereas the young subjects lost balance equally across visual conditions. The authors concluded that the older adults relied more on peripheral vision than the young adults did because when peripheral visual information was unavailable, their balance deteriorated.

Visual losses negatively affect motor skills, but severe losses of vision, which often occur in the oldest old (85–100 y), make it difficult to carry out even the motor skills necessary for activities of daily living. Not surprisingly, poor visual acuity has been related to increased incidences of falling in the elderly (Tobis et al., 1981, 1985).

Exercise Effects on Vision. The eye, because it has a variety of tissues, is an exquisite and unique organ. Worthen (1978) pointed out that "its intrinsic muscles respond to changes in the autonomic nervous system; its dual blood supply reflects both systemic and cerebral blood flow; [and] its secretory tissue responds to shifts in blood biochemistry and hormones." The retina, which is derived embryologically from the same tissue that develops into brain, has a structural organization and physiological diversity of cellular components sufficient to be considered brain tissue (Bailey & Gouras, 1985). Just as cerebral blood flow is reduced in the aging brain (Pantano et al., 1983), blood flow to the aging retina is also diminished, and the reduced retinal blood flow can affect receptors in the retina (Landahl & Birren, 1959). Thus, it is surprising that although the eye can be a sensitive sensor of many exercise-associated physiological changes, and although visual acuity is so greatly affected by aging, little research has been conducted on the effects of acute and chronic exercise on eye physiology and visual function, in either young or old adults. Aerobic exercise should have the same beneficial effect on the blood flow to the retina that it has on cerebral blood flow (Thomas et al., 1989). Thus, it is reasonable to hypothesize that poor fitness might negatively affect retinal function, thereby impairing vision of the elderly. In addition, many older adults develop adult-onset diabetes (Type II), which is highly associated with retinopathy. In fact, diabetic retinopathy is one of the three leading causes of blindness among persons with chronic disease (Kart et al., 1992). The other two are cataract and glaucoma. Part of the treatment for slowing the progression of diabetic retinopathy is to control blood glucose, and aerobic exercise contributes to blood glucose control.

Worthen (1978), in reviewing a number of studies on the effects of aerobic and anaerobic exercise on intraocular pressure and visual field, found that exercise decreased intraocular pressure and increased arterial pressure within the eye (but less than it increased systolic blood pressure). He also reported that exercise can compromise dark adaptation, which would be an additional problem for older adults, many of whom are already experiencing an age-related reduction in their ability to adapt to the dark.

Vestibular Function. The vestibular system, located in the inner ear, provides reference information necessary to control postural sway and dynamic balance. Receptors located in the inner ear provide a static vertical reference by which the position of the head with respect to gravity is compared. Receptors in the semicircular canals of the inner ear provide information about head movement, i.e., as the head turns, afferent signals are provided that indicate the extent and direction of turning.

It has been estimated that vestibular neurons decrease in both number and in size of nerve fiber with aging, beginning about age 40 (Bergström, 1973a,b). By 70 years of age, 40% of the sensory cells of the vestibular system are lost (Rosenhall & Rubin, 1975), although researchers disagree as to the functional consequences of these losses. Some evidence is available that older adults are even more sensitive to vestibular stimuli than are the young, but other researchers have reported that vestibular function seems to be relatively unchanged by aging. Brocklehurst et al. (1982) found that only 6% of elderly adults revealed any type of functional impairment in vestibular sensitivity in an eyes-closed test in which the subjects underwent a slow tilt of 20 degrees. Bruner and Norris (1971) speculated that disparate results were found because aging first affects an area of the brain that increases the excitability of brain tissue (reticular activating system) and only later impairs the sensitivity of the peripheral receptors of the vestibular system. Thus, older individuals who are measured at relatively "younger" ages (5th or 6th decade) would appear to be hypersensitive, whereas individuals measured at a later period in the aging process would be hyposensitive to vestibular stimulation. However, Sixt and Landahl (1987) have reported that more than 60% of men and women 70 y or older experience dizziness or vertigo, the common symptoms of vestibular loss, and Horak (1992) proposed that if vestibular loss occurs gradually, significant problems can occur with postural stability even in the absence of dizziness symptoms. Woollacott's (1988) report also supports the hypothesis that either vestibular function or the central processes that integrate peripheral vestibular information, or both, are impaired in aged adults.

Proprioception. Normal movements of the body are dependent upon information about the position and movement of the body and limbs, both with respect to static-position sense and to the sensation of body and limb movements. This type of information comes from muscle and joint receptors that provide information about the mechanical displacements of muscles and joints. Both provide the sense of limb movement, or kinesthesia, that is necessary to maintain balance and to control limb and trunk movements. Although the exact source of information for proprioception is controversial, it is probable that muscle spindles, joint receptors, and cutaneous receptors contribute feedback about movement, with muscle spindles playing a predominant role for movement of proximal joints such as the hip or knee, and joint and cutaneous receptors playing a more active role in movements of the distal joints, such as at the fingers. Joint position sense, or static sense, is measured by position-matching experiments, in which a subject is asked to describe the position of his or her limb, match it to a picture of a limb position, or match it with a contralateral limb. Movement sense is measured by having blindfolded subjects or patients with joint replacements detect and describe movements of their limbs that have been controlled by the experimenter.

Several investigators have reported a reduction in proprioception with aging (Kaplan et al., 1985; Skinner et al., 1984; Stelmach & Sirica, 1986). In a position-matching paradigm in which the proximal interphalangeal joints were manipulated, the sense of finger position was less accurate in 10 relatively "young" older subjects (56.6 ± 3.2 y) when compared to 10 young subjects (23.7 ± 0.5 y) (Ferrell et al., 1992). Wyke (1979) reported a gradual loss of cervical articular mechanoreceptor functions, indicating that perceptions about the position of the neck and head may grow less accurate with aging. Conversely, Kokmen et al. (1978) concluded that joint position sense in the joints of the arms and legs does not markedly decline with aging. Skinner et al. (1984) suggested on the basis of their data that older adults may lose some ability to detect motion of their limbs when these limb displacements occur at a slow speed, but when changes of limb position occur rapidly, age differences are much less apparent. Because most movements that occur in activities of daily living require moderate levels of speed, age-related differences in position sense therefore may not be functionally important. However, proprioception is a highly complex system in which many age-related changes occur. Small differences in one or more components of the system may accumulate so that overall proprioceptive function is impaired. It is possible, too, that age-related differences in the ability to perceive motion of the joints are subtle, and they may be observed only when the extremes of age groups are compared to each other.

Vibration sensitivity is also used to assess proprioceptive acuity. Receptors in the skin (Pacinian corpuscles) and the muscle (the dynamic response of the primary Ia afferents of the muscle spindles) provide information about vibration. Pacinian corpuscles, present in skin, subcutaneous tissue, and deep tissue, are sensitive to changes in tissue position, and receptors in muscle are highly sensitive to changes in muscle length. The perception of changes in tissue position and muscle length play a role in the perception of limb position, providing instant information that subtle changes in leg position have occurred. Muscles spindles thus contribute to the control of postural sway (Brocklehurst et al., 1982). They also provide information that is crucial for dynamic balance when the base of support is struck or moved significantly. The ability to detect the frequency of a vibrating stimulus reflects the sensitivity with which the receptors can "track" a stimulus and thus the accuracy that they may have in detecting limb position. Vibration sensitivity is measured by placing a vibrator over a bony area such as the wrist, ankle, or knee and determining the lowest intensity at which vibration can be detected.

Vibration sense declines with aging (Skinner et al., 1984; Whanger & Wang, 1974), the decline being seen as early as the first to second decade by some researchers (Frisina & Gescheider, 1977; Verrillo, 1979) and by the fifth decade by others (Kenshalo, 1986). Losses were greater in the legs and feet than in the arms and hands (Kenshalo, 1986). Older adults, compared to young adults, underestimated the magnitude of vibrotactile stimulation over a 40–250 Hz range of stimulus intensities, with the loss being greater at the higher frequency of vibrations. Older adults also were not as sensitive to low levels of stimulus intensity (Kenshalo, 1986; Verrillo, 1982). Furthermore, the neural activity associated with Pacinian stimulation persists over a longer period of time, causing an overlap of information from different receptors that can be construed as noise in the system (Verrillo, 1993). Both persistence and adaptation are profoundly affected by aging (Verrillo, 1993). Persistence, sometimes called enhancement, is a term that describes the lingering of the first stimulus impulse so that the second stimulus "feels" more intense (Gescheider et al., 1992). Adaptation is the process of recovery from stimulation.

Sensation of Force. The perception of muscular force produced is one of the most difficult perceptions, and for that reason has been studied infrequently. How individuals perceive the amount of force they produce in a given task is a matter of controversy. One hypothesis is that the conscious sensation of force occurs when corollary discharge of central nervous system motor outflow is simultaneously directed to the sensory cortex; thus, no peripheral input is used in the sensation of force (von Holst, 1954). The earliest hypothesis was that the perception of force may be described as a "sense of effort," which is supplied by an interpretation of information from skin, joint, muscle, and tendon receptors (Sherrington, 1900). Cafarelli and Bigland-Ritchie (1979) suggested that the conscious sensation of force from muscle contraction depends primarily on the central command to muscle but that it can be slightly modified by feedback from peripheral receptors. Whatever the mechanism is by which force is detected and programmed, older adults are differentially less accurate than young individuals. Cole (1991) found that unlike young adults, elderly women (71–92 y) produced at least two times more force than was necessary to grasp and hold a small rod-like device, and the force that the old subjects produced was more variable from trial to trial. He hypothesized that the production of excessive force may have been an effort to compensate for decreased tactile sensibility so that the old subjects maintained a higher safety margin against dropping the object by providing the greatest amount of force needed for all lifting conditions, regardless of the weight or amount of friction provided by the object. Findings by Spirduso & Choi (1993) also suggest that older subjects produce more force than is necessary for a task. In their study, women 60–83 y of age had much more difficulty tracing a template by using force control than they did when they had access to the directional cues provided by a joystick (Spirduso & Choi, 1992). These results support Cole's (1991) suggestion that because the production of excessive force increases variability (Schmidt et al., 1978), decreased sensitivity to tactile and force cues contribute to decreased accuracy in force control in the elderly.

Tactile Sensitivity. The sense of touch provides information that contributes not only to the control of movement but to understanding and experiencing the environment. Because tactile receptors provide such important information, the desire to touch things is instinctive and difficult to suppress. "Please do not touch" signs in gift shops, art galleries, and museums attest to this desire. Tactile receptors provide information about texture, which is used in planning movements and determining the parameters necessary to execute a movement designed to grasp, manipulate, or lift an object. Meissner's corpuscles, Merkel's receptors, Pacinian corpuscles, and Ruffinian corpuscles are the tactile receptors that respond to mechanical stimuli. The rapidly adapting mechanoreceptors are the Meissner's corpuscles, located in glaborous hairy skin, and the Pacinian corpuscles, located in the skin and subcutaneous tissue. The slowly adapting receptors are the Ruffinian corpuscles, which are also located in skin and subcutaneous tissue.

Aging is not kind to the skin. Throughout life, the skin is the interface or barrier between the body and the environment. As such, it suffers the insults of thermal extremes, ultraviolet radiation, and traumatic impact. Mechanical properties of skin change dramatically with aging (Kligman & Balin, 1989). Skin loses elasticity and resilience, remaining deformed from pressure longer. The epidermal ridges of the fingers become smooth with increased age, so that traction in holding and manipulating objects is more difficult. These mechanical changes in skin and subcutaneous tissue, as with visual losses, begin relatively early in life, in the mid-40s. The changes compromise the function of tactile receptors and impair tactile spatial acuity. Tactile perception, at least as measured by two-point discrimination, deteriorates dramatically with aging (Axelrod & Cohen, 1961; Gellis & Pool, 1977; Stevens, 1992). Two-point discrimination tests are usually made by placing the two blunted points of a contractor together on the skin. When the points are together, they feel as one point to a blindfolded subject. The research gradually increases the gap between the two points to such an extent that the subject recognizes the existence of two points. These age-related changes are much more drastic in the hands and toes than in other parts of the body, such as the arm (Bolton et al., 1966; Stevens, 1992). Age-related impairment in tactile acuity is probably due to a loss of tactile receptors, changes in skin characteristics, or both.

Kenshalo (1986) has reported that a decrease in the number of mechanoreceptors, Meissner's corpuscles, Pacinian corpuscles, and Ruffinian cylinders accompanies aging, and many receptors that remain are deformed. From microscopic observation, the capsule of old Meissner's corpuscles appeared enlarged, coiled, and irregular in shape. However, Bolton et al. (1966) argued that although Meissner's corpuscles were dramatically less dense in older subjects, they were not less functional.

Exercise Effects on the Sense of Body Position and Movement. Very little is known about the effects of exercise on these perceptions. Neither cross-sectional nor intervention studies have been reported in which acute or chronic direct exercise effects on vestibular function have been assessed. Era et al. (1986) found that elderly (71–75 y) subjects who reported exercising regularly were more sensitive to vibration than a similarly aged sedentary group. The 31–35-year-old and the 51–55-year-old exercise and control groups were not, however, more sensitive to vibration than the oldest group. These findings have been the only ones suggesting that chronic exercise may play a role in maintaining vibration sense in the elderly. It has been hypothesized, however, that chronic exercise may indirectly help maintain vibrotactile thresholds in the aging through its role in preventing or postponing systemic diseases such as diabetes (Whanger & Wang, 1974). Although Era et al. (1986) found that the vibration thresholds of older healthy exercisers were more similar to those of young subjects, they failed to find a negative association between vibration threshold and chronic disease in a small subset of their subjects. The authors suggested that a more systematic study of vibration threshold with a larger number of chronically diseased subjects must be conducted before the relationship between health, exercise, and vibration sensitivity can be determined.

Although no studies on the direct effects of chronic exercise on the acuity of other proprioceptive and tactile receptors have been reported, these receptors may benefit indirectly from the contribution that chronic exercise makes to the prevention of chronic diseases such as diabetes and peripheral neuropathy.

Basic Mechanisms of Motor Control

The Motor Unit. The motor unit, which includes the motor neuron, the axon, the neuromuscular junctions, and the muscle fibers innervated by that neuron, is the basic functional element of the motor system. Motor units vary in the size of the soma (neuron cell body), the velocity with which neural impulses travel across the axon, and the number and size of their muscle fibers. They also differ in the functional muscle characteristics of peak-twitch tension, contractile speed, and resistance to fatigue and in the neural characteristics of firing rates and activation patterns. Large motor units have large innervation ratios, i.e., many muscle fibers are innervated by the neuron. The recruitment of motor units throughout a muscular contraction of increasing force, barring rare exceptions, follows the size principle of Henneman et al. (1965). The order of activation is from small motor units that exhibit low twitch-force and slow twitch-speed and are fatigue-resistant, to large motor units characterized by high twitch-force, fast twitch-speed, and easy fatigability.

The number of active motor units decreases with aging (Rogers & Evans, 1993), and the largest decrease is in large motor units with large innervation ratios (Campbell et al., 1973). Because there appears to be a more homogeneous grouping of fiber types in older cadaver muscles (Lexell et al., 1986: Lexell & Taylor, 1991), and because the fiber density of motor units in old muscle was increased, Stålberg & Fawcett (1982) proposed that the smaller, surviving Type I collateral nerve fibers go through a process of sprouting and reinnervation of the muscle fibers abandoned by lost Type II motor neurons (Figure 3-2). Therefore, smaller, low-threshold, fatigue-resistant motor units that have larger innervation ratios are observed in aged muscle. Thus, although the percentages of specific fiber types such as slow-oxidative and fast-glycolytic are not lost preferentially (Coggan et al., 1992), the neurological innervation and capacity to recruit appears to be spared more in slow, small motor units than in large, fast motor units (Desypris & Parry, 1990).

Unlike the dearth of information regarding the effect of age and exercise on sensory function as it relates to movement, substantial evidence exists that motor unit function, even in the elderly, can be affected by acute muscular exercise, chronic aerobic exercise, and by chronic muscular training. In this section, the focus is on neurological and control changes in motor unit behavior that are influenced by exercise, rather than on changes in muscle tissue. The effects of aging and exercise on muscle fiber structure, number, and type are discussed in more detail in Chapter 4 of this volume (White, 1995).

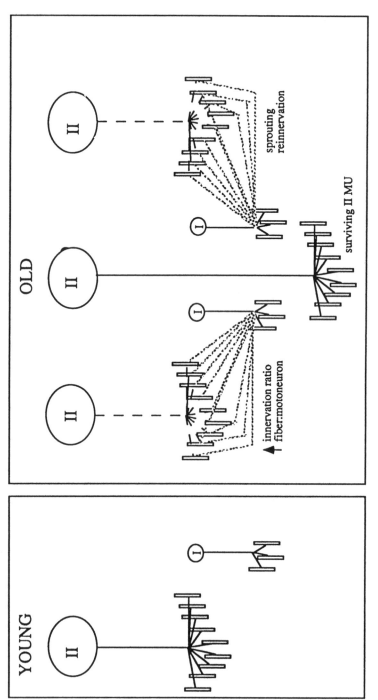

FIGURE 3-2. *Hypothesized age-related changes in motor unit innervation ratios of Type I and Type II motor units.*

Chronic Exercise Effects. Chronic muscular and aerobic training may influence motor unit control by evoking neurological adaptations or by increasing or maintaining peripheral blood flow to the muscles. One neurological adaptation is that early in a strength training program the number and size of the motor units recruited (as reflected by integrated electromyographical activity) increase, even though muscle hypertrophy has not yet occurred (Komi, 1986; Moritani & deVries, 1979). The early neurological adaptations compared to the later muscle hypertrophy are shown in Figure 3-3. Isometric strength training also enables both small and large motor units to maintain consistency in their firing rates at lower firing frequencies, but high-repetition, dynamic training decreases motor unit firing rate consistency (Sale, 1987). Furthermore, resistive exercise appears to enable the muscle to activate all of the motor units in a muscle during a maximal voluntary contraction (Sale, 1988).

It has also been proposed that one of the functions of training is to improve the "stiffness" of muscle (Komi, 1986), i.e., the force-length relationship of muscle. However, the type of training may determine the direction of stiffness changes. Endurance training has been shown to increase stiffness of the soleus muscle in rats (Goubel & Marini, 1987), whereas strength training decreased active stiffness of the plantar flexors in hu-

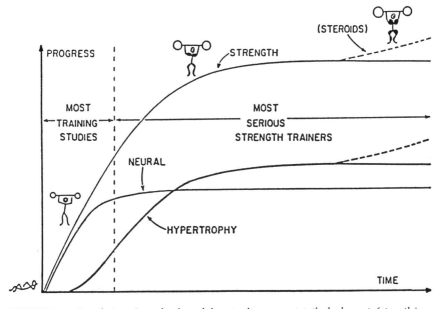

FIGURE 3-3. *Contributions of neural and muscle hypertrophy components to the development of strength in a strength training program. In the early phases of the training program, increased strength is due largely to neural adaptation. In later stages of training, strength gains are derived primarily by muscular hypertrophy.* From Sale (1988). Reprinted with permission.

mans (Blanpied & Smidt, 1993). Blanpied and Smidt (1993) found no evidence for age differences in either stiffness or the effects of strength training on stiffness, although because their age groups were not measured at similar absolute torques, they could not say conclusively that age differences did not exist.

Another example of neurological adaptation is an exercise-related change in the motor unit recruitment pattern. When muscular contraction is analyzed by recording simultaneously from intramuscular and surface electrodes, motor units are generally observed to fire independently of each other. However, Milner-Brown et al. (1975) showed that motor units in the hands of workers (manual laborers) or weightlifters who frequently exerted large, brief forces were more synchronized than the motor units commonly observed in randomly selected subjects. Furthermore, after the control group subjects trained the first dorsal interosseus muscles of the hands for 6 wk to exert maximal, voluntary contractions, motor units in some of these control subjects also appeared to become more synchronized. The authors tested two possible explanations: either the connections from sensory fibers to spinal motoneurons were more sensitized by the muscular training, or descending inputs from higher centers were increased. From an analysis of muscle, spinal, and cortical reflexes in these subjects, they concluded that supraspinal connections direct from the motor cortex may have become trained to cause better synchronization of motor units. The authors suggested that prolonged muscular training, as occurs in weightlifting or other occupations requiring repeated bursts of large muscle activity, results in the synchronization of motor unit activity. They further suggested that synchronization may result from strengthening reflex pathways involving a fast, lemniscal route to the cortex and a somewhat slower route via cerebellar connections. Synchronized motor unit activation does not, however, increase either the peak force of a voluntary muscular contraction or the rate of force development (Sale, 1987). The functional significance of increased synchronized motor unit activation as a result of training is unclear.

Some exercise-related changes in motor unit behavior may be due to the influence of exercise on muscular blood flow. The mean amplitude and firing frequency of motor units of six male subjects increased significantly when they made repeated intermittent isometric contractions (2-s contraction followed by 2-s rest period) at 20% of their maximum voluntary contraction force, for 4 min (Moritani et al., 1992). Force development was unimpaired, indicating that 1) additional motor units were recruited to maintain the contractions, 2) the firing frequency of the active motor units was increased, or 3) the contractile duration was lengthened (as in half-relaxation time). When the blood supply was interrupted by arterial occlusion for 1 min, large and progressive increases in motor unit amplitude and firing frequencies were observed during the occlusion.

The increase in frequency did not return to baseline until the last 30 s of the 4-min protocol.

The size principle of Henneman et al. (1965) states that the force and speed of contraction dictate the recruitment pattern and firing rate of motor units; however, the data of Moritani et al. (1992) leave open the possibility that oxygen availability may also influence the recruitment of high-threshold motor units. Moritani et al. speculated that when the contractility of some motor units is reduced due to the occlusion-produced reduction in oxygen supply and intramuscular glycogen stores, the muscle spindles and the Golgi tendon organs signal for the recruitment of more motor units. Although not directly applicable, these results do suggest that extremely sedentary older adults who suffer circulation impairment in their extremities might be forced to recruit more and larger motor units to execute a specific task than would a younger person. Using larger motor units would result in greater muscle fatigue, movement variability, and error. Conversely, chronic aerobic exercise markedly improves peripheral blood flow and is associated with increased capillarization in the extremities (Hagberg et al., 1985). The peripheral circulatory adaptation to exercise training occurs rather quickly. This was evident when previously sedentary elderly subjects achieved the same peripheral blood flow responses within a few months of training as were exhibited by highly trained, older road racing cyclists (Martin et al., 1990). Increased capillarization and blood flow may contribute to the ability of old muscle to retain the contractility of fibers and therefore maintain more youthful motor unit recruitment and firing rate patterns throughout aging.

Another effect of chronic exercise on motor unit function is that nerve conduction velocity may be maintained with chronic exercise. Retzlaff and Fontaine (1965) found that the nerve conduction velocity of rats that had exercised daily on a treadmill was faster than that of sedentary rats, and Samorajski & Rolsten (1975) showed that tibial nerve fibers were larger (and thus faster conducting) in chronically exercising mice. Similarly, aerobic exercise seems to influence positively the function of neuromuscular junctions in young mice and also to counter several negative age-related changes that occur in the function of presynaptic, but not postsynaptic, neuromuscular junctions of old mice. Fahim (1993) reported that the release of acetylcholine was increased 25% in the synaptic junctions of extensor digitorum longus of young aerobically trained mice (10 mo), and the acetylcholine release of the old mice (28 mo) was also improved. No postsynaptic changes, such as the number and distribution of junctional acetylcholine receptors, muscle input resistance, muscle fiber diameter, and membrane capacitance were reported. The authors concluded, therefore, that physical activity at any age can modulate the structure and function of presynaptic but not postsynaptic neuromuscular junctions in mice.

Not only do most older adults fail to exercise, but many also avoid even moderate exertion in their activities of daily living. This pattern of physical inactivity begins for most individuals very early, i.e., in their mid-30s, and continues throughout their lives. Activity avoidance behaviors include circling parking lots searching for convenient parking spots, watching television for many hours a day, and taking elevators instead of using stairs. Disuse of muscles, however, also has some consequences for motor unit function. During disuse (as occurs in bed rest or immobilization of limbs) the amount of motor unit activation and synchronization decreases, and firing frequencies of motor units become more variable (Sale, 1987). Inconsistency of motor unit firing patterns makes it more difficult to control a slow, graded muscular contraction, as might occur in some fine motor skills. Thus, older sedentary adults, because of muscle fiber atrophy and peripheral blood circulation impairments, may be required to recruit larger motor units than do young individuals to perform the same task. In addition, the firing rates and patterns may be less consistent than those of young adults. All of these factors would impact upon the neuromotor coordination necessary to perform skilled tasks.

Reflexes. The control of movement is based to a great extent on the hierarchical control of spinal reflexes, which are neural circuits in the spinal cord that link contractions of many muscles together so that they act as a unit. These reflexes are sets of elementary patterns of integration that are activated or modified by sensory stimuli and/or descending influences from the brain stem or cerebral cortex. Reflex hierarchical control involves controlling the actions of individual muscles, the coordination of muscles around a joint, and the coordination of muscles at several joints. These reflexes operate to provide a postural support system for static and dynamic actions. Some examples of simple and complex reflexes that provide a basis for the control of movements are extensor reflexes, stretch reflexes, flexor withdrawal reflexes, crossed extensor reflexes, and righting reflexes. Combinations of these reflexes with connections to brain stem and cerebral cortex make up neurosynergies, which provide more complex reflexive coordination of many muscles across several joints. Both simple and complex reflexes, and neurosynergies, can be modified by descending influences such as visual, vestibular, or cognitive commands.

The reflex that has been studied in humans more than any other is the myotatic reflex (patellar tendon and Achilles' tendon reflex), perhaps because it is the only monosynaptic reflex in humans and because it can be measured noninvasively. The myotatic reflex contributes to the control of sway during standing and to the control of balance during locomotion and other movements. On the basis of what is known about aging effects on sensory and motor unit function and nerve condition velocity, it might seem that spinal reflex latencies would be longer in older adults. Some investigators have indeed found age-related differences in monosynaptic reflexes (Laufer & Schweitz, 1968; Vandervoort & Hayes, 1989). Carel et al. (1979), for example, reported that in 9,774 subjects, the length of time that lapsed between the onset of the stimulus and the appearance of the Achilles' tendon reflex was related to age. But others have suggested that reflex mechanisms may be maintained much longer, perhaps throughout the entire life span (Hugin et al., 1960; Smith & Greene, 1962). Clarkson (1978) re-analyzed the relationship between age and Achilles' total reflex reported by Laufer and Schweitz (1968) and found no difference in reflex latency between 21–28-year-old and 61–68-year-old groups. Reinfrank et al. (1967) found a small difference of only 5% in the half-relaxation time of Achilles' reflexes of a group ranging from 15–64 y and an older group ranging from 67–76 y. The contradictions in results from these studies may be due to the fact that investigators of most of these studies made little effort to control for health, fitness, and neurological pathology. Additionally, in almost all studies, the latency of the response, rather than the magnitude of the response, was studied.

What is the functional significance of slow and weak monosynaptic spinal reflexes? Although such reflexes in themselves are not likely to be the mechanisms that prevent falling, they represent the neural integrity of the reflexive hierarchy. For example, delayed reflex reactions to perturbations of stability around the ankle joint were associated with a higher risk for ankle sprains, injuries, and falling (Konradsen & Ravn, 1991). Slower monosynaptic reflexes may also fail to provide counter-responses to changes in sway rapidly enough, so that the sway exceeds stability levels and evokes the larger more functional neurosynergistic response to avoid a loss of balance. In addition, because the muscular responses are weaker in older individuals, who have a loss of muscle fiber mass, the reflex may not be forceful enough to counter an excessive sway that could lead to a perturbation of balance.

Age-related differences in amplitude of a complex reflex have been observed in animal research. The auditory startle reflex is a complex reflex involving whole-body muscle activation in response to afferent information from auditory receptors. Wallace et al. (1980) observed that although startle reflex latencies were not different, the amount of displacement (amplitude) of a force-plate following a loud noise was significantly less in old than in young rats. Although the application of these findings to human behavior is perilous, it might be proposed that young individuals respond to a perturbation with reflexes that are both rapid and of sufficient magnitude to enable them to counteract a fall. Older adults may respond both more slowly and less vigorously. The more the body falls outside its base of support, the greater the muscular response needed to counteract the fall.

Disuse may play an important role in the deterioration of basic reflexes because neuromuscular mechanisms that are not frequently used are most impaired by aging. The monosynaptic reflex, which signals changes in muscle length and is active in all movements, might be expected to be maintained. On the basis of this hypothesis then, even a minimal level of physical activity would activate spinal reflexes, making them among the last mechanisms to be affected by aging (Clarkson, 1978).

Acute Exercise Effects on Reflexes. Both acute and chronic exercise appear to modify spinal reflexes. In an early study, Brown (1925), using the kymograph and string to measure the height of the patellar reflex kick, found that acute exercise, so long as it was not fatiguing, enhanced the amplitude of the patellar tendon reflex, but primarily in physically fit men. In untrained men it was either unchanged or decreased in amplitude. These results were later confirmed by several others who also studied the reflex latencies of quadriceps femoris and triceps surae (Brown, 1925; Fearing, 1928; Francis & Tipton, 1969; Kamen, 1979; Lombard, 1887; Tipton & Karpovich, 1966; Tuttle, 1930). However, as reviewed by Kroll & Clarkson (1977), acute exercise to fatigue lengthens total reflex time by as much as 11%. Fractionation techniques revealed that the longer total reflex times were due to a lengthening of the contractile component of the reflex (Kroll, 1974). Hortobagyi et al. (1991) failed to find differences in patellar tendon reflex latency after their young subjects completed 50 consecutive depth-vertical jumps, but they did find that the reflex time increased 6%, the compound muscle action potential lasted longer (6%), and the peak-to-peak amplitude of the reflex increased 23.3%. The authors proposed that the subjects compensated for the loss of voluntary force by lengthening the activity and/or enhancing muscle spindle sensitivity. Others have also proposed that fatiguing, acute exercise decreases the height of the reflex. A mechanism that has been suggested to explain the lengthening of total reflexes immediately following acute exercise is that the gamma system operating in spinal reflexes is adjusted during exercise (Chaffin, 1973; Hayes, 1975; Marsden et al., 1972). Activation of the gamma system increases the stiffness of the muscle (Komi, 1986).

Chronic Exercise Effects on Reflexes: Aerobic Training. Several researchers have observed that reflexes were faster in trained or aerobically exercised young groups than in sedentary groups (Table 3-1; Petajan & Eagan, 1968; Tuttle, 1930; Wickwire et al., 1938). In a more detailed study, Koceja et al. (1991) compared the means for peak isometric force, contraction time, and half-relaxation time of the Achilles' reflex of highly trained, national-caliber dancers to those for a group of sedentary, untrained subjects. In response to tendon taps, the trained dancers produced less unilateral isometric force and a longer half-relaxation time than did the untrained subjects. The two groups were also very different in their responses to a conditioned reflex, which consisted of contralateral tendon taps at varied time intervals prior to the tested stimulus tap. The conditioning taps produced more pronounced changes in the response to the stimulus tap in the trained than in the untrained group. The contralateral tendon tap affected the motoneuronal pool for approximately 150 ms following that tap and provided an indication that training affected input-output properties of the spinal cord as well as the segmental organization of specific crossed-spinal reflex pathways. The contralateral conditioning stimulus caused an inhibition of the contralateral homologous muscle group that was more pronounced in the trained dancers. The authors suggested that intensive training may change either the amplitude of the electromyographic (EMG) activity and the force produced by muscle tissue in the reflex response, or the compliance of the tendon tissue, inasmuch as several investigators have found that chronic exercise is associated with changes in tendon characteristics (for review, see Bloomfield (1995)).

The latency of the patellar tendon reflex of physically active older adults, but not the total reflex time or the contractile component, is also similar to that of young college students (Hart, 1986). Reflex latency is defined by the first onset of EMG activity, and contractile time is the duration of the muscular contraction preceding the reflex latency, as measured by the release of a mechanical switch. Clarkson (1978), however, found no differences in total patellar reflex latency, contractile time, or total reflex time of old subjects categorized either by age or physical activity level. Her conclusion was that the entire patellar stretch-reflex apparatus and the system of alpha-gamma linkage is unaffected by aging and the level of physical activity, perhaps because these spinal reflexes are used on a constant basis in static and dynamic postural adjustments throughout every day activities. It is possible that Hart's and Clarkson's subjects, who self-reported that they exercised aerobically at least three times a week, were not as physically trained as those younger subjects of earlier mentioned studies, and they certainly were not as highly trained as the dancers in the study reported by Koceja et al. (1991). It is also possible that an interaction between aging and chronic exercise occurs only in more complex spinal reflexes, such as crossed-extensor or conditioned reflexes, and not in monosynaptic reflexes.

Chronic Exercise Effects on Reflexes: Weight Training. Systematic weight training seems to have a beneficial effect on spinal reflexes. Some investigators have reported that in young men, patellar reflex times (Francis & Tipton, 1969) and triceps surae reflex times (Reid, 1967) were shorter after a strength training program of at least 6 wk. Tipton and Karpovich (1966) found that an 8-wk exercise program shortened the mean patellar reflex latency of six middle-aged adults from 100.6 ± 11.55 ms to 85.4 ± 5.3 ms. The decrease in posttraining mean latency, although not statistically significant, placed them at the same level of reflex latency as observed in young college students. Kamen et al. (1981) found that power-trained subjects had quicker tendon reflexes and faster tibial nerve conduction velocities. After holding a voluntary isometric contraction three times at 50% of maximum voluntary force for as long as possible, however, the contractile times of the power-trained subjects were longer (19.9%) following the exercise training, but the endurance-trained athletes' contractile times were not affected by the exercise. The authors noted that the 50% holding task generated a substantial amount of lactic acid and suggested that because lactate is re-utilized by slow-twitch fibers, and aerobically trained runners have proportionately more slow-twitch fibers, the runners may have been able to utilize the accumulated lactate better than the power athletes. Thus, runners were able to prevent a loss of contractile strength.

Neurosynergies. Anticipatory and postural neurosynergies are an elegant integration of spinal reflexes, righting reflexes, and longer-latency, more complex reflexes that serve to control posture. In these synergies, information from muscle spindles, Golgi tendon organs, joint receptors, cutaneous receptors, and from visual and vestibular receptors is integrated. It has been proposed that a central command center opens and closes spinal reflex circuits in a coordinated fashion, and that the center is activated from a standing posture by long-latency reflexes triggered by the rotation of the ankles during movement. These response synergies are evoked when balance is suddenly perturbed, and they are also integrally involved in the preparation, planning, and execution of willful movement.

Aging impacts neurosynergistic postural control mechanisms in several ways (Table 3-1). In an often-cited paper, Woollacott (1990) observed that neurosynergistic responses to postural perturbation by older adults differed from those of their young adults in at least four ways. First, the responses of the tibialis anterior but not of the gastrocnemius muscles of the older adults were slightly slower, indicating that the *postural* responses of foot flexors were more affected than those of foot extensors (Inglin & Woollacott, 1988). The forces encountered by the leg musculature during daily walking may have provided greater resistance for ankle extensors than for ankle flexors, and thus the functional integrity of the extensors was better maintained; plantar flexors were also chronically involved in tonic activity during standing, another mechanism by which they may have been maintained. In contrast, Vandervoort and McComas (1986) found that, although the absolute loss of strength was greater in plantar flexors, the relative loss was the same. Nevertheless, in Woollacott's (1990) work, the reflexes depending upon ankle extension were maintained, whereas those depending upon ankle flexion were degraded.

Second, the pattern of muscle activation in the early trials of older adults was occasionally different from that of the young adults. Older adults sometimes used a "hip strategy," in which they activated the stronger muscles of the hip prior to those of the thigh (Woollacott et al., 1988). This enabled them to recruit larger muscles sooner to compensate for

TABLE 3-1. *Neurosynergistic postural responses of older adults.*

Age Effects	Hypothesized Explanations	Source
Responses triggered by foot flexors (e.g., tibialis anterior) are more delayed than those triggered by foot extensors (e.g., gastrocnemius)	extensor strength is maintained by walking	Inglin & Woollacott, 1988
Response patterns of different hips may be activated before thighs	larger muscles of hips are activated sooner to compensate for loss of muscle mass	Woollacott et al., 1988
Response amplitudes within a synergy are less tightly coupled	aging central nervous system is more variable	Woollacott et al., 1986 Woollacott, 1990 Stelmach et al., 1989
Co-contraction is more prevalent	to reduce number of limb segments to be controlled to maintain balance	Woollacott, 1990 Manchester et al., 1989
Reactions from standing position are slower than from sitting	the integration of postural stabilizing mechanisms with voluntary motor programs is a key source of slowing	Stelmach, 1990
Preparations for fast responses are impaired; time between preparatory response and voluntary movement is shorter	problems with hierarchical organization of movement	Man'kovski et al., 1980 Rogers et al., 1992 Stelmach et al., 1990
Functional coordination of postural reflexes with voluntary is impaired	problems with hierarchical organization of movement	Stelmach et al., 1989

age- or disuse-related losses of muscle mass. Third, the relative *amplitude of specific muscle activation* within the synergistic response was more variable within the older subjects. Fourth, older subjects frequently employed a strategy of co-contraction, presumably to reduce the number of possible limb segments that must be controlled to maintain balance. This strategy is not unique to older adults, as subjects of all ages resort to a co-contraction mode when balance is severely threatened, as occurs in novel tasks at which they are unskilled or in high risk challenges to balance (walking on icy sidewalks or on a high wire). But older adults co-contract sooner and more than young adults in conditions that are less precarious. Although co-contraction provides a more stable balance, it is less energy efficient and does not mediate free-flowing, goal-directed movement.

Feedforward, anticipatory, neurosynergistic postural adjustments precede movement and are specific to the movement to be made. The type of postural adjustment to be made is dependent upon initial posture, the type of task (e.g., pushing or pulling), and the integrity of the CNS (e.g., the nerve-conduction velocity and the condition of the muscle mass). Voluntary responses are not initiated until postural balance has been stabilized; e.g., it is necessary to attain balance on the left foot before the right foot can be activated for a kick. It is thought that a central command system yokes the anticipatory postural adjustment to the muscle activation command. Neurosynergistic postural preparations for a slow response seem not to be affected by aging, but the preparations for fast responses are more impaired (Man'kovskii et al., 1980; Rogers et al., 1992; Stelmach et al., 1990). The time between the preparatory responses and the voluntary movement was shorter in the older subjects. In fact, in the very old subjects the preparatory response seemed to displace the voluntary response to make it slower. Some anticipatory postural reflexes, indicated by EMG recording, actually overlapped the voluntary responses. Delays in the onset of the voluntary response may have occurred because the neurosynergistic preparation was slow to develop, and the stable relationship between the preparatory activity in several involved muscles and the voluntary response was degraded.

Stelmach et al. (1990) suggested that the reason older subjects' reaction times are slower when made from a standing position than when made from a sitting position is that they have an impaired integration of postural stabilizing mechanisms with the voluntary response initiation. Similarly, Inglin and Woollacott (1988) found in a reaction-time experiment that, although the differential anticipatory postural adjustments to pushing or pulling a handle were primarily the same in young and old adults, there were some differences in the EMG patterns of the older adults. The functional coordination of postural reflexes with voluntary sway was age-impaired even in the simple task of leaning forward from the ankles (Stelmach et al., 1989). These few investigators have shown that latencies, muscular patterns, and pre-movement postural adjustments are different in old and young adults under some conditions, for some types of movements, and especially in unexpected or early trials of experimentally produced perturbations. With repeated trials, when perturbations are not extraordinary, the postural adjustment patterns normalize (Woollacott et al., 1986). Nevertheless, individuals rarely have an opportunity to practice adjusting to sudden and unexpected perturbations; thus, these age-related anticipatory postural differences provide at least some explanation for many of the functional differences seen in the movements of old and young individuals. Much remains to be determined, however, about the effects of aging on the integration of neurosynergistic and voluntary movement, as well as the overall contribution to and the precise nature of age-related postural slowing to the slowing of voluntary responses in the elderly.

Chronic Exercise Effects. Few investigations of exercise training effects on neurosynergistic control have been reported, with the exception of a study by Sale et al. (1979), in which they indicated that strength training may potentiate long-loop reflexes.

POSTURAL CONTROL, BALANCE, AND FALLING

For the elderly, an extremely significant functional outcome of the integration of sensory information, basic motor mechanisms, and neuro-synergies is the maintenance of balance and the prevention of falling. Balance can be arbitrarily categorized as the maintenance of stability in stationary positions (static balance) and during locomotion or other types of movement (dynamic balance).

Static Postural Control

Although the mechanisms by which postural neurosynergies operate to control balance are not fully understood, it is clear that older adults on average have poorer static postural control than do young adults (Stelmach & Sirica, 1986; Woollacott et al., 1982, 1986). Static postural control, measured in the laboratory by analyzing the extent and pattern of postural sway on a force platform, or in the clinic as the length of time that balance can be maintained on one or two feet, deteriorates with aging (Hasselkus & Shambes, 1975; Hayes et al., 1985; Murray et al., 1975; Overstall et al., 1977; Sheldon, 1963). Explanations for increased body sway are that the visual and vestibular contributions to balance are compromised with aging and/or that older adults may have more difficulty detecting weak sensory information from the extremities (Horak et al., 1989; Woollacott et al., 1982, 1986). In addition, the ability of older adults to balance with reduced or conflicting sensory information is also compromised (Woollacott et al., 1986).

Postural sway is an important marker of age-related changes in balance because excessive sway, particularly lateral sway under blindfolded conditions, is a moderately accurate predictor of the risk of falling (Maki et al., 1994; Wolfson et al., 1986). Postural sway has been reported to be greater in women than in men, possibly due to sex differences in the ratio of body weight to muscle mass (Overstall et al., 1977). These authors also found body sway to be more predictive of falling in women than in men.

Although static balance as measured by standing on one leg is not normally a movement that older adults choose to make, there is a moment in every stride of walking in which the full weight of the body must be balanced on one foot, and there are many instances in the ordinary activities of daily living when balance is momentarily lost and the body weight is thrown quickly onto one foot in order to prevent a fall. The one-foot balance task, therefore, is a significant predictor of falling (Fernie et al., 1982; Kirshen et al., 1984; Sheldon, 1963).

Chronic Exercise Effects on Static Balance. Substantial evidence is available that remaining physically active is associated with better balance in older adults, although it should be recognized at the onset that some balance problems, particularly those mediated by pathology of the vestibular system, are probably irreversible. Nevertheless, Myers and Hamilton (1985) proposed that the amount of exercise in an individual's life is a good predictor of balance. The performances of masters athletes and physically fit older adults are more similar to that of young subjects in clinical and functional tests of balance than to that of the older adults' sedentary peers (Brown & Mishica, 1989; Manchester et al., 1989). Other investigators have cross-sectionally compared physically active older groups to sedentary groups and found that performance on the one-foot balance test was correlated significantly but at low levels with vital capacity ($r = 0.38$), forced expiratory volume ($r = 0.38$) (Stones & Kozma, 1987), and postural sway (Era & Heikkinen, 1985). Although it may seem surprising that balance was even slightly related to pulmonary function, it is probably because these two measures of pulmonary function are frequently found to be weak but significant predictors of health status and functional age in the elderly.

Performance on single-leg standing balance tests, with and without vision, and on heel-to-toe walking, was also superior in nine old tai chi practitioners compared to nine old non-tai chi practitioners (Tse & Bailey, 1992). The men were better than women in both groups on the same three tests. Rikli and Busch (1986) compared performance in a one-foot, eyes-open balance test of women who were classified as young-active (22.2 y), young-inactive (21.1 y), old-active (68.7 y), or old-inactive (68.9 y). In their study, active was defined as having vigorously exercised three times per week for at least 3 y prior to the study. No differences existed between the young active and inactive women, but large differences existed between the old active and inactive women. In fact, the old-active group balanced more than twice as long as the old-inactive group (47.73 ± 19.15 s, compared to 20.13 ± 19.31 s). Rikli followed this cross-sectional study with a 3-y intervention study of community-dwelling, healthy women in their 60s and 70s and found that the exercise intervention had beneficial results on static balance (Rikli & Edwards 1991; Stones & Kozma, 1987).

Other investigators, who measured body sway, provided shorter exercise programs, or tested older subjects, failed to find improvements in balance with an exercise training intervention. Crilly and colleagues (1989) analyzed the postural sway of 50 elderly women (82 y) living in supervised retirement apartments, retirement homes, or rest homes. They participated three times each week in 12 wk of exercise designed to increase postural stability. Subjects were randomly assigned to an exercise or control group. Exercise duration started at 15 min and increased to 35 min in programs led by physical therapists within the subjects' residences. Exercises included activities challenging balance on one or both legs, coordination, flexibility, antigravity strength, trunk strength, ankle strength, and relaxation. The program was designed more to improve balance than to develop generalized fitness. Although it was expected that the postural sway of these subjects living in protected and caregiving facilities would be similar to that of recurrent fallers (adults who have fallen several times), the sway characteristics of the subjects were only slightly worse than those of a normal, independently living population of elderly. Lateral sway with eyes closed of both the control and experimental groups deteriorated over the course of the study, whereas only the anteroposterior sway with eyes closed deteriorated in the exercised group. However, no significant improvement in postural sway that could be attributed to an exercise effect was found.

Barry et al. (1966) reported that 13 elderly men and women (72 y) failed to improve in one-foot balance after a 3-mo controlled study, even though many of the exercises were designed to improve balance and flexibility. Finally, a 10-wk exercise program designed to improve the balance and stability of 15 women and one man (62–84 y) resulted in no change in balance (Bassett et al., 1982). None of these investigators determined the relative contributions of proprioceptive acuity, leg strength, visual impairment, or vestibular integrity to their subjects' balance capabilities.

Even though several researchers have failed to find a relationship between fitness levels and balance, it should be emphasized that an aerobic exercise program increases lower limb strength and endurance, both of which should contribute to better balance and decrease the risk for falling. For example, an exercise program that is successful in decreasing total body weight and body mass also contributes to the maintenance of balance by making the balancing task easier for the neuromuscular system (Era & Heikkinen, 1985). The causes of falling are multiple and complex. Other contributions of fitness to balance control are that fitness may reduce postural hypotension, enable the older adult to take less medication, increase self-confidence, and enhance sleep, all of which could contribute to a reduced incidence of falls (Figure 3-4). These activity-related physical enhancements may also act to reduce the severity and consequences of a fall if it does occur (Nevitt et al., 1991).

One-foot balance-test performance also improves with mental practice (Fansler et al., 1985) and with practice of the balance task (Heitmann et al., 1989). Improvements in the balance performance of older subjects on one-foot balance tasks are likely due both to increases in leg strength and to neuromotor learning. Older individuals who are physically active challenge the balance system frequently, thereby providing daily practice opportunities for balance mechanisms. Participating in physical activity on a daily basis also increases the self-confidence of older people in their

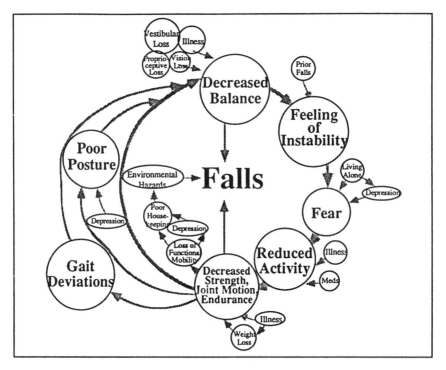

FIGURE 3-4. *Factors affecting the risk of falling in the elderly.* This diagram depicts a "vicious cycle" in which age-related changes in physiological mechanisms of balance, psychological factors, and environmental hazards interact to increase the risk of falling. The figure (reprinted with permission) was developed by Stephen Allison, Ph.D., P.T., while a graduate student at The University of Texas at Austin, 1993.

physical abilities, which in turn improves their balance and mobility (Overstall, 1980; Roberts & Fitzpatrick, 1983).

Dynamic Postural Control and Locomotion

Just as older people respond more slowly to environmental stimuli, plan and execute coordinated movements more slowly, and carry out job skills more slowly, they also have slower gaits. In the Himann et al. (1988) study of self-selected walking speeds (slow, normal, and fast), a change in the rate of slowing seemed to occur at age 62. Before the age of 62, preferred walking speeds were 1–2% slower per decade. After 63, women's preferred walking speed was 12.4% slower each decade and men's was 16.1% lower per decade (Himann et al., 1988). These gait speeds were cross-sectionally derived because gait speed has not been measured longitudinally. Himann et al. (1988) also reported that older women walk with slower velocity, higher cadence, and shorter step length than men, although these values were not corrected for height. The flexed posture that many elderly assume during walking to reduce the risk of falling may lead to earlier fatigue, decreased joint excursion, and eventually to a decreased stride and gait speed. A large amount of the variance (44%) in the walking speed of men has been attributed to lower leg strength, height, and the presence of health problems, whereas in women, 42% of the variance is contributed by height, leg strength, step-test scores, and mobility-limiting leg pain (Bendall et al., 1989).

Not only is self-selected walking speed slower, but the gait pattern of people older than 65 y is also different. Older adults use shorter and broader stride dimensions, more limited ankle movement, and lower swing-to-stance time ratios so that the period of double support is increased (Ferrandez et al., 1988; Hageman & Blanke, 1986; Murray et al., 1969). Age-related differential gait patterns can be attributed almost solely to the self-selected walking speed of older people, however. When young and old subjects with no neurological or neuromuscular pathologies walked at similar speeds, the differences in gait pattern were minimal (Ferrandez et al., 1990). Differences in gait were also minimal when stride length was equalized across ages (Elble et al., 1991). In order to increase gait speed, older adults tend to increase stride frequency, whereas younger adults tend to increase stride length (Larish et al., 1988). Older adults may favor increasing stride frequency because they are less flexible or because long strides compromise their balance. As stride length increases, the amount of double-support time decreases, which in turn is more challenging to their balance (Figure 3-5). The elderly tend to prolong the double-support phase of the gait cycle in order to enhance their balance (Gillis, et al., 1986). Another explanation is that older adults prefer slower walking speeds because these are most economical for their body structure, weight, muscular strength, flexibility, and many other variables. They may, therefore, use the strategy of increasing stride frequency over length because it also maximizes economy of motion (Larish et al., 1988). Shorter strides would also maximize endurance of the weaker musculature of the legs of older adults. A slower gait provides an older walker a longer time period in which to monitor the environment so that anticipatory adjustments in gait can be made to avoid the need for reactive responses. Slower walking speed, in addition to requiring less energy, also provides more time for adaptation in basic reflexive stride and support patterns, postural and equilibrium control, and information processing necessary to adapt to unexpected changes in the environment. Basically, however, changes in the walking gait pattern during normal aging are minimal in healthy individuals and are more related to health status (Engle, 1986), physical inactivity (Larish et al., 1988), or pathological conditions (Imms & Edholm, 1981) than to chronological age.

The strategies used by older adults to approach obstacles and negotiate them are slightly different from those used by young people. The

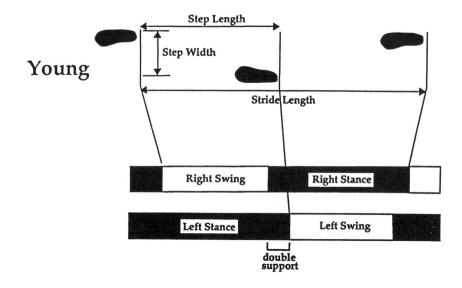

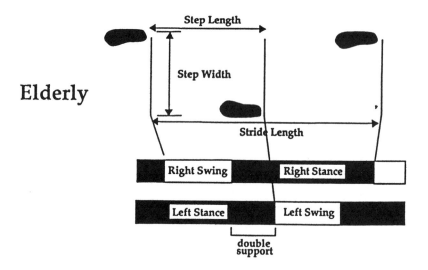

FIGURE 3-5. *The gait cycle in the young and elderly.* One cycle is the time required for the stance (support phase) and swing of one foot. The blackened areas depict stance time, and the non-blackened areas depict swing time. Periods where both feet are on the ground (bracketed) provide double support for balance. Periods where only one foot is on the ground (during the swing phase of one foot) provide only one base of support. Modified from Chao, E.Y.S. (1986). Biomechanics of the human gait. In: G.W. Schmid-Schonbein et al. (eds.) *Frontiers in Biomechanics.* New York: Springer-Verlag, 1986, p. 226 and reprinted with permission from Spirduso, W.W. (1995).

minimum foot-swing clearance over wooden blocks ranging in height from 25–152 mm was not age-related, but older adults crossed over obstacles more conservatively (Chen et al., 1991). They slowed crossing speed, reduced step length, and shortened the distance from the rear edge of the obstacle to the heel of the swing foot at heel strike. They also crossed the obstacle so that it was 10% further forward in the crossing step. Although none of the older adults actually tripped while crossing over an obstacle, they made more mistakes. Seventeen percent of them stepped on the obstacle while attempting to cross over it (Chen et al., 1991). More obstacle contact increases the risk of tripping or falling while negotiating the obstacle.

Chronic Exercise Effects on Locomotion. Decreased leg strength is a major contributor to the loss of walking speed, which presents a problem to an older adult who needs to cross a street within a short pedestrian stop light, or who might need to avoid an oncoming automobile by speeding up his or her gait. The strength of the gastrocnemius, when combined with height and poor health, accounts for almost half of the variance associated with walking speed (Bendall et al., 1989). It is not surprising, therefore, that aerobic exercise programs that enable an older adult to maintain high levels of fitness have been associated with improved walking speed (Cunningham et al., 1982). Exercise probably contributes to the maintenance of gait speed and the prevention of falling in several ways. Falling has been attributed to many factors: muscular weakness, inflexibility, degradation of neuromotor postural synergies, cardiovascular disease, obesity, vestibular and visual deterioration, and environmental hazards (Spirduso, 1995). Although high levels of aerobic fitness cannot have much effect upon vestibular and visual disease and environmental hazards, an improvement in fitness can be an effective strategy to reduce the probability of falling by improving strength and flexibility and by reducing the susceptibility to cardiovascular disease and obesity.

Several efforts have been made to determine the contribution of leg strength to balance and to determine the effect of a strength training program on static and dynamic balance. An age- or disuse-related loss of lower leg strength is probably not a primary contributor to age-related increased postural sway because muscle activity in the lower legs during quiet standing is minimal. Lower leg strength is a factor in one-foot balance testing, however, and is important in maintaining dynamic balance and walking (DiPasquale et al., 1989; MacRae et al., 1989). Aging and disuse substantially degrade the muscles that provide stabilization about the ankle joint and exert force against the ground during walking (Vandervoort & Hayes, 1989). The strength of the ankle dorsiflexors of fallers was 7.5 times lower than that of a control group of nonfallers (Whipple et al., 1987). Weak leg musculature may affect balance in several ways. Low strength in the muscles that support the knees is associated with a greater incidence of falling (Tinetti et al., 1986)). Age-related decreases in strength could limit an older adult's ability to lift the foot high enough in the swing phase of walking to completely clear an obstacle. Older adults place the landing heel closer to the obstacle as they step over it (Chen et al., 1991), but this may also increase the risk of tripping. Weak leg muscles also force older individuals to use a bent hip strategy that incorporates more and larger leg and body muscles to maintain balance when a supporting surface becomes unstable (McCollum et al., 1984). This strategy may increase their balance, but it does so at a greater cost of fatigue.

Both static and dynamic postural control benefit from the considerable redundancy that exists among the neuromuscular systems to maintain balance. Information from the visual, vestibular, and somatosensory systems is available for every physical movement, and spinal, righting, and neurosynergistic reflexes, by definition, work in concert to implement planned movements. Individuals with all systems intact have ample information and control systems to operate, and those who have impairments in one or two systems, such as occurs in younger individuals with genetic disorders or disease- or trauma-induced damage, can function reasonably well by relying more heavily on the remaining systems. When vision is lost, for example, individuals become more adept at using proprioceptive information to maintain balance. If vestibular function deteriorates, balance can be maintained somewhat by a greater reliance on vision. The problem that many elderly individuals face is that, unlike most younger handicapped adults, older adults have a more difficult time adapting to the lost information and compensating with another system (Manchester et al., 1989; Woollacott et al. 1986). In addition, the elderly face a gradual decline of not one but several systems simultaneously. Vision may be greatly impaired, the vestibular system may be compromised, and the somatosensory system may also have become less sensitive. In addition, the central integrative processes may be operating more slowly. Thus, even though system redundancy is a marvel of human engineering that works beautifully in the maintenance of balance and locomotion in normal young adults, the relentless effects of aging result in a more fragile balance, a less stable base of support for planned coordinated movements, and a higher risk of falling in the old and oldest-old population.

REACTIVE AND PLANNED COORDINATED MOVEMENT

This chapter began with the basic idea that the control of movement, either simple or complex, reactive or planned, visual or motoric, is required to accomplish any goal during the act of daily living. To this point in the chapter, the assimilation and integration of sensory information, the fundamental mechanisms, and the postural support systems necessary to control movements have been addressed. In this section, some basic categories of movements that must be programmed by the CNS will be discussed. A complete discussion of all the factors involved in controlling the force, direction, and velocity of learned complex movements is well outside the scope of this chapter. The emphasis in the following section is on those types of movements, i.e., reactive and fast movements, and complex coordinated movements, in which the CNS control processes may be most affected by aging and exercise. The section concludes with a discussion of the effects of chronic exercise on these types of movements and the potential mechanisms by which these effects might be enacted.

Reactive and Fast Movements

Slowed reactions and slowed movements are among the most visible characteristics of aging. Even the simplest reaction to the simplest stimulus, such as one simple movement (lifting a finger) in response to one simple stimulus (onset of a green light), is affected by aging. The more complex the stimulus and the more complicated the motor response, the greater the slowing of reaction time with advancing age (Spirduso, 1995; Spirduso & MacRae, 1990; Spirduso et al., 1988). The motor response parameters, such as peak velocity, duration, and amplitude of initial movements, may be minimally changed with aging, but the parameters, such as information-processing speed or motor programming, that are related to sensory information or mapping of sensory information onto motor functions are significantly impaired (Warabi et al., 1986). Clearly, the primary site of age-related slowing is in the CNS processing that is necessary to integrate goal-related sensory information, to select a motor program, and to execute it. This has been impressively shown in all of the EMG studies in which a reaction is fractionated into visual-evoked potentials, motor potentials, premotor latencies, contractile time, reaction time, and movement time (Spirduso, 1982). Accordingly, although sensory deficits and decrements in musculoskeletal integrity contribute to the slowing of a psychomotor reaction, the predominant source of slowing is in central processing.

In almost all tests of movement speed measured independently of reaction time, such as the velocity of arm movement from one target to another, age is inversely related to speed (Spirduso et al., 1988). In general, increased complexity in a task decreases the speed with which it can be performed for all ages. A task is made more complex if it requires changes in direction, multiple movements, or the coordination of more than one limb (Light & Spirduso, 1990). Although increasing complexity increases reaction time, increased complexity does not seem to amplify age differences in movement speed independent of reaction time (Stern et al., 1980). Thus, at any age reacting to a stimulus with a movement that requires a change in direction is initiated more slowly than reacting with a unidirectional movement. But once the multidirectional movement has been initiated, the speed with which it can be executed is not different from that for a unidirectional movement.

Several factors exacerbate the differences between young and old in reactive and fast movements. In addition to the complexity factor mentioned above, Chodzko-Zajko and Moore (1994) have proposed that the more effortful (versus automatic) the processing, the greater the age difference. A task that demands effortful processing requires continued attention, responds to training, is influenced by strategy use and imagery, and requires memory capacity. A task that can be accomplished through automatic processing requires only the encoding of frequency information and spatial location and can be processed simultaneously with another. Also, age-associated differences are greater the more novel the task, the more compatible the stimulus and response, and the less practiced the subjects (Spirduso, 1994).

Chronic Exercise Effects. It has been well established for some time that the primary source for slowing in reactive and fast movements is in the CNS processing and programming of the response movements, not in peripheral neuromuscular events (Botwinick & Thompson, 1966; Weiss, 1965). If even one of the physiological adaptations that occur as a result of chronic exercise positively influences CNS processing, therefore, habitual exercise could play a significant role in the maintenance of cognition in the elderly. Retention of cognitive function is so important to quality of life, that many researchers have been actively studying this topic to determine how and by what mechanism aerobic fitness may be related to CNS processing. Based upon some relatively indirect comments made by Botwinick and Thompson (1966), Spirduso (1975) developed a paradigm to compare the reaction and movement times of young and old physically fit and unfit subjects. She found that the older fit subjects were not significantly different in their reaction times from young subjects, regardless of the young subjects' fitness status. Since that time, 15 research studies on reaction time have been conducted using the same or a similar paradigm, and 22 intervention studies have also been completed (Spirduso, 1994).

As reviewed by Chodzko-Zajko & Moore (1994), Dustman et al. (1995), and Spirduso (1980), the general pattern of findings is that when cross-sectional research designs are used, aerobic fitness appears to be moderately related to fast reactions and movements, but when an intervention design is used, the improvement of aerobic fitness does not always result in an improvement in behavioral speed. Of 15 cross-sectional studies, the investigators in 14 found that physically fit older subjects reacted faster than their unfit cohorts, whereas only one failed to find a difference (Figure 3-6). But of the 22 intervention studies, only 13 (59%) found improvements following an exercise intervention. Those who failed to find effects of exercise on behavioral speed suggested that the primary

Cognition-Fitness Studies
Human Research

Not Related   Related

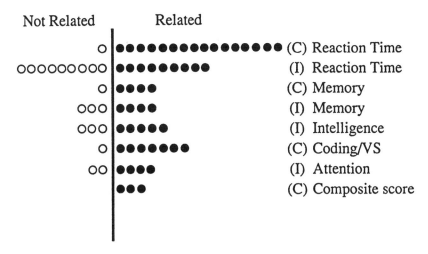

O	●●●●●●●●●●●●●●●●●● (C) Reaction Time
OOOOOOOOO	●●●●●●●●●● (I) Reaction Time
O	●●●● (C) Memory
OOO	●●●● (I) Memory
OOO	●●●●● (I) Intelligence
O	●●●●●●● (C) Coding/VS
OO	●●●● (I) Attention
	●●● (C) Composite score

FIGURE 3-6. *Studies of the relationship between physical fitness and cognition.* This figure summarizes 72 studies of human subjects on the relationship between aspects of cognition and physical fitness. The figure is divided by the vertical line into two sets: studies in which fitness and cognition were unrelated (solid filled circles) and studies in which they were (dotted filled circles). C = cross-sectional study; I = intervention study (before and after exercise training). The cognitive variable analyzed in each row of studies is labeled in the right column, e.g., the first row represents 16 cross-sectional studies in which reaction time was the dependent variable, and the results supported a positive relationship between fitness and cognition. The results from only one cross-sectional study of reaction time failed to support the cognition-fitness relationships. (Reprinted with permission from Spirduso (1994).

reason that cross-sectional comparisons of fitness and information processing in older subjects have been positive is that profound socioeconomic and psychosocial characteristics also differ between fit and unfit adults, and that these can account for the differences in behavioral speed.

Researchers who have found a relationship between fitness and processing speed argue that the reason that some interventions have failed to find this relationship is that the subjects in these interventions are at such a low level of fitness that the short-term exercise interventions have not brought the subjects to a level of fitness comparable to that of the subjects of cross-sectional studies (Spirduso, 1995). Also, physical fitness has not been measured adequately and consistently, stable measures of reaction time have not been obtained, samples have been small, and the distribution of ages within groups has not been homogeneous. Notwithstanding the few studies in which a relationship among health, fitness, and behavioral speed failed to materialize, the majority of findings from both human and animal studies suggest that exercise does positively affect CNS function and that these positive effects are reflected in faster behavioral speed.

The largest differences between chronic exercisers and nonexercisers is in the central component of the response, i.e., the premotor time (PMT), rather than in the peripheral component, the muscle fiber contractile time (CT). This can be clearly seen in Figure 3-7, in which the physically active old subjects of Kroll and Clarkson (1977) were 13% faster in PMT but only 5% faster in CT.

Coordination

Coordination and skill deteriorate with aging, but the specific mechanisms by which this deterioration occurs have not yet been identified. The study of age-related changes in coordination has been very slow to develop, perhaps because older adults find so many ways to compensate for coordination losses that the changes in coordination have not been viewed by researchers as a critical problem to address. In addition, age-related changes in coordination, being very gradual and subtle, are difficult to detect.

In general, tasks that require the control of multiple sequences of movements rather than a single movement are performed less well by ag-

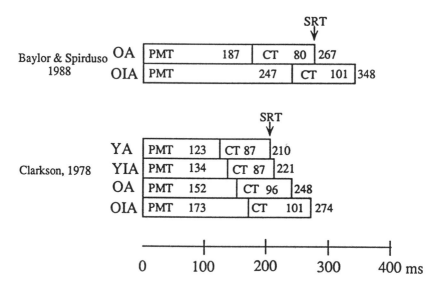

FIGURE 3-7. *Fractionated reaction time in young and old subjects who differ in physical activity history.* YA = young active subjects (18–25 y), YIA = young inactive, OA = old active subjects (>60 y), OIA = old inactive subjects. Active is defined as having exercised at a moderate level of intensity at least three times per week for at least 30 min duration for at least 3 y previous to the study. PMT = premotor time; CT = contractile time; SRT = simple reaction time. Figure adapted from Kroll and Clarkson (1977).

ing adults. Some available information indicates that older adults have less ability to initiate and terminate bilateral movements simultaneously to a stimulus and to modify motor commands during response execution (Stelmach et al., 1988).

By far the biggest impact of aging on coordination, however, is the impact of slowed processing speed on neuromuscular integration. Older people preprogram, program, and reprogram discrete movements in the same way that young adults do, only more slowly. They also learn laboratory psychomotor tasks at the same rate as young subjects, but they do not perform them as well because they usually perform them more slowly (Carnahan et al., 1992). Part of this difference in speed is that they choose to move more slowly; i.e., they trade speed for accuracy. They also may move more slowly in order to sample proprioceptive and external feedback more frequently.

Effects of Chronic Exercise on Coordinated Movement. The effects of chronic aerobic exercise and/or weight training on the control of coordinated movements have not been addressed, except in studies of achievement on neuropsychological tests that involve a substantial motor performance component. Examples are the Digit Symbol Substitution Test (DSS) and Trailmaking (TM), both of which require handwriting and the control of line drawing. In the DSS test, subjects copy a symbol into a box underneath its matching number. In TM, subjects draw with a pencil a line that connects targets labeled sequentially by alphabet or number (1,A,2,B,3,C, etc.) as quickly as possible. As reviewed by Spirduso et al. (1988, 1994a), results from studies of these two types of test have been mixed, with some finding that physically fit adults perform these tasks better and others detecting no such relationship. However, the evidence seems positive that enhanced physical fitness has a beneficial effect on many types of CNS function, such as attention, short-term memory, and information-processing speed (Chodzko-Zajko & Moore, 1994; Dustman et al., 1995; Spirduso, 1980; Vercruyssen et al., 1990). All of these cognitive functions are necessary for the successful execution of many coordinated, planned movements.

Proposed Mechanisms by Which Physical Fitness May Affect Reactive and Planned Movements

Several mechanisms have been proposed to support a relationship between physical fitness and CNS processing to control movements. Three of the most discussed mechanisms can be categorized as exercise-related enhancements of cardiovascular and cerebrovascular integrity, brain morphology, and neurotransmitter function. These mechanisms have been extensively discussed in several reviews (Dustman et al., 1995; Spirduso, 1975; Vercruyssen et al., 1990); thus, they will only be summarized in this chapter.

Cardiovascular and Cerebrovascular Mechanisms. The role that exercise plays in maintaining normal blood pressure in aging adults contributes also to the maintenance of CNS function.

Prevention of Hypertension. Long-term hypertension reduces cerebral blood flow, but medication-induced decreases in hypertension increase cerebral perfusion. Systematic exercise has also been used in many cases to reduce high blood pressure to normal levels (Tipton, 1984), thereby reversing the decline in cerebral blood flow (Meyer et al., 1985). Significant correlations have been shown between hypertension and several types of neuropsychological function (Waldstein et al., 1991). Performance on several of the subtests of the Wechsler Adult Intelligence Scale, particularly those that put a premium on psychomotor and neuropsychological performance (e.g., the Categories test, the Trials B test, the Digit Symbol Substitution test, and the Block Design test) have also been related to hypertension (Elias et al., 1990). The correlations between hypertension and CNS function, and the relationships between hypertension and performance on these psychomotor tasks, are observed throughout the range of blood pressures (Elias et al., 1990).

Maintenance of Cerebral Blood Flow. Adequate cerebral blood flow (CBF) is essential for normal brain function and, thus, normal control of planned movements. Even mild arteriosclerosis can produce a relative cerebrovascular insufficiency and brain tissue hypoxia, conditions known to contribute substantially to age-related decline of brain function (Smith, 1984). Another contribution that cardiovascular fitness can make to cortical function, therefore, is its action on CBF, which gradually decreases with increasing age (Frackowiack et al., 1980, 1983; Lenzi et al., 1981; Pantano et al., 1983; Shaw et al., 1984). Rogers et al. (1990) measured the CBF of older individuals each year for 4 y and found that it declined more in those who retired and became inactive than in those who retired but stayed active or in those who continued to work. They also found that the maintenance of CBF was related to cognitive function. This relationship is interesting, but it does not alone provide evidence that habitual physical activity can maintain CBF. Those retirees who were sedentary and had poorer CBF might have retired because they were not healthy. Yet, exercise has been shown to enhance CBF in several ways. Physical activity activates the brain, thus increasing regional metabolic demands and thereby increasing CBF in those metabolically active regions. Aerobic exercise reduces the risk factors for atherogenesis, heart disease, decreased CBF, and stroke (Haskell, 1986) and lowers triglycerides in hypertriglyceridemic patients (Meyer et al., 1988; Rogers et al., 1989). Although not causally related, these lower triglyceride levels were associated with improved CBF and cognitive performance. Chronic exercise also inhibits platelet aggregability, thereby enhancing CBF and decreasing the risk of stroke (Rauramaa et al., 1986; Wolf & Kannel, 1982).

Angiogenesis. In addition to increased cerebral blood flow, Black et al. (1987) found that vigorous physical activity induced angiogenesis, the development of new capillaries, in some brain areas of middle-aged rats. Exercise and enriched environments also increased capillary density in the motor cortex of gerbils. The capillary volume fraction was 50% greater, the amount of capillary per synapse was greater, and there was additional capillary branching (Black et al., 1987, 1989). Their results indicated that significant plasticity in the brain vascular system can occur after developmental years, but that exercise-induced angiogenesis may be age-limited. Angiogenesis occurred in middle-aged rats, but not in old rats.

The Oxygen Hypothesis. This hypothesis has been strongly supported by Dustman et al. (1984, 1995) and is a corollary of the cerebral blood flow hypothesis. Reduced cerebral blood flow may restrict the delivery of oxygen to brain tissue. As individuals age and cerebral blood flow decreases, a condition of cerebral hypoxia occurs, and CNS function suffers. Diseased patients who have been experiencing oxygen deficits and who have shown signs of intellectual deterioration for several years were improved by treatments with hyperoxygenation (Jacobs et al., 1969). However, the work of Thompson and colleagues (1976) contradicted that finding, and they suggested that results from hyperoxygenation probably depend on the type of brain deterioration. Hyperbaric oxygen might be effective in patients with cerebrovascular disease, cardiovascular insufficiency, or brain ischemia, but it is unlikely to be effective in patients with stabilized neurologic deficits or irreversible ischemic damage. Aerobic exercise might be beneficial, therefore, for the patients with cerebrovascular problems because exercise can increase the cerebral blood flow to motor and sensory cortex, cerebello-cerebral cortex, and corticospinal and ascending spinal tracts (Gross, 1980). Thomas et al. (1989) also reported that moderate exercise ($\sim$50% $\dot{V}O_2$max) significantly increased cerebral blood flow by 31–58%.

The results from studies of healthy elderly have not been as supportive of the oxygen hypothesis. One of the difficulties associated with studying this problem is that no one has demonstrated that chronic exercise increases oxygen extraction in brain tissue. This critical step is necessary for the validation of the oxygen hypothesis.

Exercise-induced Morphological Changes. Yet another mechanism that has been proposed to explain beneficial effects of exercise on information processing is exercise-induced morphological changes in brain tissue. The brains of rats and primates housed in an enriched environment that included opportunities for physical activity revealed substantial morphological differences from the brains of animals housed in laboratory cages (Floeter & Greenough, 1979; Pysh & Weiss, 1979). The cerebellar areas of the paraflocculus, nodulus, and uvula from active animals had longer dendritic branches, increased dendritic spine density, and larger, more complex Purkinje cells. The plasticity of the brain is not as great for old animals as it is for young ones, however (Black et al., 1989, 1991). The implications of this are that the older brain is less plastic and might not respond as much to exercise, so that an exercise program initiated at 70 y of age might not benefit cognitive functions as much as one initiated at 50 y of age. This line of study is, however, in its infant stage.

Neurotransmitter Mechanisms. Neurotransmitters provide a biochemical interface between neurons in the central nervous system and are key components in communicating sensory, motor, and integrative neuronal messages. Impaired neurotransmitter function delays synaptic transmission, which in turn slows the processing of information. As will be discussed below, aging is associated with changes in the characteristics of several neurotransmitters and/or with the balance among neurotransmitters.

Researchers have shown that exercise and training are associated with changes of neurotransmitters in a direction counter to age-associated changes. For example, aging seems to decrease the numbers of transmitter receptors and the concentrations of neurotransmitters in the catecholamine system, particularly in the dopaminergic neurons in the pars compacta of the substantia nigra, which is highly related to motor control (McGeer & McGeer, 1978). Yet, animals that exercised for 8 wk had more dopamine receptors and a greater binding affinity (de Castro & Duncan, 1985; Gilliam et al., 1984; MacRae et al., 1987). As reviewed by Spirduso (1983 a, b), these neurotransmitter changes were also associated with faster behavioral reaction times. Other investigators have also found aerobic exercise to be associated with higher levels or faster turnover of biogenic amines, such as norepinephrine (Ebert et al., 1972; Gordon et al., 1966) and serotonin (Barchas & Freedman, 1963; Brown et al., 1979). Exercise might influence brain function by acting directly or indirectly on neurotransmitters that influence the reticular activating system and consequently influence a behavior such as reaction time.

Exercise also might conceivably affect neurotransmitters through its role in glucose regulation. Saller and Chiodo (1980) reported that daily fluctuations of glucose within normal levels influence the activity of dopaminergic neurons in the basal ganglia, a brain area that is critical to motor control.

Among other potential effects of exercise on neurotransmitter function are the relationships among aging, exercise, and cholinergic dysfunction. One of the hypotheses to explain age-related memory dysfunction is that aging leads to a cholinergic deficit. In many elderly patients who exhibit memory losses, substantial cholinergic deficits are found, particularly in the hippocampus, which is the major brain area for learning and memory. Deficits have been found in the number of hippocampal cholinergic neurons; in acetylcholine synthesis; in the activity-dependent, high-affinity cholinergic uptake (HACU); in acetylcholine release upon stimulation; and in postsynaptic muscarinic-receptor sites. Conversely, both acute and chronic exercise can increase acetylcholine release, HACU, and muscarinic-receptor density (Fordyce & Farrar, 1991a, 1991b). Once again, the exercise-induced alterations may be age-limited, because plasticity was shown in middle-aged but not in old rats.

Practice Effects on Reactive and Coordinated Movement

A major source of the contradictions that exist in the findings of studies of chronic exercise and reactive and coordinated movement is that age- or exercise-related differences in motor skills must always be experimentally isolated from age-related differences in practice as well as potential age-related differential learning. Practice makes a dramatic difference in the ability of older adults to maintain motor skill performance. As an example, older typists who practice the majority of their work days can type as rapidly as much younger typists, even though their reaction times in making individual key strokes are slower than those of young typists (Salthouse, 1984). The author proposed in this case that the older typists were able to compensate for age effects and to anticipate the necessary key strokes by reading ahead.

Practice effects may also transfer from one task to another, as was shown when older subjects improved in a two-choice reaction time task after practicing playing video games (Clark et al., 1987; Dustman et al., 1992). In these tasks, the performance of older adults was slower and also not as accurate as that of younger subjects.

In laboratory tests of reactivity, such as reaction time, in which relatively few trials are ever provided (compared to real-world motor skills), greater age-related decrements are many times seen in the first few trials. Thereafter the effects of practice are similar for old and young (Clarkson, 1978), even though the performance of the young continues to be better than that of the old adults. Similarly, older adult performance in terms of speed and accuracy on laboratory psychomotor tasks is almost always slower, less accurate, and more variable, especially in more complex tasks, than that of young adults, but the rate and learning style of older adults is not significantly different from that of young adults (Carnahan et al., 1992; Salthouse & Somberg, 1982; Swanson & Lee, 1992).

NUTRITIONAL EFFECTS ON MOTOR CONTROL

Evidence from experimental and epidemiological research indicates that nutritional factors and dietary patterns can substantially influence the aging process and the onset and progression of many diseases leading to morbidity and mortality (Kannel, 1989). Not surprisingly, an inadequate diet can also impair the function of muscles and the CNS. For example, an abnormally low dietary intake of protein detrimentally affects muscle tissue, producing low RNA and glycogen concentrations, increased muscle fatigue, and an altered pattern of muscle contraction and relaxation (Young et al., 1989). Inadequate nutrition, therefore, by causing detrimental changes in muscle tissue and CNS function, can accelerate normal age-related declines in motor control. Recently, attention has also been directed toward the potentially beneficial effects on CNS function that might be provided by an enhanced diet, as well as by dietary supplements such as vitamins and minerals.

The topic of nutritional influences on motor control, although important, is so broad that it cannot be dealt with adequately in this chapter. Also, the topic of nutrition and motor control in the healthy elderly is relatively new, and few researchers have directly addressed this topic. However, a few examples are provided of how nutrition might interact with aging to influence motor control. These examples include the effects of diet on brain neurotransmitters, the effects of fluctuating blood glucose on cognitive function as it may be expressed in processing fast movements, the role of vitamin supplements in brain function (Figure 3-8), and the effects of restriction of dietary energy on motor behavior.

Nutrition, Neurotransmitters, and Brain Function

Normal CNS function is dependent upon the proper function of neurotransmitters that are synthesized from amino acid precursors. Just as it was suggested earlier in this chapter that exercise may alter the levels and function of some neurotransmitters crucial to motor control, another area of recently heightened interest has been the role diet can play in the enhancement of elderly CNS function.

Neurotransmitter synthesis and release can be influenced by dietary fluctuations and manipulations if three conditions are met: 1) the plasma levels of transmitter precursors must vary in proportion to the amount of dietary precursor; 2) the brain, because of its inability to make adequate quantities of neurotransmitter, must rely on uptake of the precursor from the blood by an unsaturated transport system; and 3) the precursor must be converted to the neurotransmitter by an enzyme that is also unsaturated with its substrate (Growdon, 1989). Three neurotransmitter precursors meet these conditions: tryptophan, which can be converted to serotonin; tyrosine, which can be converted to dopamine and norepinephrine; and choline, which can be converted to acetylcholine. All four of these transmitters—serotonin, dopamine, norepinephrine, and acetylcholine—are crucial to motor control.

Increased intake of foods containing high levels of these precursors can be particularly helpful to individuals suffering from metabolic or neurologic diseases (Wurtman, 1982), and a large body of literature has ac-

NUTRITIONAL EFFECTS ON MOTOR CONTROL

Diet-produced increases in circulating precursors

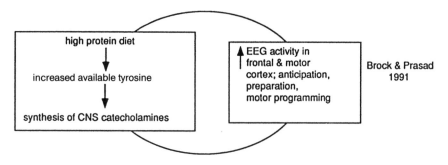

Dietary Fluctuations of Blood Glucose and Brain Function

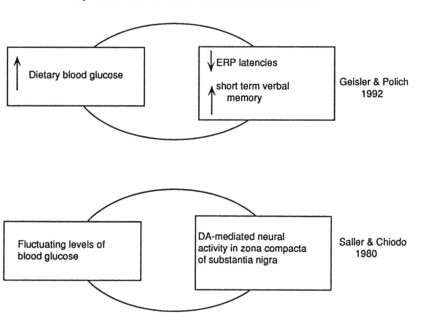

FIGURE 3-8. *Hypothetical nutritional effects on motor control.* Findings of three studies in which dietary manipulations of neurotransmitters or glucose were related to changes in brain function. EEG = electroencephalographic; ERP = EEG event-related potential; DA = dopamine. Information for diagram from Brock and Prasad (1991), from Geisler and Polich (1992), and from Saller and Chiodo (1980).

cumulated on the use of nutritional manipulation as a form of therapy for these individuals. For example, tryptophan has shown some promise in suppressing myoclonus in a few patients with posthypoxic intention myoclonus (Growdon, 1979), and a diet containing increased levels of L-tyrosine seemed to increase dopamine turnover in Parkinson's patients (Growdon & Melamed, 1982). Because some successes of this type have been seen with dietary manipulation of precursors, attempts have also been made to determine whether diet-produced increases in circulating precursors could enhance neurotransmitter function in healthy animals that maintain relatively normal diets. Brock and Prasad (1991) showed in rats that high-protein diet increased tyrosine availability, which in turn increased the synthesis of CNS catecholamines. They noted that increases in dietary protein were associated with electrical activity in the frontal and motor cortex, areas that are involved in the anticipation, preparation, and issuance of motor commands. The electroencephalographic (EEG) cortical negativity responses had larger amplitudes and longer latencies in the rats that consumed the high-protein diet. Although results such as these cannot reasonably be extrapolated to elderly humans, these results do suggest the possibility that protein supplements for the elderly might be explored as a possible intervention through which the motor performances that require attention, i.e., complex thought processes and fast action, might be benefited.

Brain Function and Diet-Induced Fluctuations of Blood Glucose

As adults age, their circulating levels of blood glucose rise, but the rates of glucose utilization in local areas of the brain decline (Smith, 1980). Circulating glucose concentrations rise because aging, in addition to being associated with increased obesity and physical inactivity, independently decreases glucose tolerance (Shimokata et al., 1991). Brain utilization of glucose is decreased by changes in enzyme-mediated metabolic processes (Smith, 1984). Poor blood glucose regulation and impaired cerebral glucose utilization impact brain function. These influences are most easily seen in a disease state such as diabetes, in which the fluctuating levels of glucose are sometimes excessive.

Diabetics demonstrate cognitive deficits in some neuropsychological and psychomotor tasks. Although the performance of complex cognitive tasks was significantly impaired in elderly non-insulin-dependent diabetics (Type II), simple reaction time was not different between non-insulin-dependent diabetics and controls. In Type I diabetics, Wirsen et al. (1992) found significant losses in reactive latency and neuropsychological tests that required speed and attention. The authors suggested that Type I diabetics are more influenced by insulin-induced hypoglycemia than are Type II diabetics, perhaps because they exhibit a larger absolute decrease in blood glucose in response to insulin, or because of a cumulative effect of repeated hypoglycemic episodes. The effect of hypoglycemia on neural function may be primarily central, as suggested by the work of Tamburrano et al. (1992), who found that acute hypoglycemia did not affect peripheral nerve-conduction velocity but did slow neural conduction in some central pathways.

Within the last 20 y it has been shown that circulating glucose levels can have robust and wide-reaching effects on many neural and behavioral functions of healthy adults. The effects shown have been primarily in learning and memory (Gold, 1993). In young subjects, EEG event-related potentials (ERPs), which provide a measure of reaction latency independent of the motor behavior, were affected by food consumption-related increases in blood glucose (Geisler & Polich, 1992), although the glucose manipulation had a much greater effect on short-term verbal memory than on ERP latency. However, short-term memory is important in many motor skills. In driving an automobile, for example, the ability to remember the location and velocity of oncoming automobiles in one direction while scanning the opposite direction is important for decision making.

One mechanism by which glucose manipulation influences motor behavior is through altered dopamine-mediated activity in the brain. Saller & Chiodo (1980) found that fluctuating levels of circulating blood glucose were related to parallel changes in dopamine-mediated neural activity in the zona compacta of the substantial nigra, a brain area known to play a major role in the control of movement.

Vitamin Supplements and Brain Function

In the first half of this century the initial thrust of vitamin research was the identification of nutritional deficiencies such as rickets and beriberi and the development of diet therapies to combat them. Now some researchers are suggesting that vitamin supplements above minimum daily requirements are necessary for *optimal* health and that these higher levels may prevent chronic disease and some aging-related dysfunction. The efficacy of vitamin supplementation in young adults is far from clear. Singh et al. (1992) found that supplementation with a high-potency multivitamin-mineral supplement in a double-blind, placebo-controlled study for 12 wk did not affect maximal aerobic capacity; treadmill time to exhaustion; heart rates; rectal temperatures; plasma glucose, lactate, and adrenocorticotropin; muscle strength; and muscle endurance in young adults. In a review of other studies of the effects of vitamin supplements on maximal aerobic capacity and maximal running time, no performance benefits accrued to young athletes on well-balanced diets (Williams, 1989).

In contrast, Bonke and Nickel (1989) found that elevated intakes of vitamin B1, B6, and B12 improved the fine motor control involved in target shooting. They reported that in two experiments, the first of which was an open, controlled design, and the second of which was a double-blind design incorporating assessments over 8-wk, marksmen in vitamin-treated groups (a combination of B1, B6, and B12) were significantly more accurate than marksmen in control groups. Their conclusions were that target shooting depends heavily upon the ability to control physiological tremor and that vitamin supplements may enhance the neurological processes necessary to control tremor.

Even if vitamin supplementation were found to be of no benefit for the physical performance of young adults, it may nevertheless benefit older adults more than young individuals because older adults are at greater risk for vitamin deficiency. Many are precariously close to malnutrition because they have lost interest in food, don't use meals for social or business contacts, or don't have the energy to prepare their own meals. Age-related changes in the gastrointestinal tract and in vitamin metabolism make it difficult for older people to absorb and/or metabolize some vitamins, particularly B12, B6, and folate (Rosenberg & Miller, 1992). In addition, dietary levels of some nutrients that are adequate for young adults may be inadequate for older adults who have age-related impairments in some physiological systems. For example, almost all older adults suffer losses in night vision that impair their ability to drive an automobile at night. Vitamin A is necessary for the optimal function of night vision in all ages; supplementation might, therefore, be beneficial to older drivers who are deficient in Vitamin A, but have no effect on young drivers who are not deficient.

Dietary Energy Restriction and Motor Behavior

One of the most fascinating and robust findings in aging research is that undernutrition, as distinct from malnutrition, substantially slows the aging process in warm-blooded animals (Ingram et al., 1990). In fact, restricting dietary energy in mice and rats to approximately 60% of their *ad libitum* consumption, while at the same time maintaining the nutritional components necessary for good health, has been the only intervention shown to be effective in changing the *rate* of aging. A vast array of biochemical, physiologic, and immunologic variables are more "youthful" in energy-restricted animals than in *ad libitum*-fed animals. The contribution that restriction of energy intake makes to the maintenance of motor control has received very little attention. Ingram et al. (1987) found that mice fed ~55 kcal/wk from weaning were significantly better at tests of motor coordination and maze learning than were mice fed ~95 kcal/wk. Although the diet-restricted mice consumed less energy, their diets were identical in terms of other nutrients provided. The old mice on the relatively normal diets were significantly worse at a balance task, but the performances of the diet-restricted old mice was indistinguishable from those of the young mice. The diet-restricted old mice also performed better in a locomotor maze task. Thus, some aspects of motor performance and memory were maintained in the diet-restricted old mice. Similarly, unlike diet-restricted rats, old rats fed *ad-libitum* exhibited a deterioration in performance of a water maze task, although swimming performance *per se* was unimpaired in the old rats, regardless of diet (Pitsikas et al., 1990).

Diet-restricted old mice also maintained higher levels of spontaneous locomotive activity throughout their life spans than did mice that ate *ad libitum* (Ingram et al., 1987; Pitsikas et al., 1990; Yu et al., 1985). All of these research teams considered the possibility that it was the increased physical activity, rather than the reduction in dietary energy, that might account for the beneficial differences found between old diet-restricted and *ad libitum*-fed rodents. They rejected this hypothesis, concluding that the contribution of increased physical activity toward a reduction in aging rate is unresolved and, if significant, is dwarfed by the contribution of dietary restriction (Yu et al., 1985).

In summary, it has long been known that dysfunction in neurotransmitters and inadequate intake of neurotransmitter precursors and vitamins can cause impaired motor behavior. Exercise and nutrition work synergistically in relatively healthy individuals to help regulate the concentrations of circulating neurotransmitters, their precursors, and glucose. The pursuit of the explicit relationships among aging, exercise, and nutrition may be the next research frontier in gerontological research.

DIRECTIONS FOR FUTURE RESEARCH

Because so little is known about the role that acute aerobic or resistance exercise plays in modifying neurological function, it is important to conduct much more research on this topic. As should be apparent from the reading of this chapter, research on the effects of aging and exercise on movement-related sensory function, basic mechanisms of motor control, motor synergies, static and dynamic postural control, and planned coordinated movements is still in an infant stage. Given the growing realization of the importance of having the senior members of an aging society able to function physically and live independently, it is likely that the topic of exercise and motor control will receive more attention within the last half of this decade. Also, the increased number of masters athletes who are training harder and competing more rigorously will provide more impetus to the research effort in this field.

Some of the areas that are particularly lacking in research are the effects of aerobic and/or resistance training programs and flexibility programs on proprioceptive, tactile, and vibratory receptor function. Specifically, studies of adaptations to different types of exercise training in the nature, density, and function of sensory receptors are warranted. What is the effect of acute or chronic exercise on different aspects of visual function, muscle spindle sensitivity, or vestibular function? Why are chronically active older adults more sensitive to vibration? How do aerobic exercise and resistance training affect muscle stiffness in older adults? Similarly, other than a few studies on the effects of exercise on the monosynaptic reflex, body sway, balance, and locomotion, little work has been completed on the role of health and exercise on postural neurosynergies. How would the neurosynergistic muscular patterns of older adults who hike, mountain climb, or sail compare to those of young adults? Would a program of weight training or aerobic exercise affect these patterns? Would such a program improve the economy of walking so that gait speed would be voluntarily increased by older adults?

Another area that has not been addressed is that of the mechanisms that contribute to the loss of hand function and the role of flexibility and strength exercises in maintaining this function. Why do older adults produce more force than necessary to manipulate objects, and what is the impact of this on common household activities? Would instrumental activities of daily living, such as taking the lids off jars, opening locks, or placing boxes on shelves, be substantially improved by a weight training program targeted for upper body and hand strength?

Finally, one of the most fertile fields for future research lies in the study of age and exercise effects on the coordination of skilled movements, particularly those involving upper limb control. The effects of aging, muscle strength, and flexibility on the parameters of position, velocity, and acceleration in the instrumental movements of older adults has not been addressed.

SUMMARY

Motor control gradually deteriorates with advanced aging, especially in inactive, sedentary individuals, and may eventually become a primary limiting factor in the quality of their lives. Declines in motor control can lead to the loss of hand function and mobility, two abilities that are necessary in most cases for independent living. Aging compromises all levels of motor control—sensory reception, motor effector properties, and the integration of sensory information and control mechanisms in the central nervous system. Postural control and balance are compromised, so that older adults are at a higher risk of falling. Reactive movements are more slowly initiated, and planned, coordinated movements are impaired.

Sensory functions critical to the precise control of movement, such as vision, vestibular sense, proprioception, and touch, are impaired to different degrees and at different rates in most people as they age. Age-related changes also occur in the basic unit of motor control, the motor unit. The number of active motor units decreases with aging, and the largest decrease is in large motor units that contain the largest number of muscle fibers. A significant problem in understanding the effects of aging on motor unit behavior is that it is difficult to disentangle aging effects from the negative consequences of disuse. Among the negative effects of disuse on motor units are atrophy of muscle fibers, resulting in the production of low peak force; inconsistent firing rate; inability to recruit all the motor units in a muscle; and slower nerve conduction velocity. Chronic exercise has the potential to reverse or slow the rate of change in these characteristics.

Aging affects the magnitude of spinal reflexes more than the latency of the responses. For example, the latency of spinal reflexes such as the patellar tendon and Achilles' tendon reflex, because they are monosynaptic, are maintained well into the senior years. Chronic exercise enhances the amplitude of the reflex. More complex reflexes, which involve multiple interconnections with sensory information and descending influences, are more affected by aging. Neurosynergistic postural responses are delayed, the pattern of muscular responses is different in early trials and is more variable, the response amplitudes within a synergistic pattern are less tightly coupled, and older adults exhibit greater amounts of co-contraction.

The functional significance of age-affected spinal and neurosynergistic reflexes is that body balance is compromised in both stationary and movement conditions. Balance declines with aging, especially when one or two sensory modalities such as vision and vestibular function are impaired, but the maintenance of leg strength is associated with a decreased risk of falling.

Poor balance affects the locomotor skill of walking. Older adults walk more slowly and with a wider base of support and a shorter step length, partly so that they can maintain a double-support phase longer throughout the walking stride. Postural mechanisms also provide the stability for voluntary movements, and one of the sources of deterioration in motor function appears to be in the preparation and integration of postural reflexes with the motor programming of goal-oriented movements. Thus, problems in the hierarchical organization of anticipatory postural adjustments can result in older adults physically reacting to a stimulus more slowly in a standing position than in a sitting position.

Older adults react more slowly to environmental stimuli such as those experienced in a reaction-time paradigm, and they move more slowly once they have initiated movement. The predominant source of slowing in reactive responses is central, i.e., in the cognitive processing of the stimulus, rather than in the peripheral apparatus, the neural innervation of muscle tissue, and the contractile mechanics. Movements in the aged are slower because of decreased muscle mass and age-related changes in muscle tissue, such as decreased contraction velocity. Older adults who habitually exercise react more quickly, although it has not been resolved whether the apparent relationship between fitness and reactive speed is correlational or causal. The mechanisms that have been proposed to explain this relationship are exercise-induced increases in: a) cerebral blood flow, oxygen utilization, and the control of hypertension, b) morphological plasticity, and c) neurotransmitter function.

Although information about aging and exercise effects on coordination is relatively sparse, the speed and amplitude with which movements are made constitute the major differences in motor skill between old and young adults. Older adults appear to preprogram, program, and reprogram discrete movements in the same way that young adults do, only more slowly. In timed laboratory tasks of motor coordination, old persons learn these tasks at a similar rate; they simply perform them more slowly.

A developing research area that may have great significance for the understanding of motor control in the elderly is that of the effects of nutrition on motor control mechanisms. Some nutritional manipulations that have shown promise are the modulation through diet of some neurotransmitters, such as dopamine, that are related to motor programming, and the enhancement of cognitive function through manipulations of glucose utilization and vitamin supplementation. In addition, dietary restriction, or underfeeding, which has been shown to improve motor function and skill in rats, is a research paradigm that may provide a clearer understanding of the role of energy metabolism in the control of movement.

BIBLIOGRAPHY

Axelrod, S., and L.D. Cohen (1961). Senescence and embedded-figure performance in vision and touch. *Percep. Mot. Skills* 12:283–288.

Azar, G., and A. Lawton (1964). Gait and stepping as factors in the frequent falls of elderly women. *Gerontologist* 4:83–84.

Bailey, C.H., and P. Gouras (1985). The retina and phototransduction. In: E.R. Kandel and J.R. Schwartz (eds.) *Principles of Neuroscience*. New York: Elsevier Science Publishing Co. Inc., pp. 344–355.

Ball, K., and C. Owsley (1991). Identifying correlates of accident involvement for the older driver. *Human Factors* 33:583–595.

Barchas, J.D., and D.X. Freedman (1963). Brain amines: Response to physiological stress. *Biochem. Pharmacol.* 12:1232–1235.

Barry, A.J., J.R. Steinmetz, H.F. Page, and K. Rodahl (1966). The effects of physical conditioning on older individuals: II. Motor performance and cognitive function. *J. Gerontol.* 21:192–199.

Bassett, C., E. McClamrock, and M. Schmelzer (1982). A 10-week exercise program for senior citizens. *Geriatr. Nurs.* 3:103–105.

Baylor, A.M., and W.W. Spirduso (1988). Systematic aerobic exercise and components of reaction time in older women. *J. Gerontol.* 43:121–126.

Bendall, M.J., E.J. Bassey, and M.B. Pearson (1989). Factors affecting walking speed of elderly people. *Age Ageing* 18:327–332.

Bergström, B. (1973a). Morphology of the vestibular nerve. II. The number of myelinated vestibular nerve fibers in man at various ages. *Acta Otolaryn.* 76:173–179.

Bergström, B. (1973b). Morphology of the vestibular nerve. III. Analysis of the caliber of the myelinated vestibular nerve fibers in man at various ages. *Acta Otolaryn.* 76:331–338.

Black, J.E., W.T. Greenough, B.J. Anderson, and K.R. Isaacs (1987). Environment and the aging brain. *Can. J. Psy.* 41:111–130.

Black, J.E., K.R. Isaacs, and W.T. Greenough (1991). Usual versus successful aging: Some notes on experimental factors. *Neurobiol. Aging* 12:325–328.

Black, J.E., M. Polinsky, and W.T. Greenough (1989). Progressive failure of cerebral angiogenesis supporting neural plasticity in aging rats. *Neurobiol. Aging* 10:353–358.

Blanpied, P., and G.L. Smidt (1993). The difference in stiffness of the active plantarflexors between young and elderly human females. *J. Gerontol.: Med. Sci.* 48:M58–M63.

Bloomfield, S.A. (1995). Bone, ligament, and tendon. In: C.V. Gisolfi, D.R. Lamb, and E.R. Nadel (eds.) *Perspectives in Exercise Science and Sports Medicine, Vol. 8: Exercise in Older Adults.* Carmel, IN: Cooper Publishing Group, pp. 175–235.

Bolton, C.F., M.D. Winkelmann, and P.J. Dyck (1966). A quantitative study of Meissner's corpuscles in man. *Neurology* 16:1–9.

Bonke, D., and B. Nickel (1989). Improvement of fine motoric movement control by elevated dosages of vitamin B1, B6, and B12 in target shooting. *Int. J. Vita. Nutr. Res.* (Suppl.) 30:198–204.

Botwinick, J.E., and L.W. Thompson (1966). Components of reaction time in relation to age and sex. *J. Gen. Psychol.* 108:175–183.

Brock, J.W. and C. Prasad (1991). Motor, but not sensory, cortical potentials are amplified by high-protein diet. *Physiol. Behav.* 50:887–893.

Brocklehurst, J.C., D. Robertson, and P. James-Groom (1982). Clinical correlates of sway in old age: Sensory modalities. *Age Ageing* 11:1–10.

Brown, L.T. (1925). The influence of exercise on muscle tonus as exhibited by the knee-jerk. *Am. J. Physiol.* 72:241–247.

Brown, M., and G. Mishica (1989). Effect of habitual activity of age-related decline in muscular performance: A study of master athletes. *Gerontologist* 29:257A.

Brown, B.S., T. Payne, K. Chang, G. Moore, P. Krebs, and W. Martin (1979). Chronic response of rat brain norepinephrine and serotonin levels to endurance training. *J. Appl. Physiol.* 46:19–23.

Bruner, A., and T.W. Norris (1971). Age-related changes in caloric nystagmus. *Acta Otolaryn.* Supplement 282.

Cafarelli, E., and B. Bigland-Ritchie (1979). Sensation of static force in muscles of different length. *Exp. Neurol.* 65:511–525.

Campbell, M.J., A.J. McComas, and F. Petito (1973). Physiological changes in aging muscle. *J. Neurol. Neurosurg. Psych.* 36:174–182.

Carel, R.S., A.D. Korczyn, and Y. Hochberg (1979). Age and sex dependency of the Achilles tendon reflex. *Am. J. Med. Sci.* 278:57–63.

Carnahan, H., A.A. Vandervoort, and L.R. Swanson (1992). The influence of aging on motor skill learning. In: G.E. Stelmach and V. Hömberg (eds.) *Sensorimotor Impairment in the Elderly.* Boston, MA: Kluwer Academic Publishers, pp. 41–72.

Chaffin, D.B. (1973). Localized muscle fatigue—definition and measurement. *J. Occup. Med.* 15:346–354.

Chen, H., J.A. Ashton-Miller, N.B. Alexander, and A.B. Schultz (1991). Stepping over obstacles: Gait patterns of healthy young and old adults. *J. Gerontol: Med. Sci.* 46:M196–203.

Chodzko-Zajko, W.J., K.A. Moore (1994). Physical fitness and cognitive function in aging. In: J.O. Holloszy (ed.) *Exercise and Sport Sciences Reviews,* Vol. 22. Baltimore, MD: Williams & Wilkins, pp. 195–220.

Clark, J.E., A.K. Lanphear, and C.C. Riddick (1987). The effects of videogame playing on the response selection processing of elderly adults. *J. Gerontol.* 42:82–85.

Clarkson, P.M. (1978). The relationship of age and level of physical activity with the fractionated components of patellar reflex time. *J. Gerontol.* 33:650–656.

Coggan, A.R., R.J. Spina, D.S. King, M.A. Rogers, M. Brown, P.M. Nemeth, and J.O. Holloszy (1992). Skeletal muscle adaptations to endurance training in 60- to 70-yr-old men and women. *J. Appl. Physiol.* 72:1780–1786.

Cole, K.J. (1991). Grasp force control in older adults. *J. Motor Behav.* 23:251–258.

Crilly, R.G., D.A. Willems, K.J. Trenholm, K.C. Hayes, and L.F.O. Delaquérriere-Richardson (1989). Effect of exercise on postural sway in the elderly. *Gerontology* 35:137–143.

Cunningham, D.A., P.A. Rechnitzer, M.E. Pearce, and A.P. Donner (1982). Determinants of self-selected walking pace across ages 19 to 66. *J. Gerontol.* 37:560–564.

deCastro, J.M., and G. Duncan (1985). Operantly conditioned running: Effects on brain catecholamine concentrations and receptor densities in the rat. *Pharmacol. Biochem. Behav.* 23:495–500.

Desypris, G., and D.J. Parry (1990). Relative efficacy of slow and fast α-motoneurons to reinnervate mouse soleus muscle. *Am. J. Physiol.* 258:C62–C70.

DiPasquale, R., M. Morey, R. Sullivan, G. Crowley, P. Cowper, and J. Feussner (1989). Strength improvements in geriatric exercise: Falls history and deficits. *Gerontology* 29:39A.

Dustman, R.E., R.Y. Emmerson, L.A. Steinhaus, D.E. Shearer, and T.J. Dustman (1992). The effects of videogame playing on neurophysiological performance of elderly individuals. *J. Gerontol.:Psychol. Sci.* 47:P168–171.

Dustman, R.E., R. Hanover, and D. Shearer (1995). Physical activity, age, and cognitive/neuropsychological function. *J. Aging Phys. Act.*, in press.

Dustman, R.E., R.O. Ruhling, E.M. Russell, D.E. Shearer, H.W. Bonekat, J.W. Shigeoka, J.S. Wood, and D.C. Bradford (1984). Aerobic exercise training and improved neuropsychological function of older individuals. *Neurobiol. Aging* 5:35–42.

Ebert, M.H., R.M. Post, and F.K. Goodwin (1972). Effect of physical activity on urinary M.H.P.G. excretion in depressed patients. *Lancet* 2:766.

Elble, R.J., S.S. Thomas, C. Higgins, and J. Colliver (1991). Stride-dependent changes in gait of older people. *J. Neurol.* 238:1–5.

Elias, M.F., M.A. Robbins, N.R. Schultz, Jr., and T.W. Pierce (1990). Is blood pressure an important variable in research on aging and neuropsychological test performance? *J. Gerontol.: Psychol. Sci.* 45:P128–135.

Engle, V.F. (1986). The relationship of movement and time to older adults' functional health. *Res. Nurs. Health* 9:123–129.

Era, P. and E. Heikkinen (1985). Postural sway during standing and unexpected disturbance of balance in random samples of men of different ages. *J. Gerontol.* 40:287–295.

Era, P., J. Jokela, H. Suominen, and E. Heikkinen (1986). Correlates of vibrotactile thresholds in men of different ages. *Acta Neurol. Scand.* 74:210–217.

Fahim, M.A. (1993). Exercise affects presynaptic age-related changes at mouse neuromuscular junctions. *American Association of Aging: Abstracts* (abstract no. 8). San Francisco, CA: American Association of Aging.

Fansler, C.L., C.L. Poff, and K.F. Shepard (1985). Effects of mental practice on balance in elderly women. *Phys. Ther.* 65:1332–1338.

Fearing, F. (1928). The history of the experimental study of the knee jerk. *Am. J. Physiol.* 40:92–111.

Fernie, G.R., C.I. Gryfe, and P.J. Hollidayal (1982). The relationship of postural sway in standing to the incidence of falls in geriatric subjects. *Age Ageing* 11:11–16.

Ferrandez, A.M., J. Pailhouse, and M. Durup (1990). Slowness in elderly gait. *Exp. Aging Res.* 16:79–89.

Ferrandez, A.M., J. Pailhous, and G. Serratrice (1988). Locomotion in the elderly. In: B. Amblard, A. Berthoz, and F. Clarac (eds.) *Development Adaptation and Modulation of Posture and Locomotion.* Amsterdam: Elsevier, pp. 115–124.

Ferrell, W.R., A. Crighton, and R.D. Sturrock (1992). Age-dependent changes in position sense in human proximal interphalangeal joints. *Ageing* 3:259–262.

Floeter, M.K., and W.T. Greenough (1979). Cerebellar plasticity: Modification of Purkinje cell structure by differential rearing in monkeys. *Science* 206:227–229.

Fordyce, D.E., and R.P. Farrar (1991a). Physical activity effects on hippocampal and parietal cortical cholinergic function and spatial learning in F344 rats. *Behav. Brain Res.* 43:115–125.

Fordyce, D.E., and R.P. Farrar (1991b). Enhancement of spatial learning in F344 rats by physical activity and related learning-associated alterations in hippocampal and cortical cholinergic functioning. *Behav. Brain Res.* 46:123–133.

Frackowiak, R.S.J., G.C. Lenzi, T. Jones, and J.D. Heather (1980). The quantitative measurement of regional cerebral blood flow and oxygen metabolism in normal man using oxygen-15 and positron emission tomography: Theory, procedure and normal values. *J. Comput. Assist. Tomogr.* 4:727–736.

Frackowiak, R.S.J., R. Wise, J.M. Gibbs, and T. Jones (1983). Oxygen extraction in the aging brain. *Eur. Neurol.* 22:24–25.

Francis, P.R., and C.M. Tipton, (1969). Influence of a weight training program on quadriceps reflex time. *Med. Sci. Sports* 1:91–94.

Frisina, R.D., and G.A. Gescheider (1977). Comparison of child and adult vibrotactile thresholds as a function of frequency and duration. *Percept. Psychophys.* 22:100–103.

Geisler, M.W., and J. Polich (1992). P300, food consumption, and memory performance. *Psychophysiology* 29:76–85.

Gellis, M., and R. Pool (1977). Two-point discrimination distances in the normal hand and forearm. *Plas. Reconstr. Surg.* 59:57–63.

Gescheider, G.A., A.A. Valetutti, M.C. Padula, and R.T. Verillo (1992). Vibrotactile forward masking as a function of aging. *J. Acoustics. Soc. Am.* 91:1690–1696.

Gilliam, P.E., W.W. Spirduso, T.P. Martin, T.J. Walters, R.E. Wilcox, and R.P. Farrar (1984). The effects of exercise training on [³H]-spiperone binding in rat striatum. *Pharmacol. Biochem. Behav.* 20:863–867.

Gillis, B., K. Gilroy, H. Lawley, L. Mott, and J.C. Wall (1986). Slow walking speeds in healthy young and elderly females. *Physiother. Can.* 38:350–352.

Gold, P.E. (1993). The role of glucose in regulating brain and cognition (Abstr). *Symposium Proceedings: New dimensions in carbohydrates.* Washington, D.C: American Society for Clinical Nutrition.

Gordon, R., S. Spector, A. Sjoerdsma, and S. Udenfriend (1966). Increased synthesis of norepinephrine and epinephrine in the intact rat during exercise and exposure to cold. *J. Pharmacol. Exper. Ther.* 153:440–447.

Goubel, F., and J.F. Marini (1987). Fibre type transition and stiffness modification of soleus muscle of trained rats. *Pflügers Arch.* 410:321–325.

Gross, P.M., M.L. Marcus, and D.D. Heistad (1980). Regional distribution of cerebral blood flow during exercise in dogs. *J. Appl. Physiol.* 48:213–217.

Growdon, J.H. (1979). Serotonergic mechanisms in myoclonus. *J. Neural Trans.* (Supp.) 15:209–216.

Growdon, J.H. (1989). Nutrition and the ageing nervous system. In: A. Horwitz, D.M. Macfadyen, H. Munro, N.S. Scrimshaw, B. Steen, and T.F. Williams (eds.) *Nutrition in the Elderly.* New York: Oxford U. Press, pp. 224–233.

Growdon, J.H., and E. Melamed (1982). Effects of oral L-tyrosine administration on CSF tyrosine and homovanillic acid levels in patients with Parkinson's Disease. *Life Sci.* 30:827–832.

Hagberg, J.M., W.K. Allen, D.R. Seals, B.F. Hurley, A.A. Ehsani, and J.O. Holloszy (1985). A hemodynamic comparison of young and older endurance athletes during exercise. *J. Appl. Physiol.* 58:2041–2046.

Hageman, P.A., and D.J. Blanke (1986). Comparison of gait of young women and elderly women. *Phys. Ther.* 66:1382–1387.

Hart, B.A. (1986). Fractionated myotatic reflex times in women by activity level and age. *J. Gerontol.* 41:361–367.

Haskell, W.L. (1986). The influence of exercise training on plasma lipids and lipoproteins in health and disease. *Acta Med. Scand. (Suppl)* 711:25–37.

Hasselkus, B.R., and G.M. Shambes (1975). Aging and postural sway in women. *J. Gerontol.* 30:661–667.

Hayes, K.C. (1975). Effects of fatiguing isometric exercise upon Achilles tendon reflex and plantar flexion reaction time components in man. *Eur. J. Appl. Physiol.* 34:69–79.

Hayes, K.C., J.D. Spence, C.L. Riach, S.D. Lucy, and A.J. Kirshen (1985). Age-related change in postural sway. In: D.A. Winter, R.W. Norman, R. Wells, K.C. Hayes, and A.E. Patla (eds.) *Biomechanics IX-A.* Vol. 5A. Champaign: Human Kinetics Publ., pp. 383–387.

Heitmann, D.K., M.R. Gossmann, S.A. Shaddeau, and J.R. Jackson (1989). Balance performance and step width in noninstitutionalized, elderly, female fallers and nonfallers. *Phys. Ther.* 69:923–931.

Henneman, E., G. Somjem, and D.O. Carpenter (1965). Functional significance of cell size in spinal motoneurons. *J. Neurophysiol.* 28:560–580.

Himann, J.E., D.A. Cunningham, P.A. Rechnitzer, and D.H. Paterson (1988). Age-related changes in speed of walking. *Med. Sci. Sports. Exerc.* 20:161–166.

Horak, F.B. (1992). Effects of neurological disorders on postural movement strategies in the elderly. In: B. Vellas, M. Toupet, L. Rubenstein, J.L. Albarede, and Y. Christen (eds.) *Falls, balance, and gait disorders in the elderly.* Paris: Elsevier, pp. 137–151.

Horak, F.B., C.L. Shupert, and A. Mirka (1989). Components of postural dyscontrol in the elderly: A review. *Neurobiol. Aging* 10:727–738.

Hortobagyi, T., N.J. Lambert, and W.P. Kroll (1991). Voluntary and reflex responses to fatigue with stretch-shortening exercise. *Can. J. Sport Sci.* 16:142–150.

Hugin, F., A.H. Norris, and N.W. Shock (1960). Skin reflex and voluntary reaction times in young and old males. *J. Gerontol.* 15:388–391.

Imms, F.J., and O.G. Edholm (1981). Studies of gait and mobility in the elderly. *Age Ageing* 10:147–156.

Inglin, B. and M.H. Woollacott (1988). Anticipatory postural adjustments associated with reaction time arm movements: A comparison between young and old. *J. Gerontol.* 43:M105–M113.

Ingram, D.K., R.G. Cutler, R. Weindruch, D.M. Renquist, J.J. Knapka, M. April, C.T. Belcher, M.A. Clark, C.D. Hatcherson, B.M. Marriott, and G.S. Roth (1990). Dietary restriction and aging: The initiation of a primate study. *J. Gerontol.: Biol. Sci.* 45:B148–B163.

Ingram, D.K., R. Weindruch, E.L. Spangler, J.R. Freeman, and R.L. Walford (1987). Dietary restriction benefits learning and motor performance of aged mice. *J. Gerontol.* 42:78–81.

Jacobs, E.A., P.M. Winter, H.J. Alvis, and S.M. Small (1969). Hyperoxygenation effect on cognitive functioning in the aged. *New Engl. J. Med.* 281:753–757.

Jette, A.M., L.G. Branch, and J. Berlin (1990). Musculoskeletal impairments and physical disablement among the aged. *J. Gerontol: Med. Sci.* 45: M203–M298.

Kamen, G. (1979). Serial isometric contractions under imposed myotatic stretch conditions in high-strength and low-strength men. *Eur. J. Appl. Physiol.* 41:73–82.

Kamen, G., W.P. Kroll, and S.T. Zigon (1981). Exercise effects upon reflex time components in weight lifters and distance runners. *Med. Sci. Sports Exerc.* 13:198–204.

Kannel, W.B. (1989). Nutritional factors that influence cardiovascular functions. In: A. Horwitz, D.M. Macfadyen, H. Munro, N.S. Scrimshaw, B. Steen, and T.F. Williams (eds.) *Nutrition in the Elderly.* New York: Oxford University Press. pp. 234–259.

Kaplan, F.S., J.E. Nixon, M. Reitz, A. Rindfleish, and J. Tucker (1985). Age-related changes in proprioception and sensation of joint position. *Acta Orthopaed. Scand.* 56:72–74.

Kart, C.S., E.K. Metress, and S.P. Metress (1992). *Human Aging and Chronic Disease.* Boston, MA: Jones and Bartlett Publishers.

Kenshalo, D.R. (1986). Somesthetic sensitivity in young and elderly humans. *J. Gerontol.* 41:632–742.

Kirshen, A.J., R.D.T. Cape, K.C. Hayes, and J.D. Spencer (1984). Postural sway and cardiovascular parameters associated with falls in the elderly. *J. Clin. Exp. Gerontol.* 6:291–307.

Kligman, A.M., and A.K. Balin (1989). Aging of the human skin. In: A.K. Balin and A.M. Kligman (eds.) *Aging and the Skin.* New York: Raven Press., pp. 1–42.

Kline, D.W., T.J.B. Kline, J.L. Fozard, W. Kasnik, F. Schieber, and R. Sekuler (1992). Vision, aging, and driving: The problems of older drivers. *J. Gerontol.: Psychol. Sci.* 47:P27–P34.

Knox, C.A., E. Kokmen, and P.J. Dyck (1989). Morphometric alteration of rat myelinated fibers with aging. *J. Neuropathol. Exp. Neurol.* 48:119–139.

Koceja, D.M., J.R. Burke, and G. Kamen (1991). Organization of segmental reflexes in trained dancers. *Int. J. Sports Med.* 12:285–289.

Kokmen, E., R.W. Bossemeyer, and W.J. Williams (1978). Quantitative evaluation of joint motion sensation in an aging population. *J. Gerontol.* 33:62–67.

Komi, P.V. (1986). Training of muscle strength and power: Interaction of neuromotoric, hypertrophic, and mechanical factors. *Int. J. Sports Med.* 7 (Suppl. 1):10–15.

Konradsen, L., and J.B. Ravn (1991). Prolonged peroneal reaction time in ankle instability. *Int. J. Sports Med.* 12:290–292.

Kozma, A., and M.J. Stones (1978). Some research issues and findings in the study of psychological well-being in the aged. *Can. Psychol. Rev.* 19:241–249.

Kroll, W.P. (1974). Fractionated reaction and reflex time before and after fatiguing isotonic exercise. *Med. Sci. Sports* 6:260–266.

Kroll, W.P. and P.M. Clarkson (1977). Fractionated reflex time, resisted and unresisted fractionated time under normal and fatigued conditions. In: D.M. Landers and R.W. Christina (eds.). *Psychology of Motor Behavior.* Champaign. IL: Human Kinetics, pp. 106–129.

Landahl, H.D., and J.E. Birren (1959). Effects of age on the discrimination of lifted weights. *J. Gerontol.* 14:48–55.

Larish, D.D., P.E. Martin, and M. Mungiole (1988). Characteristic patterns of gait in the healthy old. In: J.A. Joseph (ed.) Central determinants of age-related declines in motor function. *Ann. New York Acad. Sci.* 515:18–31.

Laufer, A.C., and M.D. Schweitz (1968). Neuromuscular response tests as predictors of sensory-motor performance in aging individuals. *Am. J. Phys. Med.* 47:250–263.

Lenzi, G.C., R.S.J. Frackowiak, T. Jones, J.D. Heather, A.A. Lammertsma, C.G. Rhodes, and C. Pozzilli (1981). CMRO$_2$ and CBF by the oxygen-inhalation technique. *Eur. Neurol.* 20:285–290.

Lexell, J., D. Downham, and M. Sjostrom (1986). Distribution of different fibre types in human skeletal muscle: fibre type arrangement in m. vastus lateralis from three groups of health men between 15 and 83 years. *J. Neurol. Sci.* 72:211–222.

Lexell, J., and C. Taylor (1991). Variability in muscle fibre areas in whole human quadriceps muscle: effects of increasing age. *J. Anat.* 174:239–249.

Light, K.E., and W.W. Spirduso (1990). Effects of adult aging on the movement complexity factor of response programming. *J. Gerontol.* 45:P107–P109.

Lombard, W.P. (1887). The variations of the normal knee jerk and their relation to the activity of the central nervous system. *Am. J. Psychol.* 1:2–14.

MacRae, P.G., M. Lacarse, and R. Moldaron (1992). Physical performance measures that predict faller status in community-dwelling older adults. *J. Orthoped. Sport Phys. Ther.* 16:123–128.

MacRae, P.G., S. Reinsch, and J. Tobis (1989). Strength, muscular endurance, balance, and reaction time as predictors of faller status in the older adult. *Gerontology* 29:159A.

MacRae, P.G., W.W. Spirduso, G.D. Cartee, R.P. Farrar, and R.E. Wilcox (1987). Endurance training effects on striatal D$_2$ dopamine receptor binding and striatal dopamine metabolite levels. *Neurosci. Lett.* 79:138–144.

Maki, B.E., P.J. Holliday, and A.K. Topper (1994). A prospective study of postural balance and risk of falling in an ambulatory and independent elderly population. *J. Gerontol.: Med. Sci.* 49:M72–M84.

Manchester, D., M. Woollacott, N. Zederbauer-Hylton, and O. Marin (1989). Visual, vestibular and somatosensory contributions to balance control in the older adult. *J. Gerontol.: Med. Sci.* 44:M118–117.

Man'kovskii, N.B., A.Y. Mints, and V.P. Lysenyuk (1980). Regulation of the preparatory period for complex voluntary movement in old and extreme old age. *Human Physiol.* 6:46–50.

Marsden, C.D., P.A. Merton, and H.B. Morton (1972). Servo action in human voluntary movement. *Nature* 238:140–143.

Martin, W.H., W.M. Kohrt, M.T. Malley, E. Korte, and S. Stoltz (1990). Exercise training enhances leg vasodilatory capacity of 65-yr-old men and women. *J. Appl. Phsiol.* 69:1804–1809.

McCollum, G., F.B. Horak, and L.M. Nashner (1984). Parsimony in neural calculations for postural movements. In: J. Bloedel, J. Dichgans, and W. Precht (eds.). *Cerebellar Functions.* Berlin: Springer-Verlag, pp. 52–65.

McFarland, R.A. (1963). Experimental evidence of the relationship between ageing and oxygen want: In search of a theory of ageing. *Ergonomics* 6:339–366.

McGeer, P.L., and E.G. McGeer (1978). Aging and neurotransmitter systems. In: C.E. Finch, D.E. Potter, and A.D. Kenny (eds.) *Parkinson's Disease II. Aging and Neuroendocrine Relationships.* New York: Plenum Press, pp. 41–57.

Meyer, J.S., K. McClintic, P. Sims et al. (1988). Etiology, prevention and treatment of vascular or multi-infarct dementia. In: J.S. Meyer, H. Lechner, and J. Marshall (eds.) *Vascular and Multi-Infarct Dementia.* Mount Kisco, N.Y.: Futura, pp. 129–147.

Meyer, J.S., R.L. Rogers, and K.F. Mortel (1985). Prospective analysis of long-term control of mild hypertension on cerebral blood flow. *Stroke* 16:985–989.

Milner-Brown, H.S., R.B. Stein, and R.G. Lee (1975). Synchronization of human motor units: Possible roles of exercise and supraspinal reflexes. *Electroenceph. Clin. Neurophysiol.* 38:245–254.

Moritani, T., and H.A. deVries (1979). Neural factors vs. hypertrophy in time course of muscle strength gain. *Am. J. Phys. Med. Rehab.* 58:115–130.

Moritani, T., W.M. Sherman, M. Shibata, T. Matsumoto, and M. Shinohara (1992). Oxygen availability and motor unit activity in humans. *Eur. J. Appl. Physiol.* 64:552–556.

Moss, F.E., and V.J. Halamandaris (1977). *Too Old, Too Sick, Too Bad: Nursing Homes in America.* Germantown, MD: Aspen Systems Corporation.

Murray, M.P., P. Kory, C. Ross, and B.H. Clarkson (1969). Walking patterns in healthy old men. *J. Gerontol.* 24:169–178.

Murray, M.P., A.A. Seireg, and S.B. Sepic (1975). Normal postural stability and steadiness: Quantitative assessment. *J. Bone Joint Surg.* 57:510–516.

Myers, A.M., and N. Hamilton (1985). Evaluation of the Canadian Red Cross Society's Fun and Fitness Program for seniors. *Can. J. Aging* 4:201–212.

Nevitt, M.C., S.R. Cummings, and E.S. Hudes (1991). Risk factors for injurious falls: A prospective study. *J. Gerontol.: Med. Sci.* 46:M164–170.

Overstall, P.W., A.N. Exton-Smith, F.J. Imms, and A.L. Johnson (1977). Falls in the elderly related to postural imbalance. *Br. Med. J.* 1:261–264.

Overstall, P.W. (1980). Prevention of falls in the elderly. *J. Amer. Gerontol. Soc.* 28:481–484.

Pantano, P., J.C. Baron, P. Lebrun-Grandie, N. Duquesdnay, M.G. Bousser, and D. Comar (1983). Effects of aging on regional CBF and CMRO$_2$ in humans. *Eur. Neurol.* 22:24–31.

Petajan, J.H., and C.J. Eagan (1968). Effect of temperature, exercise and physical fitness on the triceps surae reflex. *J. Appl. Physiol.* 25:16–20.

Pitsikas, N., M. Carli, S. Fidecka, and S. Algeri (1990). Effect of life-long hypocaloric diet on age-related changes in motor and cognitive behavior in a rat population. *Neurobiol. Aging* 11:417–423.

Pysh, J.J., and G.M. Weiss (1979). Exercise during development induces an increase in Purkinje cell dendritic tree size. *Science* 206:230–231.

Rauramaa, R., J.T. Salonen, K. Seppänen, R. Salonen, J.M. Venäläinen, M. Ihanainen, and V. Rissanen (1986). Inhibition of platelet aggregability by moderate-intensity physical exercise. *Circulation* 74:939–944.

Reid, J.G. (1967) Static strength increase and its effect upon triceps surae reflex time. *Res. Quart.* 38:691–697.

Reinfrank, R.F., R.P. Kaufman, H.J. Wetstone, and J.A. Glennon (1967). Observations of the Achilles reflex test. *J. Amer. Med. Assoc.* 199:59–62.

Retzlaff, E., and J. Fontaine (1965). Functional and structural changes in motor neurons with age. In: A.T. Welford and J.E. Birren (eds). *Behavior, Aging, and the Nervous System.* Springfield, IL: Charles C. Thomas Publ., pp. 340–352.

Reuben, D.B., R.A. Silliman, and M. Traines (1988). The aging driver: Medicine, policy, and ethics. *J. Am. Gerontol. Soc.* 36:1135–1142.

Rikli, R., and S. Busch (1986). Motor performance of women as a function of age and physical activity level. *J. Gerontol.* 41:645–649.

Rikli, R. and D.J. Edwards (1991). Effects of a three-year exercise program on motor function and cognitive processing speed in older women. *Res. Quart. Exerc. Sport.* 62:61–67.

Roberts, B.L., and J.J. Fitzpatrick (1983). Improving balance: Therapy of movement. *J. Gerontol. Nursing* 9:151–156.

Rogers, M.A., and W.J. Evans (1993). Changes in skeletal muscle with aging: Effects of exercise training. In: J. Holloszy (ed.) *Exercise and Sport Sciences Reviews, Vol. 21.* Baltimore: Williams & Wilkins, pp. 65–102.

Rogers, R.L., C.G. Kukulka, and G.L. Soderberg (1992). Age-related changes in postural responses preceding rapid self-paced and reaction time arm movements. *J. Gerontol: Med. Sci.* 47:M159–M165.

Rogers, R.L., J.S. Meyer, K. McClintic, and K.F. Mortel (1989). Reducing hypertriglyceridemia in elderly patients with cerebrovascular disease stabilizes or improves cognition and cerebral perfusion. *Angiology* 40:260–269.

Rogers, R.L., J.S. Meyer, and K.F. Mortel (1990). After reaching retirement age physical activity sustains cerebral perfusion and cognition. *J. Am. Geriatr. Soc.* 38:123–128.

Rosenberg, I.H., and J.W. Miller (1992). Nutritional factors in physical and cognitive functions of elderly people. *Am. J. Clin. Nutr.* 55:1237S–1243S.

Rosenhall, U., and W. Rubin (1975). Degenerative changes in the human vestibular sensory epithelia. *Acta Otolaryn.* 79:67–81.

Rubenstein, H.S., F.H. Miller, S. Pastel, and H.B. Evans (1983). Standards of medical care based on consensus rather than evidence: The case of routine bedrail use for the elderly. *Law Med. Health Care* 11:271–276.

Russell, C. (1989). Accidents happen. *Greensboro (North Carolina) News and Record,* December, pp. A9, A11.

Sale, D.G. (1987). Influence of exercise and training on motor unit activation. In: K.B. Pandolf (ed.) *Exercise and Sport Sciences Reviews, Vol. 15.* New York: Macmillan, pp.95–151.

Sale, D.G. (1988). Neural adaptation to resistance training. *Med. Sci. Sports Exerc.* 20:S135–S145.

Sale, D.G., J.D. MacDougall, A.R.M. Upton, and A.J. McComas (1979). Effect of strength training upon motoneuron excitability in man. *Med. Sci. Sports* 11:77 (Abstract).

Saller, C.F., and L.A. Chiodo (1980). Glucose suppresses basal firing and haloperidol-induced increases in the firing rate of central dopaminergic neurons. *Science* 210:1269–1271.

Salthouse, T.A. (1984). Effects of age and skill in typing. *J. Exp. Psychol.: Gen.* 113:345–371.

Salthouse, T.A., and B.L. Somberg (1982). Skilled performance: The effects of adult age and experience on elementary processes. *J. Exp. Psychol.: Gen.* 111:176–207.

Samorajski, T., and C. Rolsten (1975). Nerve fiber hypertrophy in posterior tibial nerves of mice in response to voluntary running activity during aging. *J. Comp. Neurol.* 159:553–558.

Schmidt, R.A., H.N. Zelaznik, and J.S. Frank (1978). Sources of inaccuracy in rapid movement. In: G.E. Stelmach (ed.) *Information Processing in Motor Control and Learning*. New York: Academic Press, pp. 183–203.

Sekuler, R., and L.P. Hutman (1980). Spatial vision and aging. I: Contrast sensitivity. *J. Gerontol.* 35:292–699.

Shaw, T.G., K.F. Mortel, J.S. Meyer, and R.L. Rogers (1984). Cerebral blood flow changes in benign aging and cerebrovascular disease. *Neurology*, 34:855–862.

Sheldon, J.H., (1963). The effect of age on the control of sway. *Gerontol. Clin.* 5:129–138.

Sherrington, C.S. (1900). The muscular sense. In: E.A. Schafer (ed.) *Textbook of Physiology*. London: Pentland, pp. 1002–1025.

Shimokata, H., D. Muller, J.L. Fleg, J. Sorkin, A.W. Ziemba, and R. Andres (1991). Age as independent determinant of glucose tolerance. *Diabetes* 40:44–51.

Singh, A., F.M. Moses, and P.A. Deuster (1992). Chronic multivitamin-mineral supplementation does not enhance physical performance. *Med. Sci. Sports Ex.* 24:726–732.

Sixt, E., and S. Landahl (1987). Postural disturbances in a 75-year-old population. I. Prevalance and functional consequences. *Age Ageing* 16:393–398.

Skinner, H.B., R.L. Barrack, and S.D. Cook (1984). Age-related decline in proprioception. *Clin. Orthoped.* 184:208–211.

Smith, C.B. (1984). Aging and changes in cerebral energy metabolism. *Trends Neurosci.* 7:203–208.

Smith, C.B., C. Goochee, S.I. Rapoport, and L. Sokoloff (1980). Effects of ageing on local rates of cerebral glucose utilization in the rat. *Brain* 103:351–365.

Smith, K.U., and D. Greene (1962). Scientific motion study and aging processes in performance. *Ergonomics* 5:155–164.

Spirduso, W.W. (1975). Reaction and movement time as a function of age and physical activity level. *J. Gerontol.* 30:435–440.

Spirduso, W.W. (1980). Physical fitness, aging, and psychomotor speed: A review. *J. Gerontol.* 35:850–865.

Spirduso, W.W. (1982). Effects of physiological fitness on the aging motor system. In: J.A. Mortimer, F.J. Pirozzolo, and G.B. Maletta (eds.) *Progress in Neurogerontology, Volume III: The Aging Motor System*. New York: Praeger, pp. 120–151.

Spirduso, W.W. (1983a). Exercise and the aging brain. *Res. Quart. Exerc. Sport*, 54:208–218.

Spirduso, W.W. (1983b). Nigrostriatal dopaminergic function in aging, exercise, and movement initiation. In: T. White, D. Edington, and K. Borer (eds.) *Frontiers of Exercise Biology*. Champaign, IL.: Human Kinetics Publ., pp. 244–262.

Spirduso, W.W. (1994). Physical activity and aging: Retrospections and visions for the future. *J. Aging Phys. Act.* 2:233–242.

Spirduso, W.W. (1995). *Physical Dimensions of Aging*. Champaign, IL: Human Kinetics Publishers. (In press)

Spirduso, W.W., and J.H. Choi (1992). Age and practice effects on force control of the thumb and index fingers in precision pinching and bilateral coordination. In: G.E. Stelmach and V. Hömberg (eds.) *Sensorimotor Impairment in the Elderly*. Boston, MA: Kluwer Academic Publishers, pp. 393–412.

Spirduso, W.W., H.H. MacRae, P.G. MacRae, J. Prewitt, and L. Osborne (1988). Exercise effects on aged motor function. In: J.A. Joseph (ed.) *Central determinants of age-related declines in motor function*. *Ann. New York Acad. Sci.* 515:363–375.

Spirduso, W.W., and P.G. MacRae (1990). Motor performance and aging. In: J.E. Birren and K.W. Schaie (eds.) *Handbook of the Psychology of Aging*, 3rd Ed. Orlando, FL: Academic Press, pp. 183–200.

Stålberg, R., and P.R. Fawcett (1982). Macro E.M.G. in healthy subjects of different ages. *J. Neurol. Neurosurg. Psychiatry* 45:870–878.

Stelmach, G.E., P.C. Amrhein, and N.L. Goggin (1988). Age differences in bimanual coordination. *J. Gerontol.: Psychol. Sci.* 43:P18–P23.

Stelmach, G.E., J. Phillips, R.P. DiFabio, and N. Teasdale (1989). Age, functional postural reflexes, and voluntary sway. *J. Gerontol.: Biol. Sci.* 44:B100–B106.

Stelmach, G.E., L. Populin, and F. Müller (1990). Postural muscle onset and voluntary movement in the elderly. *Neurosci. Lett.* 117:188–193.

Stelmach, G.E., and A. Sirica (1986). Aging and proprioception. *Age* 9:99–103.

Stern, J.A., P.J. Oster, and K. Newport (1980). Reaction time measures, hemispheric specialization, and age. In: L.W. Poon (ed.) *Aging in the 1980s: Psychological Issues*. Washington, D.C.: American Psychological Association, pp. 309–326.

Stevens, J.C. (1992). Aging and spatial acuity of touch. *J. Gerontol.: Psychol. Sci.* 47:P35–P40.

Stones, M.J., and A. Kozma (1987). Balance and age in the sighted and blind. *Arch. Phys. Med. Rehab.* 68:85–89.

Swanson, L.R. and T.D. Lee (1992). Effects of aging and schedules of knowledge of results on motor learning. *J. Gerontol.:Psychol. Sci.* 47:P406–P411.

Tamburrano, G., N. Locuratolo, G. Pozzessere, O. Lostia, S. Caiola, E. Valle, F. Bianco, A. Giaccari, and P.A. Rizzo (1992). Changes in central and peripheral nervous system function during hypoglycemia in man: an electrophysiological quantification. *J. Endocrinol. Invest.* 15:279–282.

Thomas, S.N., T. Schroeder, N.H. Secher, and J.H. Mitchell (1989). Cerebral blood flow during submaximal and maximal dynamic exercise in humans. *J. Appl. Physiol.*, 67:744–749.

Thompson, L.W., G.C. Davis, W.D. Obrist, and A. Heyman (1976). Effects of hyperbaric oxygen on behavioral and physiological measures in elderly demented patients. *J. Gerontol.* 1:23–28.

Tinetti, M.E., T.F. Williams, and R. Mayewski (1986). Fall risk index for elderly patients based on number of chronic disabilities. *Am. J. Med.* 80:429–434.

Tipton, C.M. (1984). Exercise, training, and hypertension. In: R.J. Terjung (ed.) *Exercise and Sport Sciences Reviews* 12:245–306.

Tipton, C.M. and P.V. Karpovich (1966). Exercise and the patellar reflex. *J. Appl. Physiol.* 21:15–18.

Tobis, J.S., L. Nayak, and F.K. Hochler (1981). Visual perception of verticality and horizontality among fallers. *Arch. Phys. Med. Rehab.* 62:619–622.

Tobis, J.S., S. Reinsch, J.M. Swanson, M. Byrd, and T. Scharf (1985). Visual perception dominance of fallers among community residing older adults. *J. Am. Geriatr. Soc.* 33:330–333.

Transportation Research Board (1988). Transportation in an aging society: Improving mobility and safety for older people. Washington, DC.: Transportation Research Board.

Tse, S.K., and D.M. Bailey (1992). T'ai chi and postural control in the well elderly. *Am. J. Occup. Ther.* 46:295–300.

Tuttle, W.W. (1930). The effect of exercise on the Achilles-jerk. *Arbeitphysiologie* 2:367–371.

Vandervoort, A.A., and K.C. Hayes (1989). Plantarflexor muscle function in young and elderly women. *Eur. J. Appl. Physiol.* 58:389–394.

Vandervoort, A.A., and A.J. McComas (1986). Contractile changes in opposing muscles of the human ankle joint with aging. *J. Appl. Physiol.* 61:361–367.

Vercruyssen, M., M.T. Cann, J.E. Birren, J.M. McDowd, and P.A. Hancock (1990). Effects of aging, physical fitness, gender, neural activation, exercise, and practice on CNS speed of functioning. In: M. Kaneko (ed.) *Fitness for the Aged, Disabled, and Industrial Worker.* Champaign, IL: Human Kinetics Books, pp. 61–67.

Verrillo, R.T. (1979). Change in vibrotactile thresholds as a function of age. *Sensory Processes* 3:49–59.

Verrillo, R.T. (1982). Effects of aging on the suprathreshold responses to vibration. *Percep. Psychophys.* 32:61–68.

Verrillo, R.T. (1993). The effects of aging on the sense of touch. In: R. T. Verrillo (ed.) *Sensory Research: Multimodal Perspectives.* Hillsdale, N.J.: Lawrence Erlbaum, pp. 285–298.

von Holst, E. (1954). Relations between the central nervous system and the peripheral organs. *Brit. J. Anim. Behav.* 2:89–94.

Waldstein, S.R., S.B. Manuck, C.M. Ryan, and M.F. Muldoon (1991). Neuropsychological correlates of hypertension; Review and methodologic considerations. *Psychol. Bull.* 110:451–468.

Wallace, J.E., E.E. Krauter, and B.A. Campbell (1980). Motor and reflexive behavior in the aging rat. *J. Gerontol.* 3:364–370.

Warabi, T., H. Noda, and T. Kato (1986). Effect of aging on sensorimotor functions of eye and hand movements. *Exp. Neurol.* 92:686–697.

Weiss, A.D. (1965). The locus of reaction time change with set, motivation, and age. *J. Gerontol.* 20:60–64.

Whanger, A.D., and H.S. Wang (1974). Clinical correlates of the vibratory sense in elderly psychiatric patients. *J. Gerontol.* 29:39–45.

Whipple, R.H., L.I. Wolfson, and P.M. Amerman (1987). The relationship of knee and ankle weakness to falls in nursing home residents: An isokinetic study. *J. Am. Geriatr. Soc.* 35:13–20.

White, T.P. (1995). Skeletal muscle structure and function in old mammals. In: C.V. Gisolfi, D.R. Lamb, and E.R. Nadel (eds.) *Perspectives in Exercise Science and Sports Medicine, Vol. 8: Exercise in Older Adults.* Carmel, IN: Cooper Publishing Group, pp. xxx–xxx.

Wickwire, G.C., H.L. Terry, R. Krouse, W.E. Burge, and C.D. Monsson (1938). Further study on threshold of knee-jerk: An index to physical fitness. *Am. J. Physiol.* 123:213–214.

Williams, M.H. (1989). Vitamin supplementation and athletic performance. *Int. J. Vita. Nutr. Res.* (Suppl.) 30:163–191.

Wirsen, A., G. Tallroth, M. Lindgren, and C.D. Agardh (1992). Neuropsychological performance differs between type 1 diabetic and normal men during insulin-induced hypoglycaemia. *Diabet. Med.* 9:156–165.

Wolf, P.A., and W.B. Kannel (1982). Controllable risk factors for stroke: Preventative implications of trends in stroke mortality. In: J.S. Meyer, and T.G. Shaw (eds.) *Diagnosis and Management of Stroke and TIAs.* Menlo Park, CA: Addison-Wesley, pp. 25–61.

Wolfson, L., R. Whipple, P. Amerman, and A. Kleinberg (1986). Stressing the postural response: A quantitative method for teaching balance. *J. Am. Geriatr. Soc.* 34:845–850.

Woollacott, M.H. (1990). Changes in posture and voluntary control in the elderly: Research findings and rehabilitation. *Topics Geriatr. Rehab.* 5:1–11.

Woollacott, M., A. Shumway-Cook, and L. Nashner (1982). Postural reflexes and aging. In: J.A. Mortimer, F.J. Pirozzolo, and G.J. Maletta (eds.) *The Aging Motor System*. New York: Praeger, pp. 98–119.

Woollacott, M., A. Shumway-Cook, and L. Nashner (1986). Aging and posture control: Changes in sensory organization and muscular coordination. *Int. J. Aging Human Dev.* 23:97–114.

Woolacott, M.H., B. Inglin, and D. Manchester (1988). Response preparation and posture control in the older adult. In: J. Joseph (ed.) *Central determinants of age-related declines in motor function*. New York: New York Academy of Sciences, pp. 42–51.

Worthen, D.M. (1978). Effects of exercise on the visual system. *Med. Sport* 12:38–46.

Wurtman, R.J. (1982). Nutrients that modify brain function. *Sci. Am.* 246:50–59.

Wyke, B. (1979). Conference on the ageing brain. Cervical articular contributions to posture and gait: Their relation to senile dysequilibrium. *Age Ageing* 8:251–257.

Young, V.R., H.N. Munro, and N. Fukagawa (1989). Protein and functional consequences of deficiency. In: A. Horwitz, D.M. Macfadyen, H. Munro, N.S. Scrimshaw, B. Steen, and T.F. Williams (eds.) *Nutrition in the Elderly*. New York: Oxford University Press, pp. 65–84.

Yu, B.P., E.J. Masaro, and C.A. McMahan (1985). Nutritional influences on aging of Fischer 344 rats. I. Physical, metabolic, and longevity characteristics. *J. Gerontol.* 6:657–670.

DISCUSSION

EDGERTON: When we study aging-related changes in motor control, we are analyzing a complex combination of aging effects and compensatory actions. For example, age-related changes in neurovestibular control of posture can be affected both by aging and by the ability of the individual to compensate for a given deficiency. As soon as there is an age-induced loss of function, there will be some compensation; the real challenge in trying to pinpoint the direct effects of aging is to separate out the compensatory effects. Unfortunately, there is very little information on this phenomenon.

SPIRDUSO: That's a good point. In addition, systems age at different rates. When one system ages at a more accelerated rate than another system, it may place an additional burden on remaining systems. The elderly find themselves having to compensate with systems that are also being compromised by aging.

EDGERTON: Another clear example is age-related changes in walking. The way locomotion is modified as one ages is not necessarily a reflection of what the person can no longer do, but how the gait is modified to decrease the chance of injury. People often modify walking patterns so they have increased periods of double support, shorter step cycles, and wider stance. These are compensatory mechanisms, not the direct effect of the age-induced perturbation itself.

SPIRDUSO: In fact, even the posture that older individuals adopt is to some extent compensatory. They adopt a posture in which the weight is more forward, perhaps to avoid the possibility of falling backward. When they adopt a forward leaning posture, however, they maintain balance by continuous contractions of extensor muscles rather than by reaching a more balanced posture directly over the center of gravity. This compensatory forward leaning posture may prevent falling backward, but it does so at the cost of greater fatigue of the extensor muscles.

EDGERTON: Given that the larger muscles around the hip are perhaps the most important in maintaining balance, do individuals who have had double hip replacements fall more frequently than their peers?

SPIRDUSO: I'm not aware of any statistics on that point. Interestingly, the fact that people with hip replacements, who have had all joint receptors removed, show little change in the ability to position and sense the position of that limb, clearly indicates that joint receptors are not the primary receptors involved in position sense.

EDGERTON: Gandevia and his colleagues showed very specifically that sensitivity to changes in muscle length is the primary sensory component of postural regulation. Thus, it would seem that maintaining balance would be a serious problem for hip-replacement patients. However, there may well be compensatory actions for the loss of sensory input.

Pain could also have a tremendous effect on one's willingness, ability, or desire to be active. The processes involved in pain itself may induce changes in muscle, in connective tissue, or in other tissues. Are there any reports of gender-related differences in pain tolerance related to participation in physical activity?

SPIRDUSO: I don't know that anyone has studied gender effects on the role of pain in the elderly's motivation to be active. It may be that women have a much lower pain tolerance than do men. Alternatively, because elderly women are weaker than men, perhaps they actually experience more lower leg pain. Certainly many women aged 60–70 y have little tolerance to pain associated with exercise. In fact, many of them don't even like to sweat profusely. In their view, when they start sweating, it is time to stop. But I think that attitude is a function of the particular cohort. When the current 20-, 30-, and 40-year-olds reach their 60s, they may have an entirely different subjective view of pain.

CLARKSON: You have nicely outlined the simple motor control tasks such as reaction time and reflex time. For those tasks, one can get a handle on where the age-related dysfunction is located. With reaction time, the dysfunction seems to be in central processing because reflex times are less impaired by aging than are reaction times. What do the studies of proprioceptive tasks tell us? You suggest that there is a decrease in sense of force or joint position sense, which might be interpreted to mean that proprioceptors themselves may be dysfunctional in some way. I don't think this is the case. The proprioceptors could be sending messages appropriately, but the brain perhaps can't interpret the messages. For example, in a force-matching test, one limb may not be able to match the position of the contralateral limb, but in a unilateral test it can match its own position just fine. In other words, the proprioceptors are sending the correct message, but the brain can't interpret the message correctly. When interpreting force-matching tasks, we need to examine whether they are bilateral tasks, which increases the integration required by the brain, or unilateral. I predict that unilateral tasks will show fewer or less severe age-related changes in proprioception than do the bilateral tasks because I think that the greatest age-related change is in the central processing components. Please comment on this idea.

SPIRDUSO: I think you are probably correct. In fact, my guess is that the greater the involvement of the brain in a given task, the more that aging affects processing. Stelmach suggests that it is in the hierarchical organization of postural reflexes with intentional movement that the elderly have the greatest difficulty. We have completed some studies recently in which individuals trace with a cursor a template on a computer screen by using the synergistically controlled precision grip. There is very little actual movement in this task, so that most of the control is accomplished by a sense of force output and pressure sensation. We have set it up so that the task requires a symmetrical application of force to trace one side of a triangle, but on the second side of the triangle, this neurosynergistic precision grip has to be decoupled so that the index finger moves in one direction while the thumb moves in the same direction. These two fingers almost always work in opposition. In our task, for that one side, the subject has to voluntarily override synergistic control of the precision grip. We found that older individuals are almost 12 times worse at decoupling this synergistic control, and they are only about 2 times worse on the side of the template that requires symmetrical gripping. At least in this situation, it seems that when older individuals have to voluntarily override some kind of synergistic control mechanism, they have serious problems.

NADEL: How accurately can one separate the sensory from the motor and central integration changes that occur with aging? Among other events associated with aging, two-point discrimination ability is dramatically reduced, indicating that the transfer of sensory input from the skin deteriorates with age. Also, there are fewer neurons in the olfactory and auditory systems, the motor unit innervation of skeletal muscle decreases, and there is a marked decline in brain cell mass with age. How can one determine the true cause of the decrease in function with advancing age when all of these other phenomena are changing concurrently?

SPIRDUSO: It is extremely difficult. One could use the typical measures of sensory sensitivity and motor control, perhaps single motor-unit control, and measure these on the same subjects or measure the subjects' abilities on some type of functional task. You could then statistically analyze the contribution of each of these abilities to performance of the tasks. Unfortunately, the measures chosen may have little relevance to the functional task.

BAR-OR: I'll borrow from my experience in the pediatric area and try to look at two aspects of aging and motor control. One is regarding the energy cost of locomotion. There are two groups who expend energy excessively during the gait cycle—the elderly and young children. We just completed an experiment with prepubescent, pubescent, and late pubescent girls and boys in which we found that concurrent with a high energy cost of locomotion, there was a higher co-contraction of agonist and antagonist muscles in the prepubescents, compared with the older adolescents. Perhaps the same may occur in elderly people who cannot synchronize their agonists and antagonists, thereby requiring excessive energy during locomotion.

SPIRDUSO: There is a substantial amount of co-contraction that occurs in elderly, not only during locomotion, but also in the control of movements in general. Part of the reason for this is that co-contraction is a strategy used by those of all ages to reduce the risk of movement error. In the case of the elderly, the consequences of movement errors may be much greater because such errors can lead to falling. When one cannot predict what the outcome of movement is going to be, co-contraction is a safer strategy. If the outcome is predictable, and that is part of the process of learning a skill, one can move from a co-contraction strategy to an agonist-antagonist strategy. But there is always a greater risk of movement error with the agonist-antagonist strategy. It is highly probable that older individuals use a co-contraction strategy that will reduce the degrees of freedom within the movement that must be controlled.

BAR-OR: People have suggested that the rating of perceived effort (RPE) depends to some extent on proprioceptive information from the periphery. We examined a group of children who had a whole array of neuromuscular diseases such as muscular dystrophy, spastic cerebral palsy, and advanced rheumatoid arthritis. We assumed that they would not be able to rate their perceived exertion accurately because of presumably disrupted proprioceptive cues. We were therefore very surprised to find a very tight relationship between the RPE and percentage of maximal aerobic power. We then hypothesized that maybe such children compensate by using some sort of a feedforward mechanism, rather than feedback through proprioceptors, to gauge how hard they are exercising. Can such a compensatory process occur in the elderly?

SPIRDUSO: Probably. I don't recall having seen any reports on such a question, but I can't think of any reason why the elderly would differ in this respect from younger people.

BALDWIN: I would like you to contrast the young versus the old in terms of the ability to recruit motor units for force generation. When older people gain strength after resistance training, is the enhancement in strength primarily one of neurological adaptation versus inducing the accumulation of contractile proteins in the muscle fibers? Does the aged individual have a lesser capacity to experience a hypertrophic adaptation to resistance training relative to the younger individual?

SPIRDUSO: Bill Evans can answer this better than I. Early increases in strength are neurologically mediated, followed later by hypertrophy. Moritani and deVries in the late 1970s proposed that the strength increases in old adults were more dependent on neurological changes, whereas increases in strength seen in younger subjects were due to hypertrophy. I believe that more recent research has indicated that the processes are the same in both age groups. Older individuals can activate all the motor units in a muscle, just as young individuals can. Disuse is probably a more potent factor than aging—at least up to the age of the mid-70s.

EVANS: We measured isokinetic force production, muscle mass, and fat-free mass in subjects aged 45–80 y. We saw that force production was directly related to muscle mass. On the other hand, strength training caused a 100–200% increase in strength with only a 10–15% increase in muscle size. So the early adaptations must be neurologic in nature. Thus, the strength adaptations that older people exhibit don't seem to be much different than those observed in young people.

SPIRDUSO: So the loss of strength with aging is greater than the loss of muscle mass?

EVANS: No. Our data indicate that the strength loss is directly related to loss in muscle.

TERJUNG: Does this mean that the characteristic way in which an elderly person sits down (i.e., holding on to the arm supports of a chair, bending at the knees, and dropping to the seat) is solely due to a loss of strength, or is slower central processing a contributor?

SPIRDUSO: That part of the task of sitting down would more likely be attributed to the loss of muscle strength.

MORA: It is very difficult, when talking about deterioration of motor control during aging, to know which component is more important, the deterioration of the neural circuits in the central nervous system responsible for the control of motor behavior or the peripheral elements of the motor system that execute the motor act. I believe that a main component, if not the most important one, is the deterioration of the neurochemical systems that code for control of specific motor patterns. In the past 2–3 y there have been advances in knowledge that have changed our perspective of this topic. For instance, the deterioration of the nigrostriatal system during aging is accepted as being responsible for the motor deficits found in elderly people. However, the discovery that blockade of glutaminergic receptors in the striatum can, in part, ameliorate the effects produced by lesions of the nigrostriatal dopamine system has provided a different perspective on mechanisms and may have therapeutic potential in the control of motor behavior during aging. So I would like to emphasize the importance of considering not simply a single neurochemical system or a single neurotransmitter in relation to motor control (in particular during aging) but rather the interaction of different neurochemical systems and the interplay of several neurotransmitters.

SPIRDUSO: Your point is well taken.

4

Skeletal Muscle Structure and Function in Older Mammals

TIMOTHY P. WHITE, Ph.D.

INTRODUCTION

The reduction in the ability to produce and sustain muscular power is an age-related phenomenon of profound importance and consequence. Physical frailty, i.e., a severe impairment in strength, mobility, balance, and endurance (Hadley et al., 1993), is an inevitable consequence of a long life. These impairments are driven, in large measure, by neuromuscular declines. Strength of the arms, legs, and back declines at approximately 8–10% per decade after about age 30 (Asmussen, 1980), and these muscular impairments affect ordinary activities, such as the maintenance of posture and locomotion and the ability to perform life's daily activities in the home or workplace. Neuromuscular impairments are also likely to contribute to the increased incidence of falls and muscle injury and to a reduced regenerative capacity in aged muscle.

Aging Affects on Performance by Elite Athletes

The age-associated declines in muscular strength, contractile speed, power, and endurance also adversely affect the performances of elite competitors in sport and dance activities that require these attributes. World-class running performances provide simple yet elegant evidence of intrinsic age-associated change in skeletal muscle. Elite performers are highly motivated, have often trained for a large percentage of their adult lives, and are likely to be free of significant neuromuscular, cardiovascular, and pulmonary disease. However, maximal running velocities for sprint and endurance events decline from the third to eighth decade of life by approximately 8% per decade (Moore, 1975), and similar results are seen in swimming (Hartley & Hartley, 1986). This rate of decline is similar to the rate of decrease in muscle mass, which in humans is about 7% per decade after the third decade of life (Grimby & Saltin, 1983). Granted, human performance is not solely a function of the neuromuscular system, but decrements in muscle function clearly play a major role in the age-associated changes in athletic performance.

Gender Differences. Joyner (1993) noted a gender difference for age-associated declines in 10,000 m records. The decline for men is 6% per decade from the mid-20s to the mid-late 50s, with an increasing rate of decline thereafter. For women, the rate of decline is 9% per decade into the late 50s, and after age 60, their performances worsen at an ever increasing rate. At all ages, 10,000 m times for women exceed those for men. The gender-specific declines likely reflect some biological factors related to body weight and percentage fat, as well as factors associated with differences in the oxygen-carrying capacity of blood. In addition, one cannot overlook the impact of cultural factors that have, more so historically than today, limited the opportunities for women to train and compete. It will take at least a generation of performances to ameliorate any cultural attenuation of record performances. In conclusion, gender differences in age-related changes in performance are partially explained by differences in muscle mass, but other equally important factors are also involved.

Primary versus Secondary Effects of Aging

One of the major problems in studying the phenomenon of aging and skeletal muscle is distinguishing inherent aging processes from adaptations that occur secondary to changes in habitual physical activity and other confounding variables. Skeletal muscle is a highly plastic tissue, capable of adapting its structure and function to a variety of stimuli ranging from altered neural recruitment and mechanical loading patterns to trauma, altered levels of neuroendocrines, insufficient energy intake, and pharmacological interventions. Adaptive responses in muscle structure and function to aging demonstrate several parallels to adaptations to decreased physical activity. The parallels have prompted many to hypothesize that the consequence of aging is merely a reflection of reduced use. Indeed, in studies of lifetime activity patterns in laboratory animals (which are less confounded by social and cultural factors than are human studies), Goodrick (1980) and Vailas et al. (1985) showed 90% and 70% decreases, respectively, in daily voluntary running distance with age. In some circumstances and for some variables, reduced physical activity may contribute to the age-associated decline in muscle structure and function, but this is by no means the predominant explanation.

The evidence described in this chapter leads to the unambiguous conclusion that there are inevitable age-associated intrinsic changes in skeletal muscle and its component molecules, cells, and organelles, the cause(s) of which is(are) unknown. The intrinsic aging factors predominate over those that can be ascribed to physical inactivity. Furthermore, the functional deficits in aged humans and animals are associated with, but often exceed, the decrease in skeletal muscle mass (i.e., muscle atrophy) that is caused in large measure by a decrease in myofibrillar protein.

Relevance to Exercise Science and Sports Medicine

Exercise scientists, sports medicine clinicians, and fitness practitioners need to understand the beneficial effects and the limitations of physical activity for improving the fitness and health of older people and for improving the quality of life. The plasticity of skeletal muscle provides an opportunity for exercise professionals to delay the rate and onset of some age-associated impairments that might otherwise occur. A lifetime of activity, however, does not provide a total prophylaxis to the age-associated declines. Athletes at any age have performance capacities that exceed their age-matched sedentary counterparts; nonetheless, as a group they exhibit declines in muscular structure and performance (Moore, 1975; Schultz & Curnow, 1988; Stones & Kozma, 1981). For example, when the strength performance of untrained individuals categorized by age is expressed as a percentage of strength achieved at age 30 y (Brooks & Faulkner, 1994), the pattern of strength loss with age is almost identical to the pattern of age-related decline in world-record 200 m sprint velocity.

Appropriate exercise is also indicated in therapeutic circumstances surrounding partial or full recovery from disease and traumatic injuries. Thus, it is important to gain further understanding of minimal and optimal training protocols to achieve specific objectives in older people, as most training programs have been established on the basis of studies of young adults. Mobility, with the independence it provides, is also of major importance for quality of life, particularly for the old. Adequate neuromuscular function is, obviously, one essential factor for maintaining adequate mobility in older persons.

AGE-RELATED CHANGES IN SKELETAL MUSCLE STRUCTURE AND FUNCTION

Experimental Models

The explanatory power of many human studies of the aging process is compromised to some extent. If the study design is cross-sectional, interpretation of the results is problematic due to the heterogeneity of genotype and to the confounding influences of potential differences in physical activity habits, nutrition, and other lifestyle factors. Access to sufficient and representative samples of tissue is also an issue with humans, although contemporary magnetic resonance imaging techniques that provide noninvasive or minimally invasive measurements of metabolism, coupled with judicious use and interpretation of needle biopsy data, can yield meaningful results.

Nevertheless, much of what informs our thinking about aging and muscle comes from animal models, primarily studies with rodents. Mice and rats are excellent models for research into the fundamental aspects of aging, the relationship between aging and disease, and the influence of environmental factors, such as exercise, on aging processes (Hollander & Burek, 1982). The life span of a rodent is relatively short, and sufficient tissue is accessible to permit definitive measurements. One must be cautious, however, in selecting the appropriate animal strain, stock, and gender, as there is wide variability in age-associated pathology, even within the same strain of different stock (Anver & Cohen, 1979). As a point of reference, a 24-mo rat is considered aged because 24-mo is the median life span for most colonies of sedentary rats fed *ad libitum* (Caccia et al., 1979; Goodrick, 1980). The use of the median life span is the best recognized and accepted criterion for an aged animal (Hollander & Burek, 1982).

Mass and Protein Content

Grimby and Saltin (1983) estimated that by age 65, muscle mass in human beings decreases by approximately 25–30% from peak values of the third decade. Frontera et al. (1991) estimated muscle mass loss from the fifth to seventh decade to be about 11%. Muscle mass values of rats and mice drop by 10–30% from peak values in young adults to those in old animals (Brooks & Faulkner, 1988; Daw et al., 1988; Faulkner et al., 1990; Fitts et al., 1984). Net growth or the maintenance of muscle mass occurs as a result of the balance between protein synthesis and degradation. The rates of skeletal muscle protein synthesis decline in aged animals and contribute to muscle atrophy (Florini, 1978; Makrides, 1983; Pluskal et al., 1984).

Although muscle atrophy is inevitable if life is continued long enough, the rate of atrophy varies. The variations reflect differences in species and strain of animals studied, the particular muscle(s) studied, the age of the animal in relation to that colony's median and maximum expected life span, and the habitual level of physical activity. Likewise, not all skeletal muscles are affected equally by the aging process (Grimby et al., 1982; Klitgaard et al., 1990a, 1990b). Indeed, some have reported no change (Pettigrew & Gardiner, 1987) or increased mass (Larsson & Edstrom, 1986) for some muscles with age. With respect to the confounding effects of physical activity, one must recognize that muscles within an organism vary in level of habitual use. For example, comparison between the diaphragm muscle and the extensor digitorum longus muscle (EDL) in a sedentary organism is, in fact, comparing a relatively endurance-trained muscle (the diaphragm) with a sedentary one. This comparison can be even more dramatic than comparing the same limb muscle between trained and untrained animals.

As an example, we studied soleus and EDL muscles in adult (12 mo) and old (27 mo) rats (Daw et al., 1988). Some rats were cage sedentary, and others were involved in treadmill running 5 d/wk since age 3 mo. At 27 mo, the masses of soleus and EDL muscles of sedentary control rats were 83% and 70%, respectively, of 12-mo values (P < 0.05). In the trained animals, the age-associated decrease in soleus mass was only half that found in sedentary rats. In contrast, the degree of atrophy of the EDL muscles was unaffected by training and was twofold greater than the atrophy of the soleus muscles in the sedentary rats (Table 4-1). The difference between muscles likely reflects inherent distinctions in neuronal recruitment and mechanical loading. In a sedentary existence, a rat will use the soleus more than the EDL during movement around the cage because the soleus, unlike the EDL, is a plantarflexor and supports the body weight of the rat. With daily running, the soleus muscle is recruited even more, whereas the small increase in recruitment of the EDL muscle, an ankle dorsiflexor, is insufficient to induce similar adaptations. This simple experiment demonstrates rather eloquently the complexity that "physical activity" brings to the study of aging and skeletal muscle.

The impact of age-associated muscle atrophy extends beyond neuromuscular function. For example, Fleg and Lakatta (1988) concluded that a large portion of the age-related decline in $\dot{V}O_2$max in untrained individuals is explicable by the age-associated loss of muscle mass. This issue is especially important if, as hypothesized by Booth (1989), and Comfort (1979), maximum life span is the age at which $\dot{V}O_2$max reaches the value of resting or basal $\dot{V}O_2$.

Another example of the potential wide-ranging impact of muscle atrophy is that it may contribute to impairments in protein metabolism that are often seen in old people. Such impairments can adversely affect the ability of the older person to resist or recover from traumatic stress and disease (Jeevanandam et al., 1990). In this regard, Rosenberg (1989) suggested that muscle atrophy may have a direct deleterious effect on immunocompetence and functional capacity that influences survival in acute and chronic disease and starvation.

Motor Unit Remodeling and Reinnervation

The remodeling of motor units is an inevitable consequence of aging. Aging of skeletal muscle is associated with a combination of changes in nerve and muscle cells, resulting in weakened neural influences and a shift toward "functional denervation" concomitant with senile muscle atrophy (Frolkis et al., 1976; Gutmann & Hanzlikova, 1972, 1976). Terminal sprouting is a mechanism that maintains neuromuscular contact and is persistent throughout life (Barker & Ip, 1966; Haimann et al., 1981). This process decreases with advancing age in rats and is associated with

TABLE 4-1. *Body and skeletal mass of F-344 rats at 12 and 27-mo age. Values are mean ± SE, number of rats are parentheses. * significantly different from sedentary at same age; • significantly different from 12-mo values in same group (Data from Daw et al., 1988, with permission).*

Variable	12-mo		27-mo	
	Sedentary	Trained	Sedentary	Trained
Body mass (g)	442 ± 8 (9)	358 ± 5 (8)*	332 ± 9 (9)•	330 ± 5 (8)•
Soleus mass (mg)	138 ± 5 (9)	152 ± 3 (8)	115 ± 4 (9)•	130 ± 4 (8)*•
EDL mass (mg)	166 ± 4 (9)	153 ± 2 (8)*	116 ± 5 (8)•	120 ± 3 (8)•

senile muscle atrophy (Pestronk et al., 1980). Motor endplate associated choline acetyltransferase (a marker enzyme for synapse integrity) and acetylcholinesterase (which is necessary for transmitter breakdown) activity also decline with age (Berman and Decker, 1985; Frolkis et al., 1976). Brown et al. (1981) suggested that the age-associated motor unit remodeling is a consequence of alterations in the normal turnover of synaptic junctions that results from a cycle of denervation, axonal sprouting, and reinnervation. In young adults, the turnover occurs without any alteration in the type of innervation reaching fibers. With age, however, it is common to observe an aggregation of Type I fibers. This age-associated change reflects some denervated Type II fibers becoming reinnervated by axonal sprouting from adjacent innervated Type I fibers (Brown et al., 1981). There is also evidence that some loss of alpha-motoneurons occurs at the ventral root (Larsson, 1994). Although incomplete, there is subsequently some degree of reinnervation of surviving motoneurons that leads to rearrangement of motor units in their preexisting territory. Any loss in fibers presumably occurs from a population of the Type II fibers not being reinnervated and thus atrophying (Grimby & Saltin, 1983). Alternatively, Desypris and Parry (1990) have suggested that both Type I and II fibers denervate with similar propensity but that Type I motoneurons are more effective in reinnervating fibers.

Nerve injury or degradation might, in some cases, lead to many of the age-associated impairments of muscle structure and function. However, it is clear that the deficits can develop without any known injury. For example, the experiments of Campbell et al. (1973) showed a reduced twitch-force after 60 y in human extensor digitorum brevis muscle that correlated with reduced number of motor units. However, the results might be influenced by injury, as the common peroneal nerve is susceptible to injury, even in young persons. Motor unit remodeling was a focus of a study by Doherty et al. (1993), who examined the relationship between strength and motor unit number in proximal muscles whose nerves are likely to have been unaffected by repeated trauma over time. These investigators studied the biceps brachii and brachialis muscles in men and women of two age groups: 24 persons ranged from 22–38 y, and 20 persons were from 60–81 y. The quotient of the amplitude of the maximum compound muscle action potential to the single motor unit action potential (S-MUAP) yielded an estimate of the number of motor units. The number of motor units declined 47% with age, as the older subjects had 189 ± 77 compared with 357 ± 97 in the younger adults (mean $\pm$ SD), with comparable decreases in both genders (Table 4-2, Figure 4-1). The size of the S-MUAPs increased 23% in the old persons, and twitch-force, as well as maximum voluntary contraction force, declined by 33%.

Similar remodeling occurs in rat limb muscles (Pettigrew & Gardiner, 1987). Edstrom & Larsson (1987) and Kanda & Hashizume (1989) found

TABLE 4-2. *Results of electrophysiological and muscle contractile strength studies in young and older subjects.*

	Young	Older
Age, yr		
M	30±5	69±6
F	26±4	68±6
MF	29±8	69±6*
Maximum M-potential, m V		
M	16.2±3.9	11.4±2.7
F	11.7±2.3	7.8±1.4
MF	14.5±4.0	9.6±2.8*
Means S-MUAP size, μ V		
M	46.4±11.5	55.3±18.0
F	36.5±13.1	56.1±18.9
MF	42.7±12.8	55.7±18.0†
Estimated number of motor units		
M	363±99	224±79
F	347±99	153±61
MF	357±97	189±77*
Maximum twitch contraction, N m		
M	6.4±2.4	4.5±1.8
F	2.8±0.8	1.9±0.3
MF	4.8±2.6	3.2±1.8‡
Time to peak tension, ms		
M	64.9±5.7	71.1±8.7
F	71.4±9.8	76.0±16.9
MF	67.8±8.2	73.6±13.3
One-half relaxation time, ms		
M	132.7±38.1	124.3±13.0
F	127.2±22.2	133.7±19.3
MF	129.7±31.2	128.9±16.7
Maximum voluntary contraction, N m		
M	81.8±16.9	57.8±8.1
F	39.6±9.9	27.2±5.3
MF	63.1±25.6	42.5±17.0*

Values are means ± SD. Maximum M-potential, maximum compound muscle action potential; S-MUAP, surface-recorded single motor unit action potential; M, male; F, female; MF, male and female combined. Young vs. Old: * $P < 0.001$; † $P < 0.01$; ‡ $P < 0.05$. From Doherty et al., (1993); with permission.

reductions of approximately 30% in the total number of motor units in medial gastrocnemius and soleus muscles and increases in the size of slow motor units. The number of fibers and the total fiber area in a given motor unit also increased. There was a 30% drop in maximum force of Type II motor units in old compared with adult rats, with a 2.5-fold increase in force values for Type I motor units (Kanda & Hashizume, 1989). Furthermore, Shorey et al. (1988) found an increased percentage of Type I fibers in the soleus, with no change in fast-twitch muscle. In conclusion, even in the absence of known nerve injury, there is significant remodeling of motor units with age.

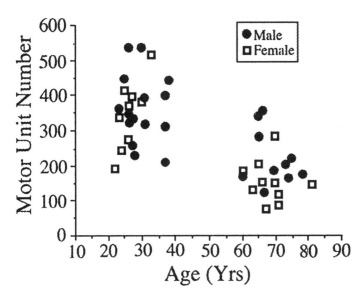

FIGURE 4-1. *Relationship between estimated number of motor units (MUE) and age in young and older men and women.* There was a significant reduction in the number of motor units with age ($P < 0.001$). From Doherty et al. (1993) with permission.

Change in innervation patterns of skeletal muscle that occur due to physical inactivity are similar to those associated with aging. For example, collateral sprouting occurs in the viable motor nerves of a partially denervated muscle (Betz et al., 1980) and in muscles of senescent animals (Pestronk et al., 1980). Moreover, increased physical activity increases motor end plate size and terminal sprouting proportional to changes in fiber diameter in young animals (Appell, 1984; Granbacher, 1971) and old animals (Smith & Rosenheimer, 1982; Stebbins et al., 1985). The adaptations are specific to individual types of muscle fibers. These data give rise to the possibility that neural traffic, associated with volitional exercise or some other means, might facilitate reinnervation.

The neuronal axons of old animals are less able to regenerate or reinnervate motor endplates (MEPs) following various perturbations than are young animals (Pestronk et al., 1980). For example, with cross-reinnervation in young adult and old rats there was an age-associated decrease in the reinnervation of muscle (Clark & White, 1991). In this study, adaptations of MEPs and muscle fibers to the reinnervation of extensor digitorum longus (EDL) muscle by the EDL nerve (i.e., self-reinnervation) or the nerve ordinarily supplying the soleus (i.e., cross-reinnervation) was examined. There was an age-associated decrease in the reinnervation of muscle following nerve section, as evidenced by an increased number of noninnervated MEPs and by decreased neuronal contact with innervated MEPs (Table 4-3). The conversion of fiber type following cross-reinnervation

TABLE 4-3. *Morphological data for MFP and terminal nerve parameters in control and experimental EDL and SOL muscles from rats at 12 and 29 mo of age.*

Exptl Group	No. of Terminal Nerves	Terminal Nerve Length, μm	MEP Area, μm²	Terminal Nerve Length/MEP Area, μm/μm²	Noninnervated MEPs, % of total
			Rats at 12 mo of age		
Control EDL	8.2±0.7 (6)	133.7±11.4 (6)	995.2±67.8 (6)	0.147±0.01 (6)	1.4±0.6 (6)
Self-reinnervated EDL	8.1±0.7 (9)	140.6±12.0 (9)	724.0±55.3* (9)	0.199±0.01* (9)	15.8±1.8* (9)
Cross-reinnervated EDL	7.1±0.7 (9)	142.0±12.7 (9)	861.9±107* (9)	0.182±0.01* (9)	17.4±1.9* (9)
Control SOL	11.1±0.6 (6)	148.0±12.1 (6)	1,091.5±83 (6)	0.136±0.01 (6)	1.1±0.2 (6)
Self-reinnervated SOL	10.2±0.8 (9)	157.7±9.7 (9)	942.2±92 (9)	0.162±0.01* (9)	19.1±3.4* (9)
			Rats at 29 mo of age		
Control EDL	6.3±0.5* (6)	110.4±10.2* (6)	499.9±47.2* (6)	0.228±0.01* (6)	6.2±1.2* (6)
Self-reinnervated EDL	3.4±0.4† (9)	61.9±6.1† (9)	610.0±64.1 (9)	0.112±0.01† (9)	43.6±12.0† (9)
Cross-reinnervated EDL	3.7±0.6† (9)	71.2±9.1† (9)	415.3±26.3‡ (9)	0.167±0.02†‡ (9)	48.1±6.3† (9)
Control SOL	13.2±0.5 (6)	162.4±9.8 (6)	1,150.0±64.1 (6)	0.141±0.2 (6)	4.4±2.0* (6)
Self-reinnervated SOL	5.2±0.6† (9)	110.2±15† (9)	806.7±67† (9)	0.137±0.13 (9)	50.6±9.3† (9)

Values are means ± SE; nos. in parentheses indicate no. of muscles. EDL, extensor digitorum longus; SOL, soleus. For control groups 20 motor end plates (MEPs)/muscle were sampled; for experimental groups 30 MEPs/muscle were sampled. Values are significantly different ($P \leq 0.05$) from the following: * 12-mo control; † 29-mo control; ‡ age-matched self-innervated value. From Clark and White (1991); with permission.

correlated closely with the number of innervated MEPs, suggesting that innervated fibers in old rats are capable of adapting to a new stimulus.

Fiber Number

There is a wide variety of claims regarding the magnitude of fiber loss associated with aging. Much of the controversy exists because studies on humans are based on indirect approaches and employ cross-sectional designs, which can easily lead to imprecise results. In studies of experimentally inbred rats, these difficulties can be circumvented by direct and complete counts and can provide evidence in these models that hypoplasia makes a relatively small contribution to muscle atrophy.

Daw et al. (1988) studied skeletal muscle mass and fiber number in male Fischer-344 rats. At ages 12 mo and 27 mo, the soleus and EDL muscles were excised and weighed, and the numbers of fibers were counted following nitric acid digestion of the surrounding connective tissue. At 27 mo the weights of soleus and EDL muscles of sedentary control rats were 83% and 70%, respectively, of 12 mo values. Fiber number for soleus muscle declined 5.6% from 2,678 ± 47 at 12 mo to 2,528 ± 24 at 27 mo. For EDL muscles, fiber number declined with age by 4.2%, from 5,246 ± 68 at 12 mo to 5,027 ± 64 at 27 mo. To analyze further the role of fiber number in dictating mass, linear regression analyses were conducted. Insignificant correlations between fiber number and mass were observed for soleus and EDL muscles. The evidence in this study indicates that with aging, hypoplasia can account at most for approximately 25% of the observed skeletal muscle atrophy. Comparing soleus and EDL muscles of rats aged 6 mo to 24 mo with direct fiber counts, Brown (1987) found that fiber number did not change. Other investigators who have counted fibers in cross-sections or used other indirect techniques have concluded that hypoplasia occurs in rodents. As but one example, Klitgaard (1989a) reported an 11% decrease in fiber number of rat soleus muscle from 9 mo to 24 mo and a further reduction of 26% from 24 mo to 29 mo. The difficulty in obtaining valid counts in cross-section has been described previously (Maxwell et al., 1974).

An early report by Grimby and Saltin (1983) suggested an approximate 25% drop in fiber number from adult through old age in humans. These estimates were based on measuring fiber cross-sectional area from percutaneous needle biopsy samples and then calculating fiber number based on muscle cross-sectional area as determined by computer tomography scans. Lexell et al. (1988) studied muscle morphometrics in whole vastus lateralis muscle obtained at autopsy in persons ranging from 15 y to 83 y. Total fiber number was estimated from the product of the total cross-sectional area of the muscle and the number of fibers in samples of known area (i.e., fiber density). As seen in Table 4-4, muscle atrophy commences in the third decade of life, as evidenced by muscle cross-

TABLE 4-4. *Estimates of muscle area, total number of fibers, perecentage Type I, and fiber cross-sectional area for Type I and Type II fibers from autopsy study of whole human vastus lateralis muscle. Values are means (SD). (Adapted from Lexell et al., 1988, with permission)*

Age (yr)	Number of Subjects	Muscle Area (mm²)	Total Fiber Number	Percent-age Type I	Fiber Area (um²) Type I	Type II
19 (3)	9	3,648 (480)	648,000 (164,000)	50 (5)	3,554 (1,242)	3,589 (1,528)
32 (4)	9	3,600 (432)	599,000 (85,000)	50 (4)	3,724 (326)	4,054 (547)
51 (3)	8	3,312 (528)	579,000 (173,000)	52 (15)	2,988 (684)	3,223 (433)
73 (2)	9	2,688 (912)	380,000 (70,000)	52 (6)	3,560 (840)	2,699 (855)
82 (1)	8	2,064 (432)	323,000 (79,000)	55 (11)	3,653 (789)	2,728 (645)

sectional area declining 43% from an average age of 25.5 y to 82 y. Muscle atrophy was explained primarily by a 48% decrease in fiber number over the age range. Across all ages, the slow and fast fibers each represented about 50% of the total number. Interestingly, the total cross-sectional area of Type I fibers did not differ across the ages, whereas the area of Type II fibers decreased by 28%.

The conclusion from the available human studies regarding the underlying cause of muscle atrophy is opposite to that from studies of rats; hypoplasia appears to be a major mechanism of muscle atrophy in humans. There are numerous technical problems in obtaining credible human data on this variable, including the fact that the results are necessarily obtained from cross-sectional studies and thus compare persons of different genotype, age, and cause of death. Nonetheless, even if one acknowledges a fudge factor, hypoplasia in older humans seems to be a real phenomenon. The explanation may in part be that the old persons studied had some type of neurological disease that led to fiber loss. This and other hypotheses that may resolve the disparity between evidence from rats and that from humans remain untested.

Fiber Diameter

It is generally accepted that a decrease in muscle size can occur when fibers atrophy after undergoing denervation and/or as a consequence of disuse. In addition, the concentration of carnitine is lower in aged muscles (Costell et al., 1989), and this decrease can cause fiber atrophy by unknown mechanisms (Spagnoli et al., 1990). In the young, carnitine-insufficiency-induced atrophy is reversible; whether this is the case in old animals awaits further study.

In humans, the fiber diameter in limb muscles remains relatively constant, at least through age 70 y (Grimby et al., 1982; Larsson, 1978, 1983; Lexell et al., 1988; Overend et al., 1992a, 1992b). The human autopsy data of Lexell et al. (1988) demonstrated atrophy in Type II fibers from subjects who died in their 70s and 80s (Table 4-4), and Coggan et al. (1992a) described atrophy in both IIa and IIb fiber subgroups in older subjects. On the other hand, Aniansson et al. (1992) followed changes in muscle morphology (vastus lateralis muscle) and strength (knee extension) for 11 y in 9 men who were aged 69.3 ± 0.3 y at the onset of study and 80.4 ± 0.3 y on the last occasion. Fiber diameters did not change between 69 y and 76 y and actually increased in both Type I and Type II fibers from 76 to 80 y, despite an overall decrease in total muscle size. The isokinetic strength performance declined 25–35% over the 11-y period. The authors interpreted the fiber hypertrophy, in the face of overall muscular atrophy, to be a compensatory adaptation to the presumed loss of motor units in these persons.

In rats, fiber diameters of various muscles are affected differently by age, apparently because of differences in habitual use (Lexell, 1993; Lexell & Taylor, 1991). For example, in a comparison of the fiber cross-sectional areas of the diaphragm muscle and three limb muscles, there is an age-associated cellular hypertrophy of the former and cellular atrophy of the latter (White & Clark, 1995). Tissues for this study were obtained at intervals from female F-344 rats as they aged from 9 mo to 27 mo. The muscles studied have a diversity of characteristic recruitment and loading patterns, even in sedentary rats. In the limb muscles, fiber areas remained relatively constant through 18 mo, and then declined. In comparing fiber areas in muscles of rats aged 9 mo with those of rats aged 27 mo, there were decreases for soleus, EDL, and plantaris muscles of 25%, 22%, and 29%, respectively. In contrast, the average fiber area in the diaphragm increased by 25%. The cellular hypertrophy of the diaphragm compared to cellular atrophy in limb muscles likely reflects the different usage patterns among these muscles (Gutmann & Melichna, 1972; Husain & Pardy, 1985). Data from rats and humans indicate that age-related alterations in the compliance of the lungs and chest wall necessitate a 20% increase in muscular work in order to overcome rigidity during normal breathing (Masora, 1975; Turner et al., 1968). Furthermore, with age-associated decreases in the capacity of the rib cage to expand, the diaphragm may contribute a greater percentage of the total force needed to increase lung volume upon inspiration (Rizzato & Marazzini, 1970); increased mechanical loading is known to increase fiber cross-sectional area (Faulkner & White, 1990).

Myosin Phenotype

In the early literature, there is lack of agreement regarding whether the proportion of Type II fibers declines with age or remains stable. There is consensus, however, that the diameter of Type II fibers decreases with age (Aniansson, et al., 1981; Clarkson et al., 1981; Grimby et al., 1982, 1984; Larsson & Karlsson, 1978; Larsson et al., 1978; Lexell & Downham, 1991, 1992). Some of the ambiguity may reflect sampling problems (Nygaard & Sanchez, 1982). More recent work, however, suggests that in the absence of disease, myosin phenotype, at least Type I and Type II, is stable throughout adult and old age in well-controlled studies of muscles from barrier-raised rodents.

In the mid 1980s, Florini and co-workers undertook an extensive experiment that was based on the belief from published literature that myosin phenotype did change with age; namely, there was a presumed decrease in fast fibers. He and his colleagues were determined to see if treatment of rats with growth hormone, clonidine, and insulin-like growth factor (to restore circulating somatomedin levels in old animals to levels found earlier in life) could reverse the anticipated age-associated decrement of fast fibers, particularly late in life (Florini & Ewton, 1989). The principal conclusion of this work was that there was no age-associated change in the fiber composition or myofibrillar myosin ATPase activity of EDL, soleus, and diaphragm muscles of F-344 rats.

The investigators indicated the rationale for studying these muscles was that they are primarily fast, slow, and mixed (both fast and slow fibers) in their phenotype, respectively. The then-surprising results are consistent with work from other labs that also studied barrier-protected, specific-pathogen-free rats (Eddinger et al., 1985, 1986; McCarter & McGee, 1987; White & Clark, 1995) and are inconsistent with the earlier work of rats housed in conventional colonies. The specific reason for differences in myosin phenotype between rats raised in barrier and conventional colonies is unknown. Most gerontologists would agree, however, that barrier facilities provide the most appropriate environment for the study of aging, i.e, one as free as possible from intervening pathologies.

Recently, Lars Larsson discussed his observation of an increase in Type IIx myosin (at the cost of decreased IIb) in the EDL and anterior tibialis muscles, but not in the soleus muscles, of non-barrier raised rats (Larsson, 1994). In earlier experiments, this increase in the IIx phenotype may have been undetected because neither monoclonal antibodies nor electrophoretic conditions that could detect this protein were used. Larsson found that the IIx motor units, either pure or co-expressed with a different isoform, become the predominant fiber type in selected muscles of the old rats. Type IIx motor units have functional properties intermediate to those of Type IIa and IIb units.

Coggan et al. (1992a) published a comprehensive and carefully controlled study of healthy but inactive young adults and old men and women (Table 4-5). The non-smoking subjects were carefully screened for relevant diseases. The results of histochemical analyses of their lateral gastrocnemius muscles, sampled by percutaneous needle biopsy, are presented in Table 4-6. The percentages of Type I, IIa, and IIb fibers did not differ with age. Because Type IIa and IIb fibers had cross-sectional areas that were 13–31% smaller in the old compared to young adults, the relative muscle area comprised of Type I fibers increased with age (60.6 ± 2.6% versus 53.6 ± 2.0%). These results are consistent with prior work on human vastus lateralis muscles (Aniansson et al., 1981; Essen-Gustavsson & Borges, 1986; Lexell et al., 1983; Stalberg et al., 1989). Indeed, in 68-year-old sedentary Scandinavians compared to subjects 28 y of age, Klitgaard et al. (1990b) found a 27% greater content of Type I myosin heavy chain (MHC) and a 39% greater content of slow-myosin light-chain-2 in vastus lateralis muscles. Similar differences were found in biceps brachii muscles, but because histochemical fiber typing and immunocytochemical co-expression of Type I and II MHC isoforms were not different between ages, the increase in slow MHC content with aging is attributable to a relative increase in the total area of Type I fibers, induced by preferential atrophy of Type II fibers.

There is no consensus in regard to age-associated change in skeletal muscle myosin phenotype in humans, and definitive research is needed. In humans, compared to barrier-raised rodents, more profound myosin changes may occur as a result of selective denervation of fast motor units due to human aging *per se* or to the susceptibility of humans to disease and trauma. The estimates of motor unit denervation in some (Campbell et al., 1973) but not all (Doherty et al., 1993) studies of humans are twofold to threefold greater than in studies of rodents (Edstrom & Larsson 1987; Kanda & Hashizume, 1989).

Functional Properties

Strength of Muscle Groups. Arm, leg, and back strength decline at an overall rate of 8% per decade, starting in the third decade of life (Asmussen, 1980). The rate of decline is not linear but is slightly lower early in the decline and greater late in life. In one of the major investigations of this phenomenon, Kallman et al. (1990) studied the role of muscle atrophy in the age-related decline of grip strength. These investigators studied 847 healthy persons aged 20–100 y as part of the Baltimore Longitudinal Study of Aging. Their imaginative study combined cross-sectional data with longitudinal data obtained from individuals in each age-group over the subsequent nine years. The muscle mass data were estimated from forearm circumference measurements and from urinary creatinine, an often-used index of total muscle mass (Heymsfield et al., 1983). There is necessarily some imprecision in these data. For example, using decreased creatinine excretion to indicate a decrease in muscle mass would overestimate the muscle loss by whatever degree protein turnover is slowed in old age (Florini, 1978; Makrides, 1983; Pluskal et al., 1984). Nevertheless, the results are informative.

TABLE 4-5. *Physical characteristics of the subjects (Mean ± SE).*

	Young Men	Old Men	Young Women	Old Women	Age Effect	Gender Effect
Age (yr)	26 ± 1	64 ± 1	23 ± 1	63 ± 1	$p < .001$[a]	n.s.[a]
Height (cm)	180 ± 1	181 ± 2	165 ± 5	166 ± 2	n.s.	$p < .001$
Weight (kg)	74.7 ± 3.2	84.5 ± 2.4	63.2 ± 3.7	61.3 ± 2.0	n.s.	$p < .001$
Body fat (%)	17.4 ± 1.3	27.1 ± 1.5	24.5 ± 1.8	36.1 ± 1.7	$p < .001$	$p < .001$
Fat-free mass (kg)	64.1 ± 2.1	61.4 ± 1.5	47.6 ± 2.6	39.3 ± 1.3	$p < .05$	$p < .001$
$\dot{V}O_2$max (L/min)	3.44 ± 0.12	2.34 ± 0.13	2.22 ± 0.12	1.40 ± 0.06	$p < .001$	$p < .001$
$\dot{V}O_2$max (mL/kg/min)	46.2 ± 1.1	27.7 ± 1.4	35.3 ± 1.3	22.7 ± 0.9	$p < .001$	$p < .001$

[a]p-values refer to significant main effects identified by two-way (age by gender) ANOVA. See text for details. n.s. = not significant.
From Coggan et al., (1992 A); with permission.

TABLE 4-6. *Skeletal muscle fiber type distribution and fiber areas (Mean ± SE).*

	Young Men	Old Men	Young Men	Old Women	Age Effect	Gender Effect
Type I (%)	59.2 ± 2.8	59.8 ± 3.5	57.4 ± 3.0	61.9 ± 3.6	n.s.	n.s.
Type IIa (%)	20.2 ± 2.9	21.4 ± 2.4	22.1 ± 2.5	19.8 ± 2.5	n.s.	n.s.
Type IIb (%)	20.6 ± 2.9	18.8 ± 2.3	20.6 ± 3.3	18.3 ± 2.8	n.s.	n.s.
Type I area (μm^2)	4,696 ± 393	4,770 ± 308	3,546 ± 304	3,150 ± 159	n.s.	$p < .001$
Type IIa area (μm^2)	5,960 ± 630	5,193 ± 348	4,020 ± 347	3,052 ± 155	$p < .05$	$p < .001$
Type IIb area (μm^2)	6,444 ± 659	5,055 ± 505	3,935 ± 421	2,743 ± 160	$p < .01$	$p < .001$

From Coggan et al., (1992 A); with permission.

Both cross-sectional and longitudinal results indicated that grip strength increased into the fourth decade of life and declined at an ever-increasing rate thereafter (Table 4-7, Figure 4-2) (Kallman et al., 1990). On average, grip strength declined 37% from 35 y to 83 y of age, an overall rate of 7.3% per decade. Interestingly, during the 9-y follow-up, grip strength was stable in 48% of persons less than 40 y of age, in 29% of those aged 40–59 y, and in only 15% of those older than 60 y. The smaller percentages of each older age cohort that could maintain strength over the 9 y likely reflect in part the progressively declining habitual physical activity levels within the older cohorts; nevertheless, this age-associated decline in strength is apparently inevitable.

The roughly parallel age-related declines of mass and function has led some to prematurely conclude that it is the decrease in mass that determines the decrease in strength and that intrinsic differences do not exist in functional attributes of old muscle compared to young or adult (Frontera et al., 1991; Grimby & Saltin 1983; McCarter & McGee, 1987). It is true that grip strength is correlated with muscle mass (r = 0.60, P<0.001); however, multiple regression analysis shows a stronger relationship between strength and age than between strength and mass, leading Kallman et al. (1990) to conclude that muscle atrophy is only a partial explanation for decreased strength. However, when one compares the actual grip strength to that estimated based on forearm circumference (Kallman et al., 1990), and even acknowledging the deficiency of measuring muscle mass by this approach, one is left with the impression that strength exceeds that predicted from age 25 y to 55 y and is less than predicted thereafter (Figure 4-3). Thus, from loose approximations of muscle mass from creatinine excretion and anthropometric measurements, the conclusion may be drawn that unknown factors in addition to a loss of muscle mass must explain the age-associated loss of strength. Kallman et al. (1990) suggest that changes in muscle fiber composition and/or motoneuron disease are likely explanations.

Valid measurements of muscle cross-sectional areas in humans are problematic. Even modern imaging techniques require knowledge of the architecture of the muscle(s) contributing to the force production. Also, the lever systems translate muscle force to joint moments, thereby complicating interpretations of force measurements at a given joint. These complexities exist particularly for muscles causing movements at the ankle, knee, hip, elbow, or shoulder, but are much less of an issue for the adductor pollicis muscle. This fact, along with the ability to isolate force measurements and manage contraction conditions such as the interpolation of twitch and tetanic contractions, has led to the study of the adductor pollicis muscle in classical (Merton, 1954) and contemporary studies (Narici et al., 1991; Phillips et al., 1992). Despite the technical limitations previously mentioned, many investigators studying muscles of humans

TABLE 4-7. *Cross-sectional and longitudinal analysis of grip strength**.

	Cross-sectional Results			Longitudinal Results				
Age Group	N†	Mean Age (yr)	Mean Grip Strength (kg)	N†	Mean Age (yr)	Mean Grip § Strength (kg)	Mean Follow-up (yr)	Mean slope (kg/yr)
20–29	55	27.2	100.2 ± 1.97	5	---	---	---	---
30–39	115	34.7	104.3 ± 1.56	24	36.8	103.9 ± 2.70	8.5	0.33 ± 0.23
40–49	130	45.8	101.0 ± 1.28	90	45.6	100.7 ± 1.36	8.7	-0.31 ± 0.12
50–59	187	55.0	95.2 ± 1.03	105	54.8	97.1 ± 1.17	9.3	-0.65 ± 0.11
60–69	158	64.4	88.0 ± 1.00	71	64.6	88.2 ± 1.58	9.2	-0.78 ± 0.15
70–79	155	74.6	75.4 ± 1.04	40	74.5	77.9 ± 1.43	8.8	-1.27 ± 0.21
80–89	42	83.2	66.0 ± 1.56	5	---	---	---	---

*Summed grip strength (left- + righthand grip).
†Data are not reported when $n = 5$ or less. Cross-sectional data are not shown for one 19-year old subject. 3 subjects in their 90s, and one 100-year old subject. Data for all 847 cross-sectional subjects are shown in Figure 4-2.
‡Decade mean of each subject's average age during the period he was followed.
§Decade mean of each subject's average grip strength during the period he was followed.
Mean value ± standard error of the mean.
From Kallman et al., (1990); with permission.

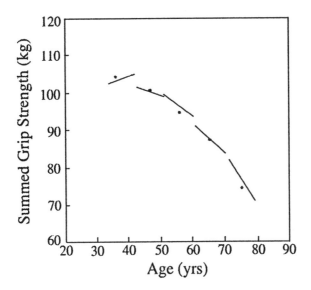

FIGURE 4-2. *Comparison of cross-sectional age differences and longitudinal age changes in grip strength.* The dots represent the mean values for each decade obtained from cross-sectional data. Line segments represent the longitudinal results and indicate the decade means of the rate of change of grip strength for each individual as determined by regression analysis. Lines are drawn with the midpoints at the mean grip strength for each age decade, and with their lengths, along the abscissa, representing the mean time span over which the longitudinal data were collected for each age group (see Table 4-7). From Kallman et al. (1990), with permission.

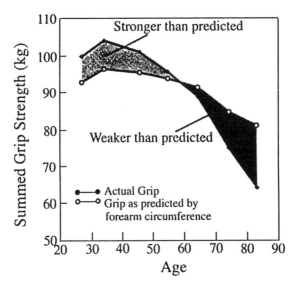

FIGURE 4-3. *Comparison of decade means of actual grip strength and grip strength as predicted from forearm circumference (cross-sectional)* (N = 608). From Kallman et al. (1990), with permission.

SKELETAL MUSCLE STRUCTURE **133**

conclude that force declines with age at a rate greater than that predicted by muscle atrophy (Bruce et al., 1989; Davies et al., 1986; Phillips et al., 1992; Vandervoort & McComas, 1986).

Muscle Force. Similar to the age-related decline of strength in humans, decreases of 20–35% in absolute values for maximal, isometric, tetanic force occur in both fast and slow limb muscles of old mice and rats (Brooks & Faulkner, 1988; Larsson & Edstrom, 1986; Larsson & Salviati, 1989).

When force is normalized to total muscle cross-sectional area, i.e., *specific force*, one can gain insight into intrinsic alterations in muscle contractile capacity that extend beyond any factor(s) due to changes in muscle mass *per se*. *Specific weakness* is defined as a decrease in specific force of a rested (nonfatigued) muscle fiber, muscle, or muscle group. Age-associated decrements of specific isometric force of approximately 20% have been detected in rodent limb muscle studied *in situ* or *in vitro* (Brooks & Faulkner, 1988; Fitts et al., 1984; Larsson & Edstrom, 1986). Thus, the general consensus among well-conducted studies with humans and rodents is that the capacity to generate force declines with age (Bassey et al., 1992; Borges, 1989; Brooks & Faulkner, 1988; Häkkinen & Häkkinen, 1991; Harries & Bassey, 1990; Stanley & Taylor, 1993; Young et al., 1984, 1985) and that the decline is greater than what is expected based on the degree of muscle atrophy.

One possible explanation for the observed specific weakness with age would be, of course, that the old were less able to fully activate their existing muscle mass, due possibly to reflex inhibition or less inclination to generate maximum force. To address this issue as a possible cause of specific weakness, Phillips et al. (1992) investigated the adductor pollicis muscle in a group of 53 young adult men and women (29 ± 1.1 y) and in 39 healthy old men and women (80 ± 0.7 y). Muscle cross-sectional areas and maximal voluntary forces were measured in all persons. The results indicated an age-associated decline in specific force, i.e., a specific weakness with age, as these workers have indicated previously (Bruce et al., 1989). The ratio of maximal voluntary force to cross-sectional area was 26 ± 3% lower in the older than in the younger adults (Table 4-8). In a subset of the young and old, a twitch interpolation technique was used to determine if full recruitment occurred in both age groups. There is unequivocal evidence that the young adults were able to fully recruit their adductor pollicis muscles; i.e., when muscles were electrically stimulated during maximal voluntary contractions, the stimulation evoked no additional force (Figure 4-4) (Phillips et al., 1992). A strict statistical interpretation is that full voluntary recruitment also occurred in the old. However, one is compelled to note that the mean intercept for the old occurred at about 85% of the maximal voluntary force; because the sample size was so small (n = 3) the 99% confidence limits indicated that this 85% value was not

TABLE 4-8. *A summary of MVF and CSA data for young and elderly male and female subjects.*

		n	MVF (N) (mean ± SEM)	CSA (mm) (mean ± SEM)	Age (yrs) (mean ± SEM)
Young	Females	27	61.0 ± 2.1	439.9 ± 18.9	26.6 ± 1.4
	Males	26	81.6 ± 3.4	612.7 ± 24.9	29.6 ± 1.6
	All	53	71.1 ± 2.4	524.6 ± 19.5	28.0 ± 1.1
Elderly	Females	17	40.0 ± 2.7	401.1 ± 27.2	80.8 ± 0.7
	Males	22	55.0 ± 3.8	555.6 ± 30.8	79.9 ± 1.1
	All	39	48.5 ± 2.7	488.3 ± 24.2	80.3 ± 0.7

From Phillips et al., (1992); with permission.

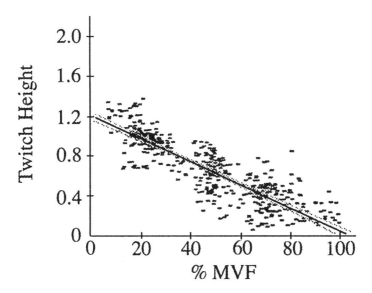

FIGURE 4-4. *The relationship between [normalized twitch height]$^{0.66}$ and percentage of maximum voluntary force (MVF) from eight young subjects.* Regression line (---) and 99% confidence limits (—) of the population regression line are shown. From Phillips et al. (1992), with permission.

statistically different from 100% (Figure 4-5). Vandervoort and McComas (1986) also found with twitch interpolation at maximal voluntary force that most old subjects could maximally activate their ankle musculature. Accordingly, incomplete recruitment of innervated muscle appears not to be a cause of specific weakness in the old, at least with the caveat noted above. In preliminary work, Woledge (1994) found that hormone replacement therapy in postmenopausal women can delay, but not prevent, the development of specific weakness; this work holds promising insight for the cause of specific weakness.

The limit to the approach described in the preceding paragraphs is

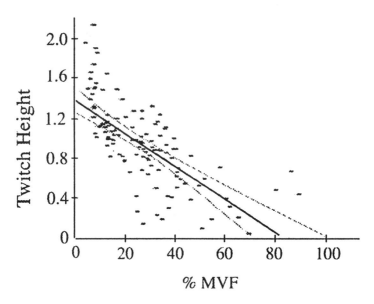

FIGURE 4-5. *The relationship between [normalized twitch height]$^{0.66}$ and percentage of maximum voluntary force (MVF) from three old subjects with low MVF per muscle cross-sectional area.* From Phillips et al. (1992), with permission.

that any denervated fibers present in the muscle would contribute to the measurement of cross-sectional area but would not contribute to force, either during voluntary contractions or by twitch interpolation, because the site of denervation is at the terminal axon level, well-distal to the site of electrical stimulation. This may explain why the deficit in specific force with humans is marginally greater, e.g., 26% in Phillips et al.(1992), than that reported from mouse muscle studied *in vitro*, e.g., 20% in Brooks and Faulkner (1988). In the *in vitro* model, the muscle fibers are stimulated directly; whether they are denervated or not, they will be activated and will contribute to the power or force developed.

No studies have tested hypotheses regarding possible architectural changes that could lead to specific weakness; it is known, however, that fiber lengths do not change with age (McCarter & McGee, 1987), and this suggests that angle of pennation (and therefore sarcomere packing) likely do not vary appreciably with age. Investigation of changes in muscle-tendon junctions may hold promise for discovery of age-related changes that might contribute to specific weakness of whole muscles and/or the propensity for injury (Tidball, 1991). Muscle-tendon junctions are the specialized areas at the end of each muscle fiber that transmit the force of myofibrils to the tendon. In old mice (30 mo), the macroscopic structural features of these junctions are unchanged by age (Trotter et al., 1987). However, the ratio of the area of force-transmitting membrane to force-generating myofibrils is reduced by up to 30% in muscles of the old compared to those of younger adults. Whether or not this morphological difference relates to specific weakness is subject to further study.

It is reasonable to postulate that in whole muscle preparations *in vitro*, the site of age-associated impairment in specific isometric force is in part within single fibers. The age-associated, specific isometric weakness might reflect, singularly or in combination, an alteration in the number of attached crossbridges in strong binding states, the number of crossbridges strongly bound in parallel per half sarcomere, or the force developed per crossbridge. Other intracellular changes that would be consistent with decreased specific force include elevated phosphate concentrations or lowered pH in cells of the old compared to young, as these factors are known to adversely affect force (Brandt et al., 1982; Edman & Mattiazzi, 1981; Metzger & Moss, 1987). However, the provocative result of Phillips et al. (1991), in which specific force during pliometric contractions did not decline with age as it does for isometric and miometric contractions, contradicts any hypothesis that reduced force is due to less contractile material per unit of cross-sectional area. There is evidence that specific force during pliometric contractions in humans is also age-independent (Vandervoot et al., 1990). Thus, of the options described above, it is unlikely that the number of crossbridges differs in limb muscles of old and young mammals.

The demonstration of specific isometric weakness of whole muscles (Brooks & Faulkner, 1988) led Susan Brooks and co-workers to hypothesize that such weakness was caused by intracellular changes. To test this hypothesis, she compared forces generated during miometric, isometric, and pliometric contractions of single permeabilized fibers isolated from limb muscles of young adult and old mice (Brooks, 1994). There was a rightward shift with age in the curve describing the relationship between isometric force and pCa, indicative of decreased calcium sensitivity with age (i.e., fewer bound calcium-binding sites on troponin). During miometric and isometric contractions, there were no differences in maximal specific force with age, but during pliometric contractions, the specific force of single fibers of the old was actually greater than in the young adult. This increased specific force in single fibers undergoing pliometric contractions is consistent with the observation of Phillips et al. (1991) that specific force during pliometric contractions of whole soleus muscles of mice was unaffected by age when force was expressed as a percentage of age-specific maximal isometric force (P_o). Brooks speculated that age-associated increases in force during a pliometric contraction may be caused by a relatively minor increase in the number of crossbridges attached during lengthening and a relatively large increase in force developed per attached crossbridge as a result of extension of the crossbridge (i.e., the crossbridge being strained to a greater degree). Brooks reconciled the observations at the levels of whole muscle and single fiber in the following way.

There appear to be two processes occurring concurrently, one intrinsic to myofibrils and the other extrinsic. During pliometric contractions, the increase in specific force in old single fibers is masked at the whole muscle level by a second process that decreases force production. The decrease is evident during isometric and miometric contractions in whole muscles, when specific weakness is evident. Brooks hypothesized that: 1) the presence of unknown inhibitory or excitatory factors in the cytosol *in vivo* may be affected by age, thereby resulting in differential activation, or 2) the electrical recruitment of fibers in whole muscles does not result in adequate calcium release, which leads to incomplete activation of the crossbridge cycle.

Velocity. The force-velocity relationship during miometric contractions of muscles of homogenous myosin phenotype is essentially unaffected by age. In limb muscles of rodents, the maximum velocity of shortening and the curvature of the entire hyperbolic force-velocity relationship during shortening contractions do not change with increasing age (Brooks & Faulkner, 1988; Fitts et al., 1984; Phillips et al., 1991). The fact that maximum velocity does not change, even though there is an increase in Type I MHC content due to Type II fiber atrophy, may reflect the fact that the fastest of the Type II fibers dictate the unloaded shortening velocity (Claflin & Faulkner, 1985). Alternatively, because the muscles typically studied *in vitro* are predominately of one myosin phenotype, the effect of a selective denervation of fast fibers would have little impact on maximal velocity of shortening. In strips of diaphragm muscle of hamsters, there is evidence that maximal and submaximal velocities of shortening do decline with age (Zhang & Kelsen, 1990). It is unknown if this difference between limb and diaphragm muscle is a function of the more heterogeneous myosin phenotype of diaphragm compared to the homogeneous soleus and EDL muscles, or is caused by the more chronic recruitment and loading pattern of diaphragm compared to limb muscles.

For humans, there is a paucity of studies on maximal velocity of shortening and age, in part because of the difficulty in making valid measurements. Nevertheless, Grimby and Saltin (1983) and Larsson et al. (1979) concluded that maximal speed of human muscle contraction is insensitive to advancing age.

The absence of an aging effect on contractile velocity studied in isolated muscles *in vitro* and in muscle groups *in situ* is in contrast to the previously described declines in human running speed of about 8% per decade after the third decade of life. Thus, it is clear that factors other than inherent velocity properties of muscle underscore the performance declines of the whole organism.

Power and Endurance. Brooks and Faulkner (1991) published an elegant paper on maximal and sustained power (i.e., endurance) in EDL muscles of immature, young adult, and old C57BL/6 mice. Maximal power of EDL muscle in old mice was about 30% less than that of young adults. Approximately one third of this decline was explained by atrophy, while the balance reflected intrinsic changes in the muscle fibers. These investigators established a progressive exercise test with the EDL muscle *in situ*, consisting of repeated contractions with progressive increases in duty cycles. (A duty cycle is the fraction of time that a muscle is active during repeated bouts of contraction.) In their study, the maximal absolute power (W) and the normalized power (W/kg) during single contractions were 20–30% less for immature mice and old mice, compared to the young adults (Figure 4-6). The ability to sustain absolute and normalized power at any given duty cycle was greatest for EDL muscles of immature mice, intermediate for young adults, and least for the old mice (Figure 4-7). Furthermore, the muscles of the immature mice could tolerate higher duty cycles than could muscles of the young adults; such tolerance was poorest in muscles of the old mice.

A prolonged relaxation time in muscles of old rodents is typically (Fitts et al., 1984; Gutmann & Syrovy, 1974; Phillips et al., 1991), but not always (Larsson & Edstrom, 1986), reported. This is likely mechanistically related to the reduced sustainable duty cycles in the old, described in the preceding paragraph. Vince Caiozzo (personal communication) has shown that the ability of the muscle to relax is one rate-limiting factor in the capacity of muscle to carry out cyclic work; with aging it may be that the impaired relaxation characteristics lead to a loss in the ability to extract positive work out of a muscle during cyclic behavior.

The capacity to sustain a given power output may also depend on the capacity of the involved musculature to buffer the metabolic acids that are produced during intense contractions. Spriet et al. (1991) examined the effect of aging on the *in situ* buffering capacity of fast-twitch muscles in rats. Ankle dorsiflexor muscles were stimulated according to a standardized protocol in young adult (10 mo) and old (24 mo) animals. Both hydrogen ion release and buffering capacity were found to be lower in the tibialis anterior muscles, but not in the EDL muscles, of the older rats. Most of the decrease in buffering capacity was due to a reduced capacity for buffering by proteins. It is interesting that muscle pH was unaffected by age at rest and following contractions. Although work performance was not measured by Spriet et al. (1991), it is possible that pH was unaffected by age because the muscles of the old rats produced less work than did the younger ones. Indeed, (Campbell et al, 1991) described an age-associated decrease in tetanic tension produced by ankle plantarflexor muscles subjected to standardized contractile protocols *in situ*; this decrease was linked to a decrease in anaerobic energy production in older muscles.

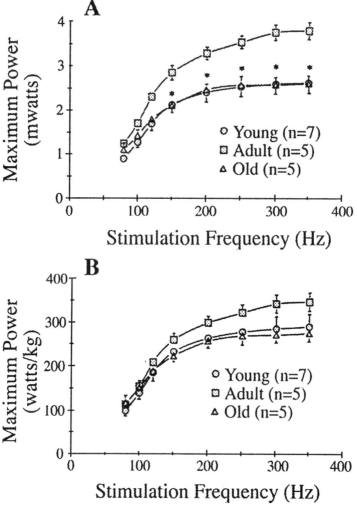

FIGURE 4-6. *Relationship of stimulation frequency (Hz) and (A) absolute maximal power (mW) and (B) normalized maximum power (W/kg) developed by EDL muscles in immature (O), young adult (□), and old (△) mice. Error bars are shown whenever the SE is larger than the symbol for the mean. The asterisks indicate values for muscles in immature and old mice that are different from the values for muscles in young adult mice (P <0.05). From Brooks and Faulkner (1991), with permission.*

Metabolic Pathways and Energy Flux

The impact of age-associated changes in muscle on metabolic processes requires at least three considerations. First, because there is significant muscular atrophy in old muscle, exercise performed at a given absolute intensity will be performed at a higher percentage of maximal exercise capacity. This establishes a relatively greater metabolic stress, thereby al-

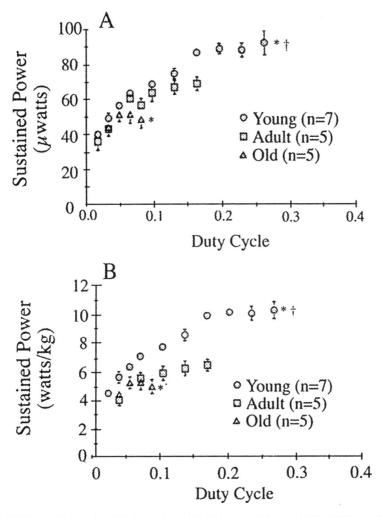

FIGURE 4-7. *Relationship of the duty cycle and (A) absolute sustained power (μW) and (B) normalized sustained power (W/kg) for EDL muscles in immature (O), young adult (□), and old (△) mice.* Error bars are shown whenever the SE is larger than the symbol for the mean. The asterisks indicate that the maximal values for muscles in immature and old mice are different from the maximal value for muscles in young adult mice, and the crosses indicate that the maximal value for immature mice is also greater than that for the old mice ($p < 0.05$). From Brooks and Faulkner (1991), with permission.

tering the integration among substrate pathways and systemic responses. Second, there is good evidence of an age-related impairment of glucose transport in skeletal muscle. This change will affect substrate availability and integration of metabolic pathways during exercise. Third, there is the potential for phenotypic change in the enzymes and substrates that support the diversity of metabolic pathways within muscle cells.

Muscle Atrophy. Sustained muscular performance requires an integrated response of substrate pools of glucose, glycogen, amino acids, free-fatty acids, and lactate in blood, muscle, adipose tissue, and liver. For example, the crossover concept (Brooks & Mercier, 1994) suggests that the pattern of substrate utilization at a given instant will reflect the interaction between the relative exercise intensity (greater intensity increases the use of carbohydrate) and the effect of any endurance training, which promotes lipid oxidation. Thus, with the inevitable decrease in muscle mass in older organisms, a given absolute intensity of exercise will represent a greater relative intensity compared to that in younger animals, and this effect seems likely to evoke greater carbohydrate utilization in the old. Likewise, an additional impetus for older mammals to utilize more carbohydrate during exercise will presumably occur secondary to the reduction in habitual physical activity that typically occurs.

Muscle atrophy with age leads to less available tissue mass for the conversion of one substrate moiety to another, as well as to an increase in the relative intensity of a given absolute level of exercise. These two factors will likely influence the dynamics of the Lactate Shuttle and Glucose Paradox. During exercise, lactate turnover is integral to the transfer of potential energy among cells within and between tissues. Carbon flux through the exchangeable lactate pool, i.e., the Lactate Shuttle, provides energy and supports blood glucose homeostasis (Brooks, 1985). A substantial portion of dietary carbohydrate is converted first to lactate, which is a gluconeogenic precursor that leads indirectly to storage of carbohydrate as liver glycogen, a concept termed the Glucose Paradox (Foster, 1984). Sites of conversion of dietary carbohydrate to lactate include skeletal muscle, intestine, red blood cells, liver, and white adipose tissue.

Glucose Uptake. If substrate availability is altered for any reason, the interaction among substrates will be affected. Since the observation of Spence in 1920, it has been recognized that glucose tolerance is impaired in persons over 60 y. Age-associated insulin resistance is primarily due to defects in skeletal muscle (Barnard et al., 1992). Numerous investigators have found in a variety of skeletal muscles that levels of Glut-4 protein, the insulin-regulated glucose transporter in plasma membranes, decrease in skeletal muscle during maturation but not during aging. For example, there is a decrease in Glut-4 in skeletal muscle between 2–3 mo and 12–13 mo, with no further change thereafter (Barnard et al., 1992; Cartee et al. 1993; Gulve et al., 1993; Kern et al., 1992). Although the pool of intracellular transporters does not change with age, Barnard et al. (1992) demonstrated that there is an age-associated decline in the insulin-receptor signaling system. Specifically, these investigators discovered a down-regulation of tyrosine kinase activity of the insulin receptor, which explains why there is an age-associated reduction in the translocation of transporters from the intracellular compartment to the sarcolemmal membrane.

Enzyme Activity. Age-associated differences were not apparent in enzymes of glycolysis (phosphorylase, phosphofructokinase, and lactate dehydrogenase) in the lateral gastrocnemius muscle of young adult (24 ± 1 y) and old (64 ± 1 y) men and women (Coggan 1992a). However, the mitochondrial enzymes studied (succinate dehydrogenase, citrate synthase, and β-hydroxyacyl-CoA-dehydrogenase) were approximately 25% lower in the old compared to the young adult. Obviously, interpretation of these biochemical changes in oxidative enzymes is complicated by the possibility that the older persons used their gastrocnemius muscles less than did the young and by the fact that the mitochondrial enzymes readily adapt to increased or decreased use (Faulkner & White, 1990). Others have reported a variety of associations between age and enzyme activities in specific fiber types (Borges & Essen-Gustavsson, 1989). Indeed, Coggan et al. (1990) reported that the activities of mitochondrial respiratory enzymes in skeletal muscles of endurance-trained master athletes were similar to or greater than those of young athletes with whom they were matched based on amount and intensity of habitual exercise.

McCully et al. (1993) studied skeletal muscle *in vivo* by magnetic resonance spectroscopy (MRS) in persons aged 29 y and 66 y during plantar-flexion exercise and *in vitro* by analyzing muscle samples obtained by needle biopsy during cycle ergometer exercise. They demonstrated an age-related impairment in muscle metabolism, as indicated by a decreased rate of phosphocreatine (PCr) repletion following a 5-min bout of standardized exercise that decreased PCr values to 50% of the initial resting value. This study also demonstrated a good correlation between *in vivo* and *in vitro* measurements of oxidative metabolism.

Using muscle biopsies and ^{31}P-MRS to study lateral gastrocnemius muscle metabolism during graded plantar flexion exercise in young (25 ± 2 y) and older (63 ± 3 y) untrained men, Coggan et al. (1993) found that the old men exhibited a greater metabolic stress during exercise than did the young. This interpretation was based on the older men's 50% greater rate of increase in the Pi-to-PCr ratio during graded increases in power output. After correcting for the 15% lesser plantarflexor muscle mass in the old, the rate of Pi-to-PCr increase was still 25% greater in the old subjects. Citrate synthase activity was about 20% less in the muscles of the old compared to the young. Thus, the authors attributed the age-associated difference in exercise response to a decrease in respiratory capacity and to muscle atrophy.

Mitochondrial DNA. Interest in the possibility that multiple mitochondrial DNA (mtDNA) deletions may occur in aging skeletal muscles has been spurred by a variety of human case study reports indicating that such deletions increase in aged tissues, as well as by the suggestions that mitochondria are mechanistically involved in the aging process (Wallace, 1992). Arnheim & Cortopassi (1992) acknowledged that the physiological impact of the deletions was unknown but also indicated that the deletions appeared to be only the "tip of the mutational iceberg." Lee et al. (1993) studied quadriceps muscles of 14 rhesus monkeys aged 6–27 y. (Note that the maximal life span of these animals is poorly characterized and is likely to be 40–45 y.) In young animals, DNA deletions were undetected, whereas a variety of deletion patterns was detected at progressively greater frequencies as the age increased beyond 13 y. Finally, evidence has also been found that mitochondrial DNA deletions accumulate with age in skeletal muscle of human subjects (Cortopassi et al., 1992). Thus, although the work is very preliminary, this approach may give insight into mechanisms of muscular deficits in the old.

Blood Flow and Capillarity

Sustained muscular performance requires a proper balance between energy supply and demand. Worsening endurance capacity of muscle from aged individuals likely reflects decreased blood flow (Irion et al., 1987) and decreased oxidative capacity (Cartee & Farrar, 1987; Farrar et al., 1981), possibly impairing energy balance (Dudley & Fleck, 1984). In human lateral gastrocnemius muscles, capillary density was approximately 25% lower in men and women whose average age was 64 y than in 26-year-old subjects (Coggan et al., 1992a) (Table 4-9). The reduced capillary density appeared to be due to an actual reduction in the total number of capillaries, as both capillary-to-fiber ratio and the number of capillaries in contact with each muscle cell were 19–40% lower in the aged. The reduction in capillarity has major importance for the ability of muscle to sustain power output over time (Faulkner & White, 1990).

The work of Coggan et al. (1992a) conflicts with other studies demonstrating a maintenance of capillarity with age. The comparisons in these other studies may be flawed, however, because they did not study appropriate young control subjects (Aniansson et al., 1981; Grimby et al., 1982) and because they compared *active* old to *inactive* young (Denis et al., 1986; Jakobsson et al., 1990). Parizkova et al. (1971) detected a plasticity in capillarity, and therefore the ease of confounding influences, when she demonstrated that the capillary-to-fiber ratio was similar in sedentary young men and very active old men, yet was low in sedentary old men. This is significant because, as described earlier, muscle atrophy occurs even in active adults.

Perfusion of muscle, of course, depends not only on the morphology of the microvasculature but also on its functional reactivity. In this vein, Cook et al. (1992) studied the microvasculature of the cremaster muscle in adult (12 mo) and old (24 mo) F344 male rats. These investigators found that the average capillary diameter did not differ between age groups, nor did the tortuosity index. However, the segmental lengths

TABLE 4-9. *Skeletal muscle capillarization (Mean ± SE).*

	Young Men	Old Men	Young Women	Old Women	Age Effect	Gender Effect
Capillary density (cap/mm²)	308 ± 16	228 ± 13	328 ± 19	248 ± 12	$p < .001$	n.s.
Capillary/fiber ratio	1.72 ± 0.14	1.39 ± 0.13	1.56 ± 0.15	0.94 ± 0.07	$p < .001$	$p < .01$
Capillaries in contract with each muscle fiber	4.39 ± 0.28	3.55 ± 0.30	3.96 ± 0.35	2.67 ± 0.16	$p < .001$	$p < .05$

From Coggan et al., (1992 A); with permission.

(i.e., the distance between adjacent branches) increased with age by 25–30%, resulting in statistical trends in 1st and 2nd order vessels and in significant differences in 3rd order vessels. When pharmacological agents were applied topically *in vivo*, the degree of vasoconstriction produced by norepinephrine was unaffected by age. The vasodilation produced by adenosine (10^{-3} M) was 74% less in 1st and 2nd order vessels with advancing age. Thus, it appears that the increase in vascular resistance in skeletal muscle during contraction in old rats can be explained on both morphological and functional bases. Because Proctor and Duling (1982), among others, showed that adenosine is partly responsible for exercise hyperemia, the reduced dilation in response to extracellular adenosine (Cook et al., 1992) could contribute to the increased vascular resistance. This in turn could impair muscle blood flow, as is observed in working skeletal muscle of aging rats (Irion et al., 1987, 1988). The reduced muscle blood flow was associated with impaired work capacity.

Nutritional Considerations in Age-Associated Neuromuscular Change

In terms of adaptations of skeletal muscles to endurance or resistance training, the effects of either undernutrition or of supplements beyond daily nutrition requirements have not been adequately studied. Nutritional status can have a profound, albeit secondary, effect if poor nutrition renders an organism unable to train at the desired intensity (Conlee, 1987). For example, diet-induced reductions in muscle and liver stores of glycogen might prevent the performance of an endurance activity at sufficient intensity and duration to allow adaptive changes. Neither short-term starvation (Parsons et al., 1982) nor lifetime dietary restriction of animals affects muscle fiber number (Daw et al., 1988), but each can cause muscle atrophy. Consequently, following dietary restriction, refeeding reverses muscle wasting by inducing fiber hypertrophy.

There is an interesting adaptation in the muscles of rats subjected to lifetime dietary restriction. In 12-mo-old rats that were raised in a specific pathogen-free barrier facility, the mass of soleus and EDL muscles was 21% and 23%, respectively, less than that of age-matched *ad libitum*-fed counterparts (Daw et al., 1988). However, at 27 mo there were no differences between food-restricted and *ad libitum* fed rats, not because the muscle mass in the food-restricted animals increased but rather because the muscle mass in the *ad libitum* fed rats decreased. Similar results were observed by Boreham et al., (1988) in a colony reared in conventional facilities. The convergence of values may reflect a decrease in the volitional dietary intake of rats as they age or an intrinsic age-associated change of unknown mechanism in the skeletal muscle.

MUSCLE ADAPTATIONS TO TRAINING IN THE OLD

Our understanding is emerging, at least at a descriptive level, of the role of chronic exercise training and the inherent potential for adaptation of skeletal muscle to changes in habitual activity concomitant with aging. Some studies with humans and animals suggest that the rate of adaptation of several variables to training is diminished with developing age (Skinner et al., 1982, Steinhagen-Thiessen et al., 1980); this has not been demonstrated unequivocally (Kovanen, 1989; Larsson, 1982). When training is of high intensity, the old adapt in a manner comparable to that of the young (Coggan et al., 1992b). Indeed, Cartee (1994) concluded in a review of exercise training in the old that the adaptability of muscle remains robust even in very old age.

Gutmann and Melichna (1972) noted that the age-associated changes in speed of contraction and in the frequency of spontaneous release of neuromuscular transmitter occurred later in life in the chronically recruited diaphragm muscle than in other skeletal muscles. Brown (1987) reported that daily forced training maintained the cross-sectional areas of Type I fibers in soleus muscles of rats aged 18 and 24 mo at values seen at 12 mo in control animals. These observations underscore the potential of regular physical activity to attenuate some of the age-related deficits in skeletal muscle.

Training Continuum

Muscular activity is determined by the interaction between the frequency of recruitment and the mechanical load during the contraction (Faulkner & White, 1990). Physical activity constitutes a continuum from very low levels during bed rest and limb immobilization, through nominal levels in sedentary individuals, to high levels in physically active persons. Toward the high end of the continuum, a dichotomy arises as endurance performers primarily increase the frequency of recruitment with minimal increase in mechanical load, whereas strength and power performers principally increase load at a relatively low frequency.

Adaptations in skeletal muscle result from habitual changes in the intensity, duration, and frequency of physical activity (Booth & Thomason, 1991; Faulkner & White, 1990; Roy et al., 1991). The adaptations are evidenced by changes in morphological, biochemical, and molecular properties that alter functional attributes of specific motor units. The criterion for an adaptive response is a qualitative or quantitative alteration in one or more specific muscle proteins: contractile, regulatory, structural, metabolic, or transport. Adaptations range from a diminished capacity to generate or maintain power in response to reduced physical activity, to an enhanced capacity to develop maximal power or maintain power following strength training and endurance training, respectively. Strength and endurance adaptations may occur independently or concurrently if appropriate training programs are used (Hickson et al., 1988).

Structure-Function Adaptations to Resistance Training

A 1988 study of resistance training of the legs of older men demonstrated convincingly that concomitant muscle enlargement, muscle fiber hypertrophy, and performance improvements can occur (Frontera et al., 1988). In this study, men aged 60–72 y increased by 110% the force they could develop during a one repetition maximum (1 RM) contraction of the knee extensors following a 12-wk strength training program (Figure 4-8). The increase in performance was accompanied by increases in quadriceps area (9%) (Figure 4-9) and in the cross-sectional area of Type I (34%) and Type II (28%) fibers in vastus lateralis muscle (Figure 4-10). For two groups of individuals ages 18–26 y and 67–72 y, Moritani and de Vries (1980) reported comparable strength gains of 30% and 22%, respectively. The gains in performance were accompanied by an overall increase in arm girth of 9% in the young and no change in the arm girth of the old. These results do not resolve whether the age-associated difference in the adaptive response was due to differences in the training stimulus (e.g., the young training at a higher percentage of maximal capacity than the old) or

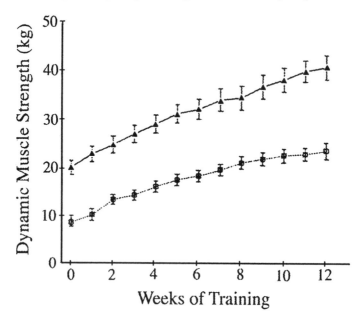

FIGURE 4-8. *Weekly measurements of dynamic muscle strength (1 repetition-maximum) of left knee extensors (- Δ -) and flexors (- □ -). Results are means ± SE. From Frontera et al. (1988), with permission.*

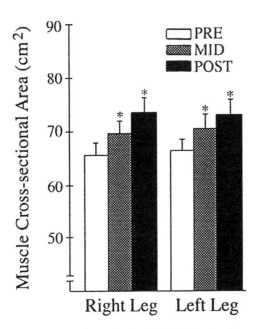

FIGURE 4-9. *Changes in cross-sectional area of right and left quadriceps muscles as calculated from planimetric analysis of computerized tomography scans.* Results are means ± SE. *Different from pretraining measurements (P < 0.005). From Frontera et al. (1988), with permission.

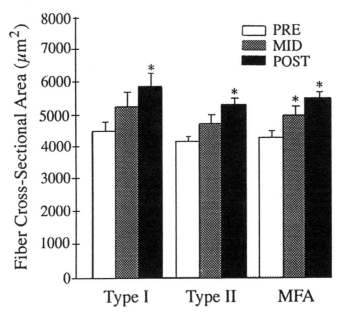

FIGURE 4-10. *Effects of strength training on areas of Type I and Type II fibers of vastus lateralis muscle of left leg.* Results are means ± SE. *Different from pretraining measurements (P < 0.005). From Frontera et al. (1988), with permission.

due to neuromuscular mechanisms underlying a gain in strength. Indeed, neural adaptations are evident in the response to training (Sale, 1988). Many studies have demonstrated positive adaptations to strength training in the old (Brown et al., 1990; Frontera et al., 1990; Greig et al., 1993; Grimby et al., 1992). Some have focused on resistance training in older women (Charette et al., 1991), including septuagenarians (Cress et al., 1991); others have focused on adaptations in the elbow flexors of old men (Roman et al., 1993), high-intensity strength training in nonagenarians (Fiatarone, et al., 1990), resistance training effects on regional bone mineral density (Menkes et al., 1993), and year-long resistance programs in old men and women (Pyka et al., 1994), to name just a few. The overall results of these investigations underscore the conclusion that old humans have a tremendous capacity to adapt to resistance training that leads to an increased capacity for physical performance. The interested reader is referred to Rogers and Evans (1993), who recently provided an excellent review of this literature.

In rodent studies, Klitgaard et al. (1989b) demonstrated that strength training (but not swimming) attenuated the age-associated atrophy of soleus and plantaris muscle. Tomanek and Woo (1970) induced growth in plantaris muscle in young (1.5 mo) and old adult (19 mo) rats by partial denervation of the gastrocnemius muscle coupled with treadmill walking. Plantaris muscle mass increased 39% in young rats and 25% in the old adult rats. However, this study is difficult to interpret because the gastrocnemius will reinnervate following partial denervation; thus, the "exercise" stimulus to the plantaris will change with time, probably at different rates in old and young animals.

The plasticity of soleus and plantaris muscles in 15-mo and 28-mo F344 rats was studied by examining the adaptive response to myectomy of synergist muscles (White et al., 1988). Hypotheses were tested regarding mass, muscle and fiber cross-sectional areas, and function. Following myectomy of synergists in 15-mo-old rats, average soleus muscles mass was 106% of the control value, whereas maximal isometric force (P_o) was not different from the control value. In 28-mo-old rats, mass and P_o were 133% and 150% of the respective control values. In 15-mo-old rats, plantaris muscle mass was 119% of the control value, while P_o was not different. In 28-mo-old rats, mass and P_o were 175% and 213% of the control values. While there was a trend toward increased fiber area due to myectomy of synergists, the high variability obviated significant differences. Adaptation to myectomy of synergists was greater in soleus and plantaris muscles from 28-mo compared to those from 15-mo rats.

Structure-Function Adaptations to Endurance Training

Some studies that evaluated training-induced muscular adaptations in the old have observed minimal adaptive responses. A question emerges about where the deficit falls in the dose-response equation. Is it because the training stimulus is less in the old, or is it a result of a diminished adaptive response to an equivalent stimulus in the old? In a relatively intense training program, Coggan et al. (1992b) trained 23 men and women (64 ± 3 y) for 9–12 mo at 80% of maximal heart rate for 45 min/d, 4 d/wk. The $\dot{V}O_2$max increased 23%. Biopsies of lateral gastrocnemius muscle revealed no change in percentage of Type I fibers but a small decrease and increase in Type IIb and IIa, respectively. The training increased the cross-sectional areas of Type I and IIa fibers by about 11%. Capillary density increased 20% with training; capillary-to-fiber ratio and number of adjacent capillaries per fiber also increased. Training decreased lactate dehydrogenase activity by 21% and increased activities of measured mitochondrial enzymes by 24–55%. These authors compared their results with those from young subjects and concluded that given an adequate stimulus, the skeletal muscles of old men and women adapt to endurance training in a fashion similar to that in the young.

Alterations in the recruitment patterns of skeletal muscle can also be approached experimentally by providing atypical innervation to a skeletal muscle, in studies of so-called cross-innervation (more properly called cross-reinnervation). In experiments of this type, the nerve to a muscle such as the EDL is cut, and the nerve to another muscle, such as the soleus, is implanted in the EDL. Because the nerves have different habitual levels of recruitment frequency, the reinnervated muscle fibers will be stimulated to adapt their morphological and functional properties. The formerly fast EDL muscle, which normally receives periodic, high-frequency recruitment stimuli, now receives chronic, low-frequency stimulation via the slow nerve that previously supplied the soleus. Clark and White (1991) used this approach to test hypotheses regarding the adaptive response of the EDL muscle of 12-mo and 29-mo rats following denervation and cross-reinnervation by the soleus nerve. The adaptive response to cross-reinnervation of myosin heavy-chain phenotype in *innervated* fibers was similar at both ages. However, there was an age-associated decrease in the ability of neurons to reinnervate the motor endplate area after nerve section. This was indicated by a marked increase in the number of non-innervated motor endplates in cross-reinnervated muscles of the old compared to the young adult rats, as well as by a decreased neuronal density in the innervated motor endplates of the old compared to the young adults.

Metabolic Adaptations in Skeletal Muscle to Endurance Training

Phospoglycerate kinase (PGK) is one of several glycolytic enzymes in skeletal muscle and other tissues that become more resistant to heat inactivation as animals age (Sharma et al., 1980). Rothstein (1985) concluded that the structural modifications of PGK with age are purely conformational, and this was confirmed by Yuh and Gafni (1987) when they reported that the heat lability of PGK in muscles of the old became fully rejuvenated to that seen in muscles of young animals when the protein structure of the enzyme was unfolded and refolded.

Zhou et al. (1990) tested the hypothesis that aging of PGK in knee extensors and flexors of old rats may be attenuated by a lifetime of treadmill training, i.e., from 2–22 mo; the study included control groups of untrained rats aged 4.5 mo (young untrained) and 22 mo (old untrained). The results showed the expected decrease in heat lability of PGK from 4.5 mo to 22 mo in the untrained rats, whereas the values for the old trained rats were essentially unchanged from those of the young untrained animals. This training-induced maintenance of PGK in the young form shows that adaptation to endurance training can occur at the molecular level. It remains for further experimentation to address whether this PGK adaptation stems from an enhanced enzyme turnover (i.e., a given PGK molecule is retained in the cell for too brief a time to allow aging modifications to develop), or from increased protection against oxidation, which is the first step in PGK aging.

Sanchez et al. (1983) found that muscles of old rats that had been trained exhibited a marked increase in the activities of several glycolytic enzymes that ordinarily decline with age. In young rats, on the other hand, endurance training effects on glycolytic enzymes are either negative, absent, or moderately positive (Baldwin et al., 1973), whereas training did enhance the activities of respiratory enzymes of young rats (Baldwin et al., 1972). Examining training-induced adaptations in other variables, Steinhagen-Thiessen et al. (1980) found that forced running by CWI mice aged 27 mo induced negative adaptations in creatine kinase activity, soluble protein content, and total DNA, whereas with younger mice the adaptations were positive.

Mitochondrial function was studied in plantarflexor muscles of untrained rats and of rats trained for endurance over their life spans (Farrar et al., 1981). The amount of intermyofibrillar mitochondrial protein decreased with age, whereas training increased the mitochondrial protein contents of both intermyofibrillar and subsarcolemmal fractions of muscle extracts, and enhanced state-3 respiration, i.e., the oxidative capacity of mitochondria when substrate is unlimited.

In a study of the metabolic response of the lateral gastrocnemius muscle to graded plantar flexion exercise in men aged 25 y and 63 y, Coggan et al. (1993) found that old trained men demonstrated less metabolic stress during exercise than did old untrained men. The lesser stress was evidenced by a training-induced decrease in the rate of increase in the Pi-to-PCr ratio during standardized graded exercise protocols. However, this rate of increase in the Pi-to-PCr ratio in the old trained was still about 10% and 75% greater than in untrained and trained young men, respectively. These conclusions hold for the absolute data, as well as when data were corrected for age-associated differences in muscle cross-sectional area, muscle volume, and peak power. Thus, it is evident that training status attenuated, but did not prevent, the age-associated decrements in these variables.

Microcirculatory Adaptations to Training in the Old

Yang et al. (1994) showed that old animals (21-mo F-344 rats) with experimentally induced peripheral arterial insufficiency will develop improvements in muscular performance with endurance training that are unrelated to an increase in peak muscle blood flow. These investigators subjected the old rats to bilateral stenosis of the femoral arteries. The stenosis impaired exercise hyperemia, but not resting muscle blood flow. Half of the animals trained by walking twice a day on a treadmill for 8 wk under modest exercise conditions (20 m/min; 15% grade), whereas, the other rats were cage-sedentary for the 8-wk period. The treadmill performance capacity of the trained rats increased fourfold over that of the untrained rats. When hind limb muscles were studied *in situ*, those of the trained rats demonstrated an enhanced endurance performance and peak $\dot{V}O_2$ relative to the untrained. The training-induced improvements were due to increased oxygen extraction, which was attributed to the enriched capillarity and mitochondrial content of trained muscles. Blood flow was unaffected by the training. Similar training-induced adaptations have been noted in adult rats (Erney et al., 1991; Yang et al., 1991).

Implications for Normal and Elite Human Performance

It is evident that the trained, at any age, have the capacity for enhanced physical performance compared to the untrained, and that age-associated declines in performance exist for all individuals. However, with increased habitual physical capacity, life's daily activities are carried out at a lower percentage of one's maximal capacity. This is advantageous, not only for neuromotor control, but also for reducing the chance of injury. Indeed, the higher the relative force generated during activity, the greater the chance for muscle injury (McCully & Faulkner, 1985, 1986).

A study by Coggan et al. (1990) on young and old endurance athletes demonstrates how skeletal muscle adaptations can partially or fully compensate, at least from an exercise performance perspective, for other systemic age-associated declines, such as a decrease $\dot{V}O_2$max. The study matched masters athletes (63 ± 6 y) with young runners (26 ± 3 y) on the basis of the intensity and volume of training and on performance times for 10,000 m ($42:03 \pm 2:57$ and $41:41 \pm 3:36$ min for old and young, respectively). Despite comparable performance times, the $\dot{V}O_2$max was greater in the young age-matched runners when compared to the old runners in absolute (L/min, + 18%) and relative terms (mL·kg^{-1}·min^{-1}, + 13%). Fiber type profiles did not differ, with both groups having about

60% Type I fibers and few Type IIb fibers. Activities of succinate dehydrogenase and β-hydroxyacyl-CoA dehydrogenase were 31% and 24% higher, respectively, in the old athletes than in the young, whereas lactate dehydrogenase activity was 46% lower in the old athletes. The capillary-to-fiber ratio was 31% greater in the old athletes. However, the numbers of capillaries per mm^2 of muscle cross-sectional area were similar in the two groups, owing to the 34% larger area of Type I fibers in the old athletes. The different phenotype of skeletal muscle in master athletes compared to the young may explain the comparable performance times and ability to compete at higher percentages of $\dot{V}O_2$max.

MEDICAL AND CLINICAL CONCERNS

Neuromuscular Contributions to Falls in Older Persons

Falls occur in 30–50% of the American population over age 65 at a rate of one or more per year (Tinetti et al., 1986), and these falls often result in fractures and other injuries. Furthermore, the fear of falling is enough to functionally disable many individuals (Hagberg, 1994; Maki et al., 1991). Adequate strength, flexibility, and balance are important for traversing stairs and curbs, for avoiding clutter, and for decreasing the proneness for injury (Baker & Harvey, 1985; Nevitt et al., 1989; Tinetti et al., 1988). Although the evidence falls short of establishing a causal relationship, the inverse association between muscular strength and propensity for falls is highly suggestive that strength is, at a minimum, a major contributing factor to falls (Lipsitz et al., 1991; Robbins et al., 1989). Although age-induced alterations in sensory function clearly contribute to impairments in balance and to the increased incidence of falls (Whipple et al., 1993), there is also evidence that old persons with a propensity for falls possess lower strength in knee and ankle flexors and extensors than do the old who fall less often (Whipple et al., 1987). Falls, in turn, dramatically increase the risk for fracture, leading often to premature morbidity and mortality (Hadley et al., 1993).

Lipsitz et al. (1991) studied ambulatory frail old (87 y) people, of which 70 were recurrent fallers and 56 were not. Because many associations were described, it is impossible to identify one or two as the cause of falling, but it is interesting to note that the fallers of both genders could not stand up from a chair without pushing off, implying insufficient development of strength in the lower extremities.

Specific training programs can be designed to remedy balance and flexibility inadequacies. Brown and Holloszy (1991) demonstrated in persons aged 60–71 y who had balance deficits that a 3-mo program of activities for flexibility, balance, gait, and strength improved hip range of motion and one-legged balance, with eyes either open or closed. Three months of flexibility exercises can produce average improvements of 22% in range of motion of most major joints (Munns, 1981). Hu and Woollacott (1994a, 1994b) have demonstrated that multisensory balance-training programs can optimize the postural responses of older adults to perturbations in balance. While these improvements are expected to reduce the incidence of falls, follow-up studies have not yet been published to verify such a reduction.

Nevitt et al. (1991) found that the risk of minor injury during an accidental fall was increased in persons with slower hand-reaction times and decreased strength, as indexed by grip strength. In regard to the prophylaxis for falls, one positive correlate to endurance training is occasional improvement in reaction time and other motor skills, as well as increased strength of the involved musculature (Dustman et al., 1984; Sherwood & Seider, 1979; Sipila & Suominen, 1991a, 1991b, 1993; Spirduso & Clifford, 1978). However, the correlated improvement in neurocognitive function is not found in all training studies. For example, reaction times were unaltered in a 6-mo endurance training intervention involving persons aged 70–79 y (Panton et al., 1990). Also, it should be noted that increased strength is not normally a correlate of endurance training in younger populations; strength adaptations induced by exercise occur only when the challenge is of sufficient intensity relative to the muscle's current strength. In the old, exercise performed at a low absolute intensity may be at high relative intensity, thereby inducing muscle hypertrophy. Similar parallels were seen in studies of regenerating rat muscle, which grew as an adaptation to moderate running (White et al., 1984), whereas such an adaptive growth in response to endurance training is not seen in normal rat muscle.

As described earlier, resistance exercise training causes marked improvements in the muscular strength of older persons. For example, Frontera et al. (1988) and Fiatarone et al. (1990) found 107%–227% increases in strength of knee extensors and flexors in men aged 60 y to 96 y as a result of 2–3 mo of specific resistance training. Thus, it is clear that if strength is a factor in an older individual's propensity to fall, then specific remediation will be successful and should be part of the person's exercise prescription.

Mobility and Activities of Daily Life

The hypothesis that physical frailty is fully preventable or reversible, although honorable and understandable in its intent, is unsupported by the scientific evidence. As frailty has multiple domains, in addition to physical structure and function, any attempt to distinguish the physical from other overlapping domains is inherently flawed. By way of example, Guralnik and Simonsick (1993) noted that impairments in daily function may arise from physical, cognitive, and/or sensory dysfunction, and that frail people frequently have difficulty in multiple domains. The potential of exercise training as a prophylactic or therapeutic tool to enhance muscle function can only be realized if: 1) adequate muscle fibers are innervated, 2) the person is willing and able to recruit and mechanically load the motor units, and 3) joint pain or other impairments do not prevent persons from engaging in a sufficient exercise stress to induce the desired adaptations. Even if one meets these criteria, it will not be possible to fully reverse or permanently prolong the age-associated decline in muscular function.

In 1987, it was estimated that more than 2 million non-institutionalized persons over the age of 65 y had difficulty in rising from or lowering into a chair or bed, an alarming 8% of the aged population (National Center for Health Statistics, 1987). The reasons for this include the amount of muscle strength that can be coordinated to the task, relevant joint flexibility, and ultimately the biomechanics of the movement. Wheeler et al. (1985) found that exaggerated trunk and knee flexion, as well as greater knee extensor muscle EMG activity, was required by healthy older women who otherwise had no obvious difficulty in rising. However, as years pass and muscle mass and strength decline, the enhanced reliance on muscle power *per se* will require a greater percentage of the muscle's capacity and will increase the risk of injury, the incidence of failure to perform the task, or both.

Alexander et al. (1991) conducted a sophisticated biomechanical analysis of chair rising in young (23 y) and older subjects who were either *able* (72 y) or *unable* (84 y) to rise without the use of armrests. Even the *able* old, who required the same total time to rise as did the young, spent a greater fraction of the rise-time in the first phase of rising (longer time of leg, thigh, and trunk rotation) when not using their hands, and in thigh rotation when using their hands. The old *unable* subjects (who were required to use their hands to rise) took longer to rise, extended their thighs less, and flexed their trunks more than the *able* old subjects did when they used their arms voluntarily. Also, the *unable* old used much larger ratios of armrest-force to body weight, implying that the relative stress to existing musculature was greater during rising from a chair than it was for the *able* old.

There is a hypotensive adaptation to resistance training that has positive implications for avoiding cerebrovascular accidents. McCartney et al. (1993) examined the effect of 12 wk of resistance training on the strength of older males (66 ± 1 y), and found that training increased the 1 RM by 24% in legs and 54% in arms. Moreover, after training, there was a marked attenuation of heart rate and arterial pressure during exercise when subjects lifted the same absolute loads. After training, the heart rate and blood pressure responses for the same relative loads (greater absolute loads after training) were the same as those recorded before training. This experiment shows that appropriate physical training can reduce the exertion-induced elevation of blood pressure that occurs when older people perform their daily routine activities, such as rising from chairs.

Muscular Injury in Active Older Adults

In laboratory animals, degeneration of skeletal muscle fibers and subsequent regeneration follows from widespread damage to the fibers that can be caused by a variety of insults, including free grafting operations, other mechanical and chemical trauma, ischemia, exposure to extreme heat and cold, and some diseases (White & Devor, 1993). Subtle and focal areas of degeneration-regeneration in skeletal muscle can result from excessive stretch, specific types and duration of exercise, particularly those emphasizing eccentric contractions (Armstrong, 1990), and denervation or mild compression. An ongoing presence of a population of regenerating skeletal muscle fibers may be an inevitable and normal consequence of an active lifestyle.

The potential for contraction-induced muscle injury leading to degeneration and regeneration is increased in older mammals (Brooks & Faulkner, 1990). In mice, repeated eccentric contractions induce more injury in muscles of old rodents, compared to young adult and immature rodents (Zerba et al., 1990). Similarly, when injury is induced to the same degree, muscles in old mice recover less well than those of immature and young adult mice (Brooks & Faulkner 1990).

It is generally accepted that the restorative capacity of mammalian organs declines with age (Sidorova, 1976). An early study by Gutmann and Carlson (1976) showed that freely transplanted muscle into old rats regenerates poorly compared to muscle transplanted into young rats. Also, in a qualitative histological study, Sadeh (1988) found that regeneration following bupivacaine-induced degeneration was threefold slower in 24-mo rats compared to 3-mo rats. Furthermore, Carlson and Faulkner (1989) demonstrated that muscles of either young or old rats grafted into young host rats regenerated better than muscles from animals of either age grafted into old rats, as evidenced by a twofold increase in mass and a threefold increase in maximal isometric force by 60 d. This study led to the conclusion that the poor regenerative capacity of muscles in old animals is a function of the environment for regeneration provided by the old host organism.

With aging there is a diminished response of axons to regenerate or reinnervate motor endplates (MEPs) following perturbation (Clark & White, 1991; Pestronk et al., 1980). Impaired ability for reinnervation in old hosts is one factor contributing to the decline in capacity for regeneration with age (Carlson & Faulkner, 1988). Obviously, the consequence of impaired reinnervation concomitant with transplantation would reduce nerve-muscle fiber interaction and impair the ability to generate and maintain power.

A single 45-min bout of "eccentric" exercise on a cycle ergometer at a power eliciting 80% $\dot{V}O_2$max in untrained young (24 ± 1 y) and old men (61 ± 1 y) produced similar increases in whole-body protein breakdown (Fielding et al., 1991). However, there is evidence that myofibrillar proteolysis may have contributed more to whole-body protein breakdown in the older group.

Pollock et al. (1991) reported injury rates coincident with training of the old (ages 70-79 y). In a walk/jog training program, only one of nine injuries occurred during the first half of the study, when walking alone was used as the training mode. An additional 8 injuries occurred in the 14 subjects who began walk/jog intervals at the mid-point of the study, giving an injury rate of 57% for this phase of training. This compares unfavorably with results for younger groups in similar studies, in which training elicited injury rates of only 18% and 41% in those aged 20-35 y and 49-65 y, respectively (Pollock et al., 1976, 1977). There was a significant risk of injury when subjects underwent tests of maximal strength, but not when they participated in resistance training. There also appeared to be a greater incidence of exercise-induced injury in older women, compared to old men (Carroll et al., 1992), the basis of which is unclear.

Although the etiology of injury is a complex matter, it appears that the vast majority of injuries can be assigned to the high forces associated with ground impact (Carroll et al., 1992). These observations in the field with human subjects are correlated with findings in rodents that the high force associated with pliometric muscle contractions is the primary factor in inducing the sequelae of degeneration and regeneration (McCully & Faulkner, 1986).

DIRECTIONS FOR FUTURE RESEARCH

Applied Research Needs

To the extent that age-associated declines are related to physical inactivity, appropriate training programs need to be developed that provide necessary physiological stimuli as well as the proper psychological components to augment adherence and to accommodate the unique social and cultural needs and expectations of the old. In addition to the high or low loading during contractions and the short or long duration of the periods of activity, training variables include the frequency of the training sessions per week and the total duration of the training sessions in months and years. However, because it is clear that there are unavoidable intrinsic age-associated impairments in muscle structure and function that are unexplained by physical inactivity, it is unreasonable to aspire to a goal of full compensation for age-associated muscular deficits. We can learn from history and empirical evidence that no matter how trained one is, there are deficits in the muscular structure and function of the old compared to their younger counterparts. However, there is a great need to focus experimental and clinical work more on the elementary physical activities routinely employed in domestic, occupational, and recreational tasks and less on peak elite human performance applicable to only a few persons. To identify and implement achievable training protocols that forestall the development of frailty to the point of dependence, or to intervene with acute training to push an individual back over the threshold between impaired mobility and dependence to sufficient mobility and independence is a worthwhile goal.

Much of the current research on training-induced muscular adaptations in the old are "high end" interventions or studies of athletes. Research needs to be directed, particularly in light of the demographics of an aging population in the United States, to identify optimal and minimal interventions to elicit useful improvements in neuromuscular structure and function.

The implications for muscle structure and function derived from cross-sectional studies showing differences between young and old muscle, should provoke more definitive studies to identify the causal relationships. For example, the reductions in Type II area, capillarization, and activities of mitochondrial respiratory enzymes seem related, yet it is not clear if one of these variables starts the entire cascade of decline. Are there interventions that can minimize the onset of, or orchestration of, decline? How do the age-associated changes affect the ability to generate and maintain power under a variety of loading and velocity conditions, and how do they integrate with the cardiovascular system and with other systems to sustain human performance? At what point are deficits so great that dependence on others is necessary and independence is lost?

Basic Research Needs

Generally, a mechanistic understanding of why cells age is of fundamental importance. Furthermore, the extent of hypoplasia needs to be studied further in humans. Definitive studies are difficult to design with humans, but the existing data indicate a significant loss of fibers, particularly in the later years (Lexell et al., 1988). This is unlike the case in rodents, where hypoplasia can explain only 25% of muscle atrophy. The discrepancy between models needs attention, and the identification of exercise or pharmacological interventions to slow the rate of denervation and enhance the rate of reinnervation seems worthy.

The cause(s) of specific weakness of skeletal muscle requires further delineation. Particularly, an understanding of the relationships among neural, endocrine, and muscular factors is needed.

Many morphological and physiological changes associated with aging have been described. Indeed, sufficient evidence exists to encourage hypotheses about the mechanisms underlying motor unit remodeling, for example. However, the field has followed somewhat of a reverse hierarchical approach. Early studies were focused at the whole organism, with respect to muscular capacity and adaptive responses to training. With time, investigations have focused on the whole limb, the muscle, motor units, and single fibers. Each level of organization brings unique insights, but each further reduction in level of organization increases the loss of integration of biological processes. Nevertheless, an area of promising direction remains at the molecular level, which is a frontier insufficiently explored with respect to skeletal muscle, aging, and plasticity. Other well-designed studies, at cellular through organismal levels, must endeavor to go beyond the descriptive and identify causal relationships and genuine mechanisms. For example, greater insight into mitochondrial DNA deletions, as well as determining the potential for similar events in other contractile regulatory, structural, metabolic, and transport proteins in skeletal muscle, may help explain the inevitable development of physical frailty, at least with respect to the ability to generate and sustain muscular power.

With regard to plasticity, i.e., the capacity to adapt to stimuli, we need to learn more about protein turnover, protein synthesis, and protein degradation mechanisms, transcriptional and translational processes, etc. These investigations should be targeted, at least initially, on the regulation of gene products involved in the regulation of muscle contraction and relaxation and of energy metabolism. It is unclear whether muscle of aged organisms has the same capacity or cellular machinery to adapt to precise stimuli of known magnitude and duration as does muscle of young organisms. Moreover, little is known regarding the mechanistic impact of factors in addition to physical activity on muscle plasticity of the aged. Areas that hold promise for discovery include possible reductions in growth factors or in muscle responsiveness to growth factors, as well as changes in anabolic hormones and other hormones that impact metabolism. Applications of this more experimental work will follow, for example, in tailoring physical activity paradigms to the inherent adaptive potential of any given individual or population subset.

SUMMARY

There is an inevitable reduction with age in the ability to produce and sustain muscular power. This age-associated phenomenon is of profound importance and consequence for the maintenance of posture, locomotion, and the ability to perform life's daily activities in the home or workplace. The age-associated decline in muscular strength and endurance also affects the performance capacity of recreational and elite performers in sport and dance. Neuromuscular impairments are likely to contribute to an increased incidence of falls and muscle injury and to a reduced regenerative capacity of muscle.

In some circumstances and for some variables, physical inactivity may contribute to the age-associated decline in muscle structure and function, but this is by no means the predominant explanation. There are inevitable age-associated changes intrinsic to skeletal muscle and its component molecules, cells, and organelles. The cause(s) of the intrinsic changes is(are) unknown. The intrinsic aging factors predominate over those that can be ascribed to physical inactivity.

Physical training of the appropriate intensity, duration, and frequency can induce adaptations in skeletal muscle of older mammals. In many cases, the magnitudes of the adaptations are similar to those observed in the young. However, it will not be possible to fully reverse or permanently prolong the age-associated decline in muscular function. If one lives a long life, the neuromuscular declines are inevitable.

ACKNOWLEDGMENTS

The author thanks Keith Baar, Steve Devor, and Ron Gomes for their review of earlier drafts of this chapter and reviewers Ken Baldwin, Ron Terjung, and Larry Spriet for their thoughtful critiques.

BIBLIOGRAPHY

Alexander, N.B., A.B. Schultz, and D.N. Warwick (1991). Rising from a chair: effects of age and functional ability on performance biomechanics. *J. Gerontol.* 46:M91–M98.
Aniansson, A., G. Grimby, and M. Hedberg (1992). Compensatory muscle fiber hypertrophy in elderly men. *J. Appl. Physiol.* 73:812–816.
Aniansson, A., G. Grimby, M. Hedberg, and M. Krotkiewski (1981). Muscle morphology, enzyme activity and muscle strength in elderly men and women. *Clin. Physiol.* 1:73–86.
Anver, M.R., and B.J. Cohen (1979). Lesions associated with ageing. In: H.J. Baker, J.R. Lindsey, and S.H. Wersbroth (eds.) *The Laboratory Rat, Vol. 1.* New York: Academic Press, pp. 378–399.
Appell, H.J. (1984). Proliferation of motor endplates induced by increased muscular activity. *Int. J. Sports Med.* 5:125–129.
Armstrong, R.B. (1990). Initial events in exercise-induced muscular injury. *Med. Sci. Sports Exerc.* 22:429–435.
Arnheim, N.A., and G. Cortopassi (1992). Deleterious mitochondrial DNA mutations accumulate in aging human tissues. *Mutat. Res.* 275:157–167.
Asmussen, E. (1980). Aging and exercise. In: S.M. Horvath, and M.K. Yousef (eds.) *Environmental Physiology: Aging, Heat and Altitude (Sec. 3).* New York: Elsevier, North Holland, pp. 419–428.
Baker, S.B., and A.H. Harvey (1985). Fall injuries in the elderly. *Clin. Geriatr. Med.* 1:501–508.
Baldwin, K.M., G.H. Klinkerfuss, R.L. Terjung, P.A. Mole, and J.O. Holloszy (1972). Respiratory capacity of white, red and intermediate muscle, adaptive response to exercise. *Am J. Physiol.* 222:373–378.
Baldwin, K.M., W.W. Winder, R.L. Terjung, and J.O. Holloszy (1973). Glycolytic enzymes in different types of skeletal muscle: adaptation to exercise. *Am. J. Physiol.* 225:962–966.
Barker, D., and M.C. Ip (1966). Sprouting and degeneration of mammalian motor axons in normal and de-afferentated skeletal muscle. *Proc. Roy. Soc. (Biol.)* 163:538–554.
Barnard, R.J., L.O. Lawani, D.A. Martin, J.F. Youngren, R. Singh, and S.H. Scheck (1992). Effects of maturation and aging on the skeletal muscle glucose transport system. *Am. J. Physiol.* 262:E619–626.
Bassey, E.J., M.A. Fiatarone, E.F. O'Neill, M. Kelly, W.J. Evans, and L.A. Lipsitz (1992). Leg extensor power and functional performance in very old men and women. *Clinical Science* 82:321–327.
Berman, H.A., and M.M. Decker (1985). Changes with aging in skeletal muscle molecular forms of butrylcholinesterase and acetylcholinesterase. *Fed. Proc.* 44:1633 (abstract).

Betz, W.J., J.H. Caldwell, and R.R. Ribchester. (1980). Sprouting of active nerve terminals in partially inactive muscles of the rat. *J. Physiol.* 303:281-297.

Booth, F.W. (1989). Letter to the editor. *J. Appl.Physiol.* 67:1299-1300.

Booth, F.W., and D.B. Thomason (1991). Molecular and cellular adaptation of muscle in response to exercise: perspectives of various models. *Physiol. Rev.* 71:541-585.

Boreham, C.A.G., P.W. Watt, P.E. Williams, B.J. Merry, G. Goldspink, and D.F. Goldspink (1988). Effects of aging and chronic dietary restriction on the morphology of fast and slow muscles of the rat. *J. Anat.* 157:111-125.

Borges, O. (1989). Isometric and isokinetic knee extension and flexion torque in men and women aged 20-70. *Scand. J. Rehab. Med.* 21:45-53.

Borges, O., and B. Essen-Gustavsson (1989). Enzyme activities in type I and II muscle fibres of human skeletal muscle in relation to age and torque development. *Acta Physiol. Scand.* 136:29-36.

Brandt, P.W., R.N. Cox, M. Kawai, and T. Robinson (1982). Regulation of tension in skinned muscle fibers: effect of cross-bridge kinetics on apparent calcium-sensitivity. *J. Gen. Physiol.* 70:997-1016.

Brooks, G.A. (1985). Glycolytic end product and oxidative substrate during sustained exercise in mammals—the "lactate shuttle." In: R. Gilles (ed.) *Circulation, Respiration and Metabolism: Current Comparative Approaches.* Berlin:Springer-Verlag, pp. 208-218.

Brooks, G.A., and J. Mercier (1994). The balance of carbohydrate and lipid utilization during exercise: the "crossover" concept. *J. Appl. Physiol.* 76:2253-2261.

Brooks, S.V. (1994). Single muscle fibers: intrinsic changes in mechanical properties. Symposium paper, 1994 annual meeting of the American College of Sports Medicine. Indianapolis, IN: American College of Sports Medicine.

Brooks, S.V., and J.A. Faulkner (1988). Contractile properties of skeletal muscles from young adult and aged mice. *J. Physiol. (Lond.)* 404:71-82.

Brooks, S.V., and J.A. Faulkner (1991). Maximum and sustained power of extensor digitorum longus muscles from young, adult, and old mice. *J. Gerontol.: Biol. Sci.* 46:B28-33.

Brooks, S.V., and J.A. Faulkner (1990). Recovery from contraction-induced injury to skeletal muscles in young and old mice. *Am. J. Physiol.* 258:C436-C442.

Brooks, S,V., and J.A. Faulkner (1994). Skeletal muscle weakness in old age: underlying mechanisms. *Med. Sci. Sports Exerc.* 26:432-439.

Brown, A.B., N. McCartney, and D.G. Sale (1990). Positive adaptations to weight-lifting training in the elderly. *J. Appl. Physiol.* 69:1725-1733.

Brown, M., and J.O. Holloszy (1991) Effects of a low intensity exercise program on selected physical performance characteristics of 60- to 71-yr-olds. *Aging* 3:129-139.

Brown, M.B. (1987). Change in fiber size, not number, in ageing skeletal muscle. *Age Ageing* 16:244-248.

Brown, M.C., R.L. Holland, and W.G. Hopkins (1981). Motor nerve sprouting. *Ann. Rev. Neurosci.* 4:17-42.

Bruce, S.A., D. Newton, and R.C. Woledge (1989). Effect of age on voluntary force and cross-sectional area of human adductor pollicis muscle. *Quart. J. Exp. Physiol.* 74:359-362.

Caccia, M.R., J.B. Harris, and M.A. Johnson (1979). Morphology and physiology of skeletal muscle in aging rodents. *Muscle Nerve* 2:202-212.

Campbell, C.B., D.R, Marsh, and L.L. Spriet (1991). Anaerobic energy provision in aged skeletal muscle during tetanic stimulation. *J. Appl. Physiol.* 70:1787-1795.

Campbell, M.J., A.J. McComas, and F. Petito (1973). Physiological changes in ageing muscles. *J. Neurol. Neurosug. Psychiatry* 36:74-182.

Carlson, B.M., and J.A. Faulkner (1989). Muscle transplantation between young and old rats: age of host determines recovery. *Am. J. Physiol.* 256:C1262-C1266.

Carlson, B.M., and J.A. Faulkner (1988). Reinnervation of long-term denervated rat muscle freely grafted into an innervated limb. *Exper. Neurol.* 102:50-56.

Carroll, J.F., M.L. Pollock, J.E. Graves, S.H. Leggett, D.L. Spitler, and D.T. Lowenthal (1992). Incidence of injury during moderate- and high-intensity walking training in the elderly. *J. Gerontol.* 47:M61-M66.

Cartee, G.D. (1994). Aging skeletal muscle: response to exercise. In: J.O. Holloszy (ed.) *Exercise and Sport Sciences Reviews,* Vol. 22. Baltimore, MD: Williams & Wilkins, pp. 91-120.

Cartee, G.D., C. Briggs-Tung, and E.W. Kietzke (1993). Persistent effects of exercise on skeletal muscle glucose transport across the life span of rats. *J. Appl. Physiol.* 75:972-978.

Cartee, G.D., and R.P. Farrar (1987). Muscle respiratory capacity and $\dot{V}O_2$max in identically trained young and old rats. *J. Appl. Physiol.* 63:257-261.

Charette, S.L., L. McEvoy, G. Pyka, C. Snow-Harter, D. Guido, R.A. Wiswell, and R. Marcus (1991). Muscle hypertrophy response to resistance training in older women. *J. Appl. Physiol.* 70:1912-1916.

Claflin, D.R., and J.A. Faulkner (1985). Shortening velocity extrapolated to zero load and unloaded shortening velocity of whole rat skeletal muscle. *J. Physiol. (London)* 359:357-363.

Clark, K.I., and T.P. White (1991). Neuromuscular adaptations to cross-reinnervation in 12- and 29-month Fischer 344 rats. *Am. J. Physiol.* 260:C96-C103.

Clarkson, P.M., W. Kroll, and A.M. Melchionda (1981). Age, isometric strength, rate of tension development and fiber type composition. *J. Gerontol.* 36:648-653.

Coggan, A.R., A.M. Abduljalil, S.C. Swanson, M.S. Earle, J.W. Farris, L.A. Mendenhall, and P.-M. Robitaille (1993). Muscle metabolism during exercise in young and older untrained and endurance-trained men. *J. Appl. Physiol.* 75:2125–2133.

Coggan, A.R., R.J. Spina, D.S. King, M.A. Rogers, M. Brown, P.M. Nemeth, and J.O. Holloszy (1990). Histochemical and enzymatic characteristics of skeletal muscle in masters athletes. *J. Appl. Physiol.* 68:1896–1901.

Coggan, A.R., R.J. Spina, D.S. King, M.A. Rogers, M. Brown, P.M. Nemeth, and J.O. Holloszy (1992a). Histochemical and enzymatic comparison of the gastrocnemius muscle of young and elderly men and women. *J. Gerontol.* 47:B71–76.

Coggan, A.R., R.J. Spina, D.S. King, M.A. Rogers, M. Brown, P.M. Nemeth, and J.O. Holloszy (1992b). Skeletal muscle adaptations to endurance training in 60- to 70-yr-old men and women. *J. Appl. Physiol.* 72:1780–1786.

Comfort, A. (1979). *The Biology of Senescence*, 3rd Ed. New York: Elsevier, p. 85.

Conlee, R.K. (1987). Muscle glycogen and exercise endurance: a twenty-year perspective. In: K.B. Pandolf (ed.) *Exerc. Sport Sci. Rev.*, Vol. 15. New York: MacMillan, pp. 1–28.

Cook, J.J., T.D. Wailgum, U.S. Vasthare, H.N. Mayrovitz, and R.F. Tuma (1992). Age-related alterations in the arterial microvasculature of skeletal muscle. *J. Gerontol.* 47:B83–B88.

Cortopassi, G.A., D. Shibata, N.-W. Soong, and N.A. Arnheim (1992). Pattern of accumulation of a somatic deletion of mitochondrial DNA in aging human tissues. *Proc. Natl. Acad. Sci. USA* 89:7370–7374.

Costell, M., J.E. O'Connor, and S. Grisolia (1989). Age-dependent decrease of carnitine content in muscle of mice and human. *Biochem. Biophys. Res. Comm.* 161:1135–1143.

Cress, M.E., D.P. Thomas, J. Johnson, F.W. Kasch, R.G. Cassens, E.L. Smith, and J.C. Agre (1991). Effect of training on V̇O₂max, thigh strength, and muscle morphology in septugenarian women. *Med. Sci. Sports Exerc.* 23:752–758.

Davies, C.T.M., D.O. Thomas, and M.J. White (1986). Mechanical properties of young and elderly human muscle. *Acta Med. Scand. Suppl.* 711:219–226.

Daw, C.K., J.W. Starnes, and T.P. White (1988). Muscle atrophy and hypoplasia with aging: impact of training and food restriction. *J. Appl. Physiol.* 64:2428–2432.

Denis, C., J.-C. Chatard, D. Dormois, M.-T. Linossier, A. Geyssant, and J.-P. Lacour (1986). Effects of endurance training on capillary supply of human skeletal muscle on two age groups (20 and 60 years). *J. Physiol. Paris* 81:379–383.

Desypris, G., and D.J. Parry (1990). Relative efficacy of slow and fast-motoneurons to reinnervate mouse soleus muscle. *Am. J. Physiol.* 258:C62–C70.

Doherty, T.J., A.A. Vandervoort, A.W. Taylor, and W.F. Brown (1993). Effects of motor unit losses on strength in older men and women. *J. Appl. Physiol.* 74:868–874.

Dudley, G.A., and S.J. Fleck (1984). Metabolite changes in aged muscle during stimulation. *J. Gerontol.* 39:183–186.

Dustman, R.E., R.O. Ruhling, E.M. Russell, D.E. Shearer, H.W. Bonekat, J.W. Shigeoka, J.S. Woods, and D.C. Bradford (1984). Aerobic exercise training and improved neuropsychological function of older individuals. *Neurobiol. Aging* 5:35–42.

Eddinger, T.J., R.G. Cassens, and R.L. Moss (1986). Mechanical and histochemical characterization of skeletal muscles from senescent rats. *Am. J. Physiol.* 251:C421–C430.

Eddinger, T.J., R.L. Moss, and R.L. Cassens (1985). Fiber number and type composition in extensor digitorum longus, soleus, and diaphragm muscles with aging in Fischer 344 rats. *J. Histochem. Cytochem.* 33:1033–1041.

Edman, K.A.P., and A.R. Mattiazzi (1981). Effects of fatigue and altered pH on isometric force and velocity of shortening at zero load in frog muscle fibers. *J. Muscle Res. Cell Motility* 2:321–334.

Edstrom, L., and L. Larsson (1987). Effects of age on contractile and enzyme-histochemical properties of fast- and slow-twitch single motor units in the rat. *J. Physiol. (London)* 392:129–145.

Erney, T.P., G.M. Mathein, and R.L. Terjung. (1991). Muscle adaptations in trained rats with peripheral arterial insufficiency. *Am. J. Physiol.* 260: H445–H452.

Essen-Gustavsson, B., and O. Borges (1986). Histochemical and metabolic characteristics of human skeletal muscle in relation to age. *Acta Physiol. Scand.*, 123:107–114.

Farrar, R.P., T.P. Martin, and C.M. Ardies (1981). The intertaction of aging and endurance exercise upon the mitochondrial function of skeletal muscle. *J. Gerontol.* 36:642–647.

Faulkner, J.A., S.V. Brooks, and E. Zerba (1990). Skeletal muscle weakness and fatigue in old age: underlying mechanisms. In: V.J. Cristofalo (ed.) *Annual Review of Gerontology and Geriatrics*. New York: Springer, pp. 147–166.

Faulkner, J.A., and T.P. White (1990). Adaptations of skeletal muscle to physical activity. In: C. Bouchard, R.J. Shephard, T. Stephens, J.R. Sutton, and B.D. McPherson (eds.) *Exercise, Fitness and Health: A Consensus of Current Knowledge*. Champaign: Human Kinetics, pp. 265–279.

Fiatarone, M.A., E.C. Marks, N.D. Ryan, C.N. Meredith, L.A. Lipsitz, and W.J. Evans (1990). High-intensity strength training in nonogenarians: effects on skeletal muscle. *J. Am. Med. Assoc.* 263:3029–3034.

Fielding, R.A., C.N. Meredith, K.P. O'Reilly, W. R. Frontera, J.G. Cannon, and W.J. Evans (1991). Enhanced protein breakdown after eccentric exercise in young and older men. *J. Appl. Physiol.* 71:674–679.

Fitts, R.H.P., F.A. Troup, F.A. Witzmann, and J.O. Holloszy (1984). The effect of ageing and exercise on skeletal muscle function. *Mech. Ageing Dev.* 27:161-172.

Fleg, J.L., and E.G. Lakatta (1988). Role of muscle loss in the age associated reduction in $\dot{V}O_2$max. *J. Appl. Physiol.* 65:1147-1151.

Florini, J.R (1978). Biosynthesis of contractile proteins in normal and aged muscle. In: G. Kaldor and W.J. DiBattista (eds.) *Aging in Muscle*, Vol. 6. New York: Raven, pp. 49-85.

Florini J.R., and D.Z. Ewton (1989). Skeletal muscle fiber types and myosin ATPase activity do not change with age or growth hormone administration. *J. Gerontol.: Biol. Sci.* 44:B110-B117.

Foster, D.W. (1984). From glycogen to ketones and back. *Diabetes* 33:1188-1199.

Frolkis, V.V., O.A. Martynenko, and V.P. Zamostyan (1976). Aging of the neuromuscular apparatus. *Gerontology* 22:244-279.

Frontera, W.R., V.A. Hughes, K.A. Lutz, and W.J. Evans (1991). A cross-sectional study of muscle strength and mass in 45- to 78-yr-old men and women. *J. Appl. Physiol.* 71:644-650.

Frontera, W.R., C.N. Meredith, K.P. O'Reilly, and W.J. Evans (1990). Strength training and determinants of $\dot{V}O_2$max in older men. *J. Appl. Physiol.* 68:329-333.

Frontera, W.R., C.N. Meredith, K.P. O'Reilly, H. Knuttgen, and W.J. Evans (1988). Strength conditioning in older men: skeletal muscle hypertrophy and improved function. *J. Appl. Physiol.* 64:2038-1044.

Goodrick, C.L. (1980) Effects of long-term voluntary wheel exercise on male and female Wistar rats. *Gerontology* 26:22-23.

Granbacher, N. (1971) Relationship between the size of muscle fibers, motor endplates and nerve fibers during hypertrophy and atrophy. *Z. Anat. Entwickl.-Gesch.* 135:76-87.

Greig, C.A., J. Botella, and A. Young (1993). The quadriceps strength of healthy elderly people remeasured after eight years. *Muscle Nerve* 16:6-10.

Grimby, G., A. Aniansson, M. Hedberg, G.-B. Henning, U. Grangard, and H. Kvist (1992). Training can improve muscle strength and endurance in 78- to 84-yr-old men. *J. Appl. Physiol.* 78:2517-2523.

Grimby, G., A. Aniansson, A. Zetterberg, and B. Saltin (1984). Is there a change in relative muscle composition with age? *Clin. Physiol.* 4:189-194.

Grimby, G., B. Danneskiold-Samsoe, K. Hvid, and B. Saltin (1982). Morphology and enzymatic capacity in arm and leg muscles in 78-82 year old men and women. *Acta Physiol. Scand.* 115:124-134.

Grimby, G., and B. Saltin (1983). The aging muscle. *Clin. Physiol.* 3:209-218.

Gulve, E.A., E.J. Henriksen, K.J. Rodnick, J.H. Youn, and J.O. Holloszy (1993). Glucose transporters and glucose transport in skeletal muscles of 1-25-mo-old rats. *Am. J. Physiol.* 264:E319-E327.

Guralnik, J.M., and E.M. Simonsick (1993). Physical disability in older Americans. *J. Gerontol.* 48:3-10.

Gutmann, E., and B.M. Carlson (1976). Regeneration and transplantation of muscles in old rats and between young and old rats. *Life Sci.* 18:109-114.

Gutmann, E., and V. Hanzlikova (1972) Basic mechanisms of aging in the neuromuscular system. *J. Mech. Ageing* 1:327-349.

Gutmann, E., and V. Hanzlikova (1976). Fast and slow motor units in ageing. *Gerontology* 22:280-300.

Gutmann, E., and J. Melichna (1972). Contractile properties of different skeletal muscles of the rat during development. *Physiol. Bohemoslov.* 21:1-8.

Gutmann, E., and I. Syrovy (1974). Contraction properties and myosin-ATPase activity of fast and slow senile muscles of the rat. *Gerontologia* 20:239-244.

Hadley, E.C., M.G. Ory, R. Suzman, R. Weindruch, and L. Fried (eds.) (1993). Symposium of physical frailty: a treatable cause of dependence in old age. *J. Gerontol.* 48:1-88.

Hagberg, J.M. (1994). Physical activity, fitness, health, and aging. In: C. Bouchard, R.J. Shephard, and T. Stephens (eds.) *Physical Activity, Fitness, and Health: International Proceedings and Consensus Statement.* Champaign: Human Kinetics, pp. 993-1005.

Haimann, C., A. Mallart, J. Tomas, I. Ferre, and N. F. Zilber-Gachelin (1981). Patterns of motor innervation in the pectoral muscle of adult *xenopus laevis*: evidence for possible synaptic remodeling. *J. Physiol.* 310:241-256.

Häkkinen, K., and A. Häkkinen (1991). Muscle cross-sectional area, force production and relaxation characteristics in women at different ages. *Eur. J. Appl. Physiol.*, 66:555-558.

Harries, U.J., and E.J. Bassey (1990). Torque-velocity relationships for the knee extensors of women in their 3rd and 7th decades. *Eur. J. Appl. Physiol.*, 60:187-190.

Hartley, A.A., and J.T. Hartley (1986). Age differences and changes in sprint swimming performances of masters athletes. *Exper. Aging Res.* 12:65-70.

Heymsfield, S.B., C. Arteaga, C. McManus, J. Smith, and S. Moffit (1983). Measurement of muscle mass in humans: validity of the 24-hour urinary creatinine method. *Am J. Clin. Nutr.* 37:478-494.

Hickson, R.C., B.A. Dvorak, E.M. Gorostiaga, T.T. Kurowski, and C. Foster (1988). Potential for strength and endurance training to amplify endurance performance. *J. Appl. Physiol.* 65:2285-2290.

Hollander, C.F., and J.D. Burek (1982). Animal models in gerontology. In: A. Viidik (ed.) *Lectures on Gerontology*, Vol. 1, Part A. London: Academic Press, pp. 253-274.

Hu, M.-H., and M.H. Woollacott (1994a). Multisensory training of standing balance in older adults: I. Postural stability and one-leg stance balance. *J. Gerontol.* 49:M52-M61.

Hu, M.-H., and M.H. Woollacott (1994b). Multisensory training of standing balance in older adults: II Kinematic and electromyographic postural responses. *J. Gerontol.* 49:M62–M71.

Husain, S.A., and R.L. Pardy (1985). Inspiratory muscle function with restrictive chest wall loading during exercise in normal humans. *J. Appl. Physiol.* 59:826–831.

Irion, G.L., V.S. Vasthare, and R.F. Tuma (1987). Age-related change in skeletal muscle blood flow in the rat. *J. Gerontol.* 42:660–665.

Irion, G.L., U.S. Vasthare, and R.F. Tuma (1988). Preservation of skeletal muscle hyperemic response to contraction with aging in female rats. *Exper. Gerontol.* 23:183–188.

Jakobsson, F., K. Borg, and L. Edström (1990). Fibre-type composition, structure and cytoskeletal protein location of fibres in anterior tibialis muscle. Comparison between young adults and physically active aged humans. *Acta Neuropath.* 80:459–468.

Jeevanandam, M., D.H. Young, L. Ramias, and W.R. Schiller (1990). Effect of major trauma on plasma free amino acid concentrations in geriatric patients. *Am. J. Clin. Nutr.* 51:1040–1045.

Joyner, M.J. (1993). Physiological limiting factors and distance running: influences of gender and age of record performances. In: J.O. Holloszy (ed.) *Exercise and Sport Sciences Reviews* Vol. 21. Baltimore, MD: Williams & Wilkins, pp. 103–133.

Kallman, D.A., C.C. Plato, and J.D. Tobin (1990). The role of muscle loss in the age-related decline of grip strength: cross-sectional and longitudinal perspectives. *J. Gerontol.: Med. Sci.* 45:M82–M88.

Kanda, K., and K. Hashizume (1989). Changes in properties of the medial gastrocnemius motor units in aging. *J. Neurophysiol.* 61:737–746.

Kern, M., P.L. Dolan, R.S. Mazzeo, J.A. Wells, and G.L. Dohm (1992). Effect of aging and exercise on Glut-4 glucose transporters in muscle. *Am. J. Physiol.* 263:E362–E367.

Klitgaard, H., A. Brunet, B. Maton, C. Lamaziera, C. Lesty, and H. Monod (1989a). Morphological and biochemical changes in old rat muscles: effect of increased use. *J. Appl. Physiol.* 67:1409–1417.

Klitgaard, H., M. Mantoni, S. Schiaffino, S. Ausoni, L. Gorza, C. Laurent-Winter, P. Schnohr, and B. Saltin (1990a). Function, morphology and protein expression of ageing skeletal muscle: a cross-sectional study of elderly men with different training backgrounds. *Acta Physiolog. Scand.* 140:41–54.

Klitgaard, H., R. Marc, A. Brunet, H. Vandewalle, and H. Monod (1989b). Contractile properties of old rat muscles: effect of increased use. *J. Appl. Physiol.* 67:1401–1408.

Klitgaard, H., M. Zhou, S. Schiaffino, R. Betto, G. Salviati, and B. Saltin (1990b). Ageing alters the myosin heavy chain composition of single fibres from human skeletal muscle. *Acta Physiol. Scand.* 140:55–62.

Kovanen, V. (1989). Effects of aging and physical training on rat skeletal muscle. *Acta Physiol. Scand.* 135:1–56.

Larsson, L. (1983). Histochemical characteristics of human skeletal muscle during aging. *Acta Physiol. Scand.* 117:469–471.

Larsson, L. (1978). Morphological and functional characteristics of the ageing skeletal muscle in man: a cross-sectional study. *Acta Physiol. Scand.* 457:5–36.

Larsson, L. (1994). Motor units: remodeling in aged animals. Symposium at 1994 annual meeting of the American College of Sports Medicine. Indianapolis, IN: American College of Sports Medicine.

Larsson, L. (1982). Physical training effects on muscle morphology in sedentary males at different ages. *Med. Sci. Sports Exerc.* 14:203–206.

Larsson, L., and L. Edstrom (1986). Effects of age on enzyme histochemical fibre spectra and contractile properties of fast- and slow-twitch skeletal muscles in the rat. *J. Neurol. Sci.* 76:69–89.

Larsson, L., G. Grimby, and J. Karlsson (1979). Muscle strength and speed of movement in relation to age and muscle morphology. *J. Appl. Physiol.* 46:451–456.

Larsson, L., and J. Karlsson (1978). Isometric and dynamic endurance as a function of age and skeletal muscle characteristics. *Acta Physiol. Scand.* 104:129–136.

Larsson, L., and G. Salviati (1989). Effects of age on calcium transport activity of sarcoplasmic reticulum in fast- and slow-twitch rat muscle fibres. *J. Physiol.* 419:253–264.

Larsson, L., B. Sjodin, and J. Karlsson (1978). Histochemical and biochemical changes in human skeletal muscle with age in sedentary males, age 22–65 years. *Acta Physiol. Scand.* 103:31–39.

Lee, C.M., S.S. Chung, J.M. Kaczkowski, R. Weindruch, and J.M. Aiken (1993). Multiple mitochondrial DNA deletions associated with age in skeletal muscle of rhesus monkeys. *J. Gerontol.* 48:B201–B205.

Lexell, J. (1993). Ageing and human muscle: observations from Sweden. *Can. J. Appl. Physiol.* 18:2–18.

Lexell, J., and D.Y. Downham (1991). The occurence of fibre type grouping in healthy muscle: A quantitative study of cross-sections of whole vastus lateralis from men between 15 and 83 years. *Acta Neuropathol.* 81:377–381.

Lexell, J., and D.Y. Downham (1992). What is the effect of ageing on type 2 muscle fibres? *J. Neurolog. Sci.* 107:250–251.

Lexell, J., K. Henriksson-Larsén, B. Winblad, and M. Sjöström (1983). Distribution of fiber type in human skeletal muscle: effects of aging studied in whole muscle cross sections. *Muscle Nerve* 6:588–594.

Lexell, J., and C. Taylor (1991). Variability in muscle fibre areas in whole human quadriceps muscle: effects of increasing age. *J. Anat.* 174:239–249.

Lexell, J., C. Taylor, and M. Sjostrom (1988). What is the cause of the aging atrophy? Total number, size and proportion of different fibre types studied in whole vastus lateralis muscle from 15- to 83-year old men. *J. Neurolog. Sci.* 84:275-294.

Lipsitz, L.A., P.V. Jonsson, M.M. Kelley, and J.S. Koestner (1991) Causes and correlates of recurrent falls in ambulatory frail elderly. *J. Gerontol.* 46:M114-M122

Maki, B.E., P.J. Holliday, and A. K. Topper (1991). Fear of falling and potural performance in the elderly. *J. Gerontol.* 46:M123-M131.

Makrides, S.C. (1983). Protein synthesis and degradation during aging and senescence. *Biol. Rev.* 58:343-422.

Masora, E.J. (1975). An analysis of the effect of age on respiratory and digestive functions of the rat. *Exp. Aging Res.* 1:325-334.

Maxwell, L.C., J.A. Faulkner, and G.J. Hyatt (1974). Estimation of number of fibers in guinea pig skeletal muscles. *J. Appl. Physiol.* 37:259-264.

McCarter, R., and J. McGee (1987). Influence of nutrition and aging on the composition and function of rat skeletal muscle. *J. Gerontol.* 42:432-441.

McCartney, N., R.S. McKelvie, J. Martin, D.G. Sale, and J.D. MacDougall (1993) Weight-training-induced attenuation of the circulatory response of older males to weight lifting. *J. Appl. Physiol.* 74:1056-1060.

McCully, K.K., and J.A. Faulkner (1986). Characteristics of lengthening contractions associated with injury to skeletal muscle fibers. *J. Appl. Physiol.* 61:293-299.

McCully, K.K., and J.A. Faulkner (1985). Injury to skeletal muscle fibers of mice following lengthening contractions. *J. Appl. Physiol.* 59:119-126.

McCully, K.K., R. A. Fielding, W.J. Evans, J.S. Leigh, Jr., and J.D. Posner (1993). Relationships between *in vivo* and *in vitro* measurements of metabolism in young and old human calf muscles. *J. Appl. Physiol.* 75:813-819.

Menkes, A., S. Mazel, R.A. Redmond, K. Koffler, C.R. Libanati, C.M. Gundberg, T.M. Zizic, J.M. Hagberg, R.E. Pratley, and B.F. Hurley (1993). Strength training increases regional bone mineral density and bone remodeling in middle-aged and older men. *J. Appl. Physiol.* 74:2478-2484.

Merton, P.A. (1954). Voluntary strength and fatigue. *J. Physiol. (Lond.)* 123:553-564.

Metzger, J.M., and R.L. Moss (1987). Greater hydrogen ion-induced depression of tension and velocity in skinned single fibres of rat fast than slow muscles. *J. Physiol. (Lond.)* 393:727-742.

Moore, D.H. (1975). A study of age group track and field records to relate age and running speed. *Nature* 253:264-265.

Moritani, T., and H.A. deVries (1980). Potential for gross muscle hypertrophy in older men. *J. Gerontol.* 35:672-682.

Munns, K. (1981). Effects of exercise on the range of joint motion in elderly subjects. In E.L. Smith and R.C. Serfass (eds.) *Exercise and Aging.* Hillside, NJ: Enslow Publishers, pp. 167-178.

Narici, M.V., M. Bordini, and P. Cerretelli (1991). Effect of aging on human adductor pollicis muscle function. *J. Appl. Physiol.* 71:1277-1281.

National Center for Health Statistics (1987). Aging in the eighties. Functional limitations of individuals age 65 and over. Advance Data from Vital and Health Statistics. Dept. Health & Human Services Publication Number 133, (PHS) 87-1250. Hyattsville, MD: U.S. Government Printing Office.

Nevitt, M.C., S.R. Cummings, and E.S. Hudes (1991). Risk factors for injurious falls: a prospective study *J. Gerontol.* 46:M164-M170.

Nevitt, M.C., S.R. Cummings, S. Kidd, and D. Black (1989). Risk factors for recurrent nonsyncopal falls: a prospective study. *J. Am. Med. Assoc.* 261:2663-2668.

Nygaard, E., and J. Sanchez (1982). Intramuscular variation of fiber types in the brachial biceps and the lateral vastus muscles of elderly men: How representative is a small biopsy sample? *Anatomical Record* 203:451-459.

Overend, T.J., D.A. Cunningham, J.F. Kramer, M.S. Lefcoe, and D.H. Paterson (1992b). Knee extensor and knee flexor strength: cross-sectional area ratios in young and elderly men. *J. Gerontol.* 47:M204-M210.

Overend, T.J., D.A. Cunningham, D.H. Paterson, and M.S. Lefcoe (1992a). Thigh composition in young and elderly men determined by computed tomography. *Clin. Physiol.* 12:629-640.

Panton, L.B., J.E. Graves, M.L. Pollock, J.M. Hagberg, and W. Chen (1990). Effect of aerobic and resistance training on fractionated reaction time and speed of movement. *J. Gerontol.* 45:M26-M31.

Parizkova, J., E. Eiselt, S. Sprynarova, and M. Wachtlova (1971). Body composition, aerobic capacity, and density of muscle capillaries in young and old men. *J. Appl. Physiol.* 31:323-325.

Parsons, D., M. Riedy, R.L. Moore, and P.D. Gollnick (1982). Acute fasting and fiber number in rat soleus muscle. *J. Appl. Physiol.* 53:1234-1238.

Pestronk, A., D.B. Drachman, and J.W. Griffin (1980). Effects of ageing on nerve sprouting and regeneration. *Exper. Neurol.* 70:65-82.

Pettigrew, F.P., and P.F. Gardiner (1987). Changes in rat plantaris motor unit profiles with advanced age. *Mech. Ageing Dev.* 40:243-259.

Phillips, S.K., S.A. Bruce, D. Newton, and R.C. Woledge (1992). The weakness of old age is not due to failure of muscle activation. *J. Gerontol.: Med. Sci.* 47:M45-M49.

Phillips, S.K., S.A. Bruce, and R.C. Woledge (1991). In mice, the muscle weakness due to age is absent during stretching. *J. Physiol. (Lond.)* 437:63–70.

Pluskal, M.C., M. Moreya, R.C. Burini, and Y.R. Young (1984). Protein synthesis in skeletal muscle of aging rats. *J. Gerontol.* 39:385–391.

Pollock, M.L., J.F. Carroll, J.E. Graves, S.H. Leggett, R.W. Braith, M. Limacher, and J.M. Hagberg (1991). Injuries and adherence to walk/jog and resistance training programs in the elderly. *Med. Sci. Sports Exerc.* 23:1194–1200.

Pollock, M. L., G.A. Dawson, and H.S. Miller et al. (1976). Physiologic responses of men 49 to 65 years of age to endurance training. *J. Am. Gerontol. Soc.* 24:97–104.

Pollock, M.L., L.R. Gettman, C.A. Milesis, M.D. Bah, L. Durstine, and R.B. Johnson (1977). Effects of frequency and duration of training on attrition and incidence of injury. *Med. Sci. Sports* 9:31–36.

Proctor K.G., and B.R. Duling (1982). Adenosine and free-flow functional hyperemia in striated muscle. *Am. J. Physiol.* 242:H688–H697.

Pyka, G., E. Lindenberger, S. Charette, and R. Marcus (1994). Muscle strength and fiber adaptations to a year-long resistance training program in elderly men and women. *J. Gerontol.: Med. Sci.* 49:M22–M27.

Rizzato, G., and L. Marazzini (1970). Thoracoabdominal mechanics in elderly men. *J. Appl. Physiol.* 28:457–460.

Robbins, A.S., L.Z. Rubenstein, K.R. Josephson, B.L. Schulman, D. Osterweil, and G. Fine (1989). Predictors of falls among elderly people. *Arch. Intern. Med.* 149:1628–1633.

Rogers, M.A., and W.J. Evans (1993). Changes in skeletal muscle with aging: effects of exercise training. In: J.O. Holloszy (ed.) *Exercise and Sports Sciences Reviews*, Vol. 21. Baltimore, MD: Williams & Wilkins, pp. 65–102.

Roman, W.J., J. Fleckenstein, J. Stray-Gundersen, S. E. Alway, R. Peshock, and W.J. Gonyea (1993). Adaptations in the elbow flexors of elderly males after heavy-resistance training. *J. Appl. Physiol.* 74:750–754.

Rosenberg, I.H. (1989). Summary comments: epidemiologic and methodologic problems in determining nutritional status of older persons. *Am. J. Clin. Nutr.* 50:1231–1233.

Rothstein, M. (1985). The alteration of enzymes in aging. *Mod. Aging Res.* 7:53–67.

Roy, R.R., K.M. Baldwin, and V.R. Edgerton (1991). The plasticity of skeletal muscle: effects of neuromuscular activity. In: J.O. Holloszy (ed.) *Exercise and Sport Sciences Reviews*, Vol. 19. Baltimore, MD: Williams & Wilkins, pp. 269–312.

Sadeh, M. (1988). Effects of aging on skeletal muscle regeneration. *J. Neurol. Sci.* 87:67–74.

Sale, D.G. (1988). Neural adaptation to resistance training. *Med. Sci. Sports Exerc.* 20:S135–S145.

Sanchez, J., C. Bastien, and H. Monod (1983). Enzymatic adaptations to treadmill training in skeletal muscle of young and old rats. *Eur. J. Appl. Physiol.* 52:69–74.

Schultz, R., and C. Curnow (1988). Peak performance and age among superathletes: track and field, swimming, baseball, tennis, and golf. *J. Gerontol.* 43:P113–P120.

Sharma, H.K., H.R. Prasanna, and M. Rothstein (1980). Altered phosphoglycerate kinase in aging rats. *J. Biol. Chem.* 255:5043–5050.

Sherwood, D.E., and D.J. Seider (1979). Cardiorespiratory health, reaction time, and aging. *Med. Sci. Sports* 11:186–189.

Shorey, C.D., L.A. Manning, and A.V. Everitt (1988). Morphometrical analysis of skeletal muscle fiber aging and the effect of hypophysectomy and food restriction in the rat. *Gerontology* 34:97–109.

Sidorova, V.F. (1976). Age and the regenerative ability of organs in mammals (Russian). Moscow: Meditsina, pp. 202.

Sipila, S., and H. Suominen (1991a). Ultrasound imaging of the quadriceps muscle in elderly athletes and untrained men. *Muscle Nerve* 14:527–533.

Sipila, S., and H. Suominen (1991b). Quadriceps muscle mass and structure in elderly trained and untrained women. *Med. Sci. Sports Exerc.* 23:555.

Sipila, S., and H. Suominen (1993). Muscle ultrasonography and computed tomography in elderly trained and untrained women. *Muscle Nerve* 16:294–300.

Sipila, S., J. Viitasalo, P. Era, and H. Suominen (1991). Muscle strength in male athletes aged 70–81 yrs and a population sample. *Eur. J. Appl. Physiol.* 63:399–403.

Skinner, J.S., C.M. Tipton, and A.C. Vailas (1982). Exercise, physical training and the aging process. In: A. Viidik (ed.) *Lectures on Gerontology*, Vol 1, Part B. London: Academic Press, pp. 407–439.

Smith, D.O., and J.L. Rosenheimer (1982). Decreased sprouting and degeneration of nerve terminals of active muscles in aged rats. *J. Neurophysiol.* 48:100–109.

Spagnoli, L.G., G. Palmieri, A. Mauriello, G.M. Vacho, S. D'Iddio, G. Giorcelli, and M. Corsi (1990). Morphometric evidence of the trophic effect of L-carnitine on human skeletal muscle. *Nephron* 55:16–23.

Spence, J.W. (1920). Some observations on sugar tolerance, with special reference to variations found at different ages. *Quart. J. Med.* 14:314–326.

Spirduso, W.W., and P. Clifford (1978). Replication of age and physical activity effects on reaction and movement times. *J. Gerontol.* 33:26–30.

Spriet, L.L., C.B. Campbell, and D.J. Dyck (1991). Effect of aging on the buffering capacity of fast-twitch skeletal muscle. *Mech. Ageing Dev.* 59:243-252.

Stalberg, E., O. Borges, M. Ericsson, B. Essen-Gustrasson, P.R.W. Fawcett, L.O. Nordesjo, B. Nordgren, and R. Uhlin (1989). The quadriceps femoris muscle in 20-70 year old subjects: relationship between knee extension torque, electrophysiological parameters, and muscle fiber characteristics. *Muscle Nerve* 12:382-389.

Stanley, S.N., and N.A.S. Taylor (1993). Isokinematic muscle mechanics in four groups of women of increasing age. *Eur. J. Appl. Physiol.* 66:178-184.

Stebbins, C.L., E. Schultz, R.T. Smith, and E.L. Smith (1985). Effects of chronic exercise during aging on muscle and endplate morphology in rats. *J. Appl. Physiol.* 58:45-51.

Steinhagen-Thiessen, E., A. Reznik, and H. Hilz (1980). Negative adaptation to physical training in senile mice. *Mech. Ageing Dev.* 12:231-236.

Stones, M.J., and A. Kozma (1981). Adult age trends in athletic performances. *Exper. Aging Res.* 7:269-280.

Tidball, J.G. (1991). Myotendinous junction injury in relation to junction structure and molecular composition. In: J.O. Holloszy (ed.) *Exercise and Sport Sciences Reviews*, Vol. 19, Baltimore, MD: Williams and Wilkins, pp. 419-445.

Tinetti, M.E., M. Speechley, and S.F. Ginter (1988). Risk factors for falls among elderly persons living in the community. *N. Engl. J. Med.* 319:1701-1707.

Tinetti, M.E., T.F. Williams, and R. Mayewski (1986). Falls risk index for elderly patients based on number of chronic disabilities. *Am. J. Med.* 80:429-434.

Tomanek, R.J., and Y.K. Woo (1970). Compensatory hypertrophy of the plantaris muscle in relation to age. *J. Gerontol.* 25:23-29.

Trotter, J.A., A. Samora, K. Hsi, and C. Wofsy. (1987). Stereological analysis of the muscle-tendon junction in the aging mouse. *Anat. Rec.* 218:288-293.

Turner, J.M., J. Mead, and M.E. Wohl (1968). Elasticity of human lungs in relation to age. *J. Appl. Physiol.* 25:664-671.

Vailas, A.C., V.A. Pedrini, A. Pedrini-Mille, and J.O. Holloszy. (1985). Patellar tendon matrix changes with ageing and voluntary exercise. *J. Appl. Physiol.* 58:1572-1576.

Vandervoort, A.V., J.F. Kramer, and E.R. Wharram (1990). Eccentric knee strength of elderly females. *J. Gerontol.: Biol. Sci.* 45:B125-B128.

Vandervoort, A.A., and A.J. McComas (1986). Contractile changes in opposing muscles of the human ankle joint with aging. *J. Appl. Physiol.* 61:361-367.

Wallace, D.C. (1992). Mitochondrial genetics: a paradigm for aging and degenerative diseases? *Science* 256:628-632.

Wheeler, J., C. Woodward, R.L. Ucovich, J. Perry and J.M. Walker (1985). Rising from a chair: influence of age and chair design. *Phys. Ther.* 65:22-26.

Whipple, R.H., L.I. Wolfson, and P.M. Amerman (1987). The relationship of knee and ankle weakness to falls in nursing home residents: an isokinetic study. *J. Am. Geriatr. Soc.* 35:13-20.

Whipple, R.H., L.I. Wolfson, C. Derby, D. Singh, and J. Tobin (1993). Altered sensory function and balance in older persons. *J. Gerontol.* (Special Issue) 48:71-76.

White, T.P., and K.I. Clark (1995). Age-associated changes in diaphragm and limb muscles of Fischer 344 rats. *J. Appl. Physiol.* in review.

White, T.P., C.K. Daw, K.I. Clark, and S.C. Kandarian (1988). Plasticity of soleus and plantaris muscles in 15- and 28-mo F344 rats. *Physiologist* 31:A132.

White, T.P., and S.T. Devor (1993). Skeletal muscle regeneration and plasticity of grafts. In: J. Holloszy (ed.) *Exercise and Sport Sciences Reviews*, Vol. 21. Philadelphia: Williams and Wilkins, pp. 263-295.

White, T.P., J.F. Villanacci, P.G. Morales, S.S. Segal, and D.A. Essig (1984). Exercise-induced adaptations of rat soleus muscle grafts. *J. Appl. Physiol.* 56:1325-1334.

Woledge, R. (1994). Whole muscle: mechanisms underlying atrophy, weakness and fatigue. Symposium presented at 1994 annual meeting of the American College of Sports Medicine. Indianapolis, IN: American College of Sports Medicine.

Yang, H.T., R.W. Ogilvie, and R.L. Terjung (1991). Low-intensity training produces muscle adaptations in rats with femoral artery stenosis. *J. Appl. Physiol.* 71:1822-1829.

Yang, H.T., R.W. Ogilvie, and R.L. Terjung (1994). Peripheral adaptations in trained aged rats with femoral artery stenosis. *Circ. Res.* 74:235-243.

Young, A., M. Stokes, and M. Crowe (1985). The size and strength of the quadriceps muscle of old and young men. *Clin. Physiol.* 5:145-154.

Young, A., M. Stokes, and M. Crowe (1984). Size and strength of the quadriceps muscles of old and young women. *Eur. J. Clin. Invest.* 14:282-287.

Yuh, K.C.M., and A. Gafni (1987). Reversal of age-related effects in rat muscle phosphoglycerate kinase. *Proc. Natl. Acad. Sci. USA* 84:7458-7462.

Zerba, E., T.E. Komorowski, and J.A. Faulkner (1990). The role of free radicals in skeletal muscle injury in young, adult, and old mice. *Am. J. Physiol.* 258:C429-C435.

Zhang, Y.L., and S.G. Kelsen (1990). Effects of aging on diaphragm contractile function in golden hamsters. *Am. Rev. Respir. Dis.* 142:1396-1401.

Zhou, J.Q., T.P. White, and A. Gafni (1990). Endurance-training induced changes in skeletal muscle phosphoglycerate kinase of old wistar rats. *Mech. Ageing Dev.* 58:163–175.

DISCUSSION

EDGERTON: Regarding the cross-reinnervation study, Tim, if I understand the situation, about 35% of the muscle fibers were not reinnervated. Were those slow units?

WHITE: No, it was the EDL muscle that was reinnervated with the soleus nerve. The vast majority of motor units were originally fast.

EDGERTON: Then it doesn't seem reasonable to assume that activity plays an important role here, because the EDL is the most active type of muscle unit. Based on these results, one would predict that training the muscle wouldn't have any effect on the success rate of reinnervation.

WHITE: The age-associated impairment was with the degree of reinnervation. Compared with young adult rats, in the old there was an increase in noninnervated motor endplates and decreased neural contact of innervated ones. But fibers that were reinnervated did adapt to the atypical innervation, as evidenced by up-regulation of slow-myosin heavy chain. This doesn't imply that training of innervated fibers would be ineffective. The diaphragm muscle, even though it's not a slow phenotype but is rather mixed, has what we all would agree is the highest usage pattern on a daily basis. Published work of others shows the least change in its motor unit size with age, although these results are from older studies and should be readdressed with more contemporary techniques. With our cross-reinnervation study, the EDL motor units were primarily fast when the nerve was cut. Reinnervation with a slow nerve will drive the myosin heavy chain of any innervated motor unit to the slow isoform. In the old there was less than half as much slow myosin as in the adult rats, but when one normalizes for the number of fibers innervated, the myosin heavy-chain response for both age groups is similar. To the extent that we can generalize to exercise training of normal muscle, I contend that innervated fibers adapt in the old in a fashion similar to that in young adults. Because there are more denervated fibers in the old, these fibers will not adapt—they are simply not recruited; however, changes in passive tension might cause some adaptations in myosin. I am unaware of credible data that addresses whether whole-organism exercise training affects the degree of innervation of locomotory skeletal muscle.

CLARKSON: Studies of denervation have shown that with aging, the extrajunctional acetylcholine receptor response is blunted. That would greatly affect reinnervation.

EVANS: The adductor pollicis test has been used by many investigators to look at skeletal-muscle function, but Kirsh Jeejeebohy has shown repeatedly that small changes in nutritional status affects adductor pollicis function. So I don't have much confidence in this test unless nutritional status can be controlled. We see, for example, that nursing-home patients who have profound vitamin D deficiency, as many very old people do, have a much prolonged relaxation time during the adductor pollicis test.

WHITE: Do you think the adductor pollicis muscle would be any more sensitive to nutritional status than any other skeletal muscle?

EVANS: Maybe not. But it is the only one that has been used *in vivo*, with the exception of the vastus lateralis. It is the one that has been seen most often to respond because it is the one that is tested the most. On another issue, Joan Bassey in Great Britain has developed a very nice test for measuring leg power. She has shown that leg power is much more closely related to function than is strength. In fact, in our nursing home population, leg power explains 90% of the variability in walking speed.

DEMPSEY: It seems to me that the advantage of the adductor pollicis test is that it is independent of volitional effort, so the investigator need not be concerned about neural phenomena affecting force production.

WHITE: That is an advantage of that test. Roger Woledge's group showed with the twitch interpolation technique that both young and old can generate maximal possible force voluntarily. Thus, with the adductor pollicis muscle one can avoid the problem of reduced force production in the old as an outcome of decreased central drive.

EDGERTON: The relaxation time of muscle increases with aging, and all the models of reduced muscular activity show that relaxation time decreases. If it is assumed that prolonging relaxation times is a disadvantage, this again causes concern about the assumption of a positive effect of increasing muscular activity. I see no reason to assume that the affect of activity would be positive, and I can easily rationalize why increased activity could be disadvantageous in attempting to minimize muscular fatigue.

TIPTON: I would like to have you discuss the time course of power change as muscle mass is lost and the relationships of those two variables to changes in balance and in the frequency of falls. To me, this is a major problem with major consequences.

WHITE: Bill Evans indicated that in their older subjects, there is a greater reliance on motor unit recruitment than on hypertrophy early in a strength training program. Once strength begins to increase more or less in parallel with increasing muscle growth, I am unaware of any major difference in adaptive response due to age, although clearly there is more variability in older subjects.

The question of the contribution of muscle strength and power to balance and the incidence of falls is an important one. Although the data are short of establishing a causal relationship, the inverse relationship between strength and falls suggests that muscular weakness is a major contributing factor. Certainly, if one has less muscle mass but the same body weight and tries to get out of a chair, the relative effort for the involved musculature is greater. In the young, such an effort may require only 10–20% of the maximal power of the involved musculature, whereas it may demand more than 100% of the available power in the old, so that moving from the chair may become impossible without assistance. Because of the redundancy of control mechanisms and one's individual ability to use a variety of compensatory mechanisms when there is an impairment, I am uncertain if one could ever conclude that decreased muscle mass and power are responsible for a specific fraction of the risk of falling.

EICHNER: There are two opposing ways to prevent hip fractures. One is to be an athlete and develop strong bones; the other is to be a couch potato and develop fat hips. A recent *New England Journal of Medicine* article reported that older women who were the most pear-shaped had the fewest hip fractures, the simplest hypothesis being that they are more padded when they fall. Also, it is not widely known that after the age of 60, many people steadily lose the ability to absorb vitamin B_{12} from food, so that serum B_{12} level drops and proprioception may be impaired before anemia occurs. This problem may contribute to falls, yet is missed by the classical Shilling test because that uses crystalline B_{12}, and people maintain the ability to absorb crystalline B_{12} longer than they do the ability to extract and absorb B_{12} from food. So if we design a sport drink for seniors, not Gatorade, but LaterAde or LaterGator, maybe we should add crystalline B_{12} to it.

DEMPSEY: The diaphragm is a wonderful muscle, isn't it? It's nice to see that we have finally recognized the only really essential skeletal muscle. I'd like to discuss an apparent dichotomy between the animal data you described for the diaphragm and some indirect information about diaphragm function in human beings. You showed that muscle fiber area in the diaphragm is probably increased in the aging rat at the same time that the size of locomotor muscle fibers is decreasing. There are some recent longitudinal data on inspiratory muscle strength for 6,000 humans that show decreasing strength of those muscles after age 35 or 40, which is opposite to the results in rats. But I think we can really be misled by these functional tests in humans because there is something else going on with aging that changes how these muscles function. That is, the lung loses elastic recoil, and when it does that, one tends to hyperinflate. This means that at the beginning of each breath, the functional residual capacity is increased slightly, which in turn means that each of the inspiratory muscles is at a shorter length. Thus, changes in muscle length might well explain *all* of the decrease in inspiratory muscle force in humans. What do you think of this interpretation I just gave? Do you think that muscle length changes can explain the muscle function test results, or would you expect the number of sarcomeres to adapt over time and change the length-tension relationship in the muscle?

WHITE: I would expect that the muscle would adapt to its new length. There is good evidence, at least in rats, that muscle will add or subtract sarcomeres in series such that they can get back to an optimal length-tension relationship. This adaptive response also occurs in the muscles of mastication in monkeys. The experimental work has been done in young adult male monkeys, but I expect the results would be similar in old animals.

DEMPSEY: That is true with the hamster model of emphysema, too. The animal hyperinflates, and the diaphragm shortens, but the number of sarcomeres increases to reestablish a more normal length-tension relationship so that there is little loss of force generation. Assuming this is occurs in rats, too, then there's got to be some other explanation for the increased cross-sectional area of the diaphragm fibers in the old rat.

WHITE: If fiber number decreased markedly in human diaphragm muscle and/or if an age-related specific weakness occurs in the diaphragm (as has been shown for human adductor pollicis muscle), this could help explain the disparate results in the two species.

SEALS: It is very important to make a distinction between epidemiological data showing how changes in physiological function are associated with age in the general population and data derived from studies that more directly seek to discover cause-and-effect associations between age and function. When we look at young and older subjects who are matched for lifestyle factors such as chronic physical activity levels, we don't see differences in maximal isometric handgrip strength. If we look at dynamic exercise that is not limited by the pumping capacity of the heart, the older subjects demonstrate the same maximal work rate and blood flow. These are examples of how age-related differences apparent in cross-sections of the general population disappear or are markedly diminished when the young and older subjects are matched on lifestyle factors.

WHITE: I agree that there is some difficulty, particularly with skeletal muscle, in differentiating primary aging effects from secondary effects due to physical inactivity, inadequate nutrition, and endocrine changes. However, I differ with you about the stability of strength across age. I contend that if one studies an old mammal relative to its life span, decays in muscle structure and function will be observed. It is conceivable, but unlikely in my opinion, that no decay in function will occur over the 40-y period between ages 20 and 60 if one accounts for physical activity, nutrition, etc.; but I guarantee that decreased function will be obvious if a person aged 90 is compared to a person aged 50, even if all lifestyle factors are controlled. Even in highly motivated, world-class age-group athletes who are unlikely to have cardiovascular, pulmonary, or neuromuscular disease of any significance, athletic performances decay at rates of 8–10%

per decade. Once a human reaches age 60 or 70, it is not possible to forestall neuromuscular decline with any known intervention.

LAKATTA: The vastus lateralis in older humans exhibits a decrease in the number of fibers but an increase in the size of those fibers. In the heart, an analogous situation occurs with aging. It is not clear why certain cells die, i.e.. drop out, but the remaining ones grow larger, perhaps as a result of chronic stretch. The heart itself may enlarge or remain unchanged in size. These changes in the heart are associated with a prolonged contraction time or prolonged relaxation, which interferes with the heart's ability to respond to rapid repetitive stimuli. The prolonged contraction time is associated with a prolonged cytosolic calcium transient following excitation. This prolonged calcium transient is at least partly attributable to a decrease in the number of calcium pump sites in the sarcoplasmic reticulum, which in turn is caused by a reduced expression of the gene for the pump protein. In the heart, exercise conditioning can reverse the prolonged contraction. Does exercise training of skeletal muscle reduce contraction times? Are there are any data on older skeletal muscle to suggest that the cytosolic calcium transient is prolonged? Is the function of the sarcoplasm reticulum in old skeletal muscle abnormal? If any of these phenomena occur, does exercise conditioning tend to reverse them, as occurs for the heart?

WHITE: Contractile proteins are different in skeletal and cardiac muscle. If exercise training affects it at all, the change in the myosin heavy chain of skeletal muscle is minor, whereas in cardiac muscle there is a clearly altered gene expression leading to an increased proportion of β (slow) myosin heavy chain. I am unaware of data on training effects on sarcoplasmic reticulum function or calcium kinetics in skeletal muscle of old animals.

COYLE: Is it possible that the greater loss of muscle fibers in people compared to rats is a function of the relatively shorter time required for rodents to age? Rats take 1.5 y to move from middle age to old age, whereas people take 20–30 y. People are simply exposed to the probability of muscle injury for a longer time?

WHITE: Yes, that may be a factor.

BAR-OR: The fact that there seems to be a preferential decrease in the size and number of Type II B fibers implies that anaerobic performance may decline with aging faster than aerobic performance. This suggests that we should expand our repertoire of tests in older subjects to include evaluations of local muscular endurance and peak muscle power.

WHITE: I could not agree with you more about the need for added sophistication of muscular testing in human beings. We will also be well-served by a change in test nomenclature. Rather than naming tests based on presumed metabolism, e.g., a test of "aerobic" power, the tests should be identified from a functional point of view, e.g., a test of maximal power output. As you know, all metabolic systems operate simultaneously during exercise, just in varying proportions, depending on relative intensity, etc.

EVANS: We need to gain some insight into why older people exhibit a greater variability in muscular adaptations to training than do young people. One of our working hypotheses is that the variability is related to a concomitant variability in immune responses to stress.

WHITE: Investigators group subjects based on chronological age. The enhanced variability in measured variables in the old may be in part due to the fact that individuals are at different percentiles of their life spans, which are unknown at the time.

TERJUNG: A change in relaxation time in the heart could have a great impact on cardiac filling, because the duty cycle of the heart is a very large fraction of the total time, especially at high heart rates. In contrast, changes in relaxation time in skeletal muscle would have relatively little impact during large-muscle, whole-body activities such as cycling, swimming, or walking that don't occur at a very high duty cycle. I would expect that the impact of changes in relaxation of skeletal muscle would be fairly inconsequential.

5

Bone, Ligament, and Tendon

Susan A. Bloomfield, Ph.D.

INTRODUCTION

Scope

Bones, the ligaments between bones, and the tendons attaching muscles to bones form a functional unit providing structural support and a lever system translating muscle contraction into movement. These three tissues share a common embryonic origin from mesenchymal cells as well as common features at maturity; all are composed of an extracellular organic matrix synthesized by its constituent cells, which remain embedded within that matrix. Collagen fibers in the organic matrix of these tissues confer to them great tensile strength; in the case of bone, mineralization of the organic matrix further strengthens the tissue. Indeed, mechanical strength and resistance to injury are key functional characteristics of bone, ligament, and tendon. The manifestations of mechanical failure in these tissues range from the temporary discomfort of a soft tissue sprain to the sometimes fatal sequelae of a hip fracture. Therefore, maintaining the integrity of these tissues over the life span is crucial for maintaining mobility and independent functioning.

One of the classical theories of aging is the cross-linkage theory, which links aging changes in tissues to the increased cross-linking of constituent proteins and nucleic acids. Collagen, the structural protein common to bone, ligament, and tendon, accounts for 30% of all proteins in the mammalian body; hence, changes in its molecular structure with aging have profound consequences for the organism. Some 40 y ago, Verzár (1955) made the key observation that the collagen in rat tails increased in "stiffness" with increasing age of the rat. Subsequent research has defined the molecular mechanisms for this functional change, primarily an increased number and altered pattern of the inter- and intra-molecular cross-links of collagen fibrils. Skin elasticity commonly declines with aging and is strongly correlated ($r = 0.604$) (Viidik, 1982) with chronological age. Functional age of a tissue, however, is not necessarily linked to chronological age. It could be argued that one of the key benefits of regular physical activity for older adults is to maximize the discrepancy between functional age of some tissues and the chronological age of their owner, that is, to maintain youthful function well into our older years. At the present time only a minority of our older population regularly engages in vigorous exercise. In 1990, the Healthy People 2000 objectives stated that more than 40% of people over the age of 65 report absolutely no leisure time physical activity; only 20% of all adults over 18 y report engaging in moderate physical activity at least 5 d/wk (U.S. Public Health Service, 1990).

In this chapter I will review the evidence regarding the effects of regular physical activity on those changes in bone, ligament, and tendon normally attributed to aging; a corollary consideration is the contribution of relative inactivity or disuse to the aging process. The converse question is also important and will be discussed, i.e., does the aging process affect the ability of these tissues to adapt to chronic exercise? "Aging" is herein defined as spanning those years between young adulthood and senescence, roughly from 25 to 90 y of age. Although the emphasis is on the human condition, data from animal models are presented when they can contribute to our understanding of mechanisms for physiological adaptation. A consistent effort is made throughout this review to consider how physiological and structural adaptations in these tissues impact on their mechanical functions. Finally, a brief overview of nutritional factors important to bone health focuses on the interaction between calcium and estrogen deficiency.

Basic Biology of Bone, Ligament, and Tendon

Bone Composition and Architecture. Bone is composed of an organic matrix (primarily Type I collagen), calcium-phosphate precipitates, and a mineralized phase of hydroxyapatite (Robey, 1989). The two distinct types of bone, cortical and cancellous, are differentiated by their architecture and functional characteristics (Figure 5-1). Cortical bone, also referred to as compact bone, accounts for 75–80% of total skeletal mass but only 33% of total bone surface (Parfitt, 1988). It forms the dense outer walls of all bones but is found primarily in the shafts of the long bones. Its functional unit on the histological level is the osteon, composed of concentric layers (lamellae) of bone with its resident osteocytes centered around a vascular channel, the Haversian canal.

Cancellous (also termed trabecular or spongy) bone has a high surface:volume ratio and accounts for the remaining two-thirds of bone surface but only 20–25% of skeletal mass. Found primarily in the spine, pelvis, and in the ends of the long bones, cancellous bone forms a latticework of interconnected plates and rods called trabeculae that are continuous with the inner (endosteal) surface of the surrounding cortical bone shell. With its greater porosity and surface:volume ratio, cancellous bone has more surface area for contact with blood supply and populations of osteoblasts and osteoclasts (bone-forming and bone-resorbing cells, respectively). This fundamental structural difference between the two types

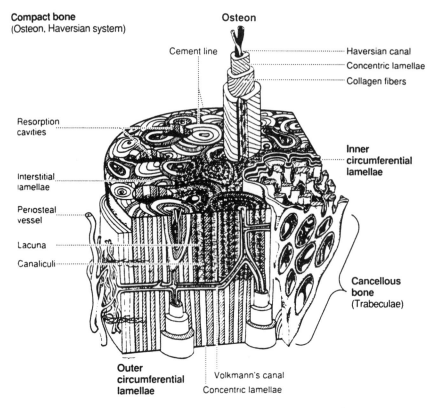

Osteon

Cement line ·· Haversian canal
·· Concentric lamellae
·· Collagen fibers

Resorption
cavities ·················

Inner
············· circumferential
lamellae

Interstitial
lamellae ·················

Periosteal
vessel ·················

Lacuna ·················

Canaliculi·················

Cancellous
bone
(Trabeculae)

Outer
circumferential
lamellae

Volkmann's canal

Concentric lamellae

FIGURE 5-1. *Schematic view of part of the proximal end of a long bone containing cortical and cancellous bone. Functional units of cortical bone are the Haversian systems, or osteons, composed of concentric lamellae surrounding a central vascular canal. Circumferential lamellae are found at the outer (periosteal) and inner (endosteal) surfaces of cortical bone; interstitial lamellae are the remains of older, remodeled osteons. Note the continuity of cancellous bone with the endosteal surface of cortical bone. Volkmann's canals provide functional connections between osteons and blood vessels and nerves at the periosteum and in the marrow cavity. More minute channels called canaliculi connect adjacent lacunae, affording communication between osteocytes and with bone cells on bone surfaces. Several resorption cavities in cortical bone are depicted. From Jee (1988) with permission.*

of bone accounts for the more rapid response of cancellous bone to changes in the endocrine milieu or in mechanical loading; for example, decrements in bone mass due to estrogen deficiency are first observed in those anatomical sites having a greater proportion of cancellous bone.

The regulation of bone mass and bone rigidity in the adult skeleton depends on the functions of three or four distinct cell populations. Integrated activity of these bone cells at the same site or anatomically distinct sites contributes to the processes of remodeling and modeling, respectively. Osteoblasts are responsible for the synthesis of organic matrix, its deposition upon existing bone surfaces, and its subsequent mineralization. It is generally presumed that some active osteoblasts are eventually surrounded by mineralized bone. These now isolated cells are termed osteocytes, and they remain in communication with cells lining bone surfaces via gap junctions (Doty, 1981) between the microprocesses of adjacent cells. These cellular extensions lie within canaliculi, the minute channels connecting osteocyte lacunae to each other and to bone surfaces (refer to Figure 5-1). The osteocytes are best situated to detect mechanical strain in bone and to communicate the amplitude of that strain signal with biochemical signals via gap junctions (and perhaps via autocrine and paracrine factors) to those cells on the bone surfaces responsible for bone remodeling.

A third type of bone cell is the osteoclast, a multinucleated cell that initiates the remodeling process by resorbing a discrete packet of mineralized bone. Osteoblasts are subsequently recruited to the remodeling site and lay down newly synthesized organic matrix, which then slowly mineralizes. The reader is referred to several excellent reviews of bone remodeling (Canalis, 1993; Parfitt, 1988; Raisz, 1988). Remodeling is active throughout the life span after the first year of life and is thought to function primarily to replace "old" bone and perhaps to repair microcracks. Modeling activity, on the other hand, is predominant during growth of the skeleton in the immature animal and is the result of coordinated activities of osteoclasts and osteoblasts at non-adjacent sites, resulting in additions or deletions of bone mass at strategic locations to improve bone strength (Frost, 1990). In this case, new bone may be formed on a quiescent bone surface without previous resorption activity at that site. Although less common in the adult skeleton than in still-lengthening bone, modeling may be the primary functional response to large increases in imposed loading on bone.

Regulation of Bone Strength and Stiffness. Functionally, we are concerned with the likelihood of bone fracture. Lowered bone mass is only one of several factors contributing to fracture risk. The geometric arrangement of bone and its intrinsic material strength are more difficult to measure than bone mass but are equally important in determining bone's resistance to fracture. A recent effective synthesis by Kimmel (1993) of control mechanisms originally described by Frost (1987), Lanyon (1987), and Turner (1991) focuses on the regulation of bone strength and stiffness, not bone mass. According to Kimmel's paradigm, the signal for a need for change in skeletal strength is cumulative deformation of bone as perceived by the osteocyte-lining cell complex. When this cumulative deformation exceeds some minimum threshold, signals are sent to the effectors in this homeostatic system: the modeling and remodeling "systems," which include the bone cells as well as the complex of largely undefined physiological signals effectively coordinating these bone cell activities. The end result is some adjustment of bone geometry and bone mass to effectively reduce those deformations below that physiological threshold.

This paradigm also accounts for the mechanisms underlying the impact of various endocrine or local factors upon bone mass by describing their individual influences upon the sensor in this system, the osteocyte-lining cell complex. For example, if an anabolic hormone decreased the rigidity of the cytoskeleton of this osteocyte-lining cell complex, previously undetectable signals would now deform this cytoskeleton, creating the perception of overload. The bone cell's response would result in an acceleration of modeling and remodeling, resulting in an increase in bone mass to stiffen the whole structure, hence reducing the deformations produced by customary loads.

Cells and Matrix of Dense Fibrous Connective Tissues. Connective tissue is well constructed to withstand tensile stress and to recover in size and shape after a load is removed. This complex tissue is made up of a mixture of collagen, elastin, ground substance, and water, the relative proportion of each varying with the type and age of the tissue. Ligaments, for example, may be slightly more metabolically active than tendons, and they contain less total collagen and more glycosaminoglycans in their ground substance (Amiel, 1984).

Collagen is the major structural protein in the matrix of all connective tissues, constituting 65–80% of their dry weight (Amiel et al., 1990); in ligaments and tendons, Type I collagen predominates. Collagen fibrils, oriented parallel to the long axis of the ligament or tendon, are composed of multiple tropocollagen units, which consist of polypeptide α-chains folded into a triple helix. These collagen fibrils range in size from 10–1500 nm in diameter; the distribution of fibril sizes varies among tissues, with age, among species (Parry et al., 1978), and perhaps with activity levels (Oakes et al., 1981). The structural stability of collagen is conferred by the formation of covalent intra- and intermolecular cross-links between adjacent tropocollagen molecules. Newly synthesized collagen has predominantly reducible cross-links, which are transformed with maturation to the more stable non-reducible cross-links. Collagen in ligaments generally has more reducible cross-links than does collagen in tendons, perhaps reflecting different functional loading of these tissues *in vivo* (Amiel et al., 1984).

The other major component of the extracellular matrix is ground substance, filling the space between collagen fibrils and around embedded cells. It is composed primarily of proteoglycans and glycosaminoglycans. These long polysaccharide chains are hydrophilic and retain a great deal of water, providing the viscoelastic properties important to the mechanical behavior of tendons and ligaments. Small amounts of fibronectin and elastin are also found in extracellular matrix. Embedded in matrix are the only cells of dense connective tissue, the fibroblasts, which are responsible for the synthesis, maintenance, and perhaps organization of the extracellular matrix. In immature tendon, some relatively large fibroblasts have long cytoplasmic processes that contact the processes of other cells (Buck-walter et al., 1987), suggesting some means of intercellular communication.

MEDICAL AND CLINICAL CONCERNS

A Consequence of Age-related Changes in Bone: Osteoporotic Fracture

Any bone will fracture if exposed to severe enough impact or tor-sional forces. So-called osteoporotic fractures occur with only mild or moderate impacts in bone of low strength, typically during a fall in elderly persons. These age-related fractures have become a major public health problem in most industrialized countries, posing a serious threat to the quality of life of an increasingly older population. Nearly one of every three women and one in every six men surviving to the age of 90 y will experience a hip fracture and its debilitating consequences. Mortality in the first year following a hip fracture ranges from 12–40% for elderly in-dividuals (White et al., 1987); many of those who survive require long-term care. Estimated annual direct costs associated with hip fractures in the U.S. alone were $7 billion in 1984 (Melton, 1988). Although less debil-itating than a hip fracture, multiple vertebral fractures can be painful and eventually impair mobility and normal pulmonary function. Each year be-tween 200,000 and 400,000 U.S. women over the age of 50 y experience new vertebral fractures (Cooper et al., 1992); almost a third of women over 65 y of age have one or more vertebral fractures (Melton, 1988). It is almost certain that imposed bed rest and reduced physical activity typical in the fracture patient exacerbate the loss of bone mass and the risk of additional fractures (Heaney, 1992). The limitations imposed by age-related fractures on independent living and physical capabilities make the main-tenance of bone strength a pivotal issue affecting the quality of life in older adults.

Consequences of Age-related Changes in Ligament and Tendon

The incidence of spontaneous ruptures of tendons in industrialized nations has increased dramatically since 1950 (Józsa et al., 1989; Kannus & Józsa, 1991). These injuries occur most often in sedentary individuals participating in occasional recreational sports activities; they appear to be the outcome of progressive histopathological changes in the tendon sub-stance itself. In biopsies from the Achilles' tendons of young individuals (mean age 38 y), 30% of collagen fibrils were abnormal; in tendons from older individuals (mean age of 66 y), there was a 50% incidence of abnor-mal fibrils (Kannus & Józsa, 1991). In light of the usual decline in habitual physical activity in the majority of older adults and the increased incidence of degenerative histopathological changes in tendons from this popula-tion, it is reasonable to presume that many older individuals are at risk for injuries to tendons and ligaments, especially with falls. Older adults are also subject to surgery more often than are young healthy adults. There is clear evidence that the recovery of injured or surgically repaired ligaments and tendons is slowed significantly by immobilization. Hence, decreased physical activity contributes to both an increased risk of injury and a protracted recovery should injury or surgery occur.

Relatively unexplored are the potential effects of age-associated reductions in tendon and ligament strength on joint kinetics and support. In addition, ligaments have an extensive number of afferent sensory fibers (Buckwalter et al., 1987), and there are documented decreases in the number of mechanoreceptor neurons from knee joints in old versus young mice (Salo & Tatton, 1993). Whether these structural changes result in a functionally important decrease in afferent feedback to the CNS during movement is unknown. These reductions in tissue strength and afferent feedback may have important implications for maintenance of normal gait and balance in the elderly.

ALTERATIONS IN BONE, LIGAMENT, AND TENDON WITH AGING

Changes in Bone Mass With Aging and Potential Mechanisms

The Decline in Bone Mass with Aging. The quantity of bone declines with age after the attainment of peak bone mass in young adulthood. This appears to be a universal phenomenon across races, geographical location, habitual activity levels, dietary habits, and historical epoch (Parfitt, 1988). These decreases in bone mass are site-specific and largely dependent upon the relative content of cancellous and cortical bone at any one anatomical site; there is also a large degree of biological variation in the rate and age at onset of loss. This loss of bone mass without any change in bone quality *per se* is termed osteopenia. Once this osteopenia becomes severe enough to result in non-traumatic fractures, it is clinically defined as osteoporosis. Bone status for most individuals over the age of 60 y is somewhere on the continuum between benign age-related osteopenia and bone loss severe enough to make fracture imminent.

Should a woman survive to 90 y of age, she will lose about 20% of her peak cortical bone mass and up to 50% of peak cancellous bone mass; the corresponding figures for men surviving to 90 y are 5% for cortical and 10–25% for cancellous bone (Riggs et al., 1982). Women tend to start losing bone earlier in life and may experience a 3–5 y acceleration of bone loss after menopause, with the effects of estrogen deficiency temporarily superimposed on age-related loss. There exists good evidence that almost half of the total bone loss in vertebral bone in women occurs before menopause, whereas cortical bone loss is generally minimal until after menopause (Riggs et al., 1986). Earlier data from the same investigative group suggest, however, that both genders experience significant bone loss at the femoral neck (approximately 25% cancellous in composition) before the age of 50 y.

More recent information derived on a large cohort of community-living women over the age of 65 y reveals continued loss of cortical bone mass into the ninth decade of life (Figure 5-2) at the femoral neck and proximal radius, as well as large decrements in bone mineral density of the calcaneus. This latter site appears to be the most sensitive to changes in weightbearing activity (see discussion below of disuse osteopenia). The much larger decrement in bone mineral density at the calcaneus versus the lumbar spine in this group of elderly women suggests that progressive declines in weightbearing activity may be contributing to this pattern of bone loss. Cross-sectional data may overestimate age-related loss of bone mineral density by as much as 13% due to increasing average adult height in cohorts with more recent birthdates (Recker & Heaney, 1990). Even so, given the strong relationship between bone mass and compressive strength ($r \geq 0.75$) (Currey, 1969; Hansson et al., 1980), it is clear that any strategy to minimize these significant decrements in bone mass with aging will greatly reduce the risk of fracture.

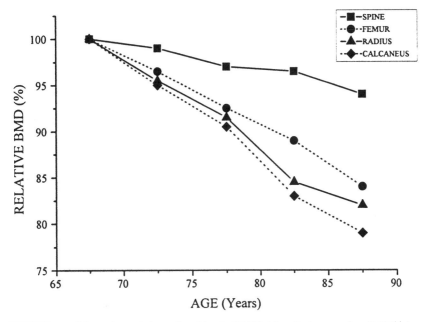

FIGURE 5-2. *Relative changes in bone mineral density (BMD) at four sites in women (n = 7,659) between 65 and 90 y of age, expressed as percent of mean BMD of women 65–69 y of age.* SPINE = lumbar spine, FEMUR = femoral neck, RADIUS = distal radius. Spine and femur BMD were assessed by dual energy X-ray absorptiometry; BMD of radius and calcaneus was estimated by single-photon absorptiometry. Adapted from Steiger et al. (1992).

It should be noted that the increase in body fat typically observed after young adulthood may attenuate some of the age-related loss of bone mass, particularly in postmenopausal women. Obese women rarely develop clinically significant osteoporosis; their risk of fractures at various sites is also lower (Kreiger et al., 1982). In the overweight individual, increased mechanical loading is imposed on the skeleton. An endocrine mechanism may play the more important role: obese women are relatively less estrogen-deficient than their thinner counterparts due to the conversion of circulating androstenedione by fat tissue to estrone (Ribot et al, 1988). What remains unanswered is the relative benefit for bone health of maintaining increased body fat stores versus the disadvantage of excess weight in maintaining high levels of physical activity, not to mention the negative impact on risk of cardiovascular disease and adult-onset diabetes.

Changes in Bone Cell Activities. Within any one macroscopic sample of bone there exist microscopic domains of bone of varying ages, with the most recently remodeled bone the youngest. The maximum life span of bone tissue has been estimated to extend years, if not decades (Frost, 1986). The life span of individual bone cells, however, is considerably shorter. Osteoblasts, after a period of active bone formation, become either inactive bone lining cells or osteocytes. Bone lining cells survive up to 3 y or until the next remodeling event occurs at that site. Osteocytes usually survive as long as the tissue surrounding them, with an upper limit of longevity estimated at 25 y (Frost, 1960).

After the age of 35 y in humans, some small net deficit of bone volume occurs at each remodeling site due to some "underfilling" of the existing resorption cavity by osteoblastic activity (Frost, 1986). This net deficit typically occurs on endosteal surfaces of cortical bone and on cancellous bone surfaces but not on the outer, periosteal surface of cortical bone, where bone formation continues, albeit slowly, throughout the life span. Studies of iliac crest biopsies in non-osteoporotic individuals provide the histological evidence for this paradigm of age-related bone loss (Meunier, 1973). Over the six decades following the attainment of skeletal maturity, there is a progressive decrease in osteoblastic activity with aging, with smaller absolute volumes of new bone tissue being deposited. Interestingly, no change with age has been documented in resorptive activity of osteoclasts. With similar resorption rates and decreased bone formation, a net loss of bone volume occurs; between the ages of 25 and 75 y, trabecular bone volume in the iliac crest declines some 19% in males and 47% in females (Meunier, 1973). The larger bone loss in females is largely due to the superimposed effect of estrogen withdrawal at menopause.

The rate of remodeling, or turnover, of bone tissue slows with age; the older individual has fewer active remodeling sites in both cortical and cancellous bone (Parfitt, 1988). The major contributor to this slowed turnover appears to be a decrease in the recruitment of osteoblast progenitor cells and/or a decrease in the activity of mature, differentiated osteoblasts. There appears to be a decreased capacity of cultured osteoblasts from human donors over 60 y old to proliferate in response to growth factors and several systemic hormones (Pfeilschifter et al., 1993). *In vivo* data from Liang et al. (1992) provide evidence for decreased responsiveness of osteoblasts to a specific physiological challenge to bone formation, the removal of bone marrow from the femur. As compared to young adult rats, mRNA in senescent rats encoding for osteoblastic proteins important in mineralization increased less in response to bone marrow ablation, coincident with a smaller bone volume formed and a lower osteoblast count. In a different model, the osteogenic response to a stimulator of ectopic bone formation is impaired in older rats (Nishimoto et al., 1985). These data are consistent with earlier findings of slower rates of mineralization of newly formed cortical bone in older humans, as well as a slower rate of organic matrix deposition (Jowsey, 1960; Ortner, 1975).

Some structural changes in osteoblasts may indirectly contribute to increases in osteoclast activity. Electron microscopy studies in senescent mice reveal degenerative changes in the ultrastructure of osteoblasts and an eventual disruption of the membrane-like arrangement of osteoblasts on periosteal surfaces (Tonna, 1978). These changes may expose the periosteal surfaces to resorptive actions of osteoclasts and thereby increase resorption rates.

Alternative possible mechanisms for slower remodeling rates in the aged individual include: 1) decreased delivery of systemic regulatory factors and/or progenitor cells due to an age-related decrease in bone blood flow (Hruza & Wachtlova, 1969); 2) changes in the mineral or organic matrix properties of aged bone that alter the transmission of strain through bone tissue and, in turn, reduce the magnitude of the osteogenic signal delivered to osteoblasts (Lanyon, 1987); 3) a decline in the available population of osteoblast progenitor cells (Meunier, 1973; Nishimoto et al., 1985); and 4) changes in the secretion or clearance of the major hormones regulating bone and calcium metabolism or changes in target cell sensitivity for these systemic hormones or for local regulatory factors.

Changes in Endocrine Regulators of Remodeling. There is increasing evidence that the parathyroid hormone (PTH)-vitamin D axis changes significantly with aging, resulting in a decline in intestinal absorption of calcium. Serum levels of intact immunoreactive PTH (iPTH) increase, and serum 1,25-dihydroxyvitamin D ($1,25\text{-}OH_2D$) decreases with age, with an acceleration of these changes noted after age 65 (Epstein et al., 1986). Normally, PTH functions to increase serum levels of $1,25\text{-}OH_2D$, the biologically active form of vitamin D, by stimulating the activity of renal α-hydroxylase (which converts relatively inactive 25-hydroxyvitamin D_3 (25OHD) to $1,25\text{-}OH_2D$. However, in some subset of individuals there may be a primary defect in the function of renal α-hydroxylase; even long-term therapy with 25OHD does not produce increases in 1,25-OH_2D in these individuals (Slovik et al., 1981; Zerwekh et al., 1983). Other contributors to the decline in intestinal calcium absorption may be an increased resistance of intestinal mucosa to the actions of 1,25-OH_2D (Francis et al., 1984) and a decline in serum levels of 25OHD (Heaney, 1988). This latter factor reflects declining solar exposure as well as vitamin D-deficient diets in the elderly. The net result in too many older adults is an endocrine milieu that favors bone loss.

There is an age-related decline in circulating growth hormone (GH) and insulin-like growth factor I (IGF-I). As important as these two factors may be to normal bone growth during maturation, it appears doubtful that age-related alterations in serum GH or IGF-I are responsible for declines in bone mass in older adults, judging from the relative ineffectiveness of replacement therapy in reversing age-related bone loss. In healthy men over 60 y old, 6 mo of treatment with hGH, which successfully elevated plasma IGF-I values to those seen in young men, produced a modest increase in bone mineral density at only one of six sites measured (Rudman et al., 1990). Although increases in serum osteocalcin, a marker for osteoblastic activity, are seen after 12 mo of hGH therapy in healthy elderly women and men, bone mineral density at the proximal femur and the spine does not change appreciably (Marcus et al., 1993). Further, serum IGF-I and IGF-II concentrations are not related to cortical bone mineral density in both healthy and osteoporotic older women (Bennett et al., 1984).

Decline in Bone Quality with Aging

Ultrastructural Changes. If indeed the primary purpose of remodeling activity is to prevent excessive aging of bone tissue, and if the remodeling rate falls with increasing age, we should expect to see an increasing proportion of "old" bone in any given unit area of mineralized bone. This has been best demonstrated with microradiographs of cross-sections from femoral shafts, which reveal an increasing proportion of hypermineralized bone from older donors (Grynpas, 1993; Jowsey, 1960).[1] Another contributing factor to this hypermineralization is osteocyte death, which occurs if the age of the surrounding mineralized tissue exceeds the normal life span of an osteocyte; the osteocyte's lacuna in which it resided becomes plugged and calcified, as can some canaliculi and Haversian canals (Frost, 1960; Jowsey, 1960). An important functional concern is the contribution of this increased mineralization to the brittleness of the tissue and therefore its decreased resistance to fracture. Currey (1979) attributed most of the threefold decrease in impact energy absorption in human cortical bone between the ages of 3 and 90 y to this hypermineralization of aging bone.

In 1981, Chatterji et al. used scanning electron microscopy to demonstrate that the particle size of apatite crystals is smaller in bone from older individuals. The decrease in particle size with age almost exactly paralleled the decline in tensile strength of whole bone specimens. With fewer smaller apatite particles, the specific surface area available for bonding with the collagen matrix decreases, thereby affecting material strength. However, more recent X-ray diffraction studies showed no change in apatite crystal size (Simmons et al., 1991); whether this opposite result is an artifact of the difference in techniques used is unclear. Age-related changes occur in the organic matrix as well. An increasing proportion of collagen fibers in tibial bone from older donors is oriented circularly rather than along the longitudinal axis of the osteon (Vincentelli, 1978). Because individual osteons with more longitudinally oriented collagen fibers have a greater tensile strength (Vincentelli & Evans, 1971), this aging change further contributes to a decline in the material strength of bone tissue.

Another ultrastructural factor potentially contributing to the age-related decline in bone material strength is the accumulation of microcracks, also termed fatigue damage, which result from repetitive loading of bone (Burr et al., 1985). This is more likely to occur in pockets of cortical bone that are far removed from remodeling surfaces. There exists a preliminary report of an exponential increase in microcracks in human cortical bone after the age of 40 (Schaffler, 1993). Whether similar microcracks accumulate in more actively remodeling cancellous bone is uncertain; no fatigue damage has been found in iliac cancellous bone (Parfitt, 1993), but there is one report of a significant accumulation of microcracks in trabeculae of the femoral neck (Fazzalari, 1993).

Alterations in Bone Geometry and Architecture. The imbalance that develops between bone formation and bone resorption with aging has a profound effect on the architecture of cancellous bone. In vertebral bodies, the best studied site, the total number of trabeculae declines as resorption sites perforate trabecular plates (Parfitt, 1984). Early studies concluded that horizontal trabeculae were preferentially lost and that the remaining vertical trabeculae underwent a compensatory thickening (Arnold, 1980; Parfitt, 1984). More direct stereological analyses have confirmed that both vertical and horizontal trabeculae are progressively resorbed with aging, with increased spacing between trabeculae and decreased connectivity (Mosekilde, 1988; Snyder et al., 1993) (Figure 5-3). These architectural changes result in trabeculae that are fewer in number, thinner, and longer and contribute to the decline in mechanical strength of vertebrae in older individuals. The 50–70% decrease observed in compressive strength of vertebral bodies between the ages of 35 and 70 y (Martin, 1993) is disproportionately larger than the decrease in bone mass.

Although bone material strength declines with age in both men and women (Burstein et al., 1976; Mosekilde & Mosekilde, 1990), redistribu-

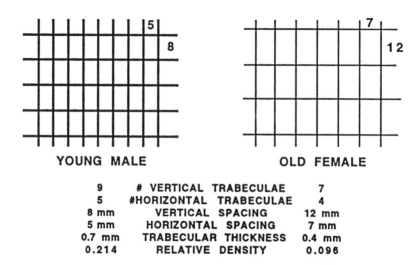

YOUNG MALE		OLD FEMALE
9	# VERTICAL TRABECULAE	7
5	#HORIZONTAL TRABECULAE	4
8 mm	VERTICAL SPACING	12 mm
5 mm	HORIZONTAL SPACING	7 mm
0.7 mm	TRABECULAR THICKNESS	0.4 mm
0.214	RELATIVE DENSITY	0.096

FIGURE 5-3. *Rectangular grids representing trabecular structure in vertebral bone for young and old subjects.* In the old subject, the number of vertical trabeculae has decreased by 22% and the number of horizontal trabeculae has decreased by 20%. More importantly, the spacing between consecutive horizontal trabeculae has increased by 50% and between consecutive vertical trabeculae by 40%. Overall, the relative density has declined 55%; 21% of this reduction is due to the decreased number of trabeculae, but an additional 43% of the decreased relative density is attributable to the thinning of remaining trabecular struts. Adapted from Snyder et al. (1993).

tion of the remaining cortical bone can compensate for this loss of material strength. In cortical bone, preferential resorption at the endosteal surfaces expands the medullary cavity throughout the life span in both genders. In men, but apparently not in women, net formation of bone continues to occur at the periosteal surface well into old age, resulting in addition of new bone to the outer perimeter (Ruff & Hayes, 1988; Figure 5-4) and a progressive increase in the cross-sectional moment of inertia (CSMI), with a constant cross-sectional area. This age-related increase in CSMI in men accounts for the maintenance of structural bending strength, whereas bending strength decreases significantly in women, who typically exhibit declines in cross-sectional area and no change in the CSMI (Martin & Atkinson, 1977; Figure 5-5).

A similar gender-related difference is noted in vertebral body structure and strength properties (Table 5-1). Continued periosteal expansion of the cortical ring of the vertebral body in men over 50 y of age results in a 15–20% larger cross-sectional area and significantly higher load at mechanical failure when compared to age-matched females (Mosekilde & Mosekilde, 1990). After the age of 75, there is no gender-related difference in load values, suggesting that thinning of the cortical ring of vertebral bodies does occur in men after the age of 75.

The vast bulk of the existing data on changes in remodeling and bone

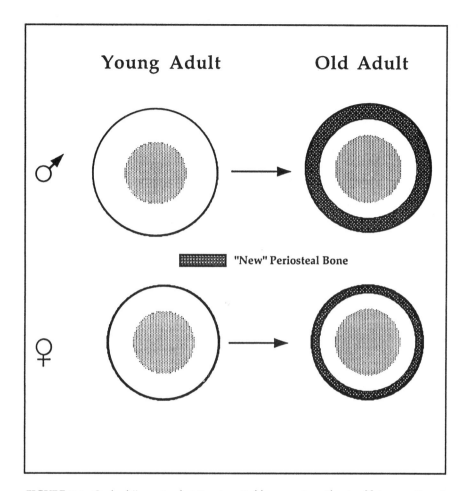

FIGURE 5-4. *Gender difference in adaptations in cortical bone geometry with aging.* Net resorption at the inner endosteal surface in both genders results in expansion of the endosteal diameter, enlarging the medullary cavity. Continued modeling activity on the periosteal surface in men results in a larger periosteal diameter and greater cross-sectional moment of inertia (CSMI) in old age. Without periosteal expansion, CSMI is reduced in women in old age and may account in part for the increased risk of cortical bone fracture in women.

strength with aging has been derived from cadaver specimens. As valuable as this information is, variations in nutritional intakes, physical activity patterns, and other lifestyle factors potentially affecting the measured variables cannot be accounted for. The development of new technologies to measure bone geometry and strength characteristics *in vivo* will allow researchers to better control for such variables and, more importantly, to pursue longitudinal studies. One recent example is the reanalysis of data derived from dual energy X-ray absorptiometry scans of the femoral neck by computer software designed to calculate CSMI along the length of the

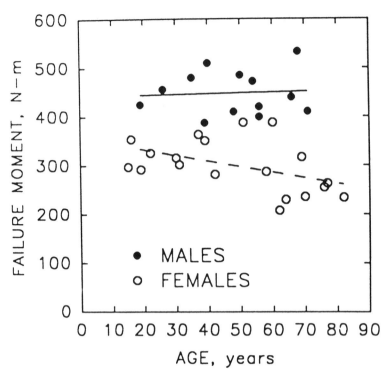

FIGURE 5-5. *Changes in strength of human femoral shafts tested in bending.* The slope of the regression line for females, but not for males, is significantly different from zero. Based on data of Martin and Atkinson (1977); reproduced from Martin (1993) with permission.

TABLE 5-1. *Comparison of vertebral ash density, size, and biomechanical competence between the genders in young and old populations.*

	Young (< 50 years)		Old (50–75 years)	
	Female	Male	Female	Male
Age (years)	28±6	30±9	66±6	64±5
Ash density (g/cm²)	0.17±0.02	0.18±0.02	0.12±0.02	0.13±0.02
Cross-sectional area (cm²)	12.28±0.74	13.68±1.31**	12.56±2.13	15.68±1.64***
Load (N)	6941±1747	8263±1583*	3257±1047	4586±1764**
Stress (MPa)	5.70±1.36	5.83±1.13	2.62±0.83	2.96±1.22

Values are means ± SD. *p<0.05, **p<0.01, ***p<0.001 female vs. male within age-group. N = Newtons, MPa = megaPascals (1MPa = 1N/mm²). Adapted from Mosekilde and Mosekilde (1990).

neck (Beck et al., 1992). Both males and females experience decreases in bone mineral density and cross-sectional area of the femoral neck with increasing age; only males demonstrate an increase in CSMI due to a small increase in periosteal diameter. In a larger sample of women, the same investigative group demonstrated 4–12% increases per decade in calculated stresses in the femoral neck in women over 50 y of age that were coincident with the decreases in bone density and CSMI (Beck et al., 1993) (Table 5-2), confirming data of earlier studies done on autopsy samples. Decreases in bone mineral density along with a less favorable bone geometry may explain the much higher rate of femoral neck fractures in elderly women than in men.

The Safety Factor in Bone

The key functional consideration relative to declines in bone mass and potential accumulation of fatigue damage is the fragility of the bone itself; i.e., how likely is it that loads typically experienced by that bone will result in a fracture? To quantify this concept, engineers employ the concept of a "safety factor," determined by the ratio of the maximum stress a structure is expected to bear to the structure's failure strength. With reference to cortical bone, it might be more relevant to consider the lower strain experienced at yield (beyond which irreversible damage accumulates rapidly) rather than strain at failure (i.e., fracture) when calculating a skeletal safety factor. Taking this more conservative approach, the safety factor for cortical bone ranges from 1.4 to 4.1 in the young adult (Figure 5-6).

Any reduction in bone mass and bone quality, as occurs with the accumulation of fatigue damage and hypermineralization of bone tissue, will result in a reduced safety factor, even when voluntary reductions in activity common in many older adults are factored in. The probability of fracture in the older population is significantly elevated, even if the safety factor remains greater than 1.0. The value of this model of a safety factor for the human skeleton rests on many assumptions that require more research, such as what level of strain is actually experienced in human bone

TABLE 5-2. *Rate of change in femoral neck BMD, geometric properties, and computed femoral neck stresses in women before and after the age of menopause*

Parameter	Premenopause (≤50 years)		Postmenopause (>50 years)	
	%Δ/decade[a]	significance[b]	%Δ/decade	significance
BMD	−3.70	0.0001	−7.05	0.0001
CSA	−2.32	0.0034	−7.62	0.0001
CSMI	0.02	NS	−4.87	0.012
Tensile Stress	−0.47	NS	8.77	0.0036
Compressive Stress	−5.36	0.002	4.18	0.046
Shear Stress	2.20	0.0013	12.57	0.0001

[a]Percent change per decade, expressed relative to the value at age 20 for premenopausal group and to the value at age 50 for postmenopausal group.
[b]Significance value from multiple linear regressions on age, weight, and height.
BMD = bone mineral density, CSA = cross-sectional area, CSMI = cross-sectional moment of inertia, NS = not significant. Adapted from Beck et al. (1993).

A. YOUNG ADULT

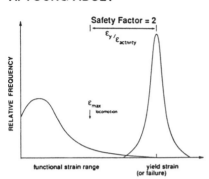

B. AGING

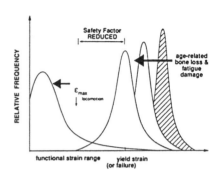

FIGURE 5-6. *(A) A schematic representation for hypothetical frequency distributions of functional strain and yield strain (representing a functional limit to bone strength) for a given population of young adults.* The safety factor is defined as the mean yield strain (ε_y) of a particular bone divided by the maximal imposed strain to which the bone is typically subjected (ε_{max}); in this illustration the safety factor is 2.0. Although during normal activity bone experiences strains below ε_{max}, some loading events may exceed this functional limit. The overlap between the two curves represents the probability of failure, i.e., when applied strain exceeds the yield strain of that bone. *(B) With age-related bone loss, accumulated fatigue damage, and other changes in material properties of bone, effective strength of the bone is decreased, shifting the distribution curve for yield strain to the left.* The widening of the yield strain distribution reflects the increasing variability of bone strength properties, resulting in part from tissue remodeling in the aging skeleton. The net result is a reduction in the safety factor and an increased risk of fracture, illustrated by increased overlap between functional strain and yield strain curves. It is likely that some of this overlap is reduced by voluntary reduction of activity in older adults. From Biewener (1993), with permission.

in vivo, assessment of variation in bone density within skeletal sites prone to fracture, and whether or not repair of microcracks by remodeling in older individuals is truly impaired (Biewener, 1993). Any agent that minimizes bone loss or maintains bone quality with aging will assure a larger skeletal safety factor throughout the life span and thereby minimize debilitating fractures. Regular physical activity may well be such an agent.

Changes in Ligament and Tendon with Aging

Morphology and Biochemical Composition. The major structural protein in all connective tissues is Type I collagen, which constitutes 65–80% of the dry weight of tendons and ligaments (Amiel et al., 1990). There are age-, tissue- and species-specific variations in the distribution of fibril diameters (Jones, 1991; Parry et al., 1978). For instance, 45% of human patellar tendon fibrils have diameters greater than 100 nm, whereas only 15% of anterior cruciate ligament (ACL) fibrils exceed 100 nm (Frank et al., 1988). In senescent animals, mean diameters of collagen fibrils are smaller than in the mature adult (Parry et al., 1978). The functional relevance of fibril size rests on the finding that larger-diameter fibrils contribute to greater tissue strength, whereas a significant number of smaller-diameter fibrils interspersed among the larger-diameter fibrils is required for optimizing tissue elasticity (Nimni & Harkness, 1988; Parry et al., 1978).

The biochemistry of collagen also contributes to the mechanical functions of the dense connective tissues. Hydroxyprolyl and prolyl residues on the α-chains of tropocollagen molecules form cross-links with adjacent proteins, giving collagen its stiffness and strength (Amiel et al., 1990). The labile reducible cross-links, i.e., dihydroxylysinonorleucine (DHLNL) and hydroxylysinonorleucine (HLNL), appear to be converted to the more stable non-reducible cross-links, e.g., pyridinoline, with normal maturation and aging. Amiel et al. (1991) documented increases of 87% and 37% in the content of pyridinoline cross-links in ACL and medial collateral ligament (MCL), respectively, in 12-mo-old rabbits as compared to younger controls. Simultaneously, the content of DHLNL and HLNL cross-links declined over the same aging period. Some of this shift in the cross-link content of aging collagen is a reflection of the decrease in collagen synthesis rates because newly synthesized collagen is stabilized almost exclusively by the reducible cross-links. Similar shifts in cross-link content occur in canine patellar tendon, with nearly 100% of cross-links in specimens from 15-y-old dogs identified as non-reducible (Haut et al., 1992). The concentration of collagen with nonreducible cross-links is positively correlated with tensile modulus (a measure of stiffness), reflecting the small increase in tensile modulus with age in these canine tendons.

Total collagen content of ligaments and tendons appears to decrease in the aging animal. The studies cited above (Amiel et al., 1991; Haut et al., 1992) both observed a decrease in collagen content (μg hydroxyproline per unit dry tissue weight) with aging. There was a significant correlation, in the case of canine patellar tendon, between collagen content and the observed decline in tensile strength with age. By contrast, Vailas et al. (1985) documented a 35% increase in collagen content in patellar tendons from 28-mo-old rats as compared to 9-mo-old rats, confirming earlier results of Tipton et al. (1978) on rat ligaments. It is unclear whether these discordant results reflect a difference in study design (e.g., the relative age of a 28-mo-old rat vs. a 36-mo-old rabbit vs. a 15-y-old dog) or a species difference.

Tendon and ligament glycosaminoglycans (GAG), the primary macromolecules of ground matrix, and particularly the galactosamine-containing GAGs, decrease in the aged rat (Vailas et al., 1985). Negative electrical charges on the long polysaccharide chains of GAGs repel each other and fill empty space; they also attract and retain water, both functions providing resistance to compression plus joint lubrication (LeVeau, 1992). Decreases in matrix GAGs account for the decrease in water content of ligaments and tendons in older animals and may contribute to some of the functional changes seen in ligament and tendon with aging.

Histologically, collagen bundle fragmentation can be seen in aged ligament, along with a decline in the density of fibroblasts (Amiel et al., 1991). The decrease in cell density may be a function of an increase in ground matrix volume rather than an absolute decrease in cell number (Ippolito et al., 1980; Tipton et al., 1978). X-ray diffraction studies confirm an increase in lateral spacing between adjacent molecules in collagen fibrils, providing evidence for structural changes consequent to an accumulation of cross-links derived from non-enzymatic glycosylation (Naresh & Brodsky, 1992). Ultrastructural changes in the fibroblasts themselves reflect the relative decline in metabolic activity; there is a loss of prominent rough endoplasmic reticulum and Golgi apparatus, and there are more vacuoles, dense bodies, and filament bundles (Amiel et al., 1991). The histology of the muscle-tendon junction s altered in 30-mo-old mice; the interfacial ratio [of surface area of force-transmitting membrane to cross-sectional area of myofibrils] is significantly reduced. Some of this reduction may be explained by a relative increase in slow-twitch fibers populations in the aging mice (Trotter et al., 1987), as interfacial ratios in predominantly slow-twitch muscles are lower than those for fast-twitch muscles in young adult mice.

Structural and Material Properties Affecting Mechanical Strength. The mechanical strength of tendons and ligaments is usually tested *in vitro* on knee-joint preparations from animal, cadaver, or amputee specimens. In discussing changes in mechanical strength of the dense connective tissues, it is critical to distinguish between 1) "structural" properties derived from testing bone-ligament-bone or bone-tendon-muscle preparations under tensile loading to failure and 2) "material" properties describing the behavior of the tendon or ligament substance itself independent of its bony insertions. When this distinction is made, it becomes clear that the physiology of insertion sites becomes very important when discussing changes with aging, exercise, or disuse because the insertion site is often the weakest link in the system.

Insertion sites of ligaments and tendons vary because of anatomical and mechanical requirements, but all share some common characteristics. The soft tissue overlying the insertion site is composed of superficial and deep fibers. Superficial fibers become continuous with the periosteum overlying bone; the deep fibers insert to bone either directly or through a zone of fibrocartilage, with a sudden transition from unmineralized to mineralized fibrocartilage. At direct insertions, the deep fibers of the soft tissue meet fibrocartilage and bone perpendicularly; at indirect insertions, superficial fibers predominate and meet the bone's periosteum at an oblique angle, blending gradually with the periosteal layers (Woo et al., 1988). Any osteopenic changes in the bone underlying either type of insertion site will compromise the structural integrity and junction strength and contribute to the risk of injury at this site.

When preparations of human anterior cruciate ligaments are tested to failure at fast strain rates (best simulating the usual conditions leading to ligament injury), a significant decline in the ultimate load or maximum force at failure is noted in specimens from older adults (age 48–86 y) when compared with those of young adults (age 16–26 y) (Figure 5-7). However, because the predominant mode of failure in the older specimens is avulsion fracture of the bone underlying the ligament insertion, the decline in ultimate load does not reflect a decline in material properties of the ligament itself, but more directly the decrease in junction strength at the insertion site (Noyes & Grood, 1976). These results may reflect the independent contribution of osteopenic changes in bone in older adults, in whom relative inactivity or other antemortem or preoperative factors may have significantly affected bone quality at insertion sites (Noyes & Grood, 1976).

By contrast, when tested at relatively slow strain rates *in situ*, junction strength in rats exposed only to cage activity continues to increase over 2 y of aging (Tipton et al., 1978). A gender difference does exist in this species. When junction strength is normalized for body weight (because larger male rats have larger ligaments), female rats have stronger junctions after the age of 1 y. This gender difference may be limited to

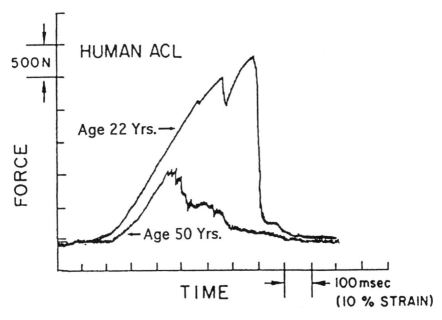

FIGURE 5-7. *Records of force vs. time from mechanical testing of anterior cruciate ligament (ACL) specimens from young and middle-aged human donors. A decrease in stiffness (initial slope of the curve) and failure at lower force and strain values is noted in the older-adult specimen. Adapted from Noyes and Grood (1976).*

those species in which the female does not experience a decline in estrogens at mid-life as do human females, because bone quality (and therefore junction strength) is highly dependent on maintenance of normal serum estrogen values.

If analysis of mechanical testing of joint preparations is limited to the prefailure region of the load-deformation curve, data describing material properties of the tendon or ligament itself can be derived. Elastic modulus is calculated from the slope of the linear range of the load-deformation curve before failure of the specimen and provides a measure of tissue stiffness (LeVeau, 1992). Elastic modulus decreases with increasing age in human ACL; similar declines in elastic modulus have been observed in ligaments from aged rats (Tipton et al., 1978), rabbits (Woo et al., 1990), and dogs (Vasseur et al., 1985). In human specimens, the ultimate load also declines significantly with age, as does strain energy (area under the load deformation curve). Similar results can be seen in rabbit MCL, although most mechanical properties do not decline until a very advanced age (Table 5-3).

Although usually presumed to be indistinguishable from ligaments, tendons appear to change less with aging, at least with regard to mechanical properties. The elastic modulus of canine patellar tendon does not decline with age, nor does its tensile strength (Haut et al., 1992). Similar findings have been documented for human palmaris longus and extensor hallucis longus tendons (Hubbard & Soutas-Little, 1984) and for human calcaneal tendons from individuals as old as 60 y (Yamada, 1970). It may be that actual physiological loads regularly imposed on patellar tendon are greater than those on ligaments or that repair of microdamage is more efficient in tendon than ligament, maintaining higher levels of tensile strength and stiffness (Haut et al., 1992; Vasseur et al., 1985).

Adaptations of Bone, Ligament, and Tendon to Disuse: A Component of Aging?

Significant declines in physical activity, whether voluntary or as a consequence of injury, are common in the elderly populations of industrialized countries (Montoye, 1975; Ramlow et al., 1987). Relative disuse can be viewed on a continuum between normal activity levels and complete immobilization. For example, intermediate decrements in junction strength of the MCL are observed in dogs limited to cage activity as compared to dogs with cast-immobilized legs (Laros et al., 1971) when the norm is defined in dogs free to exercise in large pens. The vast bulk of the literature on changes in bone, ligament, and tendon with disuse focuses on complete immobilization of a limb produced by casting or pinning. More relevant to aging issues might be those results gleaned from the mere unweighting of limbs without strict immobilization, as achieved in

TABLE 5-3. *Structural and material properties of rabbit medial collateral ligament (MCL) at different ages*

	Structural properties of FMTC			Material properties of MCL			
	Load @ failure (N)	Energy absorbed @ failure (N-m)	Linear stiffness (N/mm)	Tensile strength (MPa)	Strain at failure (%)	Modulus (MPa)
12-mo	290.4±20.2	0.77±0.15	48.2±3.1	75.8±4.8	9.4±0.7	950±80
36-mo	311.6±26.4	0.98±0.16	51.8±4.2	78.6±3.2	13.3±0.5	710±30
48-mo	267.0±26.7	0.77±0.15	50.3±2.9	68.9±4.9	11.9±1.3	520±120

Values are means ± SE; FMTC = femoral-MCL–tibia complex. Six specimens were tested at each age, except at 12 months when n=14. Adapted from Woo et al. (1990).

hindlimb suspension of rats, prolonged bedrest in healthy humans, and exposure to microgravity.

Disuse Osteopenia. The balance between resorption and formation of bone in the adult skeleton is disrupted by disuse, and particularly by the loss of weightbearing. The resulting bone loss develops at a rate 5 to 20 times greater than in common metabolic disorders of bone (Mazess & Whedon, 1983). The classic bedrest studies of Dietrick et al. (1948) demonstrated a doubling in urine calcium with 6 wk of cast immobilization and bedrest that persisted for 3 wk into a recovery period. This calcium loss is a direct reflection of increased bone resorption, and a measurable decline in bone mass, during this period of non-weightbearing. After 120 d of strict bedrest, healthy young men experience a 4–10% decrease in bone mineral density as measured by absorptiometry, with the largest loss incurred in the calcaneus (LeBlanc et al., 1990; Figure 5-8). Similar

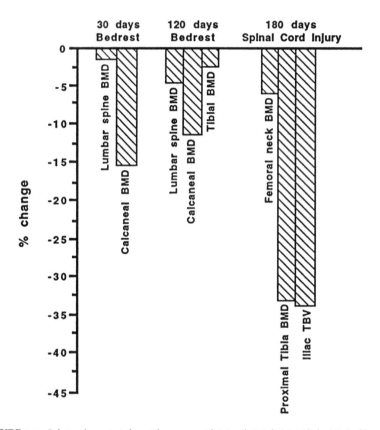

FIGURE 5-8. *Relative change in indices of bone mass with 30 and 120 d of strict bedrest in healthy young males, and at 180 d after spinal cord injury.* BMD = bone mineral density; TBV = trabecular bone volume. Based on data from Biering-Sørensen et al. (1990), LeBlanc et al. (1990), LeBlanc et al. (1987), and Minaire et al. (1974).

rates of bone mineral loss have been reported in the calcaneus following brief exposure to microgravity, where longitudinal compressive forces are greatly diminished (Rambaut & Good, 1985). Bone formation rate is suppressed as much as 60% after 120 d of bedrest (Judge et al., 1989); simultaneously, resorptive activity is either maintained (Judge et al., 1989; Palle et al., 1992) or accelerated (Vico et al., 1987). Calcium balance becomes negative and persists for the duration of bedrest or exposure to microgravity (Donaldson et al., 1970; Whedon et al., 1974) but reverses with the resumption of weightbearing activity. Much of the excess calcium found in the urine is presumed to be derived from resorbed bone, but decreases in intestinal calcium absorption during an immobilization period may also contribute to the prolonged hypercalciuria (Yeh & Aloia, 1990).

Curiously, histological analysis of iliac crest bone biopsies from healthy male volunteers taken after 4 mo of bedrest reveals no significant decrement in cancellous bone volume (Vico et al., 1987). It is possible that bone architecture is more affected than is total bone quantity, or that iliac crest bone responds differently than the long bones of the lower limb. Palle et al. (1992) found a decrease in trabecular number and a possible compensatory thickening of trabeculae after a similar period of bedrest in young males. Even if the bone loss incurred during bedrest is overestimated by noninvasive measures of bone mass (e.g., absorptiometry), it is clear that were this mismatch of resorption and formation to continue, bone mass would eventually decline. The extreme example of immobilization in humans is provided by spinal cord injury, after which 33% of iliac trabecular bone volume is lost within 6 mo (Figure 5-8). In this case, loss of muscle tone and possible changes in bone blood flow likely exacerbate the changes in bone resorption and formation activities, resulting in the more dramatic loss of bone mass.

Information derived from animal models exposed to microgravity (Morey & Baylink, 1978), hindlimb suspension (Vico et al., 1991), or immobilization (Li et al., 1990; Young et al., 1986) confirms that the lack of regular muscle contraction against normal gravitational forces produces some deficit in deposition and/or mineralization of new bone in addition to an increase in resorptive activity. Recall that the primary defect that produces age-related loss of bone mass is a decline in osteoblast activity with little or no change in the bone resorption rate. It is apparent that any period of enforced bedrest will superimpose on this decreased bone formation activity the devastating effect of increased resorption rates, hence accelerating the loss of bone mass. Apparently, however, no data exist on the effect of bedrest or immobilization on bone cell activities in aged humans.

Effect of Immobilization on Ligament, Tendon, and Junction Strength.
Chronic disuse has potent effects on connective tissue morphology, on collagen metabolism, and on junction strength, which account for the

tremendous decrements observed in the mechanical strength of the ligaments, tendons, and/or insertion sites during even brief periods of immobilization. The rate of loss of mechanical strength in these connective tissues and at insertion sites is much more rapid and the magnitude of loss far greater than the modest increases in functional strength observed with increased physical activity (Figure 5-9). The rate of recovery after a period of immobilization for the insertion site is much slower than that for the ligament or tendon itself, usually requiring up to 12 mo to regain normal architecture and strength (Woo et al., 1987). On the other hand, even with rigorous exercise training only minimal (10–15%) increases in soft tissue mass or strength and in junction strength are observed; these structures seem to be operating at or near a maximal functional limit even with average activity levels.

Without daily mechanical loading, collagen fibrils and cells lose their typical parallel organization (Akeson et al., 1984). There are metabolic consequences as well, such as an increase in collagen turnover. Because increases in degradation of old collagen exceed increases in synthesis of new collagen, net declines in collagen mass are observed (Amiel et al., 1982). Concurrently, a decline in the proportion of smaller cross-sectional area fibers and an increase in larger fibrils is noted (Binkley & Peat, 1986). Simple unweighting of the hindlimbs by tail suspension in rats produces a

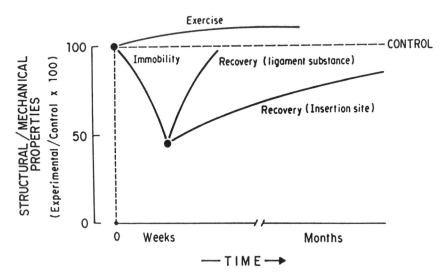

FIGURE 5-9. *Curves representing the response of the components of a ligament-bone insertion site to changes in physical activity. The response to immobilization is both more rapid and greater in magnitude than the response to increases in customary activity. The time course of recovery upon remobilization is much slower for the insertion site than for the ligament itself.* From Woo et al. (1987), with permission.

28% decrement in collagen concentration after only 4 wk as well as decreased content of uronic acid-containing proteoglycans in patellar tendon (Vailas et al., 1988). The decline of total GAGs and in dermatan sulfate-containing GAGs that is noted with immobilization (Akeson et al., 1973) echoes similar changes noted in aging patellar tendon (Vailas et al., 1985).

An increase in the proportion of reducible cross-links, reflecting the increase in newly synthesized collagen, coincides with a significant decrement in tissue stiffness (Amiel et al., 1982; Binkley & Peat, 1986; Woo et al., 1987). The load deformation curve derived from mechanical testing of the MCL (Figure 5-10) illustrates a dramatic reduction in the ultimate load at failure of the bone-ligament-bone preparation in rabbits immobilized for 9 wk. The degree of reduction in load at failure seen with immobilization resembles that seen with aging (refer to Figure 5-7). No significant change occurs in the cross-sectional area of the ligament with immobilization, hence implying that most of the reduction in tensile characteristics is due to changes in material properties of the tissue itself rather than to simple tissue atrophy (Woo et al., 1982).

Not unexpectedly, the mechanism for failure of bone-ligament-bone preparations in immobilized joints is almost always avulsion fracture of

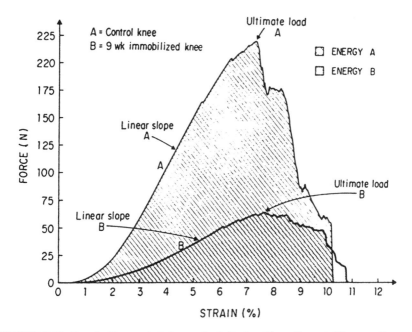

FIGURE 5-10. *Records of force vs. strain from mechanical testing of femur-ligament-tibia preparations, comparing mechanical behavior of medial cruciate ligaments from immobilized knees (curve B) and control, non-immobilized knees (curve A) in rabbits.* Note the decrease in stiffness (slope) and decreased load at failure (= "ultimate load") following 9 wk of immobilization. Reproduced from Woo et al. (1982), with permission.

the insertion site. In their classic study, Laros et al. (1971) demonstrated a 40% decline in the junction strength/body weight ratio in the MCLs of dogs that had been immobilized for 6–12 wk; this was similar to declines in load at failure noted in rabbit MCL (Woo et al., 1987) and in primate ACL (Noyes et al., 1974) after similar periods of immobilization. Histological confirmation by Laros et al. (1971) of resorption of bone at the tibial insertion sites reaffirms the importance of bony integrity in maintaining junction strength of ligaments. Interestingly, junction strength declines significantly (approximately 30%) in the contralateral, *non-immobilized* MCL. Even simple cage confinement, as opposed to free exercise conditions in large pens, produces a 17% decrement in junction strength (Laros et al., 1971). Hence, designating caged, sedentary animals as representative of normal physiology may be inappropriate when testing effects of an exercise regimen on connective tissues.

ADAPTATIONS TO EXERCISE TRAINING IN BONE, LIGAMENT, AND TENDON

Bone

Mechanisms for the Response to Increases in Mechanical Loading: Increased Modeling or Decreased Remodeling? The strength of bone depends upon both its structure (geometric arrangement in space) and the material strength of the tissue itself. The adult skeleton has two strategies, those of modeling and remodeling, to adapt its structure to new functional demands. Macroscopic changes in bone size and shape are the result of increased modeling activity; remodeling, which replaces old or fatigue-damaged bone with new bone, is primarily responsible for changes in tissue material strength (Martin, 1993). Frost's "mechanostat" theory (1987) assigns opposite roles for modeling and remodeling in the response to increases in mechanical loading. When loading of a bone is increased, remodeling is depressed. This reduction in resorptive activity reduces the creation of new resorption cavities and hence porosity of cortical bone; the slowing of bone formation activity reduces the quantity of new, less mineralized bone. Modeling may be independently stimulated to increase bone strength by changing its size or shape, e.g., by adding bone to the outer periosteal surface of a long bone. The capability of bone to adapt to increased physical activity therefore depends on how effectively one or both of these responses is activated.

"Loading" of bone with some physical activity can vary in several important factors, including the magnitude of the load (measured experimentally by strain on the bone surface) and the number of loading cycles. For example, lifting heavy weights maximizes the load magnitude on the lumbar spine with a minimum of cycles (the number of lifts performed), whereas walking for 3 miles imposes lower magnitude loads on the same bony region but maximizes the number of cycles (i.e., each step representing one cycle). Carter and colleagues (1987) have developed a mathematical model that demonstrates the relative importance of strain magnitude versus number of cycles. The total daily loading stimulus (STIM) can be expressed as

$$STIM \propto \Sigma\, n_i\, (S_i\, /S_{ult})^m$$

where the total stimulus is dependent on the total number of loading cycles (n_i), and the magnitude of each *ith* load pattern is represented as a single "effective stress" parameter, S_i, as compared to the effective stress to failure, S_{ult}. In this equation the exponent m is a weighting factor. If loading magnitude is more important than number of loading cycles, its value will exceed 1.0; if magnitude is less important, m will be less than 1.0. The best fit of this theoretical model with experimental data produces a value for m between 2 and 6, thus implying that increasing the magnitude of forces on bone more strongly affects bone mass than does increasing the number of loading cycles.

Bone mass is the best and most thoroughly studied indicator of bone functional strength, although bone geometry and material properties are also important factors. Bone mass is assessed most directly by histomorphometric measurement of bone specimens or biopsies after an experimental intervention. In human studies researchers more often have to rely on noninvasive measures of assessing bone geometry and mineral density as indicators of changes in remodeling or modeling in response to increased activity.

Although a comprehensive review of the literature in this area is outside the scope of this chapter, several thorough reviews are recommended to the reader (Forwood & Burr, 1993; Gutin & Kasper, 1992; Lanyon, 1992; Snow-Harter & Marcus, 1991). The discussion below centers primarily on those studies focusing on the bone response to loading in middle-aged and old subjects. The accumulation of literature suggests that exercise serves primarily a conservative function in the aging skeleton, that is, to slow or perhaps halt the usual loss of bone seen with aging.

Evidence for Adaptation of Bone to Increased Loading

Data from Animal Models. In mature or senescent rats subjected to endurance training on treadmills, both cortical and cancellous bone increase their mineral content (Beyer et al., 1985; McDonald et al., 1986; Silbermann et al., 1991). Increases in mouse vertebral bone mass relative to that of aging controls are maintained up to 6 mo after the cessation of training (Silbermann et al., 1991). The age at the onset of training may affect the bone response in some species; mice that begin training at midlife do not experience the increase in cancellous bone volume in lumbar vertebrae as do mice that begin a running regimen early in life (Silbermann et al., 1990). One year of treadmill running prevented the increase in bone turnover and loss of cancellous bone in the tibia seen in osteoporotic rats (Myburgh et al., 1989). Raab et al. (1991) provided histomorphometric evidence for the adaptation of cortical bone to endurance training; they detailed evidence of increased bone formation activity at the periosteum and at intra-cortical surfaces in femoral bone of adult pigs subjected to treadmill walking for 20 wk. There were no changes, however, in bone cross-sectional area and bone mineral content; the authors speculated that perhaps the intensity of the exercise was not high enough to stimulate measurable change in bone mass.

More precise information about the nature of the loading required to produce functional adaptations in bone cell activities and bone structure has been provided by several teams of researchers utilizing controlled external loading of bone in *in vivo* models. In the functionally isolated turkey ulna model of Rubin and Lanyon (1984), the ulna is surgically isolated from both joints and attached via externalized pins to a motor-driven device that delivers intermittent compressive loads. The number of cycles as well as the force delivered to the bone can be quantified precisely, because the ulna is functionally immobilized except during the externally applied loading sessions. Strain gauges applied to the bone surface can verify strain experienced at the bone surface during loading regimens.

With this model, Rubin and Lanyon verified: 1) that a dose-response relationship exists between peak strain magnitude experienced during loading and eventual change in bone mass (Rubin & Lanyon, 1985); 2) that loading must be intermittent rather than static to produce an increase in bone formation (Lanyon & Rubin, 1984); 3) that even at physiological levels of strain, a novel strain distribution, as compared to that usually experienced, is capable of producing an increase in bone mass (Rubin & Lanyon, 1985); and 4) that a single period of loading (e.g., 36 cycles) is adequate to stimulate a modeling response on previously inactive periosteal surfaces (Pead et al., 1988). Many of these results have been confirmed in a mammalian (rat) model of external loading that does not require surgery (Raab-Cullen et al., 1994; Turner et al., 1991).

Data from Humans. The information derived from animal models suggests that brief, high-intensity periods of loading (i.e., exercise), generating a diversity of strain patterns in the involved bones, will provide the maximal osteogenic response. There is certainly much cross-sectional evidence that weight-training regimens may be more effective than endurance training, which generates lower intensity muscle contractions over many more cycles (Conroy et al., 1993; Granhed et al., 1987; Nilsson & Westlin, 1971). Many other forms of exercise might be successful in minimizing age-related bone loss, as evidenced by the striking differences in bone density of the distal radius in athletic and non-athletic women over 60 y of age (Talmage et al., 1986). In the athletic women studied by Talmage et al., no significant decline in radial density was found with age (Figure 5-11). Unfortunately, little information was given about the activities of the athletic women in this study except that they exercised regularly three times per week, 9 mo/y for at least 5 y, at an intensity equivalent to playing vigorous tennis for an hour. Middle-aged long-distance runners, male and female, have 40% more mineral content in cancellous bone of the lumbar vertebrae than do age-matched sedentary controls, as measured by computed tomography (Lane et al., 1986).

Longitudinal studies in older adults have been less uniformly successful in demonstrating an absolute gain in bone mass than is implied from the cross-sectional data; see Table 5-4 for a summary of recent prospective studies involving men and women over 50 y of age. Nine months of resistance training in postmenopausal women prevents the decline in the bone mineral density of lumbar spine noted in nonexercising controls (Pruitt et al., 1992). Adding weight training to an endurance training regimen maintains bone mass but does not produce any absolute gain (Peterson et al., 1991). On the other hand, an 3% gain in bone density of the radius was noted in women who combined 2 y of low-intensity exercise with estrogen replacement therapy (Prince et al., 1991), clearly demonstrating the permissive role of estrogen on the osteogenic effect of exer-

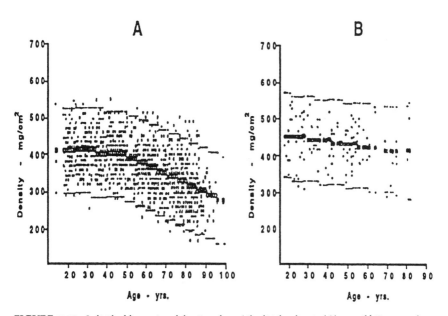

FIGURE 5-11. *Individual bone mineral density values of the distal radius in (A) non-athletic women (n = 1,105) and (B) athletic women (n = 124).* Mean regression lines from segmented regression analysis are superimposed on upper and lower 95% confidence limits. Note lack of decline in bone mineral density with age in athletic women, as compared to non-athletic women. Reproduced from Talmage et al. (1986), with permission.

TABLE 5-4. *Changes in bone with exercise interventions in older populations; prospective studies published 1987–1994*

	Sex	RT[a]	Age (years)	No. of subjects[b]	Length	Frequency (/week)	Duration (min)	Type of training	Measurement[c]	Change (%)
Beverly et al. 1989	F	N	62	57 30	6 weeks 6 months	7	0.5	Squeezing tennis balls, one hand Detraining	SPA Wrist	+3 E arm +2 C arm −3 E arm
Bloomfield et al. 1993	F	N	60	7 C 7 BE	8 months	3	50	Bicycle ergometry	DPA Spine DPA Femur	−2 C +4 BE −1 C +3 BE
Cavanaugh and Cann 1988	F	N	55 57	8 E 9 C	1 year	3	15–40	Walking (ave 3.5 mph)	QCT Spine	−6 E −4 C
Chow et al. 1987	F	Y	56	15 C 17 A 16 A-S	1 year	3	5–10 30 10–15	Stretching Weightbearing aerobic Strength training, 10 reps at 10 RM	NAA CaBI	−1 C +4 A +8 A-S
Dalsky et al. 1988	F	N	62	17 E 18 C	8 months	3	50–60	Walk, jog, stair-climbing	DPA Spine	+5 E −1 C
Hatori et al. 1993	F	Y	57	12 C 9 MI-W 12 HI-W	7 months	3	30	Walking at HR's < (= MI-W) or > (= HI-W) anaerobic threshold HR	DXA Spine	−2 C −1 MI-W +1 HI-W
Menkes et al. 1993	M	N	57	7 C 11 WT	16 weeks	3	30–60	High-intensity weight training	DXA Spine DXA Femur	0 C +2 WT 0 C +4 WT

Study	Sex		Age	Groups	Duration			Intervention	Site	Results
Nelson et al. 1991	F	N	60	9 C[e] / 9 W[e]	12 months	4	50	Walking with 3-kg weight belts	DPA Spine QCT Spine DPA Femur SPA Wrist	0 C / +2 W -7 C / +1 W +1 C / +3 W -1 C / +3 W
Peterson et al. 1991	F	N	52	19 C / 19 ED / 21 ED-WT		3 (ED) / 6 (ED + WT)	50 / 40–50	Endurance dance alone or with WT on alternate days	DPA Spine DPA Femur SPA Wrist	0 C / +1 ED / +1 ED-WT -1 C / +1 ED / +1 ED-WT 0 C / +1 ED / -2 ED-WT
Prince et al. 1991	F	Y	56	42 C / 41 E / 40 E-E_2	2 years	3	30–60	Low-impact aerobics w/arm work 1x/week; walking 2x/week	SPA Wrist	-3 C / -3 E / +3 E-E_2
Pruitt et al. 1992	F	N	54	9 C / 17 WT	9 months	3	50–60	Weight training at > 60% 1 RM[d]	DPA Spine DPA Femur SPA Wrist	-4 C / +1 WT -1 C / -3 WT -1 C / +1 WT
Rikli and McManis 1990	F	?	57–83	13 GE / 10 GEWT / 11 C	10 months	3	50 / 20	General aerobic training; Upper body strength training, free weights	SPA Radius	+1 GE / +2 GEWT / -3 C

(continued)

TABLE 5-4. *Continued.*

	Sex	RT[a]	Age (years)	No. of subjects[b]	Length	Frequency (/week)	Duration (min)	Type of training	Measurement[c]	Change (%)
Sinaki et al. 1989	F	Y	49–65	34 E 31 C	2 years	5	(5?)	10 back extensions with weights	DPA Spine	−3 E −2 C
Smidt et al. 1992	F	Y	56	27 C 22 TE	12 months	3–4	(30?)	Sit-ups, double leg raises, prone trunk extension	DPA Spine DPA Femur	−2 C −2 TE 0 C +1 TE
Smith et al. 1989	F	N	35–65	80 E 62 C	4 years	3	50	Endurance dance	SPA Radius	−3 E −7 C

[a]RT, randomized trial; N, no; Y, yes

[b]Letters refer to subject groups: E, exercise; C, control; GE, general exercise; GEWT, GE plus weight training; W, walkers; ED, endurance dance; ED-WT, endurance dance plus weight training; TE, trunk exercise

[c]NAA, neutron activation analysis; SPA, single photon absorptiometry; QCT, quantitative computed tomography; CaBI, calcium bone index; DPA, dual photon absorptiometry; DXA, dual energy x-ray absorptiometry

[d]RM, repetition maximum

[e]Experimental groups on high-calcium diet

Adapted and updated from Smith and Gilligan, 1991.

cise (Dalsky, 1990). Middle-aged men experienced a 3.8% gain in femoral neck bone density after 4 mo of a rigorous strength training program (Menkes et al., 1993); given that this time period represents only one remodeling cycle of adult bone, this result may not represent a new steady-state for bone mass.

Although weight-training regimens may be theoretically optimal, many older adults prefer other forms of activity. Two well-designed prospective studies have successfully demonstrated an absolute gain in bone mass utilizing combinations of moderate intensity aerobic dance and jogging (Chow et al., 1987) and stair-climbing and jogging (Dalsky et al., 1988) (Figure 5-12). Nonweightbearing exercise such as stationary cycling prevents age-related decrements in bone mass at the lumbar spine (Bloomfield et al., 1993). These gains in bone mass with exercise are not permanent; that is, bone mass decreases back to pre-training levels if the training stimulus is reduced (Dalsky et al., 1988; Michel et al., 1991).

There is limited evidence that there may be an upper threshold of exercise stimulus for the salutary effect of exercise on bone, beyond which decrements of bone mass may occur. For example, Michel et al. (1991) describe a select few of a study population who exercised more than 200–300 min/wk; bone density of the lumbar spine in these over-exercisers was extremely low compared to moderate and nonexercisers. This intriguing observation reflects increasing evidence from animal models that intense

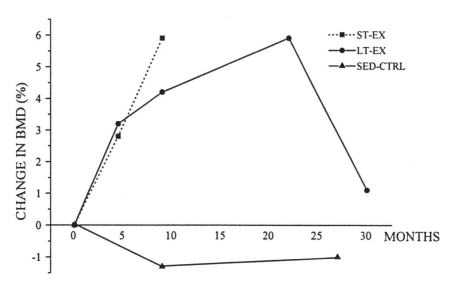

FIGURE 5-12. *Relative change in bone mineral density (BMD) in healthy postmenopausal women with short-term (ST = 9 mo) and long-term (LT = 22 mo) exercise, as compared to sedentary, age-matched control subjects.* The LT exercise group was re-scanned after 13 wk of detraining, at which time BMD had returned to within 1% of pretraining values. BMD was measured by dual-photon absorptiometry. From the data of Dalsky et al. (1988).

training can result in decreases in bone mass, even in male animals not subject to shifts in serum estrogens.

It is possible that physical activity patterns over the entire life span have a larger impact on bone status in the older adult than does current activity level, making it more difficult to demonstrate a positive effect of exercise training on bone mass. Current anthropometric and lifestyle factors (including physical activity) accounted for less than 30% of the variance in bone mineral density in 1600 Finnish perimenopausal women (Kröger et al., 1994).

There is almost no evidence for alterations in bone cell activities associated with exercise in humans, except for occasional reports of favorable changes in serum or urine markers for bone resorption and formation. One intriguing line of evidence that regular activity may stimulate modeling in aging human bone stems from comparisons between cortical bone specimens from subjects who lived in contemporary industrialized countries and archaeological samples from a pre-17th century Pecos Pueblo population. Continued periosteal expansion of femoral bone, which requires modeling activity at the bone surface, is evident in specimens from both male and female Pecos Pueblo inhabitants (Ruff & Hayes, 1983). Adding bone to the outer surface increases the cross-sectional moment of inertia and thereby resistance to bending. Hence, declines in bone material strength with age were compensated for by increased structural strength conferred by continued activity of bone-forming osteoblasts at the periosteal surface of cortical bone.

This result contrasts with findings in contemporary female specimens, which show no evidence of periosteal expansion after skeletal maturity (refer to Figure 5-4). A likely explanation for this difference in cortical modeling activity between contemporary and a Native American population of three centuries ago is the latter's habitual physical activity; ethnographic and historical records document that Pecos women shared with men equal responsibility for such tasks as building houses, carrying water, irrigating fields, and harvesting crops (Ruff & Hayes, 1983). Epidemiological data on fracture incidence in living populations support this relationship between habitual activity and maintained bone strength. Rural populations who customarily engage in hard physical labor do not experience the same age-related increase in fractures as do urban populations (Chalmers & Ho, 1970; Sernbo et al., 1988).

Is The Osteogenic Response To Exercise Impaired In Aging Bone? Given that osteoblastic activity slows with aging, it would be reasonable to hypothesize that the bone formation response to exercise or external loading of bone might also be impaired in older adults or senescent animals. Two recent publications support this concept. Using the functionally isolated turkey ulna model to quantify the response to external loading, Rubin et al. (1992) demonstrated a 30% increase in cortical bone area after 8 wk of daily loading in 1-y-old adult turkeys; the same regimen produced no measurable change in cortical area in 3-y-old turkeys (Figure 5-13). Histomorphometric analysis revealed a significant activation of bone formation at the periosteal surface (4.0 ± 0.4 μm/d) in the young animals, whereas a much lower rate (< 0.8 μm/d) of this modeling activity was detected in only one of the three old turkeys. This lack of response was not due to a global suppression of osteoblast activity because intracortical remodeling, with coordinated activity of osteoclast and osteoblast populations, was observed in the 3-y-old birds. In fact, turnover of intracortical bone appeared to be elevated after 8 wk of loading in the older turkeys, with an increase in the number of resorption cavities observed on cross-section (see Figure 5-13); the net effect is a slight but non-significant decrease in cortical area, which would be reversed as soon as osteoblasts replaced the resorbed bone.

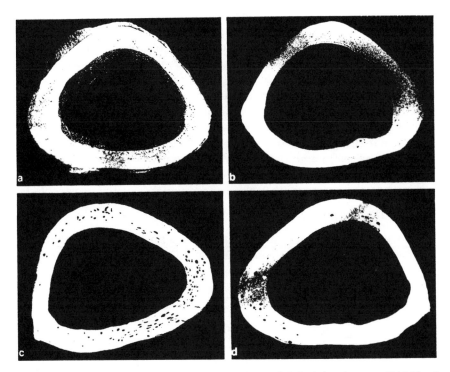

FIGURE 5-13. *Photomicrographs of 100 μm sections from mid-shaft of ulnae from 1-y-old (A,B) and 3-y-old (C,D) turkeys.* Experimental ulnae (A,C) were subjected to 8 wk of controlled external loading. Compared to their respective control ulnae (from the intact contralateral limb; B,D), substantial new bone formation, indicated by the gray stippled area, can be seen on periosteal and endosteal surfaces of the 1-y-old turkeys (A), whereas in the 3-y-old animals there was no new bone formation. Intra-cortical remodeling appears to be elevated in the loaded ulna in the older turkey, evidenced by numerous resorption cavities. From Rubin et al. (1992), with permission.

Treadmill running arguably provides a more physiological form of exercise than does external loading of fixated limb bones; using the rat as an animal model also yields information on the response of mammalian bone, which differs in some respects from avian bone. After 8 wk of treadmill training, both femoral and vertebral bone mass increases in young (4-mo-old) rats; a reduction in resorptive activity and an increase in periosteal formation both contribute to the increase in femoral bone mass (Yeh et al., 1991). Similar training of 14-mo-old rats has no effect on resorptive activity and increases bone mass only in the femur, suggesting that bone in the older animal responds less efficiently than does young adult bone to an equivalent exercise stimulus.

Interestingly, with a more vigorous treadmill protocol including running up a 15% grade, Raab et al. (1990) demonstrated improvements in mechanical properties of the femur in both young (2.5 mo) and old (25 mo) rats (Table 5-5). An increase in fat-free dry weight of femurs in the old rats after training, with no increase in moment of inertia, implies an increase in bone density. Such an adaptation would explain the increase in material strength, measured by ultimate stress, observed in the old rats. It is unclear why this latter study was able to demonstrate similar training adaptations in young and old rats, whereas the protocol of Yeh et al. (1991) did not, unless some minimal threshold of loading intensity must be surpassed to activate osteoblast populations in older animals. These intriguing results require corroboration in other models, but raise the possibility that the ability of osteoblasts to respond to an osteogenic signal may be impaired in aging animals. An alternative explanation is an impairment of some element of the signal transduction system activated by mechanical loading, resulting in a dampened signal delivered to osteoblasts.

Ligament, Tendon, and Junction Strength

Structural and Biochemical Changes. Training can induce a number of changes in the structure and biochemical constituents of connective

TABLE 5-5. *Changes in mechanical properties of the femur in young (2.5-mo) and old (25-mo) rats with endurance training*

	FFW (mg)	MI (mm⁴)	Ultimate force (kg/mm)	Ultimate stress (kg/mm²)
YC	409±8*	2.64±0.07*	41.7±1.1*	21.8±0.7*‡
YT	422±11*†	2.80±0.10*	42.9±1.8*†	21.6±0.6*‡
OC	521±8	4.10±0.32	45.7±1.1	17.4±0.8‡
OT	574±26†	3.92±0.10	53.1±3.4†	20.5±1.1‡

YC = young controls (n=10); YT = young trained (n=8); OC = old controls (n=6); OT = old trained (n=8); FFW = bone fat free dry weight; MI = moment of inertia. Ultimate force and stress determined for whole femur in three-point bending. *p<0.05 for significant age difference [(YC+YT) vs. (OC+OT)]; †p<0.05 for significant training difference [(YT+OT) vs. (YC+OC)]; ‡p<0.05 for interaction between age and training. Adapted from Raab et al. (1990).

tissues. Turnover of collagen, as measured by uptake of tritiated proline, is increased in tendon of aged mice after endurance exercise training (Heikkinen & Vuori, 1972), but it is unclear whether this increased turnover results in any net increase in collagen content. With both sprint and endurance training, rat MCL increased in wet weight normalized for ligament length, with no increase in water content, implying a net increase in tissue collagen or other matrix constituents (Tipton et al., 1975; Table 5-6). When collagen is estimated by hydroxyproline content, increases with training occur in dog ligaments (Tipton et al., 1970) and in tendons of rats (Vailas et al., 1985) and swine (Woo et al., 1980), but not in rat ligaments (Tipton et al., 1975) or in rabbit tendons (Viidik, 1967). Tipton et al. (1970) measured an increase in collagen fiber bundle diameters in ligaments from trained dogs, suggesting hypertrophy of individual collagen fibers, but this finding has not been reported in other species. In fact, there is recent evidence that chronic endurance exercise stimulates ligament fibroblasts to synthesize more smaller-diameter collagen fibrils, with a resulting decrease in mean fibril diameter, even as total collagen fibril cross-sectional area per unit area remains constant (Oakes, 1988). Glycosaminoglycan concentration increases after training in tendons of rats (Vailas et al., 1985) and rabbits (Gillard et al., 1979), which may provide one potential mechanism for observed alterations in collagen fibril size (Gillard et al., 1979; Parry et al., 1982).

Independent of any change in tissue mass, training appears to decrease the content of nonreducible cross-links in rabbit tendon (Viidik, 1986), which probably is the result of the increased turnover of collagen. Although this increased turnover is reminiscent of that occurring in immobilized connective tissue, yielding a proportional increase in newly synthesized collagen, the functional outcomes of training are diametrically opposed to those seen with disuse. An increase in collagen stiffness occurs after training (Viidik, 1967; Woo et al., 1982), corresponding to improvements in tensile strength of tendons and ligaments, as confirmed in extensor tendons in swine (Woo et al., 1980). Junction strength increases 8–24% after training in most species tested (Adams, 1966; Tipton et al., 1975), which may reflect improvements in bone as well as in ligament strength. Hypophysectomy in rats does not abolish this improved junction strength with training or the decrement in junction strength observed with immobilization (Tipton et al., 1975). Two interesting exceptions are female rats, both intact (Booth & Tipton, 1969) and ovariectomized rats on estrogen (Tipton et al., 1975), and primates (Tipton et al., 1979), in whom junction strength did not improve with training.

The specificity of training principle applies to connective tissues just as it does to bone. In particular, increased tensile and/or junction strength will occur only in those ligaments and tendons actively recruited during training and exposed to greater loading than normally experienced. The lack of increase in medial collateral ligament junction strength in the primate study of Tipton et al. (1979) may reflect the fact that the MCL is not recruited for locomotion and jumping activities in this primate as much as is the patellar tendon, in which material strength did improve with training (Tipton & Vailas, 1990). Studies of adaptations in swine tendons to endurance exercise training provide a particularly instructive example of these concepts (Woo et al., 1981). After 12 mo training, there was no change in tensile properties of digital flexor tendons, whereas a significant improvement was noted in the tensile strength of digital extensor tendons (Figure 5-14). In fact, as can be seen when comparing stress-strain curves in the unexercised control animals, extensor tendons are normally not as strong as flexor tendons. The different responses of extensor and flexor tendons may well depend upon the relative increase in daily loading of the specific tendon provided by the training protocol. In this case, it seems reasonable to presume that extensor tendons experience more of a relative overload with training and therefore a greater adaptive response.

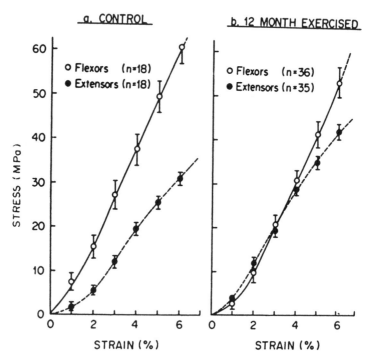

FIGURE 5-14. *Comparison of stress-strain curves derived from mechanical testing of digital flexor and digital extensor tendons from 4 sedentary control swine and 5 swine subjected to 12 mo of running. Note that in the* control animals, flexor tendons are stronger and stiffer (denoted by the steeper slope of the curve) than extensor tendons; exercise training appeared to abolish most of the difference between these two tendons. Reproduced from Woo et al. (1981), with permission.

In another example of the specificity principle, some forms of exercise appear to be more effective than others in producing functional increases in ligament strength. A training regimen for adult rats utilizing frequent sprints up a 20% grade produces increased ligament mass but no improvement in junction strength of rat MCL (Tipton et al., 1975); by contrast, endurance training elicits increases in ligament mass and improved junction strength (Table 5-6). Even an endurance training protocol must include some running up a grade to be effective. There is no improvement in *in situ* junction strength of MCL in rats performing only level running rigorous enough to produce increases in muscle cytochrome oxidase. By contrast, rats regularly trained on a graded treadmill exhibit a 12% increment in junction strength in addition to improved muscle oxidative capacity (Tipton et al., 1986), confirming earlier findings by Adams (1966). Clearly, it would be helpful to establish the actual strain generated in ligaments and tendons, in order to identify optimal training regimens.

The Response to Exercise in Older Animals. Only one study in the literature compared the response of connective tissue in young and senescent animals to a standardized training regimen. After 9 mo of voluntary running exercise in activity wheels, no increases in ground matrix proteoglycans were noted in patellar tendon of 28-mo-old rats, whereas most of these matrix constituents increased in 9-mo-old rats (Table 5-7; Vailas et al., 1985). However, because the older rats voluntarily ran only 31% of the kilometers covered by the younger rats, some of this difference may be due to the difference in total loading experienced by the patellar tendon. Interestingly, galactosamine-containing proteoglycan concentration in the 28-mo-old runners was not significantly different from that in sedentary 9-mo-old rats; exercise may prevent the age-related decline in this matrix constituent noted in the sedentary, senescent rats.

Kasperczyk et al. (1991) provided indirect evidence that chronic exercise may help minimize aging changes in ligaments with their data comparing mechanical properties of knee ligaments from young (mean age 30 y) and old (mean age 65 y) donors matched for habitual activity levels.

TABLE 5-6. *Effects of sprint and endurance training regimens on rat medial collateral ligament properties*

	% H_2O	Wet Weight/ length (mg/mm)	Separation Force (N)	Junction Strength/BW (kg/kgBW)	Elastic Stiffness (kg/mm)
SPRINT TRNG					
Untrained control	57.0±0.6	0.37±0.02	27.4±1.1	6.06±0.25	1.10±0.05
Trained	57.7±0.7	0.42±0.02*	26.3±0.9	6.09±0.26	1.05±0.04
ENDURANCE TRNG					
Untrained control	60.5±0.9	0.40±0.01	28.2±0.9	6.28±0.20	1.13±0.02
Trained	60.2±0.7	0.45±0.01*	31.4±0.9*	6.90±0.20*	1.11±0.03

*$p < 0.05$, trained vs. untrained; N = Newtons; BW = body weight; TRNG = training.
Adapted from Tipton et al. (1975).

TABLE 5-7. *Changes in rat patellar tendon dry weight, hydroxyproline and matrix constituent concentrations with age and exercise*

	28- vs. 9-mo-old[a] (sedentary)	Response to exercise 9-mo-old	Response to exercise 28-mo-old
Dry weight	NS	NS	NS
Hydroxyproline	35% ↑	NS	NS
Uronic acid	16–22% ↓	19% ↑	NS
Hexosamine	20% ↓	13% ↑	NS
Galactosamine	23% ↓	22% ↑	NS
Glucosamine	NS	NS	NS

[a][(Value in 28-mo-old)-(value in 9-mo-old)]/(value in 9-mo-old); NS = no significant change with training or aging. Adapted from Vailas et al. (1985).

Material strength properties (ultimate stress, elastic modulus, and ultimate strain) of the cruciate ligaments did not differ significantly between these two donor groups. Unfortunately, how habitual activity was assessed was not documented by the authors, but these data raise the interesting possibility that many so-called aging changes in the connective tissues are more likely due to relative disuse. Many more studies are needed in this area to determine if aging affects the adaptations of connective tissue structure and mechanical function to increased activity and, further, how regular activity might affect the aging process as expressed in connective tissues.

NUTRITIONAL FACTORS IN THE OPTIMIZATION OF BONE MASS

Calcium and Vitamin D Intake Over the Life Span

It is well accepted that a diet sufficient in calcium and vitamin D is critical to the attainment of peak bone mass. Calcium requirements are highest in infancy and adolescence, when rapid bone growth requires a positive calcium balance to proceed normally (Matkovic, 1991). When skeletal maturity is achieved, maintaining calcium balance appears to be adequate to protect bone mass. Several epidemiological studies have demonstrated a reduced fracture risk in those populations consuming more dietary calcium (Holbrook et al., 1988; Matkovic et al., 1979), although, it should be noted, the primary comparisons in these studies are between calcium-deficient and calcium-sufficient diets. Unfortunately, confounding factors such as significant variations in habitual physical activity between low- and high-calcium intake groups render some of these data inconclusive (Kanis, 1991). It would appear prudent, however, for all adults to consume 1000 mg of calcium per day and for individuals at high risk for developing significant osteopenia (including virtually all adults over the age of 65) to consume at least 1500 mg/d of calcium.

Sufficient intakes of vitamin D play a key role in assuring normal intestinal calcium absorption and hence the maintenance of calcium balance and optimal bone mass. Given the age-related decline in circulating 25-OHD and 1,25-OH$_2$D and the decreased solar exposure typical to many elderly individuals, it has been suggested these individuals should increase nutritional intake of vitamin D to well above the current RDA of 200 IU/d (Heaney, 1988).

Interactions with Endocrine Status and Physical Activity

Women experience an acceleration of bone loss for the first 1–3 y following estrogen withdrawal at menopause (Nordin et al., 1990), with an excess of calcium ions released to the circulation from resorbed bone while skeletal mass is being revised downward to a new steady-state mass. During this brief period, the need for dietary calcium is probably minimal, which explains the ineffectiveness of calcium supplementation if given during this time (Ettinger et al., 1987; Riis et al., 1987). Once a new steady-state bone mass is reached, the chronic effect of low circulating estrogens is a doubly disadvantageous one: calcium absorption efficiency is reduced (Heaney et al., 1989) and urinary calcium loss increased (Heaney et al., 1978). In this physiological state, modest increases in calcium intake (up to a total of 1500 mg/d) appear warranted and have been recommended for postmenopausal women and for men over the age of 65 y by the NIH Consensus Development Panel on Optimal Calcium Intake (1994).

Calcium-deficient diets might prove most deleterious to those individuals who are very inactive or restricted to bedrest. In at least two animal models, immobilization-related bone loss is exacerbated by calcium insufficiency, which stimulates further increases in bone resorption (Lanyon et al., 1986; Weinreb et al., 1991). Conversely, increased physical activity in growing rats increases intestinal calcium absorption (Yeh & Aloia, 1990); whether this occurs in aged animals is unknown.

DIRECTIONS FOR FUTURE RESEARCH

Most individuals in industrialized countries become increasingly sedentary over the years, despite our best public health efforts at encouraging regular exercise. All too often this reality is overlooked in the design of studies seeking to define the effect of aging in humans; the physiological and structural changes seen in connective tissues in older subjects are really the result of the interaction between chronic inactivity or outright disuse and true aging changes. If we are aiming to measure the latter, subjects (or donors, in the case of cadaver studies) must be matched for habitual activity level to control for this confounding factor. The modern-day gender difference in periosteal expansion of cortical bone over the life span, as compared to the absence of such a difference in male and female specimens from the Pecos Pueblo population, points up the need to control for activity levels when making gender comparisons as well. Of course, accurately documenting activity patterns is a thorny problem with which many researchers are still struggling, but some reasonable methods exist that should be utilized in future studies.

Recently published data suggest that genetic variation in one allele for the vitamin D receptor accounts for 50–75% of osteoporotic cases in an Australian population of both genders (Morrison et al., 1994). If indeed one gene plays such a powerful role in the development of bone fragility, future exercise trials may need to find a method for controlling for genotype when recruiting subjects.

A related design problem relevant to animal studies should be noted. Most often, caged animals are used as the baseline for comparison with trained animals to demonstrate the effect of exercise on connective tissues. We may be overestimating training adaptations with this design, for caged animals are far more likely to represent a relative disuse model. The use of "experiments of nature" might be instructive in this regard.

Researchers should recruit that fraction of our older adult population that remains vigorously active to participate in cross-sectional studies that focus on comparisons with age-matched sedentary groups, as well as with younger individuals matched for activity patterns. Iliac crest biopsy studies can reveal a wealth of data and should be pursued if we are to establish the changes in bone cell activities that are truly the result of aging *per se*. More acceptable and less risky noninvasive methods, such as that to measure bone geometry with re-analysis of bone densitometry scans (Beck et al., 1992), should be implemented whenever possible to answer relevant research questions about changes in structure. Investigators using these noninvasive techniques need to integrate awareness of the limitations of the procedure with a comprehensive understanding of bone biology. Bone densitometry, for instance, cannot reliably provide information about steady-state changes in bone mass in response to an exercise intervention until the remodeling rate has reached a new equilibrium, usually requiring at least 9–12 mo intervals between measurements (Frost, 1989)

A number of questions remain unanswered regarding the effects of exercise and aging on bone. What are the typical strains experienced by human bone during normal locomotion and sport activities? Do those strains change in magnitude in the older adult, given the changes in material properties of bone tissue with aging? We need these answers to determine the extent, if any, to which Biewener's safety factor truly does decline with aging, thereby increasing the risk of fracture. Strain in tendons and ligaments needs to be measured *in vivo* to verify that a particular training regimen does indeed stress the ligament or tendon under study, as well as to define the relative load experienced; at least one laboratory has developed a method for accomplishing this (Komi et al., 1987). The effect of exercise and disuse on ligament insertion sites has been fairly well described, but there is a dearth of data on tendinous insertions. We need to know whether microcracks really do accumulate with age in bone and if they significantly affect bone material strength. Does the capacity of remodeling to repair fatigue damage decline with age? Is this deficit specific to certain populations, such as those osteoporotic patients with low remodeling rates? How do endocrine or local factors interact with the capacity of osteoblasts to repair microcracks?

Evidence in animal models for a decreased responsiveness of osteoblasts to exercise needs corroboration in the human model, but will be almost impossible to answer without bone biopsy data. Side-by-side comparisons of old and young subjects are needed to determine if aging affects the response to disuse; there is evidence from at least one animal model that recovery of lost bone mass after immobilization is impaired with aging (Jaworski & Uhthoff, 1986). We know far more about the response of tendons and ligaments to disuse, due to the implications for recovery from surgery, than we do about their adaptations to exercise training. Much of the existing evidence in this area is 15–20 y old; the creative use of newer techniques could add substantially to our knowledge base. In particular, applications of molecular biology techniques could be helpful in deriving mechanisms for altered connective tissue cell activities.

The optimal exercise prescription for preventing age-related osteopenia and decrements in tendon and ligament strength has yet to be defined. There is some evidence that relatively high-intensity muscle contractions (such as those generated during resistance training) may be most effective, but various endurance activities are often more attractive to older adults. Is there a minimum intensity of rhythmic muscle contractions necessary to generate enough strain in these tissues to stimulate adaptive change? How important is the maintenance of muscle mass and muscle strength to effecting these responses? The creative energy of many investigators will be required to design appropriate studies to answer these questions.

SUMMARY

In aging adults a gradual decline in bone mass starts in the fourth decade; the magnitude and rate of bone loss varies by anatomical site, gender, and hormonal status. For example, cancellous bone of vertebral bodies tends to decrease in volume earlier than does cortical bone of femoral necks; the rate of bone loss accelerates for 3–5 y after serum estrogens decline precipitously at menopause in women. The mechanisms for the age-related decline in mass likely hinge on diminished activity of the bone-forming osteoblasts; increases in serum PTH and decreases in serum 1,25-vitamin D exacerbate the imbalance between resorption and formation of new bone. A decreased sensitivity of osteoblasts to endocrine regulators or local growth factors may also play a role.

Bone strength is dependent not only on bone mass but also bone quality, i.e., the material properties of bone tissue and its geometry. With a decline in the remodeling rate of normal bone in the aging adult, "older" unremodeled bone and associated microdamage accumulates, further contributing to a decrease in bone quality. A compensatory increase in cross-sectional moment of inertia, with continuing addition of new bone to the outer periosteal surface, has been observed in aging males but not in aging females. This gender difference in bone geometry probably explains the greater frequency of hip (i.e., femoral neck fractures) in older women.

We know far less about tissue-level changes with age in ligament and tendon, especially in humans. Animal data suggest that the key alteration in these connective tissues is related to the increase in nonreducible cross-links of collagen, contributing to an increased stiffness of these tissues with aging. Collagen bundle fragmentation, a decrease in density of resident fibroblasts which themselves are less metabolically active, and decreases in matrix glycosaminoglycans are seen in older animals of many species. The functional result of these ultrastructural changes is a decrease in elastic modulus and in tensile strength of ligament and tendon. In the intact animal, the insertion site of a ligament or tendon plays a key role in the functional strength of the entire structure; with osteopenic changes in underlying bone, failure at the insertion site becomes more likely in the older animal or human. Whether these changes in mechanical characteristics directly contribute to an increased risk of connective tissue injury in the elderly is unclear.

There is clear evidence that many of these aging changes are due not to aging of the tissues *per se* but to relative disuse. There is growing cross-sectional evidence that more active adults have greater bone mineral density; however, longitudinal studies lead to the conclusion that regular exercise in middle-aged and older adults acts to conserve, rather than add to, existing bone mass. Sufficient dietary calcium and vitamin D must be ingested for optimal maintenance of bone mass. Given the decline in the responsiveness of osteoblasts with aging, the response of bone to increased exercise in the older animal may be somewhat diminished, as suggested by some data from animal models. The response of ligament and tendon to exercise in humans is largely unknown; in animals, training produces an increase in tensile strength due to increases in collagen stiffness. Junction strength of insertion sites also improves. Further advances in this field will require the development and validation of noninvasive measures of bone, ligament, and tendon in humans.

ACKNOWLEDGEMENTS

I gratefully acknowledge the skill and speed with which David Hutchinson generated many figures for this manuscript. I thank Charles Tipton, David Lamb, Hugh Welch, and Steve Gregg for numerous helpful comments in revising this manuscript.

FOOTNOTE

[1]This concept of increasing mineralization of bone with aging appears to contradict the common knowledge that bone mineral density declines over the life span. The latter factor is, however, primarily a measure of bone quantity in a given unit area and includes resorption cavities and marrow space; it is expressed in grams per cm^2 or per cm^3. The mineralization profile of a discrete area of bone is a qualitative measure of the bone material itself, not including volumes occupied by space, and is independent of changes in total bone mass.

BIBLIOGRAPHY

Adams, A. (1966). Effect of exercise upon ligament strength. Res. Quart. 37:163–167.

Akeson, W.H., S.L.-Y. Woo, D. Amiel, R.D. Coutts, and D. Daniel (1973). The connective tissue response to immobility: biochemical changes in periarticular connective tissue of the immobilized rabbit knee. Clin. Orthop. Rel. Res. 93:356–362.

Akeson, W.H., S.L.-Y. Woo, D. Amiel, and C.B. Frank (1984). The biology of ligaments. In: L.Y. Hunter and F.J. Funk, Jr. (eds.) Rehabilitation of the Injured Knee. St. Louis: C.V. Mosby Company, pp. 93–148.

Amiel, D., E. Billings, and W.H. Akeson (1990). Ligament structure, chemistry and physiology. In: D.D. Daniel, W.H. Akeson, and J.J. O'Conner (eds.) Knee Ligaments: Structure, Function, Injury, and Repair. New York: Raven Press, pp. 77–91.

Amiel, D., C. Frank, F. Harwood, J. Fronek, and W. Akeson (1984). Tendons and ligaments: a morphological and biochemical comparison. J. Orthop. Res. 1:257–265.

Amiel, D., S.D. Kuiper, C.D. Wallace, F.L. Harwood, and J.S. VandeBerg (1991). Age-related properties of medial collateral ligament and anterior cruciate ligament: a morphologic and collagen maturation study in the rabbit. J. Gerontol. 46:B159–165.

Amiel, D., S.L.-Y. Woo, F.L. Harwood, and W.H. Akeson (1982). The effect of immobilization on collagen turnover in connective tissue: a biochemical-biomechanical correlation. Acta Orthop. Scand. 53:325–332.

Arnold, J.S. (1980). Trabecular pattern and shapes in aging and osteoporosis. Metab. Bone Dis. 2:297–308.

Beck, T.J., C.B. Ruff, and K. Bissessur (1993). Age-related changes in female femoral neck geometry: implications for bone strength. Calcif. Tissue Int. 53(Suppl. l):S41–S46.

Beck, T.J., C.B. Ruff, W.W. Scott, Jr., C.C. Plato, J.D. Tobin, and C.A. Quan (1992). Sex differences in geometry of the femoral neck with aging: a structural analysis of bone mineral data. Calcif. Tissue Int. 50:24–29.

Bennett, A.E., H.W. Wahner, B.L. Riggs, and R.L. Hintz (1984). Insulin-like growth factors I and II: aging and bone density in women. J. Clin. Endocrinol. Metab. 59:701–704.

Beverly, M.C., T.A. Rider, J. Evans, R. Smith (1989). Local bone mineral response to brief exercise that stresses the skeleton. Br. Med. J. 299:233–235.

Beyer, R.E., J.C. Huang, and G.B. Wilshire (1985). The effect of endurance exercise on bone dimensions, collagen, and calcium in the aged male rat. Exper. Gerontol. 20:315–323.

Biering-Sørensen, F., H.H. Bohr, and O.P. Schaadt (1990). Longitudinal study of bone mineral content in the lumbar spine, the forearm and the lower extremities after spinal cord injury. Eur. J. Clin. Invest. 20:330–335.

Biewener, A.A. (1993). Safety factors in bone strength. Calcif. Tissue Int. 53 (Suppl. 1):S68–S74.

Binkley, J.M., and M. Peat (1986). The effects of immobilization on the ultrastructure and mechanical properties of the medial collateral ligament of rats. Clin. Orthop. Rel. Res. 203:301–308.

Bloomfield, S.A., N.I. Williams, D.R. Lamb, and R.D. Jackson (1993). Non-weightbearing exercise may increase lumbar spine bone mineral density in healthy postmenopausal women. Am. J. Phys. Med. Rehabil. 72:204–209.

Booth, F.W., and C.M. Tipton (1969). Effects of training and 17-β estradiol upon heart rates, organ weights and ligamentous strength of female rats. Int. Z. angew Physiol. 27:187–197.

Buckwalter, J.A., J.A. Maynard, and A.C. Vailas (1987). Skeletal fibrous tissues: tendon, joint capsule, and ligament. In: J.A. Albright and R.A. Brand (eds.) The Scientific Basis of Orthopaedics, 2nd ed. Los Altos, CA: Appleton & Lange, pp. 387–405.

Burr, D.B., R.B. Martin, M.B. Schaffler, and E.L. Radin (1985). Bone remodeling in response to *in vivo* fatigue microdamage. *J. Biomech.* 18:189-200.

Burstein, A.H., D.T. Reilly, and M. Martens (1976). Aging of bone tissue: mechanical properties. *J. Bone Joint Surg.* 58-A:82-86.

Canalis, E. (1993). Regulation of bone remodeling. In: M.J. Favus (ed.) *Primer on the Metabolic Bone Diseases and Disorders of Mineral Metabolism*, 2nd ed. New York: Raven Press, pp. 33-37.

Carter, D.R., D.P. Fyhrie, and R.T. Whalen (1987). Trabecular bone density and loading history: regulation of connective tissue biology by mechanical energy. *J. Biomech.* 20:785-794.

Chalmers, J., and K.C. Ho (1970). Geographical variations in senile osteoporosis: the association with physical activity. *J. Bone Joint Surg.* 52-B:667-675.

Chatterji, S., J.C. Wall, and J.W. Jeffery (1981). Age-related changes in the orientation and particle size of the mineral phase in human femoral cortical bone. *Calcif. Tissue Int.* 33:567-574.

Chow, R., J.E. Harrison, and C. Notarius (1987). Effect of two randomised exercise programmes on bone mass of healthy postmenopausal women. *Brit. Med. J.* 295:1441-1444.

Conroy, B.P., W.J. Kraemer, C.M. Maresh, S.J. Fleck, M.H. Stone, A.C. Fry, P.D. Miller, and G.P. Dalsky (1993). Bone mineral density in elite junior Olympic weightlifters. *Med. Sci. Sports Exerc.* 25:1103-1109.

Cooper, C., E.J. Atkinson, W.M. O'Fallon, and L.J. Melton III (1992). Incidence of clinically diagnosed vertebral fractures: a population-based study in Rochester, Minnesota, 1985-1989. *J. Bone Miner. Res.* 7:221-227.

Currey, J.D. (1969). The mechanical consequences of variation in the mineral content of bone. *J. Biomech.* 2:1-11.

Currey, J.D. (1979). Changes in the impact energy absorption of bone with age. *J. Biomech.* 12:459-469.

Dalsky, G.P. (1990). Effect of exercise on bone: permissive influence of estrogen and calcium. *Med. Sci. Sports Exer.* 22:281-185.

Dalsky, G., K. Stocke, A. Ehsani, E. Slatopolsky, W. Lee, and S. Birge, Jr. (1988). Weightbearing exercise training and lumbar bone mineral content in postmenopausal women. *Ann. Intern. Med.* 108:824-828.

Deitrick, J.E., G.D. Whedon, and E. Shorr (1948). Effects of immobilization upon various metabolic and physiologic functions of normal men. *Amer. J. Med.* 4:3-36.

Donaldson, C.L., S.B. Hulley, J.M. Vogel, R.S. Hattner, J.H. Bayers, and D.E. McMillan (1970). Effect of prolonged bed rest on bone mineral. *Metabolism* 19:1071-1084.

Doty, S.B. (1981). Morphological evidence of gap junctions between bone cells. *Calcif. Tissue Int.* 33:509-512.

Epstein, S., G. Bryce, J.W. Hinman, O.N. Mileer, B.L. Riggs, S.L. Hui, and C.C. Johnston, Jr. (1986). The influence of age on bone mineral regulating hormones. *Bone* 7:421-425.

Ettinger, B., H.K. Genant, C.E. Cann (1987). Postmenopausal bone loss is prevented by treatment with low-dosage estrogen with calcium. *Ann. Intern. Med.* 106:40-45.

Fazzalari, N.L. (1993). Trabecular microfracture. *Calcif. Tissue Int.* 53(Suppl. 1):S143-S147.

Forwood, M.R., and D.B. Burr (1993). Physical activity and bone mass: exercises in futility? *Bone Miner.* 21:89-112.

Francis, R.M., M. Peacock, G.A. Taylor, J.H. Storer, and B.E.C. Nordin (1984). Calcium malabsorption in elderly women with vertebral fractures: evidence for resistance to the action of vitamin D metabolites on the bowel. *Clin. Sci.* 66:103-107.

Frank, C., S. Woo, T. Andriacchi, R. Brand, B. Oakes, L. Dahners, K. DeHaven, J. Lewis, and P. Sabiston (1988). Normal ligament: structure, function, and composition. In: S.L.-Y. Woo and J.A. Buckwalter (eds.) *Injury and Repair of the Musculoskeletal Soft Tissues*. Park Ridge, IL: American Academy of Orthopaedic Surgeons, pp. 103-128.

Frost, H.M. (1960). *In vivo* osteocyte death. *J. Bone Joint Surg.* 42-A:8-143.

Frost, H.M. (1986). *Intermediary organization of the skeleton*. Boca Raton: CRC Press.

Frost, H.M. (1987). Bone "mass" and the "mechanostat:" a proposal. *Anat. Rec.* 219:1-9.

Frost, H.M. (1989). Some effects of basic multicellular unit-based remodelling on photon absorptiometry of trabecular bone. *Bone Miner.* 7:47-65.

Frost, H.M. (1990). Skeletal structural adaptations to mechanical usage (SATMU): 1. Redefining Wolff's Law: the bone modeling problem. *Anat. Rec.* 226:403-413.

Gillard, G.C., H.C. Reilly, P.G. Bell-Booth, and M.H. Flint (1979). The influence of mechanical forces on the glycosaminoglycan content of the rabbit flexor digitorum profundus tendon. *Conn. Tissue Res.* 7:37-46.

Granhed, H., R. Jonson, and T. Hansson (1987). The loads on the lumbar spine during extreme weight lifting. *Spine* 12:146-149.

Grynpas, M. (1993). Age- and disease-related changes in the mineral of bone. *Calcif. Tissue Int.* 53(Suppl. 1):S57-S64.

Gutin, B., and M.J. Kasper (1992). Can vigorous exercise play a role in osteoporosis prevention? *Osteoporosis Int.* 2:55-69.

Hansson, T., B. Ross, and A. Nachemson (1980). The bone mineral content and ultimate compressive strength of lumbar vertebrae. *Spine* 5:46-55.

Hatori, M. A. Hasegawa, H. Adachi, A. Shinozaki, R. Hayashi, H. Okano, H. Mizunuma, and K. Murata

(1993). The effects of walking at the anaerobic threshold level on vertebral bone loss in postmeno-pausal women. *Calcif. Tissue Int.* 52:411–414.

Haut, R.C., R.L. Lancaster, and C.E. DeCamp (1992). Mechanical properties of the canine patellar tendon: some correlations with age and the content of collagen. *J. Biomech.* 25:163–173.

Heaney, R.P. (1988). Nutritional factors in bone health. In: B.L. Riggs and L.J. Melton III (eds.) *Osteoporosis: Etiology, Diagnosis, and Management.* New York: Raven Press, pp. 359–372.

Heaney, R.P. (1992). The natural history of vertebral osteoporosis. Is low bone mass an epiphenomenon? *Bone* 13:S23–S26.

Heaney, R.P., R.R. Recker, and P.D. Saville (1978). Menopausal changes in calcium balance performance. *J. Lab Clin. Med.* 92:953–963.

Heaney, R.P., R.R. Recker, M.R. Stegman, and A.J. Moy (1989). Calcium absorption in women: relation-ships to calcium intake, estrogen status, and age. *J. Bone Miner. Res.* 4:469–475.

Heikkinen, E., and I. Vuori (1972). Effect of physical activity on the metabolism of collagen in aged mice. *Acta. Physiol. Scand.* 84:543–549.

Holbrook, T.L., E. Barrett-Connor, and D.L. Wingard (1988). Dietary calcium and risk of hip fracture: 14-year prospective population study. *Lancet* ii:1046–1049.

Hruza, Z., and M. Wachtlova (1969). Diminution of bone blood flow and capillary network in rats during aging. *J. Gerontol.* 24:315–320.

Hubbard, R.P., and R.W. Soutas-Little (1984). Mechanical properties of human tendon and their age de-pendence. *J. Biomech. Engineer.* 106:144–150.

Ippolito, E., P.G. Natali, F. Postacchini, L. Accinni, and C. deMartino (1980). Morphological, immuno-chemical, and biochemical study of rabbit Achilles tendon at various ages. *J. Bone Joint Surg.* 62-A:583–598.

Jaworski, Z.F.G., and H.K. Uhthoff (1986). Reversibility of nontraumatic disuse osteoporosis during its active phase. *Bone* 7:431–439.

Jee, W.S.S. (1988). The skeletal tissues. In: L. Weiss (ed.) *Cell and Tissue Biology: A Textbook of Histology.* Balti-more: Urban & Schwarzenberg, pp. 212–254.

Jones, P.N. (1991). On collagen fibril diameter distributions. *Connect. Tissue Res.* 26:11–21.

Jowsey, J. (1960). Age changes in human bone. *Clin. Orthop.* 17:210–271.

Józsa, L., M. Kvist, B.J. Balint, A. Reffy, M. Jarvinen, M. Lehto, and M. Barzo (1989). The role of recrea-tional sport activity in Achilles tendon rupture: a clinical, pathoanatomical, and sociological study of 292 cases. *Am. J. Sports Med.* 17:338–343.

Judge, D.M., V. Schneider, and A. LeBlanc (1989). Disuse osteoporosis [abstract]. *J.Bone Miner. Res.* 4(Suppl. 1):S238.

Kanis, J.A. (1991). Calcium requirements for optimal skeletal health in women. *Calcif. Tissue Int.* 49(Suppl.): S33–S41.

Kannus, P. and L. Józsa (1991). Histopathological changes preceding spontaneous rupture of a tendon: a controlled study of 891 patients. *J. Bone Jt. Surg.* 73–A:1507–1525.

Kasperczyk, W.J., S. Rosocha, U. Bosch, H.J. Oestem, and U. Tscheme (1991). Alter, Aktivitat und die Belastbarkeit von Kniebandern. *Unfallchirurg* 94:372–375.

Kimmel, D.B. (1993). A paradigm for skeletal strength homeostasis. *J. Bone Miner. Res.* 8(Suppl. 2):S515–522.

Komi, P.V., M. Salonen, M. Jarvinen, and O. Kokko (1987). In vivo registration of achilles tendon forces in man. I. Methodological development. *Int. J. Sports Med.* 8(Suppl.):3–8.

Kreiger, N., J.L. Kelsey, T.R. Holford, and T. O'Connor (1982). An epidemiologic study of hip fracture in postmenopausal women. *Am. J. Epidemiol.* 116:141–148.

Kröger, H., M. Tuppurainen, R. Honkanen, E. Alhava, S. Saarikoski (1994). Bone mineral density and risk factors for osteoporosis—a population-based study of 1600 perimenopausal women. *Calcif. Tissue Int.* 55:1 –7.

Lane, N.E., D.A. Bloch, H.H. Jones, W.H. Marshall, P.D. Wood, J.F. Fries (1986). Long-distance running, bone density, and osteoarthritis. *JAMA* 255:1147–1151.

Lanyon, L.E. (1987). Functional strain in bone tissue as an objective, and controlling stimulus for adaptive bone remodelling. *J. Biomech.* 20:1083–1093.

Lanyon, L.E. (1992). Control of bone architecture by functional load bearing. *J. Bone Miner. Res.* 7(Suppl. 2):S369–S375.

Lanyon, L.E., and C.T. Rubin (1984). Static vs. dynamic loads as an influence on bone remodelling. *J. Bio-mech.* 17:897–905.

Lanyon, L.E., C.T. Rubin, and G. Baust (1986). Modulation of bone loss during calcium insufficiency by controlled dynamic loading. *Calcif. Tissue Int.* 38:209–216.

Laros, G.S., C.M. Tipton, and R.R. Cooper (1971). Influence of physical activity on ligament insertions in the knees of dogs. *J. Bone Jt. Surg.* 53–A:275–286.

LeBlanc, A.D., V.S. Schneider, H.J. Evans, D.A. Engelbretson, and J.M. Krebs (1990). Bone mineral loss and recovery after 17 weeks of bed rest. *J. Bone Miner. Res.* 5:843–850.

LeBlanc, A., V. Schneider, J. Krebs, H. Evans, S. Jhingran, and P. Johnson (1987). Spinal bone mineral after 5 weeks of bed rest. *Calcif. Tiss. Int.* 41:259–261.

LeVeau, B.F. (1992). *Williams & Lissner's Biomechanics of Human Motion*, 3rd ed. Philadelphia: W.B. Saunders Company, pp. 28–59.

Li, X.J., W.S.S. Jee, S.-Y. Chow, and D.M. Woodbury (1990). Adaptation of cancellous bone to aging and immobilization in the rat: a single photon absorptiometry and histomorphometry study. *Anat. Rec.* 227:12–24.

Liang, C.T., J. Bames, J.G. Seedor, H.A. Quartuccio, M. Bolander, J.J. Jeffrey, and G.A. Rodan (1992). Impaired bone activity in aged rats: Alterations at the cellular and molecular levels. *Bone* 13:435–441.

Marcus, R., L. Holloway, and G. Butterfield (1993). Clinical uses of growth hormone in older people. *J. Reprod. Fertil. Suppl.* 46:115–118.

Martin, B. (1993). Aging and strength of bone as a structural material. *Calcif. Tissue Int.* 53(Suppl. 1):S34–S40.

Martin, R.B., and P.J. Atkinson (1977). Age and sex-related changes in the structure and strength of the human femoral shaft. *J. Biomech.* 10:223–231.

Matkovic, V. (1991). Calcium metabolism and calcium requirements during skeletal modeling and consolidation of bone mass. *Am. J. Clin. Nutr.* 54:245S–260S.

Matkovic, V., K. Kostial, I. Simonovic, R. Buzina, A. Brodarec, and B.E.C. Nordin (1979). Bone status and fracture rates in two regions of Yugoslavia. *Am. J. Clin. Nutr.* 32:540–549.

Mazess, R.B., and G.D. Whedon (1983). Immobilization and bone. *Calcif. Tissue Int.* 35:265–267.

McDonald, R., J. Hegenauer, and P. Saltman (1986). Age-related differences in the bone mineralization pattern of rats following exercise. *J. Gerontol.* 41:445–452.

Melton, L.J. III (1988). Epidemiology of fractures. In: B.L. Riggs and L.J. Melton III (eds.) *Osteoporosis: Etiology, Diagnosis, and Management.* New York: Raven Press, pp. 133–154.

Menkes, A., S. Mazel, R.A. Redmond, K. Koffler, C.R. Libanati, C.M. Gundberg, T.M. Zizic, J.M. Hagberg, R.E. Pratley, and B.F. Hurley (1993). Strength training increases regional bone mineral density and bone remodeling in middle-aged and older men. *J. Appl. Physiol.* 74:2478–2484.

Meunier, P., P. Courpron, C. Edouard, J. Bemard, J. Bringuier, and G. Vignon (1973). Physiological senile involution and pathological rarefaction of bone: quantitative and comparative histological data. *Clin. Endocrinol. Metab.* 2:239–256.

Michel, B.A., N.E. Lane, D.A. Bloch, H.H. Jones, and J.F. Fries (1991). Effect of changes in weight-bearing exercise on lumbar bone mass after age fifty. *Ann. Med.* 23:397–401.

Minaire, P., P. Meunier, C. Edouard, J. Bemard, P. Courpron, and J. Bourret (1974). Quantitative histological data on disuse osteoporosis: comparison with biological data. *Calcif. Tissue Res.* 17:57–73.

Montoye, H.J. (1975). *Physical activity and health: An epidemiological study of an entire community.* Englewood Cliffs, N.J.: Prentice-Hall, pp. 13–28.

Morey, E.R., and D.J. Baylink (1978). Inhibition of bone formation during space flight. *Science* 210:1138–1141.

Morrison, N.A., J.C. Qi, A. Tokita, P.J. Kelly, L. Crofts, T.V. Nguyen, P.N. Sambrook, and J.A. Eisman (1994). Prediction of bone density from vitamin D receptor alleles. *Nature* 367:284–287.

Mosekilde, L. (1988). Age-related changes in vertebral trabecular bone architecture: assessed by a new method. *Bone* 9:247–250.

Mosekilde, L., and L. Mosekilde (1990). Sex differences in age-related changes in vertebral body size, density and biomechanical competence in normal individuals. *Bone* 11:67–73.

Myburgh, K.H., T.D. Noakes, M. Roodt, and F.S. Hough (1989). Effect of exercise on the development of osteoporosis in adult rats. *J. Appl. Physiol.* 66:14–19.

Naresh, M.D., and B. Brodsky (1992). X-ray diffraction studies on human tendon show age-related changes in collagen packing. *Biochim. Biophys. Acta* 1122:161–166.

Nelson, M.E., E.C. Fisher, F.A. Dilmanian, G.E. Dallal, and W.J. Evans (1991). A 1-y walking program and increased dietary calcium in postmenopausal women: effects on bone. *Am. J. Clin. Nutr.* 53:1304–1311.

NIH Consensus Development Panel on Optimal Calcium Intake (1994). NIH Consensus Conference: Optimal calcium intake. *J. Am. Med. Assoc.* 272:1942–1948.

Nilsson, B.E., and N.E. Westlin (1971). Bone density in athletes. *Clin. Orthop. Rel. Res.* 77:179–182.

Nimni, M.E., and R.D. Harkness (1988). Molecular structure and functions of collagen. In: M.E. Nimni (ed.) *Collagen. Vol.I: Biochemistry.* Boca Raton, FL: CRC Press, pp. 1–77.

Nishimoto, S.K., C.-H. Chang, E. Gendler, W.F. Stryker, and M.E. Nimni (1985). The effect of aging on bone formation in rats: Biochemical and histological evidence for decreased bone formation capacity. *Calcif. Tissue Int.* 37:617–624.

Nordin, B.E.C., A.G. Need, B.E. Chatterton, M. Horowitz, and H.A. Morris (1990). The relative contributions of age and years since menopause to postmenopausal bone loss. *J. Clin. Endocrinol. Metab.* 70:83–88.

Noyes, F.R., and E.S. Grood (1976). The strength of the anterior cruciate ligament in humans and Rhesus monkeys. *J. Bone Joint Surg.* 58-A:1074–1082.

Noyes, F.R., P.J Torvik., W.B. Hyde, and J.L. DeLucas (1974). Biomechanics of ligament failure II. An analysis of immobilization, exercise and reconditioning effects in primates. *J. Bone Joint Surg.* 56-A:1406–1418.

Oakes, B.W. (1988). Ultrastructural studies on knee joint ligaments: quantitation of collagen fibre populations in exercised and control rat cruciate ligaments and in human anterior cruciate grafts. In: J.A. Buckwalter and S.L.-Y. Woo (eds.) *Injury and Repair of the Musculoskeletal Tissues*. Park Ridge, IL: Amer. Adacemy of Orthopaedic Surgeons, pp. 66–82.

Oakes, B.W., T.W. Parker, and J. Norman (1981). Changes in collagen fibre populations in young rat cruciate ligaments in response to an intensive one month's exercise program. In: P. Russo and G. Gass (eds.) *Human Adaptation*. Sydney, Australia: Cumberland College of Health Sciences, pp. 223–230.

Ortner, D.J. (1975). Aging effects on osteon remodeling. *Calcif. Tissue Res.* 18:27–36.

Palle, S., L. Vico, S. Bourrin, and C. Alexandre (1992). Bone tissue response to four month antiorthostatic bedrest: a bone histomorphometric study. *Calcif. Tissue Int.* 51:189–194.

Parfitt, A.M. (1984). Age-related structural changes in trabecular and cortical bone: cellular mechanism and biomechanical consequences. *Calcif. Tissue Int.* 36(Suppl.):S123–S128.

Parfitt, A.M. (1988). Bone remodeling: relationship to the amount and structure of bone, and the pathogenesis and prevention of fractures. In: B.L. Riggs and L.J. Melton III (eds.) *Osteoporosis: Etiology, Diagnosis, and Management*. New York: Raven Press, pp. 45–93.

Parfitt, A.M. (1993). Bone age, mineral density, and fatigue damage. *Calcif. Tissue Int.* 53(Suppl. 1):S82–S86.

Parry, D.A.D, G.R.G. Barnes, and A.S. Craig (1978). A comparison of the size distribution of collagen fibrils in connective tissues as a function of age and a possible relation between fibril size distribution and mechanical properties. *Proc. R. Soc. Lond.* B203:305–321.

Parry, D.A.D., M.H. Flint, B.C. Gillard, and A.S. Craig (1982). A role for glycosaminoglycans in the development of collagen fibrils. *FEBS Let.* 149:1–7.

Pead, M.J., T.M. Skerry, and L.E. Lanyon (1988). Direct transformation from quiescence to bone formation in the adult periosteum following a single brief period of bone loading. *J. Bone Miner. Res.* 3:647–656.

Peterson, S.E., M.D. Peterson, G. Raymond, C. Gilligan, M.M. Checovich, and E.L. Smith (1991). Muscular strength and bone density with weight training in middle-aged women. *Med. Sci. Sports Exerc.* 23:499–504.

Pfeilschifter, J., I. Diel, U. Pilz, K. Brunotte, A. Naumann, and R. Ziegler (1993). Mitogenic responsiveness of human bone cells *in vitro* to hormones and growth factors decreases with age. *J. Bone Miner. Res.* 8:707–717.

Prince, R. L., M. Smith, I.M. Dick, R.I. Price, P.G. Webb, N. K. Henderson, M.M. Harris (1991). Prevention of post-menopausal osteoporosis: a comparative study of exercise, calcium supplementation, and hormone-replacement therapy. *N. Engl. J. Med.* 325:1189–1195.

Pruitt, L.A., R.D. Jackson, R.L. Bartels, and H.J. Lehnhard (1992). Weight-training effects on bone mineral density in early postmenopausal women. *J. Bone Miner. Res.* 7:179–185.

Raab, D.M., T.D. Crenshaw, D.B. Kimmel, and E.L. Smith (1991). A histomorphometric study of cortical bone activity during increased weight-bearing exercise. *J. Bone Miner. Res.* 6:741–749.

Raab, D.M., E.L. Smith, T.D. Crenshaw, and D.P. Thomas (1990). Bone mechanical properties after exercise training in young and old rats. *J. Appl. Physiol.* 68:130–134.

Raab-Cullen, D.M., M.P. Akhter, D.B. Kimmel, and R.R. Recker (1994). Bone response to alternate-day mechanical loading of the rat tibia. *J. Bone Miner. Res.* 9:203–211.

Raisz, L.G. (1988). Local and systemic factors in the pathogenesis of osteoporosis. *N. Engl. J. Med.* 318:818–828.

Rambaut, P.C., and A.W. Good (1985). Skeletal changes during space flight. *Lancet* (Nov. 9): 1050–1052.

Ramlow, J., A. Kriska, and R. LaPorte (1987). Physical activity in the population: the epidemiological spectrum. *Res. Q. Exer. Sport* 58:111–113.

Recker, R.R., and R.P. Heaney (1990). Letter to the editor. *J. Bone Miner. Res.* 5:307–308.

Ribot, C., F. Tremollieres, J.-M. Pouilles, M. Bonneu, F. Germain, and J.-P. Louvet (1988). Obesity and postmenopausal bone loss: the influence of obesity on vertebral density and bone turnover in postmenopausal women. *Bone* 8:327–331.

Rickli, R.E. and B.G. McManis (1990). Effects of exercise on bone mineral content in postmenopausal women. *Res. Q.* 61:243–249.

Riggs, B.L., H.W. Wahner, L.J. Melton III, L.S. Richelson, H.L. Judd, and K.P. Offord (1986). Rates of bone loss in the appendicular and axial skeletons of women. *J. Clin. Invest.* 77:1487–1491.

Riggs, B.L., H.W. Wahner, E. Seeman, K.P. Offord, W.L. Dunn, R.B. Mazess, K.A. Johnson, and L.J. Melton III (1982). Changes in bone mineral density of the proximal femur and spine with aging: differences between the postmenopausal and senile osteoporosis syndromes. *J. Clin. Invest.* 70:716–723.

Riis, B., K. Thomsen, and C. Christiansen (1987). Does calcium supplementation prevent postmenopausal bone loss? *N. Engl. J. Med.* 316:173–177.

Robey, P.G. (1989). The biochemistry of bone. *Endocrinol. Metab. Clin. N. Amer.* 18:859–902.

Rubin, C.T., S.D. Bain, and K.J. McLeod (1992). Suppression of the osteogenic response in the aging skeleton. *Calcif. Tissue Int.* 50:306–313.

Rubin, C.T., and L.E. Lanyon (1984). Regulation of bone formation by applied dynamic loads. *J. Bone Joint Surg.* 66–A:397–402.

Rubin, C.T., and L.E. Lanyon (1985). Regulation of bone mass by mechanical strain magnitude. *Calcif. Tissue Int.* 37:411–417.

Rudman, D., A.G. Feller, H.S. Nagraj, G.A. Gergans, P.Y. Lalitha, A.F. Goldberg, R.A. Schlenker, L. Cohn, I.W. Rudman, and D.E. Mattson (1990). Effects of human growth hormone in men over 60 ys old. *N. Engl. J. Med.* 323:1–6.

Ruff, C.B., and W.C. Hayes (1983). Cross-sectional geometry of Pecos Pueblo femora and tibiae—a biomechanical investigation: II. Sex, age, and side differences. *Am. J. Physical Anthropol.* 60:383–400.

Ruff, C.B., and W.C. Hayes (1988). Sex differences in age-related remodeling of the femur and tibia. *J. Orthop. Res.* 6:886–896.

Salo, P.T., and W.G. Tatton (1993). Age-related loss of knee joint afferents in mice. *J. Neuroscience Res.* 35:664–677.

Schaffler, M.B. (1993). Published discussion at NIA Workshop on Aging and Bone Quality, September 1992, Bethesda, MD. *Calcif. Tissue Int.* 53(Suppl 1):S87.

Sernbo, I., O. Johnell, and T. Andersson (1988). Differences in the incidence of hip fracture: comparison of an urban and a rural population in southern Sweden. *Acta Orthop. Scand.* 59:382–385.

Silbermann, M., B. Bar-Shira-Maymon, R. Coleman, A. Reznick, Y., Weisman, E. Steinhagen-Thiessen, H. von der Mark, and K. von der Mark (1990). Long-term physical exercise retards trabecular bone loss in lumbar vertebrae of aging female mice. *Calcif. Tissue Int.* 46:80–93.

Silbermann, M., D. Schapira, I. Leichter, and R. Steinberg (1991). Moderate physical exercise throughout adulthood increases peak bone mass at middle age and maintains higher trabecular bone density in vertebrae of senescent female rats. *Cells Mater.* (Suppl. 1):151–158.

Simmons, E.D., Jr., K.P.H. Pritzker, and M.D. Grynpas (1991). Age-related changes in the human femoral cortex. *J. Orthop. Res.* 9:155–167.

Slovik, D.M., J.S. Adams, R.M. Neer, M.F. Holick, and J.T. Potts, Jr. (1981). Deficient production of 1,25-dihydroxyvitamin D in elderly osteoporotic patients. *N. Engl. J. Med.* 305:372–374.

Smidt, G.L., S.-Y. Lin, K.D. O'Dwyer, and P.R. Blanpied (1992). The effect of high-intensity trunk exercise on bone mineral density of postmenopausal women. *Spine* 17:280–285.

Snow-Harter, C., and R. Marcus (1991). Exercise, bone mineral density and osteoporosis. In: J.O. Holloszy (ed.) *Exercise and Sport Sciences Reviews*, Vol. 19. Baltimore, MD:Williams & Wilkins, pp. 351–388.

Snyder, B.D., S. Piazza, W.T. Edwards, and W.C. Hayes (1993). Role of trabecular morphology in the etiology of age-related vertebral fractures. *Calcif. Tissue Int.* 53(Suppl. l):S14–S22.

Steiger, P., S.R. Cummings, D.M. Black, N.E. Spencer, and H.K. Genant (1992). Age-related decrements in bone mineral density in women over 65. *J. Bone Miner. Res.* 7:625–632.

Talmage, R.V., S.S. Stinnett, J.T. Landwehr, L.M. Vincent, and W.H. McCartney (1986). Age-related loss of bone mineral density in non-athletic and athletic women. *Bone Miner.* 1:115–125.

Tipton, C.M., S.J. James, W. Mergner, and T.-K. Tcheng (1970). Influence of exercise on strength of medial collateral knee ligaments of dogs. *Am. J. Physiol.* 218:894–901.

Tipton, C.M., R.K. Martin, R.D. Matthes, and R.A. Carey (1975). Hydroxyproline concentrations in ligaments from trained and non-trained rats. In: H. Howard and J.R. Poortmans (eds.) *Metabolic Adaptation to Prolonged Physical Exercise*. Basel: Birkhauser-Verlag, pp. 262–267.

Tipton, C.M., R.D. Matthes, and R.K. Martin (1978). Influence of age and sex on the strength of bone-ligament junctions in knee joints of rats. *J. Bone Jt. Surg.* 60–A:230–234.

Tipton, C.M., R.D. Matthes, J.A. Maynard, and R.A. Carey (1975). The influence of physical activity on ligaments and tendons. *Med. Sci. Sports.* 7:165–175.

Tipton, C.M., R.D. Matthes, A.C. Vailas, and C.L. Schnobelen (1979). The response of the Galago senegalensis to physical training. *Comp. Biochem. Physiol.* 63A:29–36.

Tipton, C.M., and A.C. Vailas (1990). Bone and connective tissue adaptations to physical activity. In: C. Bouchard, R.J. Shephard, R. Stephens, J.R. Sutton, and B.D. McPherson (eds.) *Exercise, Fitness, and Health: A Consensus of Current Knowledge*. Champaign, IL: Human Kinetics Books, pp. 331–344.

Tipton, C.M., A.C. Vailas, and R.D. Matthes (1986). Experimental studies on the influences of physical activity on ligaments, tendons, and joints: a brief review. *Acta Med. Scand. Suppl.* 711:157–168.

Tonna, E.A. (1978). Electron microscopic study of bone surface changes during aging. The loss of cellular control and biofeedback. *J. Gerontol.* 33:163–177.

Trotter, J.A., A. Samora, K. Hsi, and C. Wofsy (1987). Stereological analysis of the muscle-tendon junction in the aging mouse. *Anat. Rec.* 218:288–293.

Turner, C.H. (1991). Homeostatic control of bone structure: an application of feedback theory. *Bone* 12:203–217.

Turner, C.H., M.P. Akhter, D.M. Raab, D.B. Kimmel, and R.R. Recker (1991). A noninvasive, *in vivo* model for studying strain adaptive bone modeling. *Bone* 12:73–79.

U.S. Public Health Service (1990). *Healthy People 2000: National Health Promotion and Disease Prevention Objectives.* Dept. of Health and Human Services Publication #(PHS)91–50212. Washington DC: U.S. Government Printing Office.

Vailas, A.C., D.M. DeLuna, L.L. Lewis, S.L. Curwin, R.R. Roy, and E.K. Alford (1988). Adaptation of bone and tendon to prolonged hindlimb suspension in rats. *J. Appl. Physiol.* 65:373–376.

Vailas, A.C., V.A. Pedrini, A. Pedrini-Mille, and J.O. Holloszy (1985). Patellar tendon matrix changes associated with aging and voluntary exercise. *J. Appl. Physiol.* 58:1572–1576.

Vasseur, P.B., R.R. Pool, and S.P. Amoczky (1985). Correlative biomechanical and histologic study of the cranial cruciate ligament in dogs. *Am. J. Vet. Res.* 46:1842–1854.

Verzár, F. (1955). Veränderungen der thermoelastischen Eigenschaften von Sehnenfasern beim Altern. *Experientia.* 11:230.

Vico, L., S. Bourrin, V. Novikov, J.M. Very, D. Chappard, and C. Alexandre (1991). Adaptation of bone cellular activities to tail suspension in rats. *Cell Mater.* (Suppl. 1.):143–150.

Vico, L., D. Chappard, C. Alexandre, S. Palle, P. Minaire, G. Riffat, B. Morukov, and S. Rakhmanov (1987). Effects of a 120-day period of bed-rest on bone mass and bone cell activities in man: attempts at countermeasure. *Bone Miner.* 2:383–394.

Viidik, A. (1967). The effect of training on the tensile strength of isolated rabbit tendons. *Scand. J. Plast. Reconstruct. Surg.* 1:141–147.

Viidik, A. (1982). Age-related changes in connective tissues. In: A. Viidik (ed.) *Lectures on Gerontology, Volume I: On Biology of Aging.* San Diego: Academic Press, pp. 173–211.

Viidik, A. (1986). Adaptability of connective tissue. In: B. Saltin (ed.) *Biochemistry of Exercise VI.* Champaign, IL: Human Kinetic Publishers, pp. 545–562.

Vincentelli, R. (1978). Relation between collagen fiber orientation and age of osteon formation in human tibial compact bone. *Acta Anat.* 100:120–128.

Vincentelli, R., and F.G. Evans (1971). Relations among mechanical properties, collagen fibres and calcification in adult human cortical bone. *J. Biomech.* 4:193–201.

Weinreb, M., G.A. Rodan, and D.D. Thompson (1991). Immobilization-related bone loss in the rat is increased by calcium deficiency. *Calcif. Tissue Int.* 48:93–100.

Whedon, G.D., L. Lutwak, J. Reid, P. Rambaut, M. Whittle, M. Smith, and C. Leach (1974). Mineral and nitrogen metabolic studies on Skylab orbital space flights. *Trans. Assoc. Am. Physicians* 87:95–110.

White, B.L., W.D. Fisher, and C.A. Laurin (1987). Rate of mortality for elderly patients after fracture of the hip in the 1980's. *J. Bone Joint Surg.* 69A:1335–1340.

Woo, S.L.-Y., M.A. Gomez, D. Amiel, M.A. Ritter, R.H. Gelberman, and W.H. Akeson (1981). The effects of exercise on the biomechanical and biochemical properties of swine digital flexor tendons. *J. Biomech. Eng.* 103:51–56.

Woo, S.L.-Y., M.A. Gomez, T.J. Sites, P.O. Newton, C.A. Orlando, and W.H. Akeson (1987). The biomechanical and morphological changes in the medial collateral ligament of the rabbit after immobilization and remobilization. *J. Bone Joint. Surg.* 69–A:1200–1211.

Woo, S.L.-Y., M.A. Gomez, Y.-K. Woo, and W.H. Akeson (1982). Mechanical properties of tendons and ligaments II. The relationships of immobilization and exercise on tissue remodeling. *Biorheology* 19:397–408.

Woo, S., J. Maynard, D. Butler, R. Lyon, P. Torzilli, W. Akeson, R. Cooper, and B. Oakes (1988). Ligament, tendon, and joint capsule insertions to bone. In: S. L.-Y. Woo and J.A. Buckwalter (eds.) *Injury and Repair of the Musculoskeletal Soft Tissues.* Park Ridge, IL: American Academy of Orthopaedic Surgeons, pp. 133–166.

Woo, S.L.-Y., K.J. Ohland, and J.A. Weiss (1990). Aging and sex-related changes in the biomechanical properties of the rabbit medial collateral ligament. *Mech. Age. Dev.* 56:129–142.

Woo, S.L.-Y., M.A. Ritter, D. Amiel, T.M. Sanders, M.A. Gomez, S.C. Kuel, S.R. Garfin, and W.H. Akeson (1980). The biomechanical and biochemical properties of swine tendons—long-term effects of exercise on the digital extensors. *Connect. Tissue Res.* 7:177–183.

Yamada, H. (1970). In: F.G. Evans (ed.) *Strength of Biological Materials.* Baltimore, MD: Williams & Wilkins, pp. 99–101.

Yeh, J.K., and J.F. Aloia (1990). Effect of physical activity on calciotropic hormones and calcium balance in rats. *Am. J. Physiol.* 258:E263–E268.

Yeh, J.K., C.C. Liu, J.F. Aloia, and A. Foto (1991). Effect of treadmill exercise and ovariectomy on femoral and lumbar vertebrae in young and adult rats. *Cells Mater.* (Suppl. 1):159–166.

Young, D.R., W.J. Niklowitz, R.J. Brown, and W.S.S. Jee (1986). Immobilization associated osteoporosis in primates. *Bone* 7:109–117.

Zerwekh, J.E., K. Sakhaee, K. Glass, and C.Y.C. Pak (1983). Long term 25- hydroxyvitamin D3 therapy in postmenopausal osteoporosis: demonstration of responsive and non-responsive subgroups. *J. Clin. Endocrinol. Metab.* 56:410–413.

DISCUSSION

TIPTON: Woo, Akeson, Amiel and we demonstrated in dogs that the strength of ligament and tendon will decrease to 25% of normal with disuse. Moreover, the recovery time after disuse is longer with older animals. Thus, it seems likely that the older person may also take longer to recover from a period of disuse.

BOUCHARD: This area, similar to all the others that we are discussing, should also be seen in light of advances in genetics and molecular biology. In the case of osteoporosis, imaginative studies have been published by Seeman and colleagues using a co-twin design in which they compared identical twins who were discordant for physical activity, smoking, and other behavior. They showed that smoking decreased bone mass when genotype was controlled by using the co-twin as the control. Physical activity increased bone mass only when it was at high intensity, and greater fat-free mass also increased bone mass. These are powerful studies that reveal that some of the lifestyle changes, e.g., smoking cessation and regular exercise, that we commonly advocate in older persons can have a favorable impact on bone mass.

BLOOMFIELD: Smoking behavior is generally not acknowledged in discussions of relevant lifestyle factors related to bone, but it should be. There is a dearth of mechanistic information about the physiological link between smoking and bone mass. It may affect estrogen receptors or the onset of menopause. There is enough information to indicate that smoking during the ages of 20 and 50 is likely to increase a woman's risk of developing clinically significant osteoporosis.

EVANS: We recently did a cross-sectional study examining the relationship between muscle and bone and noticed that even if smoking behavior had ceased 10 y earlier, the adverse effect of prior smoking on bone mass appeared to persist. So smoking exerts a remarkably powerful effect.

BOUCHARD: But we now have to go one step further, particularly after the demonstration by Morrison et al. in *Nature* (1994) of the genetic variation in the vitamin D receptor. If one genetic polymorphism is so powerful, then the question of whether or not aging changes the response to exercise cannot be addressed in a sensible manner without controlling for that gene. The true question then is whether or not the response of bone mass to regular exercise is different if one has zero, one, or two copies of the low-bone-density allele at the vitamin receptor gene?

BLOOMFIELD: There is in a subset of our population a clear genetic predisposition to developing osteoporosis at a relatively young age. The best-designed studies of the future will try to minimize that variability in genotype when examining the effects of these other lifestyle factors.

EVANS: I would like to point out that the Dalsky study, which is frequently cited, was a non-randomized trial and that women who were taking estrogen were included in the exercise group in which she observed an increase in bone density.

BLOOMFIELD: It's a very legitimate criticism that non-randomization of subjects, even with the working goal of increasing compliance to long-term training protocols, generates the risk of selection bias. In this case, the more important criticism relates to the inclusion of some women on estrogen therapy in the group of exercisers. However, in Dalsky's study those women on estrogen constituted a small fraction of the total number of subjects. Even though their individual results may have biased the group mean in the direction of a larger increase in bone mass, there were clear increases in lumbar spine density in those subjects not on estrogen. What distinguishes Dalsky's study from most of the others was its training duration of up to 22 mo and the fact that they utilized a wide variety of exercise regimens, including stair climbing, jogging, and walking, and, I believe, cycling. Subjects even walked with weighted backpacks to increase the weight-bearing impact of the activity.

To place the study by Dalsky et al. in perspective, it is one of the very few to demonstrate an absolute increase in bone mass with exercise in post-menopausal women. The bulk of the data in older humans seem to indicate that exercise has primarily a bone-conserving effect; in other words, exercise in older populations appears to prevent or dramatically slow bone loss with aging.

As many of you are aware, the measurement error of bone densitometry is uncomfortably close to the yearly change we see in bone mass, which dictates much longer training protocols than many of us are accustomed to proposing. Secondly, accurate measurement requires the use of the latest generation of densitometers, in which reproducibility error is generally 1% or less. There are also potential problems in interpreting bone densitometry data. If investigators don't design training protocols for at least 8 or 9 mo duration, they run the risk of misinterpreting changes in bone mass that might simply reflect a transient change in remodeling activity before a new steady-state in bone mass is reached. I strongly encourage investigators to incorporate measures other than bone mineral density into their study designs. We clearly need more concurrent measures of bone metabolism, such as appropriately timed serum samples to measure endocrine factors and biochemical markers for bone resorption and formation. For example, new techniques have been developed to measure bone geometry using data collected during absorptiometry scans. A recent symposium on bone quality in aging that was sponsored by the National Institute on Aging contains a tremendous set of papers, published in a supplement to *Calcified Tissue International*, that really emphasizes the critical need to get more data on bone geometry and bone architecture. Changes in bone structure are just as important as any change in bone mass. Until now we have been limited somewhat by methodology and focused too much on bone mineral density as a single outcome variable.

There are relatively few randomized exercise intervention trials in the published literature, limiting our ability to conclude that exercise has caused the observed change in bone mass. We should insist that proposed studies use more rigorous designs. Currently, the best practical recommendation we can make for preventing osteoporotic bone changes is to participate in a wide range of physical activities and to avoid reliance on any single mode of exercise.

EVANS: We performed a randomized controlled trial of twice-weekly resistance training and observed a 1–2% increase in bone density at every site measured with dual-energy X-ray absorptiometry. Neutron activation was used to measure total body calcium, which also increased 1–2%.

Also, when we compared masters level women athletes with age-matched sedentary controls in a cross-sectional study, we observed that the 1,25-dihydroxy-vitamin D levels of the runners were much higher. It appears that regular running affects the conversion of 25-hydroxy-vitamin D to 1,25-dihydroxy-vitamin D. This effect was independent of dietary factors.

BLOOMFIELD: There are some interesting data from Norman Bell and colleagues showing increases in 1,25-OH$_2$D in males undergoing resistance training. Some of that evidence was from cross-sectional studies, but I believe they also generated some longitudinal data. All subjects had vitamin D levels within normal physiological range, so whether such increases in vitamin D translate into actual increases in intestinal calcium absorption bears further investigation.

NASH: Sue, the prevention of bone loss by physical activity is not always an option. You correctly point out that severely osteoporotic bone fails to remodel its trabecular matrix, which makes the time-course of any therapeutic intervention such as bone loading by exercise particularly important. Because one of the goals of skeletal loading is to increase bone strength, I'd like to be reassured that we are not hastening its deterioration. Are there any indices for the loss of trabecular and cortical bone that might tell us when it is safe to begin loading bone or when we ought not attempt it because of unacceptable risks associated with microtrauma or fracture?

BLOOMFIELD: You have raised a very important point. We have little information on the safety of exercise for those individuals with severe osteopenia, which elevates the risk of fracture with certain activities. Most physicians understandably err on the side of safety; if they have a patient who is severely osteoporotic, they certainly first want to "do no harm." There are clearly some individuals for whom many weightbearing forms of exercise are likely to be unsafe. For women with multiple vertebral fractures, for example, excess torsion and loading on the spine should be avoided. Furthermore, exercise might be out of the question for some individuals because of pain induced by movement. Because of ethical concerns, it will be very difficult to get prospective data on the safety of exercise for osteopenic individuals; if a creative investigator could devise a retrospective study, it would provide much needed information.

I know that you work with individuals who have spinal cord injury, which causes a very rapid loss of bone mass, particularly in cancellous bone. Those individuals who are injured in young adulthood lose the same volume of bone in the lower limbs in the first 6 mo after injury as has been lost over many years by able-bodied persons who have reached 60 years of age. However, we have good data from studies at The Ohio State University indicating that activity intervention early in the recovery process can significantly attenuate the bone loss at numerous anatomical sites. We can also minimize the negative calcium balance with contractions induced by electrical stimulation of the paralyzed muscles.

Recommendations regarding the safety of exercise should be very specific to the population being addressed. Most spinal cord-injured persons are 18–25 years of age and are quite different from the older able-bodied individual who has experienced a progressive osteopenia that develops into full-blown osteoporosis late in life.

NASH: These recommendations need to be expanded beyond spinal cord-injured patients to include the frail and very elderly, those with other neuromuscular disorders, and even post-operative patients. It is not uncommon for a previously healthy person to be immobilized for long periods after hip or spinal surgery and to thereby become osteopenic. Is there any association between measured bone-mineral density and fracture susceptibility? Have investigators looked at post-mortem bone and the stresses necessary to invoke fracture?

BLOOMFIELD: Yes, there is some information on "fracture thresholds" of bone mineral density for each anatomical site, below which the risk for fracture very much elevated. For example, the risk of vertebral fracture is dramatically elevated once lumbar-spine bone density falls below 1.00 g/cm^2. As far as I know, these fracture thresholds are determined from epidemiological data documenting an increase in statistical risk of fracture given certain bone mineral density values. The proximal tibia is another site prone to osteopenia, particularly in spinal-cord injured persons, for which there are no data on fracture threshold.

EVANS: We completed a study in which virtually all of our subjects were osteoporotic, and 30% of them had osteoporotic fractures. In this population, trying to prevent a fall is more important than trying to prevent the continued loss of bone, because it is too late to have much hope of doing the latter. These people are very weak, so high-intensity strength training causes great improvement in strength and a potential reduction in the risk of falls. Therefore, I think that a recommendation of no exercise for persons with osteoporosis is misguided.

BLOOMFIELD: I fully agree. But I believe that many physicians, when faced with a frail patient with pre-existing fractures, will err on the side of safety. Certainly the bulk of data published on human beings indicates that strength training is probably the single best form of exercise for minimizing bone loss in older individuals. The evidence from your group's training studies as well as from other labs indicates that if we can improve muscle tone and/or mass, we can improve bone mass. If we can improve muscle strength, we may be able to minimize the incidence of injurious falls and perhaps improve control of balance. We need to get the relevant information, including solid research data, to the practitioners of the medical community to convince them that there are safe and effective exercise programs for osteoporotic patients, even those with documented fractures. However, I have yet to see published studies that have documented rates of orthopedic injuries in osteoporotic subjects enrolled in exercise trials. Those investigators in charge of the larger exercise intervention trials now underway could provide a tremendous service by documenting rates of fracture and other injuries in their exercisers versus those seen in non-exercising control groups, and publishing these data in a widely read forum.

SUTTON: While high-impact exercise in those who are osteopenic may be detrimental, many forms of both weight bearing and non-weight bearing exercise improve muscle strength and bone mineral density without the negative effects of high-impact exercise. Some may wish to err on the side of caution and not prescribe exercise at all, but I believe that would be injudicious. One needs to be selective and to understand that appropriate exercise will be beneficial, not detrimental.

BLOOMFIELD: Although weight training appears to be optimal for bone health, alternate forms of exercise may be beneficial, especially for those who cannot or choose not to lift weights. A longitudinal study we performed at Ohio State demonstrated a maintenance of bone mass in the lumbar spine with stationary cycling in healthy post-menopausal women. This result suggests that even this non-weight bearing activity, given muscle contractions of at least moderate intensity, might help maintain or stimulate increases in bone mass in older populations.

The general presumption of most investigators is that, on the spectrum of all exercise activities, swimming is probably the least beneficial because it involves virtually no weight-bearing and impact forces on bone. However, for older individuals, particularly those who are arthritic or have other limitations to movement, swimming is a viable option for regular exercise. It can provide some increase in mechanical loading by increasing the force of muscle contraction. In this case, it's important to avoid including floating and passive pedaling in the definition of "swimming" and to focus on more vigorous lap swimming or the many water aerobics programs gaining in popularity. Much of the published data on the bony response to swimming focuses on young athletes who have spent many hours every week in a semi-weightless environment during those years when bone is still maturing. It is not surprising to me that those populations show average or sometimes below average values for bone mineral density. Furthermore, there is clear evidence that prolonged high-intensity exercise in immature animals can have a deleterious effect on bone mass and strength characteristics. Perhaps these lower bone density values in cross-sectional studies of swimmers reflect overtraining as much as lack of weight bearing.

SUTTON: I also maintain that it is probably going to be more beneficial on a population-wide basis to have the very inactive become a tiny bit more active than to have the moderately active become considerably more active.

BLOOMFIELD: I agree.

EICHNER: I would like to defend the medical community. At least in the Midwest, physicians widely prescribe walking, cycling, or swimming exercise for patients with osteoporosis. Many vertebral fractures are asymptomatic. In addition, we need more information on preventive factors such as calcium intake and exercise across the life span. Two recent articles in *JAMA* described data on 12-year-old girls whose calcium intake was increased from 900 to 1400 mg/d; their bone mass increased 5% over 2 y. In another study of college-age women in Omaha, a good diet and regular exercise increased bone mass up to age 30. Finally, a recent epidemiologic study in Hong Kong in the *British Medical Journal* found that regular walking protects against hip fracture in older people.

BLOOMFIELD: We do have more encouraging data on the younger populations; clearly our best chance of preventing osteoporotic factors in the future depends on the exercise and dietary practices of our daughters, granddaughters, sons, and grandsons. By the way, Barbara Drinkwater has emphasized, and rightly so, that we need to get out of the habit of regarding osteoporosis as a syndrome specific to "little old ladies." Those of you gentlemen who lead healthy lifestyles and plan to survive into your 80s or 90s run a 17% risk of experiencing a hip fracture.

TIPTON: I think there is a tendency to be a little evangelistic on this issue. There is no hard evidence that improved muscle strength is going to prevent falls. I argue that just because a person increases muscle power in old age doesn't necessarily mean that individual won't fall. There is an urgent need for appropriately designed studies to settle this question.

BLOOMFIELD: I agree. There is only suggestive evidence right now that improved muscular strength will improve balance and help prevent falls. I think the stronger evidence at present indicates that improved muscular strength will improve either reflexes or muscle strength to help minimize impact with the floor as a fall progresses. Clearly the studies of Woollacott and others on changes in postural control and tendency to fall constitute a very important area of research.

NASH: I don't want to leave the impression that we ought to oppose exercise for older individuals because of its risks. However, we probably know less about the potential harm of either judicious or injudicious exercise on the skeletal system than for any other system. The potential harm arising from vertebral damage or long-bone fracture in an elderly population or a population recovering from acute illness or disease has important consequences for the quality and quantity of life.

WHITE: Dr. Bloomfield, my question deals with hormone replacement therapy in postmenopausal women regarding bone, ligament, and tendon. Are you aware of evidence for whether hormone replacement therapy in postmenopausal women has a powerful influence for improving functional and structural variables in these three tissues? It is effective in the case of bone, but is this effect prophylactic or therapeutic and capable of reversing a decline?

BLOOMFIELD: With reference to bone, there is unequivocal evidence that estrogen replacement therapy in estrogen-deficient women prevents loss of bone mineral content and reduces the rate of fractures. Therefore, its most important effect is prophylactic, by inhibiting osteoclastic activity and reducing bone resorption. Some individuals may experience small increases in bone mass if estrogen therapy is begun within 2–3 y of the onset of menopause. The prophylactic effect can be achieved anytime, regardless of when therapy is begun relative to the onset of menopause. However, this is not a permanent effect; as soon as one goes off hormone replacement therapy, a 3–4 y period of accelerated loss occurs, just as occurs at menopause. We need more information on how estrogen replacement therapy affects bone geometry and bone architecture, which in the human model requires studying postmortem samples or creatively utilizing newer, noninvasive techniques on living subjects.

WHITE: What about hormone replacement for ligament and tendon?

BLOOMFIELD: The only data I'm aware of were published in 1969 by Booth and Tipton, documenting no effect of estradiol on ligament strength in female rats. One might speculate that estrogen replacement therapy in post-menopausal women would positively affect junction strength by minimizing osteopenic changes in bone at tendon and ligament insertion sites.

BAR-OR: I fully agree that we must focus on ways of increasing mineral bone mass of our children and grandchildren. However, is there really any evidence from human or animal research that increasing the peak bone mass early in life postpones the arrival at that dreaded osteoporotic fracture threshold?

BLOOMFIELD: To answer this question definitively would require a longitudinal study spanning some 50 y. We may never have those data. The reasonable presumption is that by increasing peak bone mass, one can delay the time at which any one bony site reaches its fracture threshold. Our best evidence to date indicates that if we can persuade our aging population to maintain regular physical activity, we can slow the rate of bone loss seen with aging. Clearly, it is hard to argue against the contention that low peak bone mass certainly puts a person at elevated risk for developing clinically significant osteopenia earlier in life. One good example is the growing concern about young amenorrheic athletics who experience bone *loss* at a time when they should be *accumulating* bone mass. This is a pertinent question because we have two important factors to be concerned with regarding any one individual's risk of experiencing osteoporotic fractures: role of peak bone mass versus the role of the *rate* of loss of bone mineral density over the adult years.

6

Aging, Exercise, and Cardiopulmonary Function

Jerome A. Dempsey, Ph.D.

Douglas R. Seals, Ph.D.

INTRODUCTION

The cardiovascular and pulmonary systems are critical for the maintenance of homeostasis at rest and under conditions of stress, such as exercise. As key components in the oxygen transport pathway, together these systems represent the crucial limiting factor for maximal aerobic work capacity which, in turn, is an important determinant of one's ability to sustain submaximal levels of physical activity. As such, reductions in the functional reserves of the cardiovascular and pulmonary systems bear primary responsibility for the age-related decline in physical work capacity that occurs even in healthy humans. Moreover, these systems are important targets of the increased prevalence of disease and other constitutional changes (e.g., obesity) that occur with advancing age, all of which exacerbate the direct effects of the aging process. Given this prominent role in physiological regulation, it is important to understand the interactions between physical activity and cardiopulmonary function in the aging human.

The purpose of this review will be to critically analyze and discuss the existing information concerning the influence of human aging on cardiopulmonary function during exercise. The primary foci will be on cardiopulmonary regulation during acute exercise, adaptations to chronic exercise (physical training), and exercise/athletic performance. The effects of aging on the cardiovascular and pulmonary systems under resting conditions also will be reviewed briefly because any such "baseline" changes can influence the responses to exercise.

We have imposed several limitations on this discussion. First, we have emphasized "adult" aging, i.e., changes that occur from early to late adulthood, rather than throughout the entire life span. Second, we have focused on findings from studies of human subjects, while supplementing this with data from animal studies. Third, we have centered our discussion primarily on healthy humans in an attempt to understand the direct effects of the aging process; thus, the complex interactions between aging and overt cardiopulmonary disease will not be addressed specifically. Finally, the we have focused on dynamic exercise performed with large muscle groups; information on the effects of aging on cardiopulmonary adjustments to isometric exercise (Ng et al., 1994a; Taylor et al., 1991) is limited and will not be discussed.

CARDIOVASCULAR FUNCTION AT REST

The age-associated changes in functions of the heart, the peripheral circulation, and the autonomic nervous system at rest have been reviewed in detail (Docherty, 1990; Folkow & Svanborg, 1993; Lakatta, 1993; Seals, 1993; Seals et al., 1994c) and will only be briefly summarized here. With regard to cardiac function and systemic hemodynamics, cardiac output appears, on average, to decline with advancing age because of a decrease in stroke volume (Brandfonbrener et al., 1955; Conway et al., 1971; Granath et al., 1964; Julius et al., 1967; Seals, 1993; Strandell, 1964). However, in healthy older subjects who have been rigorously screened for the presence of heart disease, cardiac output may not decrease significantly with aging, at least in men; cardiac output in these healthy people is unchanged because stroke volume and left ventricular end-diastolic volume (preload) are maintained or even slightly increased with advancing age (Rodeheffer et al., 1984). In contrast, left ventricular end-diastolic volume or diameter does not appear to increase with age in women (Lakatta, 1993), possibly as a result of the lack of estrogen after menopause (Giraud et al., 1993; Pines et al., 1991; Scheuer et al., 1987). There is no compelling evidence that left ventricular contractility declines with age (e.g., ejection fraction is not altered); however, there are several other age-related left ventricular changes, including increases in afterload, wall thickness, and overall mass, and a reduction in peak diastolic filling rate (Folkow & Svanborg, 1993; Lakatta, 1993). It is unclear if any observed decline in stroke volume with age is linked to a smaller total blood volume (Davy & Seals, 1994; Strandell, 1964).

Heart rate in the resting supine position does not change with age, but it appears to decline slightly in the upright position in both men and women (Docherty, 1990; Granath et al., 1964; Lakatta, 1993; Seals, 1993; Seals et al., 1994c). An increased prevalence of arrhythmias also is observed with age, but this is not necessarily clinically significant or an indication of impaired function (Lakatta, 1993).

In the general population, mean arterial blood pressure rises with advancing age, with the rate of rise especially accelerated after menopause in women (Folkow & Svanborg, 1993; Harlan et al., 1984; Imai et al., 1993; Schoenberger, 1986). In healthy, active, non-obese, older individuals, however, elevations in mean arterial pressure are either not observed or are relatively minor (Ng et al., 1993; Rodeheffer et al., 1984; Seals et al., 1985; Taylor et al., 1991), suggesting that the aging process *per se* is not responsible for the increases of arterial pressure observed in the overall population. In the healthy older adult, the primary direct effect of aging is probably a mild increase in systolic pressure, especially in women (Ng et al., 1993; Seals, 1993). The rise in systolic blood pressure, when observed, is mediated by an age-related increase in systemic vascular resistance

(Fleg, 1986; Folkow & Svanborg, 1993; Gerstenblith et al. 1976; Lakatta, 1993; Seals, 1993).

With respect to regional hemodynamics, blood flow is reduced and vascular resistance increased in several regional circulations (Folkow & Svanborg, 1993; Seals, 1993), although recent findings indicate that myocardial blood flow actually increases with age (Czernin et al., 1993). The increases in vascular resistance both systemically and in selected regions likely are mediated by a combination of structural and neurohumoral mechanisms (Bader, 1983; Fleg, 1986; Folkow & Svanborg, 1993; Gerstenblith et al., 1976; Lakatta, 1993; Seals, 1993; Seals et al., 1994c; Vaitkevicius et al., 1993). Structural changes with age consist primarily of biochemical alterations in the walls of arterial vessels (e. g., increased collagen composition) that result in reduced compliance and elasticity and increased stiffness (Bader, 1983; Fleg, 1986; Folkow & Svanborg, 1993; Gerstenblith et al., 1976; Lakatta, 1993). Sympathetic nerve activity to skeletal muscle (Morlin et al., 1983; Ng et al., 1993; Seals et al., 1994c; Sundlof & Wallin, 1978) and whole body arterial plasma norepinephrine concentrations and/or spill-over rates are elevated, even in healthy older adults free of overt cardiovascular disease (Esler et al., 1981; Goldstein et al., 1983a; Hoeldtke & Cilmi, 1985; Morrow et al., 1987; Seals et al., 1994c; Ziegler et al., 1976). However, the respective contributions of these and other neurohumoral changes versus structural changes in the age-related increases in vascular resistance and arterial pressure are unknown. Nor has the possible role of the well-documented impairments in arterial and cardiopulmonary baroreceptor function with aging been determined (Cleroux et al., 1989; Gribbin et al., 1971; Lindbald, 1977).

CARDIOVASCULAR REGULATION DURING ACUTE EXERCISE

Age-related changes in autonomic and cardiovascular function during acute exercise, especially at submaximal intensities, have been reviewed in detail (Seals, 1993). In this section, we attempt to integrate many of the observations and conclusions from such prior sources with new findings on this topic. Particular attention has been paid to changes in cardiovascular function with age during maximal exercise.

Maximal Oxygen Consumption ($\dot{V}O_2$max)

Whether expressed as the maximal attainable work rate (power output), maximal oxygen consumption ($\dot{V}O_2$max), or otherwise, the maximal capacity to perform dynamic exercise with large muscle groups declines with advancing age in humans (Figure 6-1) (Buskirk & Hodgson, 1987;

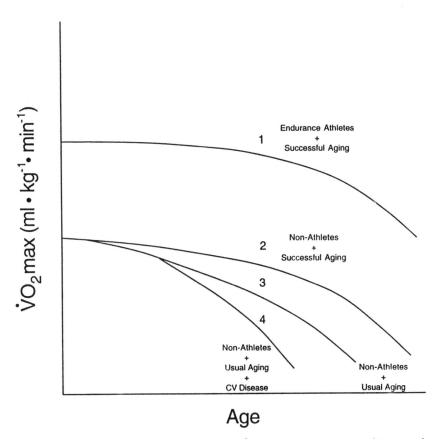

FIGURE 6-1. *Conceptualization of age-related declines in $\dot{V}O_2$max with advancing age in different populations of humans: 1) endurance athletes who remain highly active and otherwise undergo "successful" aging, i.e., they gain minimal body fat, are free of disease, and have genetic resistance to adverse effects of aging, etc. (Rowe & Kahn, 1987); 2) non-athletes who remain somewhat active and otherwise undergo successful aging; 3) non-athletes who become progressively less active and undergo "usual" aging (i.e., gradual increase in body fat, minor disease states, less aging-resistant genetic make-up, etc.); and 4) non-athletes who become progressively less active and develop serious cardiopulmonary disease (e.g., coronary heart disease with left ventricular dysfunction).*

Robinson, 1938). Using $\dot{V}O_2$max as a reflection of maximal aerobic exercise capacity, it is apparent that the rate of decline not only differs among investigations but is highly variable among individuals within a particular population (Buskirk & Hodgson, 1987). Differences among investigations are likely due to methodological factors such as use of cross-sectional versus longitudinal study designs, subject selection, and the ability to measure a "true" $\dot{V}O_2$max, especially in older subjects. Much of the variability within populations is due to constitutional (e.g., body composition), physical activity, and disease factors that modulate the rate of decline in $\dot{V}O_2$max independently of the aging process.

$\dot{V}O_2$max decreases with age in both men and women, with the most generally agreed upon average rate of decrease in $\dot{V}O_2$max in nonphysically trained subjects being ~10% per decade (Buskirk & Hodgson, 1987). The age-related decline in this population, however, appears to be curvilinear rather than linear in nature, with an accelerated reduction after age 60 (Buskirk & Hodgson, 1987). When expressed in terms of mL·kg^{-1}·min^{-1} per year, the rate of decline in $\dot{V}O_2$max has been reported to be less in women than in men (Buskirk & Hodgson, 1987).

There are both longitudinal and cross-sectional data suggesting that the rate of decrease in $\dot{V}O_2$max with age, at least in men, is up to 50% less in individuals who continue to perform vigorous aerobic-type exercise on a regular basis (Buskirk & Hodgson, 1987; Hagberg et al., 1985; Heath et al., 1981; Ogawa et al., 1992), although similar rates of declines for active and inactive subjects have also been reported (Saltin, 1986). (See below.) The results of longitudinal studies suggest that $\dot{V}O_2$max can be fairly well maintained over phases of middle age lasting 10–20 y in men who continue to train vigorously (Hagberg, 1987; Kasch et al., 1990; Marti & Howald, 1990; Pollock et al., 1987; Rogers et al., 1990); we are unaware of any corollary data in women. In contrast, the greatest rates of decline in $\dot{V}O_2$max appear to occur in highly endurance-trained subjects who subsequently stop or markedly reduce their activity (Buskirk & Hodgson, 1987; Kasch et al., 1990; Marti & Howald, 1990; Powell et al., 1987). Importantly, from an interpretation standpoint, Saltin (1986) has reported that estimation of the average decline in $\dot{V}O_2$max with age in endurance athletes is essentially the same whether evaluated cross-sectionally (the most often used approach) or longitudinally. Taken together, the available data indicate a strong, inverse relationship between the intensity and/or volume of an individual's habitual physical activity and the corresponding decline in $\dot{V}O_2$max.

There is considerable controversy regarding the mechanisms responsible for the reduction in $\dot{V}O_2$max with age. Most of the available information has been obtained from cross-sectional investigations of either nonphysically trained subjects of different ages or of highly trained masters athletes compared to young athletes; the latter have been used in an attempt to eliminate the influence of factors such as chronic physical activity and body composition that change with age in the general population. However, this model likely only minimizes such effects because older athletes cannot train at the same absolute intensities as their younger elite counterparts, nor do they all necessarily avoid changes in body composition. In some cases, the overall training volume of the masters athletes studied was only ~50–60% as great as that of the young athletic controls (Meredith et al., 1987; Rivera et al., 1989). Thus, some investigators have compared elite middle-aged and older athletes to non-elite young runners with similar levels of body fat, training volumes, and/or competitive performances (Fuchi et al., 1989; Hagberg et al., 1985). The limitation of this latter approach is that the non-elite young runners likely have inferior predispositions for endurance performance compared to the elite masters runners.

With regard to the "Fick" determinants of $\dot{V}O_2max$, i.e., maximal heart rate and stroke volume (cardiac output) and maximal arterio-venous oxygen difference (a-v O_2 D), the one consistent finding is that an age-related decrease in maximal heart rate reduces the maximal achievable cardiac output which, in turn, is a major component of the decline in $\dot{V}O_2max$ (Hagberg et al., 1985; Ogawa et al., 1992; Rivera et al., 1989). Some data in endurance-trained women and/or men indicate that the decrease in $\dot{V}O_2max$ is due solely to the decline in maximal heart rate (Hagberg et al., 1985), whereas other findings suggest a contribution of only 25–40% from this mechanism (Ogawa et al., 1992). Such discrepancies are likely the result of different approaches to estimating maximal stroke volume and/or of differences in the ages of the masters athletes studied (Ogawa et al., 1992). In studies concluding that the decline in maximal heart rate explains only a portion of the age-associated reduction in $\dot{V}O_2max$, decreases in maximal stroke volume were reported to explain up to 50% of the remaining difference (Ogawa et al., 1992). Recent findings from our laboratory indicate that: 1) total blood volume is lower in healthy older compared to young untrained men, and that these reductions are strongly related to the age-related decline in $\dot{V}O_2max$ (Davy & Seals, 1994), and 2) $\dot{V}O_2max$ and total blood volume also are directly correlated in postmenopausal women who differ in their levels of physical activity (Stevenson et al., 1994). Because total blood volume exerts an important influence on maximal stroke volume and $\dot{V}O_2max$ in young adults (Convertino, 1991; Coyle et al., 1986), the age-associated decrease in blood volume could contribute to the lower maximal stroke volume observed in older subjects. In any event, depending on the gender and chronic physical activity levels of the subjects, the reduction in maximal cardiac output produced by declines in maximal heart rate and stroke volume appears to explain between 50% and 100% of the total reduction in $\dot{V}O_2max$ with age, with the remainder due to a lower maximal a-v O_2 D (Fuchi et al., 1989; Hagberg et al., 1985; Ogawa et al., 1992; Saltin, 1986).

The influence of physical training on the age-related changes in these determinants of $\dot{V}O_2max$ is not entirely clear. Some findings indicate that the apparent lesser rate of decline in $\dot{V}O_2max$ with age in athletes who remain active is associated with smaller reductions in maximal heart rate and a-v O_2 D compared with untrained subjects (Ogawa et al., 1992; Rogers et al., 1990). On the other hand, age-related decreases in maximal heart rates have been reported to be similar in masters athletes whose activity levels decreased over time compared to those who maintained their training levels (Pollock et al., 1987; Saltin, 1986). It is interesting to speculate that the apparent lesser decline in maximal a-v O_2 D reported in highly trained older endurance athletes (Ogawa et al., 1992) is due to the maintenance of high levels of skeletal muscle oxidative capacity (Coggan et al., 1992; Rogers & Evans, 1993; Saltin, 1986).

Finally, changes in body composition appear to play an important role in the age-related decline in $\dot{V}O_2$max in at least two ways. First, independent of any change in the absolute level of whole-body $\dot{V}O_2$max (i.e., L/min), an increase in body weight with age will result in a reduction in $\dot{V}O_2$max as traditionally expressed in $mL \cdot kg^{-1} \cdot min^{-1}$. Second, at any given level of body weight, aging typically is associated with a decrease in fat-free mass in general and skeletal muscle mass in particular, as well as with an increase in body fat content (Montoye et al., 1965; Poehlman & Horton, 1990). Because the absolute $\dot{V}O_2$max is directly related to the size of the active skeletal muscle mass, these age-associated shifts in body composition will, independent of changes in cardiac pumping or peripheral oxidative capacities, cause $\dot{V}O_2$max to decline with age (Fleg & Lakatta, 1988). Although the exact magnitude of the contribution differs among studies (Booth, 1989; Fleg & Lakatta, 1988; Ogawa et al., 1992), it is clear that at least some of the age-related decrease in $\dot{V}O_2$max is due to changes in body composition, such as an increase in body fat content (Ogawa et al., 1992).

Systemic Hemodynamic Adjustments to Exercise

Heart Rate. The absolute increase in heart rate in response to the same relative exercise stress, defined here as a particular %$\dot{V}O_2$max, becomes smaller with age (Kohrt et al., 1993; Sachs et al., 1985; Seals, 1993; Taylor et al., 1992). However, this smaller heart rate elevation in older adults, frequently described as a "blunted" or "attenuated" response, appears to be appropriate for the absolute level of oxygen uptake, which is lower in the average older versus younger subject at the same relative intensity of exercise. As noted previously, maximal heart rate decreases progressively with advancing age, and there is some evidence to indicate that the rate of decline is greater in men than in women (Hossack & Bruce, 1982). An average rate of decline is difficult to determine, in part, because of the question of whether or not true maximal efforts were obtained in many studies involving older untrained subjects. For example, the maximal heart rates we reported previously in studies of untrained subjects in which a true $\dot{V}O_2$max was elicited (Seals et al., 1984b) were ~20 beats/min higher than those predicted from the traditionally-used equation of 220-age. The mechanism(s) responsible for the decline in maximal heart rate with age have not been determined. Impaired responsiveness to beta-adrenergic stimulation (Conway et al., 1971; Seals et al., 1994c; Yin et al., 1976) and a decline in the intrinsic heart rate (Lakatta, 1993) both likely contribute. The latter may be due to morphological and electrophysiological changes in the sinoatrial node and other portions of the conduction system that result in reduced conduction velocity (Saltin, 1986).

Stroke Volume and Cardiac Output. Reductions in stroke volume with age during submaximal and peak leg cycle ergometry exercise were consistently reported in early investigations using direct-Fick or indicator-dilution methodology for measuring peak cardiac output (Granath et al., 1964; Julius et al., 1967; Strandell, 1964). These were followed by a report of maintained levels of stroke volume with age during incremental cycling exercise using ventricular imaging methods in subjects rigorously screened for heart disease (Rodeheffer et al., 1984). However, recent investigations in which maximal cardiac output was determined with the acetylene rebreathing procedure during progressive treadmill exercise that elicited a true $\dot{V}O_2$max have found clear, significant reductions in stroke volume with age in both nonphysically trained subjects and highly trained endurance athletes (Ogawa et al., 1992).

With regard to the mechanisms involved, it is unclear if a reduction in left ventricular filling plays a role in the age-associated decline in maximal stroke volume. Findings of age-related increases in left ventricular end-diastolic volume (Lakatta, 1993; Rodeheffer et al., 1984) and in filling pressures (Ehrsam, 1983; Lakatta, 1993) during cycling exercise in active healthy subjects (primarily and exclusively men, respectively) do not support this concept. (It should be noted that increases in left ventricular end-diastolic volume do not appear to occur with aging in women [Lakatta, 1993]). Peak left-ventricular diastolic filling rate during both submaximal and maximal supine cycling exercise declines with age (Levy et al., 1993; Schulman et al., 1992) and is correlated with peak levels of oxygen consumption (Levy et al., 1993). However, the lower exercise heart rates of older adults may offset this reduction in peak filling rate by increasing diastolic filling time. An increase in left ventricular wall stress and afterload (which impedes emptying) may also contribute to the age-associated decline in stroke volume (Ehsani, 1987; Lakatta, 1993), especially in older subjects who demonstrate elevated levels of systolic blood pressure during exercise due to reduced arterial compliance. Moreover, it appears that left ventricular contractile reserve becomes impaired after age 60, at least in men, as indicated by an attenuated increase in ejection fraction from rest to peak cycling exercise (Lakatta, 1993; Port et al., 1980). An age-related reduction in the response to beta-adrenergic stimulation likely contributes to the impairment in both peak diastolic filling rate and systolic contractile performance (Lakatta, 1993; Schulman et al., 1992; Seals et al., 1994c; Stratton et al., 1992). Finally, an increase in left ventricular stiffness and wall motion abnormalities, as well as a prolongation of myocardial contraction and relaxation time, could play a role in these age-related changes in the left ventricular response to exercise (Ehsani, 1987; Lakatta, 1993).

The 5–6 L increase in cardiac output per liter increase in oxygen consumption each minute during incremental exercise has been reported to be unaltered with aging in healthy humans, although the absolute (L/min) level of cardiac output may be lower at the same submaximal level of oxygen consumption in older versus young subjects due to lower levels at rest (Ehrsam, 1983; Granath et al., 1964; Julius et al., 1967; Saltin, 1986; Strandell, 1964). As mentioned earlier, in the general population, peak/maximal cardiac output is reduced with advancing age because of reductions in both maximal heart rate and stroke volume (Ehrsam, 1983; Granath et al., 1964; Julius et al., 1967; Ogawa et al., 1992; Strandell, 1964). As is the case in young subjects, maximal cardiac output is lower in older women than in older men, solely because of a lower stroke volume (Ogawa et al., 1992).

Arterial Blood Pressure. The arterial blood pressure response to submaximal and maximal exercise appears to be either unchanged or greater with advancing age (Conway et al., 1971; Granath et al., 1964; Julius et al., 1967; Martin et al., 1991; Montoye, 1984; Rodeheffer et al., 1984; Seals, 1993; Strandell, 1964). Absolute levels of arterial pressure, especially systolic pressure, often are higher during exercise in older subjects as a result of their elevated resting levels. Absolute systolic pressure during maximal exercise is greater in older subjects, both men and women (Martin et al., 1991), but the magnitude of this age-associated increase appears to be greater in women than in men (Hossack & Bruce, 1982). Because maximal cardiac output is reduced with age, this elevated arterial pressure during maximal exercise must be mediated by a greater systemic vascular resistance (Gerstenblith et al., 1976; Hagberg et al., 1985; Julius et al., 1967; Ogawa et al., 1992; Strandell, 1964).

Two points deserve emphasis with regard to the regulation of arterial blood pressure during exercise with aging. First, in a recent series of investigations on autonomic-cardiovascular regulation at rest and in response to exercise and other stressors in healthy, nonobese, young and older humans with similar chronic physical activity levels (Ng et al., 1993, 1994a; Davy et al., 1995; Taylor et al., 1991, 1992), the single most consistent finding was the similarity of the regulation of arterial blood pressure in the young and older subjects. Specifically, we found that the adjustments in arterial pressures of the older adults to both brief (Taylor et al., 1992) and prolonged (Davy et al., 1995) dynamic exercise, as well as to other forms of stress (Ng et al., 1994a; Taylor et al., 1991), were similar to those observed in the young controls.

Second, when investigating age-related changes in arterial blood pressure regulation during exercise, one must consider carefully the appropriate stimulus or level of exercise at which to compare the young and older subjects. We have made our comparisons at the same relative (% maximum) exercise intensities because this appears to be the primary determinant of the arterial pressure response to exercise (Bezucha et al., 1982; Lewis et al., 1983). Assuming that this approach is appropriate, we must reexamine two prior tenets associated with the influence of age on blood pressure control during dynamic exercise. One is that the increase in the absolute level of arterial pressure during submaximal exercise is greater with age (Granath et al., 1964; Julius et al., 1967; Montoye, 1984; Strandell, 1964). These studies compared their older subjects and young controls at the same absolute submaximal exercise intensity or level of oxygen consumption, i.e., the exercise stimulus represented a higher relative intensity in the older subjects; thus, if arterial pressure were regulated appropriately, one would expect older individuals to demonstrate a greater blood pressure response.

The other concept to be reconsidered is that the capacity of the older person to undergo peripheral vasodilation (primarily in active skeletal muscle) during exercise is impaired, as indicated by an elevated systemic vascular resistance (reduced systemic vascular conductance) observed during exercise at the same %$\dot{V}O_2$max in both untrained and trained subjects (Hagberg et al., 1985; Ogawa et al., 1992; Rivera et al., 1989; Rodeheffer et al., 1984). Such observations have been attributed to factors such as the increase in arterial stiffness with age (Gerstenblith et al., 1976; Hagberg et al., 1985; Lakatta, 1993; Vaitkevicius et al., 1993). However, this elevated systemic vascular resistance may not represent an impaired response; rather it may be appropriate given the nature of the exercise stimulus employed. During exercise performed at the same absolute intensity and the same whole-body oxygen consumption and cardiac output, the older adult will be exercising at a higher percentage of peak work capacity and, therefore, will evoke a higher level of arterial blood pressure than will the young adult. Under these exercise conditions, a higher level of systemic vascular resistance must be maintained for the subject to generate the necessary level of arterial pressure. Stated more broadly, regardless of age, any individual or population with a lower peak exercise capacity *should* maintain a higher level of systemic vascular resistance during exercise performed at the same level of cardiac output.

Taken together, these observations indicate that previous conclusions regarding the influence of human aging on the arterial blood pressure responses to exercise need to be reconsidered. Differences observed with age in the healthy human appear to be appropriately adaptive, rather than maladaptive.

Regional Hemodynamic Adjustments to Exercise

Although little new information is available concerning the possible effects of age on the regulation of regional hemodynamics during exercise since our last review (Seals, 1993), two important concepts will be emphasized here. First, there is no consistent line of experimental evidence that would indicate an age-related impairment in the ability to augment blood flow to active skeletal muscle, at least during submaximal exercise. There is one report of a lower absolute levels of leg blood flow at the same absolute submaximal loads of cycling in middle-aged versus young male athletes (Wahren et al., 1974), but this observation is not supported by other findings (Carlson & Pernow, 1961; Jasperse et al., 1994). A lower *peak* level of blood flow to active muscles would be expected with age because of the declines in the maximal achievable exercise intensity, maximal cardiac output, and $\dot{V}O_2$max. However, conclusions regarding the influence of aging on blood flow to active muscles during submaximal and maximal exercise will require systematic study in the future. The ability of the aging human to properly augment coronary blood flow during exercise of various intensities is also a critical, clinically relevant issue that must be addressed.

A second point concerns the exercise-evoked adjustments in the regional circulations that undergo vasoconstriction during exercise. If older people require an elevated systemic vascular resistance (reduced systemic vascular conductance) during exercise at the same relative exercise intensity, i.e., the same %$\dot{V}O_2$max, some, if not all, of these regions might undergo greater vasoconstriction in the older individual. This is consistent with the results of a recent study in our laboratory in which older men demonstrated an augmented whole-forearm vasoconstrictor response during brief cycling exercise at the same percentage of peak oxygen consumption relative to young controls (Taylor et al., 1992). The average blood flows to forearm skin during steady-state exercise were not different in the two groups, suggesting that the greater reductions in blood flows to the forearms of the older men were mediated by correspondingly greater vasoconstriction in the non-active muscles of the forearms. This, in turn, was consistent with the augmented increases in norepinephrine concentrations in blood plasma obtained from antecubital veins of the older men during the exercise. Whether or not greater vasoconstriction occurs in other regional circulations, such as the kidneys and gut, during exercise in older humans is unknown.

Prolonged Submaximal Exercise. At the time of last review of this topic (Seals, 1993), there had been only one systematic investigation of the physiological adjustments to prolonged submaximal exercise in older humans under thermoneutral ambient conditions (Hagberg et al., 1988a). This study focused primarily on the metabolic and endocrine responses to 60 min of treadmill walking exercise at ~70% of $\dot{V}O_2$max in young and older healthy untrained men. Overall, the somewhat surprising finding was that the exercise task actually appeared to be less stressful in the older men, as indicated by smaller increases in ratings of perceived exertion and in plasma lactate and catecholamine concentrations.

Based on these findings, we postulated that older subjects may also undergo less of a loss of cardiovascular and thermal homeostasis during prolonged exercise, i.e., they may demonstrate less "cardiovascular drift." To test this hypothesis, recently (Davy et al., 1995) we studied healthy nonobese young and older men with similar chronic physical activity levels during standing rest (pre-exercise baseline) and throughout 45 minutes of treadmill walking performed at ~65% of $\dot{V}O_2$max (Figure 6-2). This relative intensity of exercise represented a much lower absolute workload and whole-body level of oxygen consumption for the older men who had lower $\dot{V}O_2$max levels than the young controls.

As in the prior study (Hagberg et al., 1988a), we observed smaller time-dependent increases in plasma lactate and norepinephrine concentrations during exercise in the older men, although there were no differences in ratings of perceived effort. Consistent with our hypothesis, the

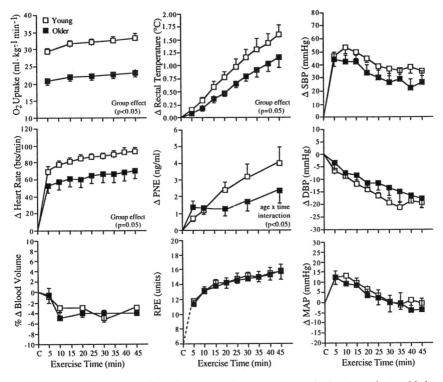

FIGURE 6-2. *Adjustments in whole-body oxygen uptake, neuro-cardiovascular function, and internal body temperature during prolonged submaximal treadmill walking exercise at ~65% $\dot{V}O_2$max in young (□) and older (■) healthy men matched for chronic physical activity levels.* After the initial 5–10 min of walking, the progressive time-dependent changes in oxygen consumption, heart rate, systolic (SBP), mean (MBP) and diastolic (DBP) arterial blood pressure, blood volume, and ratings of perceived exertion (RPE) were similar in the two groups despite much smaller increases in rectal temperature and plasma norepinephrine (PNE) levels in the older men. From Davy et al. (1995).

progressive rise in internal body (rectal) temperature throughout exercise was much smaller in the older men. In contrast, after the initial few minutes of walking, the progressive time-dependent adjustments in oxygen consumption, heart rate, arterial blood pressure, and blood volume throughout the remainder of the exercise period were similar in the young and older men. These preliminary findings indicate that during prolonged submaximal exercise performed at the same relative intensity under thermoneutral ambient conditions, older men do not demonstrate a lesser cardiovascular drift despite a smaller rise in internal body temperature. This apparent discrepancy may simply reflect a primary need to properly regulate arterial blood pressure during prolonged exercise in the older adult. If so, the older adult will evoke whatever neurocirculatory adjustments are necessary to support arterial pressure, and in so doing, the relationship between these adjustments and other central nervous system signals (internal body temperature, in this case) may be different from that observed in young adults.

CARDIOVASCULAR ADAPTATIONS TO CHRONIC EXERCISE

The reader is referred to previous reviews for detailed information on adaptations to physical training in middle-aged and older adults (Ehsani, 1987; Hagberg, 1987, 1994; Lakatta, 1993; Saltin, 1986). In this section we integrate some fundamental observations from prior work with several new findings. As mentioned earlier, both cross-sectional approaches using already highly trained older endurance athletes (primarily men) and longitudinal investigations of the effects of physical training on previously sedentary older adults provide insight into issues in this area.

$\dot{V}O_2$max

Cross-sectional Studies of Masters Athletes. Early observations of middle-aged and older male athletes (Dehn & Bruce, 1972; Dill et al., 1967; Hagberg, 1987; Heath et al., 1981) provided the first suggestion that 1) older individuals were capable of demonstrating high levels of $\dot{V}O_2$max and 2) the physiological stimulus imposed by vigorous endurance exercise training might increase $\dot{V}O_2$max in untrained older individuals. The levels of $\dot{V}O_2$max observed in these older male athletes were approximately twice as great as that of their untrained peers.

Recently, Wells and colleagues (1992) reported that middle-aged and older (35–70 y) women endurance runners also have higher levels of $\dot{V}O_2$max than those observed previously in untrained women of similar age (Kohrt et al., 1991; Ogawa et al., 1992; Seals et al., 1984b), although the differences did not appear to be as great as those reported previously in men (Hagberg et al., 1985; Heath et al., 1981; Seals et al., 1984a). We hypothesized that highly conditioned and competitive women runners of this age should demonstrate the same high levels of $\dot{V}O_2$max as the masters male athletes studied previously, relative to age- and gender-matched untrained controls. To address this, we studied a group of highly trained middle-aged and older (mean age ~54 y; range 49–67) women endurance runners (Stevenson et al., 1994). The average level of $\dot{V}O_2$max in these older women athletes was ~49 mL/kg/min, a level 20–25% greater than the highest values reported previously in women of this age (Wells et al., 1992). Moreover, the ~85% higher levels of $\dot{V}O_2$max in our middle-aged masters women runners versus the age-matched untrained controls were similar to the corresponding differences (75–95%) observed previously in men (Hagberg et al., 1985; Heath et al., 1981; Seals et al., 1984a) (Figure 6-3). Recently published data indicate that older (65–84 y) highly endurance-trained and competitive women athletes also demonstrate greater (average 67%) levels of $\dot{V}O_2$max than do sedentary women of similar age (Warren et al., 1993). Taken together, these recent findings (Stevenson et al., 1994; Warren et al., 1993; Wells et al., 1992) and those reported previously (Dehn & Bruce, 1972; Dill et al., 1967; Hagberg et al., 1985; Heath et al., 1981; Seals et al., 1984a) indicate that both older men and older women endurance athletes are capable of retaining high levels of maximal aerobic power.

Parenthetically, when the cross-sectional levels of $\dot{V}O_2$max shown in Figure 6-3 are examined closely, these data do not uniformly support the idea presented above that the rate of decline in $\dot{V}O_2$max with age is only half as great in physically trained versus untrained populations. Specifically, the % declines in $\dot{V}O_2$max per decade in this compilation of subjects age 25 versus 55 y was 9.1, 11.6, 8.4, and 7.7%, respectively, for the trained females, untrained females, trained males, and untrained males, probably because the average population values used were obtained from different studies. Alternatively, it may be that individuals who are healthy and undergo successful aging demonstrate similar rates of decline in $\dot{V}O_2$max as active athletes. Saltin (1986) has reported data in endurance trained male athletes consistent with the latter interpretation.

Longitudinal Studies of Sedentary Older Adults. Over the last decade several studies have confirmed that previously sedentary older men and women demonstrate an increase in $\dot{V}O_2$max in response to endurance training if the exercise stimulus is adequate (Hagberg, 1994; Hagberg et al., 1989; Kohrt et al., 1991; Makrides et al., 1990; Seals & Chase, 1989; Seals et al., 1984b). Older individuals can elicit a similar relative (i.e., %) increase in $\dot{V}O_2$max as can young adults when the training stimulus is sufficiently intense and prolonged, but the absolute increases (i.e., in $mL \cdot kg^{-1} \cdot min^{-1}$

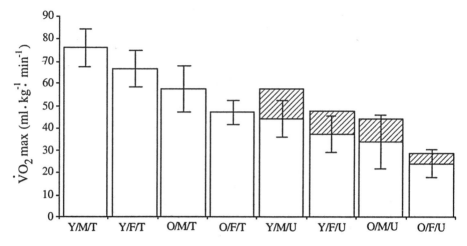

FIGURE 6-3. *Hierarchy of mean ($\pm$ 2 SD) levels of $\dot{V}O_2max$ in different populations of humans according to age (Y = young, 25 y; O = older, 55 y), gender (M = male; F = female), and state of endurance exercise training (T = highly trained endurance athlete; U = untrained subject). The cross-hatched extensions of the bars for the untrained groups represent typical improvements in $\dot{V}O_2max$ (i.e., 25% above untrained levels) achievable as adaptations to prolonged, intense endurance training. Based on data from Heath et al., 1981; Hossack & Bruce, 1982; Hagberg et al., 1985; Ogawa et al., 1992; Joyner, 1993; Stevenson et al., 1994.*

or L/min) generally are smaller; thus, the similar % increases are due to the lower pretraining baseline levels in the older subjects. Greater relative and similar absolute increases in older versus young adults, however, have been reported for peak leg cycling oxygen uptake in response to intensive training (Makrides et al., 1990).

The % increases in $\dot{V}O_2max$ observed after intense and prolonged endurance training appear to be equivalent in older men compared to older women, but the absolute increases appear to be greater in the men; again, the similar % increases are due to the lower baseline levels of the older women (Kohrt et al, 1991). The smaller $mL \cdot kg^{-1} \cdot min^{-1}$ or L/min increases in $\dot{V}O_2max$ with endurance training in older versus young adults and in older women versus men, respectively, are most likely due to lower absolute training intensities (exercise velocities, power outputs, or whole-body oxygen uptake) that are necessitated by their lower levels of $\dot{V}O_2max$ because of the fact that most people who are not competitive athletes do not voluntarily choose to exercise more intensely than ~75% of their maximal aerobic power during the training sessions.

In older adults, the magnitude of the % increase in $\dot{V}O_2max$ with endurance exercise training varies markedly among individuals. In the first study that demonstrated that regular endurance exercise could elicit physiologically significant increases in $\dot{V}O_2max$ in older healthy adults (Seals et al., 1984b), we found an average increase of 30% following 12 mo of training, with a range of 2 to 49%; Kohrt and colleagues (1991) have reported a similarly wide range of responses. The factors responsible for determining the magnitude of the increase and, thus, the large variability in $\dot{V}O_2$max with training in older adults have not been established. In older men the baseline level of $\dot{V}O_2$max, the intensity of the training pace, the reason for stopping the exercise test, and the skinfold thicknesses all correlated with the posttraining levels of $\dot{V}O_2$max, explaining 62% of the variability in the response (Thomas et al., 1985); in contrast, pretraining physical activity levels were not correlated with the increases in $\dot{V}O_2$max after training. Other findings also indicate that the intensity and length of exercise training exert a strong effect on the magnitude of the increase in $\dot{V}O_2$max observed in older adults (Hagberg, 1987; Hagberg et al., 1989; Seals et al., 1984b), as does the mode of exercise (Seals et al., 1984b). In contrast, some data do not provide support for the intensity of training as an important determinant of the increase in $\dot{V}O_2$max in older subjects (Badenhop et al., 1983; Belman & Gaesser, 1991; Foster et al., 1989). In a study reporting responses to training in young and older men and women (Kohrt et al., 1991), the % increases in $\dot{V}O_2$max were not related to age, initial (pretraining) levels, or gender. From a theoretical standpoint, it would seem that factors related to the training stimulus (i.e., mode; session intensity, duration, and frequency; and total length of the training program), the subject's initial (pretraining) levels of fitness and chronic physical activity, and genetic predisposition (Bouchard et al., 1992) should be among the critical determinants of the increase in maximal aerobic power in both healthy young and older adults.

What are the average % increases in $\dot{V}O_2$max that can be expected in older adults in response to endurance exercise training? Brief and/or very low-intensity training may produce little or no increase in $\dot{V}O_2$max in older adults (Benestad, 1965; Bouchard et al., 1992; DeVries, 1970; Foster et al., 1989; Hagberg, 1994; Niinimaa & Shephard, 1978; Seals et al., 1984b; Suominen et al., 1977; Warren et al., 1993). The largest exercise trial performed to date (Cunningham et al., 1987) reported that 1 y of moderate intensity training resulted in an average increase in $\dot{V}O_2$max of 11% in 100 men. Higher intensity training performed for periods of 6–12 mo appears to evoke increases of ~20–30% in middle-aged and older men and women (Hagberg et al., 1989; Kohrt et al., 1991; Makrides et al., 1990; Seals & Chase, 1989; Seals et al., 1984b). It should be emphasized, however, that, as in young adults, even prolonged intensive endurance training in previously sedentary, nonathletic older adults will not produce the high levels of $\dot{V}O_2$max observed in elite older endurance athletes. The latter is probably due to the combination of superior genetics, other constitutional advantages such as low body weight and body fat, and the ability to train at much higher overall exercise levels than their physically active, but non-elite, peers.

Mechanisms Responsible for the Higher $\dot{V}O_2$max in the Endurance-Trained State

Several central circulatory, peripheral oxidative, and body composition-related mechanisms appear to be responsible for the elevations in $\dot{V}O_2$max associated with endurance training in older adults.

Central Circulatory Factors. It has been reported that 50 to 100% of the higher levels of $\dot{V}O_2$max in older male endurance athletes compared to age- and gender-matched, untrained controls is due to greater maximal cardiac output, which is, in turn, solely the result of a higher maximal stroke volume because maximal heart rate is not different in the two groups (Fuchi et al., 1989; Hagberg et al., 1985; Ogawa et al., 1992; Rivera et al., 1989; Saltin, 1986). These cross-sectional data in men are consistent with data from a recent longitudinal study in which prolonged and intensive endurance training produced increases in maximal stroke volume and cardiac output that accounted for the majority of the increase in $\dot{V}O_2$max. (Maximal heart rate was either unchanged or slightly reduced after training) (Spina et al., 1993a). Similar findings have been reported for peak leg cycling stroke volume and cardiac output following intensive cycling training in older men (Makrides et al., 1990). Recent findings from both studies of older endurance athletes (Seals et al., 1994b) and longitudinal training investigations (Ehsani et al., 1991) indicate that the increase in maximal exercise stroke volume in older men after vigorous training is associated with increases in LV end-diastolic volume as well as enhanced LV systolic contractile performance during peak exercise. The increase in peak LV end-diastolic volume observed after prolonged high-intensity endurance training in men (Ehsani et al., 1991) may (Levy et al., 1993) or may not (Schulman et al., 1992), in turn, be mediated by an increase in the peak early diastolic filling rate during exercise, which is correlated with the magnitude of the increase in $\dot{V}O_2$max.

In contrast to these findings in men, recent findings indicate that the increase in $\dot{V}O_2$max in response to prolonged and intensive endurance training in older women is not associated with increases in maximal cardiac output, stroke volume, LV end-diastolic volume, or LV contractile performance (Spina et al., 1993a, 1993b). Because young women demonstrate the same endurance training-evoked adaptations in cardiac pump function during maximal exercise as young and older men (Ehsani et al., 1991; Spina et al., 1992, 1993a), and because the older (postmenopausal) women studied to date have not been on hormone replacement therapy (Spina et al., 1993a, 1993b), the apparent lack of central circulatory adaptations in these older healthy women following endurance training may be related to hormonal changes, particularly a lack of circulating estrogen (Giraud et al., 1993; Pines et al., 1991; Scheuer et al., 1987). However, less of an age-related deterioration in LV systolic function during peak exercise, which results in higher pre-training baseline levels than for men, could also have contributed to the gender-related differences in the LV adaptations to training observed in older adults (Spina et al., 1993b). It should also be noted that an augmentation in LV end-diastolic volume and stroke volume with no change in the LV ejection fraction response has been observed at the same absolute exercise cycling intensity following brief, moderate-intensity endurance training in 24 previously sedentary older adults, 18 of whom were women (Schocken et al., 1983); the hormone status of these women was not reported. The reasons for the disparate findings with regard to LV end-diastolic volume in this study and the more recent report (Spina et al., 1993b) are not clear.

Peripheral Oxidative Factors. Adaptations in the active skeletal muscles also appear to play a significant role in the endurance training-evoked increases in $\dot{V}O_2$ max in older men and women. In older men, results from both studies of masters athletes (Ogawa et al., 1992; Rivera et al., 1989) and longitudinal investigations (Spina et al., 1993a) indicate that an increase in maximal a-v O_2D can, depending on the population, account for up to 50% of the increase in $\dot{V}O_2$ max in response to endurance training. Moreover, the available data in older women suggest that their entire training-induced elevation in $\dot{V}O_2$ max is mediated by an increase in maximal a-v O_2D (Spina et al., 1993a). The elevated maximal a-v O_2D in older, endurance-trained adults is associated with increases in capillary density and oxidative enzyme activities in the trained skeletal muscles suggestive of an enhanced capacity for oxidative energy production (Coggan et al., 1990, 1992; Rogers & Evans, 1993). In addition to the increased capillary density, endurance training also appears to produce adaptations in the resistance vessels (arterioles) of the active muscles that result in an increase in peak vasodilatory capacity and peak reactive blood flow (Martin et al., 1990, 1991; Romanovska et al., 1981). These adaptations have been reported to be strongly related to the increase in $\dot{V}O_2$ max observed in response to endurance training in older adults, in some cases explaining almost 50% of the total variance (Martin et al., 1991).

Body Composition Factors. Changes in body weight and/or composition also contribute to the increase in $\dot{V}O_2$ max in older men and women with endurance training. For example, the marked differences in $\dot{V}O_2$ max between older endurance athletes and their untrained peers are substantially reduced after correction for differences in body composition (i.e., fat and fat-free masses) (Ogawa et al., 1992). More simply, any reduction in body weight in response to endurance training will result in a increase in

$\dot{V}O_2$max expressed in mL·kg^{-1}·min^{-1}, even if the absolute level of whole body (L/min) oxygen consumption is unchanged. Because endurance training often is associated with reductions in body weight and reductions in fat mass in older adults (c. f., Kohrt et al., 1991; Seals et al., 1984b), these changes likely contribute to the increases in $\dot{V}O_2$max.

Resistance Training. It should be noted that increases in $\dot{V}O_2$max have not been observed in response to resistance exercise training in middle-aged men (Hurley et al., 1984) and older (70–79 y) men and women (Hagberg et al., 1989), i.e., populations in which endurance training produces marked increases (Hanson et al., 1968; Makrides et al., 1990; Martin et al., 1991; Saltin et al., 1969; Seals et al., 1984b).

Other Cardiovascular Adaptations to Training

In general, the autonomic and cardiovascular adaptations to endurance exercise training under resting conditions and during submaximal exercise in the older adult have been shown to be similar to those observed in young adults (Ehsani, 1987; Hagberg, 1994; Lakatta, 1993).

Findings from both older athletes as well as longitudinal studies indicate that older adults demonstrate reductions in resting heart rate ("training bradycardia") and, often, in arterial blood pressure (Benestad, 1965; Cononie et al. 1991; Hagberg et al., 1985; Seals et al., 1984b; Spina et al., 1993a,b). There is experimental evidence that the decrease in resting heart rate is mediated by an increase in cardiac vagal tone and by a reduction in the intrinsic heart rate (De Meersman, 1993; Denahan et al., 1993; Seals & Chase, 1989). In older adults, plasma norepinephrine concentrations at rest generally are not different in the endurance-trained versus untrained states (Cononie et al., 1991; Kohrt et al., 1993; Ng et al., 1994), but more sensitive measures of sympathetic activity such as plasma norepinephrine appearance rates and directly recorded muscle sympathetic nerve activity actually are elevated in the endurance-trained condition (Ng et al., 1994; Poehlman et al., 1990, 1992).

Training-induced adaptations in left ventricular function and structure in older adults appear to be gender-specific. In older men, findings from studies on masters endurance athletes and longitudinal investigations indicate that endurance training is associated with increases in LV end-diastolic volume (dimension) and posterior wall thickness, with no changes in the wall thickness-to-radius ratio or indices of LV systolic contractile function under resting conditions (Child et al., 1984; Heath et al., 1981; Seals et al., 1994b). In contrast, the increase in LV end-diastolic volume at rest has not been observed even after prolonged, intense endurance exercise training in previously sedentary older women (Spina et al., 1993b). Moreover, the age-related decline in peak early diastolic filling rate at rest has been reported to be reversed by vigorous endurance training in older men (Forman et al., 1992; Levy et al., 1993; Takemoto et al.,

1992), although this has not been a uniform finding (Schulman et al., 1992). The impairment in beta-adrenergic stimulation of cardiac chronotropic and inotropic function with age, at least under resting conditions, does not appear to be affected by endurance training (Stratton et al., 1992).

At least in older men, the adaptations observed during submaximal exercise performed at the same absolute workload before and after training are similar to those documented previously in young adults, i.e., heart rate, systemic vascular resistance, and plasma catecholamine levels are lower; stroke volume is higher; and oxygen consumption, cardiac output, and a-v O_2D usually are unchanged (Seals et al., 1984b; Spina et al., 1993a). Results from cross-sectional studies on older male athletes support these findings (Hagberg et al., 1985). In contrast, recent findings in older women (Spina et al., 1993a) indicate that after training, exercise at the same absolute submaximal load is associated with the same rate of oxygen consumption, a lower level of cardiac output due to a lower heart rate and unchanged stroke volume, and a higher a-v O_2D. As mentioned earlier, the mechanism(s) responsible for the lack of increase in stroke volume with endurance training in older women is (are) unknown. In both older men and women, the lower heart rate and plasma catecholamine levels during submaximal exercise following vigorous training are related to the increases in $\dot{V}O_2max$ (Kohrt et al., 1993). This is probably because the same absolute external work load represents a progressively lower relative exercise stress with a greater training-associated increase in maximal exercise capacity. Stated more broadly, for those circulatory adjustments to acute exercise that are primarily influenced by the relative (% maximum) load, the magnitude of the training-evoked change during submaximal exercise will be in direct proportion to the increase in $\dot{V}O_2max$.

Finally, the data concerning the influence of endurance training on the regulation of arterial blood pressure during the same relative submaximal loads and during maximal exercise in older adults are somewhat inconsistent. In older men, the arterial blood pressure responses to incremental exercise have been reported to be either similar (Ehsani et al., 1991; Hagberg et al., 1985; Ogawa et al., 1992; Spina et al., 1993a) or smaller (Martin et al., 1991; Saltin, 1986; Seals et al., 1984b) in the endurance trained and untrained states. In older women, similar or only slightly lower arterial blood pressure responses to submaximal and maximal exercise have been reported in endurance trained women compared to untrained controls (Martin et al., 1991; Seals et al., 1994a) or before versus after endurance training (Spina et al., 1993a, 1993b). Preliminary evidence suggests that older women on hormone replacement therapy, however, may demonstrate lower blood pressure levels during exercise compared to controls (Martin et al., 1991; E.T. Stevenson, unpublished observations), although this observation needs to be confirmed with a larger number of subjects.

CARDIOVASCULAR FUNCTION AND HUMAN PERFORMANCE

An important practical issue in this discussion of age-related changes in cardiovascular function is the collective influence of such changes on submaximal exercise capacity. The latter can be defined either as the amount of time that a particular percentage of peak exercise capacity can be sustained or, conversely, the highest percentage of peak exercise capacity that can be sustained for a fixed period of time.

The key physiological determinants of submaximal endurance exercise capacity (performance) have been defined previously (Allen et al., 1985; Conley & Krahenbuhl, 1980; Farrell et al., 1979; Hagberg & Coyle, 1983; Joyner, 1991, 1993). It is generally considered that VO_2max is a primary determinant by establishing the upper limit of the individual's ability for maximal energy production through oxidative pathways. Another important factor is the exercise velocity or level of oxygen consumption at which blood lactate concentration begins to rise exponentially during incremental exercise, the so-called "blood lactate threshold," which is highly correlated with endurance exercise performance (Allen et al., 1985; Farrell et al., 1979; Hagberg & Coyle, 1983; Joyner, 1993). Finally, exercise "economy" (mechanical efficiency) or the oxygen cost of performing endurance exercise at a particular velocity, is thought to determine the exercise velocity that can be performed at the submaximal level of oxygen consumption associated with the lactate threshold (Allen et al., 1985; Conley & Krahenbuhl, 1980; Hagberg & Coyle, 1983; Joyner, 1991; Joyner, 1993).

Age-related changes in submaximal exercise capacity have been assessed primarily by studying the performance of endurance athletes of various ages. Changes in endurance exercise performance with age and alterations in the physiological determinants of performance that explain these changes were reviewed in detail recently (Joyner, 1993) and will only be discussed briefly here. The data compiled by Joyner, results from experimental studies (Fuchi et al., 1989), and recent data collected by our laboratory (Evans et al., 1994) indicate that endurance performance in running events (10 km to marathon) changes little until the mid-to-late 30s and then decreases relatively modestly (~6-9% per decade) up until the mid-to-late 50s; thereafter, the rates of decline become exponential with advancing age (Figure 6-4). This pattern appears to be similar for both non-elite and elite endurance athletes (Joyner, 1993). Moreover, our data (Evans et al., 1994) and those of Joyner (1993) indicate that from ~age 40 on, the rates of decline in performance are greater in women than in men (Figure 6-4). It is unknown if these gender differences are due to sociological factors, biological factors, or a combination of both (Joyner, 1993); undoubtedly, sociocultural factors contribute significantly.

The exact contributions of the physiological determinants described

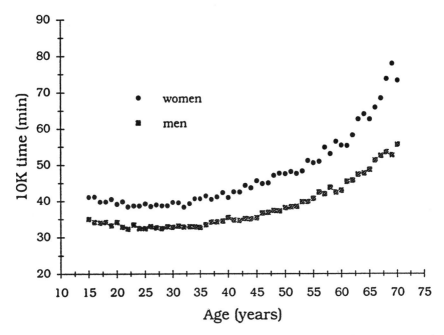

FIGURE 6-4. *Average first place 10 km times for highly trained men and women distance runners, aged 15–73 y, who completed a major U.S. road race, the 1991–1993 Bolder Boulder. After age 35, run time increases (performance decreases) with age in a curvilinear manner in both genders. The rate of increase is 1.3–2.9-fold greater in women compared to men over any particular age range, with the largest differences observed above age 60. From Evans et al., 1994.*

above to the age-related decline in endurance performance are unknown. It is clear that the progressive reduction in $\dot{V}O_2$max, which appears to accelerate above the age of 60 y (Buskirk & Hodgson, 1987) (see Figure 6-1), is a key mechanism underlying the age-associated reduction in performance (Allen et al., 1985; Fuchi et al., 1989; Joyner, 1993). In a study of male endurance athletes aged 30–80 y, the decline in 10 K run times was similar to the 6–7% decrease per decade observed for $\dot{V}O_2$max (Fuchi et al., 1989); a similar relationship was observed in male endurance athletes studied both cross-sectionally and longitudinally by Saltin and colleagues (1986). Age-related reductions in $\dot{V}O_2$max also have been reported in women distance runners (Wells et al., 1992). Findings on highly trained and competitive male runners indicate that declines in endurance performance with age also are closely related to reductions in the running velocity associated with the lactate threshold (Allen et al., 1985); recent data from our laboratory on women distance runners are consistent with this observation (Evans et al., 1995). The minimal available data suggest that decreases in exercise economy do not contribute importantly to the age-related declines in performance (Allen et al., 1985; Evans et al., 1995; Wells et al., 1992).

Joyner (1993) has speculated that constitutional factors including genetic make-up and the ability to sustain an intensive level of physical training are likely to be key influences in the rate of decline in endurance performance with age. The latter is consistent with the results of longitudinal studies of middle-aged athletes indicating that those individuals who are able to maintain training intensity and/or volume over time demonstrate little or no decline in $\dot{V}O_2$max (Hagberg, 1987; Kasch et al., 1990; Marti & Howald, 1990; Pollock et al., 1987; Rogers et al., 1990). There is some evidence that, in general, the absolute levels of training intensity or volume decrease with age in both male and female masters athletes (Pollock et al., 1987; Rogers et al., 1990; Evans et al., 1995) and non-competitive men who continue to exercise throughout middle age (Kasch et al., 1990). An increased prevalence of injuries, as well as reduced levels of motivation, may contribute to these declines in training activity (Joyner, 1993).

Recent findings from longitudinal studies indicate that endurance exercise training also can produce increases in submaximal exercise capacity in previously untrained older adults. Submaximal exercise time at the same absolute intensity was increased by 180%, on average, in men following a endurance exercise program that evoked an average increase in $\dot{V}O_2$max of only ~10% (Poulin et al., 1992). The magnitude of the increase in endurance time in these subjects was related to increases in both $\dot{V}O_2$max and ventilatory threshold. In addition, high-intensity leg cycling training that produced a 38% increase in peak cycling oxygen consumption in men 60–70-y-old also increased their capacity for total work performed in 30 s and attenuated their rate of fatigue (Makrides et al., 1990). Thus, endurance training appears to have the ability to produce marked increases in submaximal exercise capacity in older adults. These increases seem to be greater than that attributable to the associated elevation in $\dot{V}O_2$max, suggesting that other adaptations, such as elevations in the oxidative capacities of the trained muscles (Coggan et al., 1992; Rogers & Evans, 1993), contribute by increasing the lactate threshold.

PULMONARY SYSTEM STRUCTURE AND FUNCTION AT REST

The role of the pulmonary system in gas transport and exercise performance is a critical one—representing the first and last lines of defense in the regulation of the O_2 and CO_2 contents in arterial blood and the blood and tissue acid-base status. In turn, this gas exchange function at rest and especially during exercise is dependent upon the precise integration of several functions and structures, including: 1) mechanical characteristics of lung parenchyma, airways, and chest wall; 2) the strength and endurance of the respiratory musculature; 3) the neurochemical regulation of respiratory motor output and alveolar ventilation; and 4) the regulation of alveolar to arterial O_2 transport by diffusion and by the ventilation: perfusion ($\dot{V}_A$:Q) distribution. Normal healthy aging exerts significant and highly variable effects primarily on the first of these functions, i.e., lung and chest wall mechanics. Limited evidence suggests a significant but less consistent effect of aging on alveolar to arterial gas exchange, an even smaller effect on respiratory muscle function, and no substantial effect on the control system *per se*. We will now briefly outline the structural changes in the lung, chest wall, and pulmonary vasculature that underlie the age-related determinants of pulmonary function and gas transport.

Pulmonary System Structure

The major age-related changes in pulmonary system structure are a reduced elastic recoil of the lung and a stiffening of the chest wall. The lung connective tissue consists of elastin, collagen, and proteoglycans, cross-linked in a unique fashion to provide the lung with most of its elastic recoil. Unfortunately, it has been very difficult to specify precisely what structural changes occur in the aging lung because total elastin and collagen in the lung parenchyma and the length and diameter of elastic fibers remain unaltered with aging (Thurlbeck, 1991). Alveolar surface forces produced primarily by lung surfactant are another major source of the lung's elastic recoil, but there is no evidence that those forces change with the normal aging process. Thus, by exclusion, or perhaps because of unavailability of more definitive measurements, it is generally proposed that elastic recoil of the lung is reduced because of changes in the spatial arrangement of cross-linking of the elastin and collagen fibers.

Alveolar-capillary surface area of the lung declines with age from about 70 m^2 at age 20 y to 60 m^2 at age 70–80 y, and the total proportion of the lung formed by lung parenchyma declines about 30% over the same period. Not surprisingly, the major source of lung capillarization and the alveolar surface area are the alveolar septa; with aging these decline in number, and the air space diameter increases (Brody & Thurlbeck, 1985). Calcification and a reduced compliance of the pulmonary arteries also occur fairly consistently with aging (Reeves et al., 1989). The stiffening of the chest wall occurs as consistently with the aging process as does the increasing compliance of the lung. In fact, the chest wall changes probably dominate, so the compliance of the total respiratory system may fall slightly with age. The rigidity of the rib cage increases with age, perhaps in response to other changes associated with age, including: costal cartilage calcification, changes in rib to vertebral articulations, a narrowing of intervertebral discs, and a change in the shape of the chest as antero-posterior diameter increases (Brody & Thurlbeck, 1985; Crapo, 1993).

Age-associated alterations in the respiratory muscle structure have received some limited attention in animal studies. As with locomotor muscles (Kallman et al., 1990), the aging diaphragm also has a tendency to reduce its muscle mass through a reduction in the diameter of Type II fibers (Gosselin et al., 1994), but these changes are highly variable and have not been determined in humans.

Translation of Structural Changes to Age-related Pulmonary Function at Rest

The major and most consistent age-associated change in lung function is an increased limitation to expiratory flow, as shown by the concave "scooping" effect in the maximum flow:volume loop, especially at lower lung volumes (Figure 6-5). Flow limitation occurs in the intrathoracic airway during forced expiration when positive pressure outside the airway exceeds that inside, thereby causing airway narrowing or closure. Because the lung's elastic recoil pressure is a major contributor to intra-airway pressure, the loss of this recoil pressure with aging explains the increased

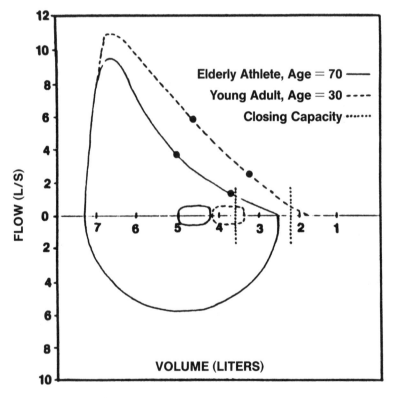

FIGURE 6-5. *Effects of healthy aging on the maximum flow:volume loop and on lung volumes.* Note the increased "scooping," i.e., flow limitation, for the expiratory flow:volume loop in the average 70-y-old, the increased functional residual capacity (FRC), and the increased closing capacity of the lung, i.e., the lung volume at which airways begin to close (adapted from Johnson & Dempsey, 1991).

tendency for airway closure at higher lung volumes than is experienced in the young. This age-dependent effect is also reflected in the more routinely measured decline in the forced expiratory volume in one second ($FEV_{1.0}$). The forced vital capacity declines in a parallel fashion with expiratory flow limitation, in part due to the increased stiffness of the chest wall and in part due to increased airway closure at lower lung volume during forced expiration. Both of these spirometric measures show an increase through the early 20s, a plateau during the mid-late 20s and often into the early 30s, and then a gradual decline thereafter (Burrows et al., 1983).

The age-dependent susceptibility to small airway closure also increases airway resistance at low lung volumes, thereby causing residual lung volume to increase with aging, whereas in the young, residual lung volume is primarily determined by the balance struck between expiratory muscle power and elastic recoil of the chest wall. Also shown in Figure 6-5 is the older individual's higher "closing capacity" of the lung, or that lung volume at which small airways close at the level of the terminal bronchioles. By the sixth decade this closing capacity volume reaches the level of the normal functional residual capacity (FRC), which may cause maldistribution of inspired ventilation and impaired gas exchange. These age-dependent reductions in expiratory flow and vital capacity, as well as increases in residual lung volume and closing volume, have significant implications for the response to exercise in terms of breathing pattern, respiratory muscle function, and gas exchange, as we shall see in the next section.

Estimations of respiratory muscle maximum force in humans use the test of maximum inspiratory pressure (MIP) at a fixed lung volume, usually residual volume. The use of this index to estimate an aging effect is fraught with problems, including the dependence of the test on volitional effort and "motor learning," the critical dependence on inspiratory muscle length (as reflected in changes in lung volume), and the fact that the measures are only static ones and do not consider important changes in velocity of muscle shortening, the latter being a key factor in respiratory muscle function during exercise hyperpnea. Understandably, results from MIP tests in the literature are highly variable across a wide age range (Black & Hyatt, 1969; McElvany et al., 1989). A recent large population study in the healthy elderly claims a systematic 15% reduction in MIP and, therefore, in inspiratory muscle strength from the sixth to the eighth decade (Enright et al., 1994). While these indices are a useful guide for clinical assessment of the capability for maximum inspiratory and expiratory muscle effort, they are not sufficiently well controlled to offer a specific evaluation of the changes in respiratory muscle strength that are associated with aging. For example, most of the observed reductions in MIP with age might be attributed to the coincident age-dependent rise in residual lung volume and, therefore, reduction in inspiratory muscle length. Recent estimates of dynamic pressure development by the inspiratory muscles across a broad range of lung volumes (muscle lengths) and flow rates (velocity of shortening) showed only negligible differences among small groups of healthy subjects aged 30 y and 70 y (Johnson & Dempsey, 1991; Johnson et al., 1991b).

Diffusion capacity of the lung, as determined by routine clinical tests of carbon monoxide diffusion ($D_L CO$), falls with age in proportion to the reduction in internal surface area of the lung (Georges et al., 1978; Murray, 1986). A reduction in pulmonary capillary blood volume is especially obvious after age 60. Limited evidence also suggests a variable yet significant increase in the nonuniformity of $\dot{V}_A$:Q distribution with healthy aging. Resting PaO_2 falls an average of 5–10 mm Hg from age 25 y to 75 y due to a doubling of the A-a DO_2. Thankfully, these "imperfections" in the aging lung are relatively small and are of negligible consequence to resting arterial oxyhemoglobin (HbO_2) saturation or O_2 content at any age.

Pulmonary arterial pressure and pulmonary vascular resistance tend to show small age-related increases at rest, reflecting the reduced compliance of the pulmonary arteries. These measurements require invasive right heart catheterization; therefore, the data to date are understandably limited (Davidson & Fee, 1990; Ehrsam et al., 1983).

There are several sources of uncertainty and marked inter-individual variability in these estimates of aging effects on pulmonary function. Almost all of these estimates are derived from cross-sectional studies with the implicit assumption that the age-associated effects are the same *as if* the *same* people are studied at different ages. Of course, this assumption is frequently violated, primarily because of the so-called "cohort effect" of selective mortality, whereby the fitter subjects (presumably with the least aging effects on organ system function) survive longer, thereby underestimating the actual aging effect. Longitudinal data are just beginning to accumulate in large multicenter studies.

The data of Ware and colleagues (1990) comparing cross-sectional with longitudinal data suggest that the annual rate of loss of pulmonary function in a longitudinal analysis is much greater than in the cross-sectional data. For example, at age 45 versus age 25, the average annual rate of decline in $FEV_{1.0}$ increased by 60% in the cross-sectional data and by 350% in the longitudinal data. The longitudinal data showed two "critical" decades, the 50s and the mid-to-late 60s, where $FEV_{1.0}$ fell disproportionately when compared to earlier decades. Women showed similar age-dependent trends; however, their rate of decline in any decade was consistently 15–30% less than in men. Furthermore, aging effects on pulmonary function are confounded to a very large extent by smoking history, which varies not only with magnitude and duration, i.e., pack-years, but also has substantial inter-individual variability in its long-term effect.

Finally, we note that normal lung function values are now known to differ significantly in minority populations in the United States. For example, at all ages African-American subjects exhibit values for most lung volume subdivisions and for flow rates that are significantly lower by an average of 7–12% than those manifested in Caucasians (American Thoracic Society, 1991). These differences persist after adjustments for age, stature, smoking, and other factors.

PULMONARY SYSTEM REGULATION DURING ACUTE EXERCISE

Key Responses/Mechanisms in the Young, Untrained Adult

The airways, lung, and muscular chest wall are truly "over-built" with respect to the functional demands for ventilation and gas exchange imposed by exercise in the young, untrained, healthy adult ($\dot{V}O_2$max ~35–55 mL·kg^{-1}·min^{-1}). In addition, the *regulation* of the pulmonary system *within* its broad structural limits is also near optimal in terms of mechanical efficiency. The key responses to acute exercise in young adults has been reviewed in detail (Dempsey & Johnson, 1992; Dempsey et al., 1985; Younes, 1989, 1991), and the important responses are summarized below.

1. Alveolar ventilation increases in near-exact proportion to increasing CO_2 production with increasing work rate, so that **alveolar PO_2 and PCO_2 are maintained near normal.** This precise regulation occurs because of a multifaceted neurochemical control system that combines at least two high-gain "primary" inputs to the medullary respiratory controller, one descending from the higher central nervous system (CNS) and another ascending from working skeletal muscle, together with precise chemoreceptor "error detectors" from the periphery.

2. **During heavy exercise** ($> 65\%$ $\dot{V}O_2$max) **alveolar ventilation increases out of proportion to CO_2 production;** therefore, alveolar and arterial PCO_2 fall, whereas alveolar PO_2 rises. This hyperventilatory response is important to partially compensate for metabolic acidosis and to prevent arterial hypoxemia. The range of the hyperventilatory response varies widely among normal subjects of both similar and widely different fitness levels.

3. **Ventilation is increased both by increased breathing frequency and increased tidal volume (VT_T),** with V_T increasing primarily at the lower work rates and frequency increasing at the higher work rates. V_T is **increased by "encroaching" on both inspiratory and expiratory reserve lung volumes.** Thus, end-expiratory lung volume (EELV) falls with increasing exercise. This is beneficial because it permits tidal volume to be limited to the linear, most compliant portion of the pressure:volume rela-

tionship of the lung and thorax; furthermore, increased intra-abdominal pressure lengthens the diaphragm, placing it on a more advantageous position on its length-tension relationship.

4. **Limits of the maximum expiratory flow:volume loop are not reached** even at maximum exercise ($\dot{V}_E$max ~110–125 L/min) because a) structural capacity of the airways exceeds the demand for flow rate, and b) airway resistance is minimized and elastic recoil pressure is high, so that intraluminal pressure stays high. Therefore, transmural pressure across the airway stays positive throughout expiration, i.e., dynamic compression of the airways does not occur during exercise hyperpnea.

5. The dynamic capacity for pressure generation by the inspiratory muscles (P_{CAP_i}) falls during exercise because velocity of shortening and end-inspiratory lung volume increases. Nevertheless, only **50–60% of the maximum available dynamic capacity for pressure generation is reached by the inspiratory muscles at the** $\dot{V}_E$ reached during maximum exercise in the untrained. This is true because of a) the relatively high capacity for power generation by the inspiratory muscles, b) the recruitment of many so-called accessory inspiratory and expiratory muscles to share the work load during exercise, and c) the regulation of near optimal length of the inspiratory muscles throughout exercise (Henke et al., 1988).

6. The **oxygen cost of breathing** increases out of proportion to the increased ventilation during strenuous exercise but still requires only 8–11% of the total body $\dot{V}O_2$max at maximum exercise (Aaron et al., 1992a, 1992b). Finally, **fatigue of the diaphragm** does **not** occur in short-term maximal exercise but does occur frequently in healthy subjects of all fitness levels during prolonged strenuous endurance exercise (Johnson et al., 1993).

7. **Afferent and efferent neural pathways** controlling the breathing pattern and the pattern of inspiratory and expiratory muscle recruitment are probably regulated by feedback from mechanoreceptors in the lung (pulmonary stretch receptors), chest wall, and diaphragm. These pathways and sensory inputs may also be responsible for the cortical perception of respiratory muscle effort. Little is known concerning the sensitivity of these mechanoreceptor feedback mechanisms in the human, nor do we understand at all the role played by the feed-forward "learned" response in this optimization of breathing mechanics.

8. The **structures of the terminal gas exchange unit and the pulmonary vasculature** are ideal to accept all of the increase in cardiac output during exercise and to ensure adequate gas exchange across the lung (i.e., a constant PaO_2 and only a 2–3-fold widening of the A-a DO_2), despite the reduced mixed-venous O_2 content and reduced time for oxygen equilibrium in the pulmonary capillaries. Key features of these structures include: a) an easily distensible, low-resistance, high-compliance vasculature, which allows pulmonary capillary blood volume to increase 3–4-fold to its

morphometric maximum during maximal exercise; b) a thin but strong blood-gas barrier; and c) a lymphatic "storm sewer" with substantial capacity for drainage of the interstitial fluid space.

9. **Pulmonary vascular resistance** falls during exercise as pulmonary arterial pressure (P_{pa}) increases slightly more than twofold. The turnover of plasma water into the interstitial fluid space increases during exercise as the surface area for gas exchange increases; however, no accumulation of extravascular water occurs in the lung.

10. **The increased alveolar-to-arterial PO_2 difference in exercise** results from: a) an imperfect $\dot{V}_A/Q$ distribution and a slight increase in this nonuniformity during exercise in the face of a reduction in mixed-venous O_2 content ($C\bar{v}O_2$), and b) a very small (~1% of total cardiac output) venous admixture from anatomical shunt in the face of a reduced $C\bar{v}O_2$ with exercise. At normal $\dot{V}O_2$max it is unlikely that alveolar-capillary diffusion limitation contributes significantly to the widening of the alveolar-arterial PO_2 difference.

A surprising characteristic of these responses and mechanisms is how uniform they are among young, healthy adults, especially in the age range of adolescence through 35–45 y of age. This uniformity in response has been widely used for diagnostic purposes in assessing normalcy and disability, especially with regard to the constancy of arterial blood gases at resting levels during even heavy exercise, the absence of dyspneic sensations, and the use of only about one-half or less of the ventilatory "capacity" during maximal exercise. It is only at higher altitudes that significant alterations in these "standard" responses to exercise in health occur. We now make the point that it is also very important that the normal aging factor in lung and chest wall structure and function receive attention in evaluating the "normalcy" of the response of the pulmonary system to exercise.

Aging Effects on Pulmonary System's Acute Response to Exercise

The structural and functional changes in the aging lung are manifested most clearly in response to the increased metabolic requirements of exercise. We will now briefly examine this response with specific reference to a group of 30 healthy, active subjects whose mean age was 69 (range = 61–79) and who had greater than average but variable fitness levels ($\dot{V}O_2$max = 44 ± 2 mL·kg^{-1}·min^{-1}, range = 25–62 mL·kg^{-1}·min^{-1}; i.e., 199 ± 9% (range 116%–300%) of age-predicted normal values for $\dot{V}O_2$max (Johnson et al., 1991a, 1991b). These subjects are emphasized here because of the comprehensive analysis of their pulmonary response to exercise; however, several other sources of data are also cited. The following are important age-related changes in the pulmonary response to exercise that may be compared with the list of key mechanisms underlying the exercise response in younger adults.

1. **Expiratory flow limitation occurs at lower exercise intensities with aging.** Given the reduced size of the maximum expiratory flow:volume loop envelope with aging, it is likely that the older, healthy individual will experience significant flow limitation during exercise. That this does indeed occur is shown in Figure 6-6A, which contrasts young (30 y) versus healthy old subjects (69 y) across a wide range of steady-state work rates. Younger subjects of normal fitness show expiratory flow limitation that was less than 10–15% of their tidal volumes (V_T) up to 100 L of minute ventilation ($\dot{V}_E$) and may approach 20% of V_T at $\dot{V}O_2$max, with $\dot{V}_E$ ~120 L/min. On the other hand, older subjects, whose mean expiratory flow rate for 50 s (MEF_{50}) is reduced to 60–70% of that for 30-year-olds, begins to experience significant expiratory flow limitation even during moderate exercise, i.e., at $\dot{V}_E$ ~50 L/min. This limitation increases progressively up to $\dot{V}_E$max to the extent that 25–35% of the V_T will be flow limited at a $\dot{V}_E$max of 70–80 L/min in the normally fit 70-year-old (who has a $\dot{V}O_2$max of 25–30 mL·kg^{-1}·min^{-1}), and greater than 50% of V_T may be flow limited at a $\dot{V}_E$ of 110–120 L/min in the highly fit (whose $\dot{V}O_2$max is 40–45 mL·kg^{-1}·min^{-1}). Also shown are flow:volume loops reached in the highly fit younger persons. Many of them do reach flow limitations comparable to those in some older subjects, but this occurs at ventilatory

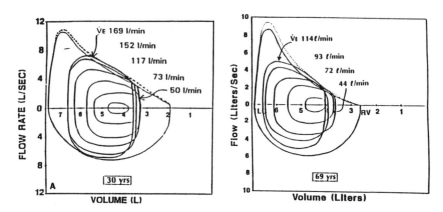

FIGURE 6-6A. *Maximum flow:volume and tidal flow:volume loops generated during exercise in the healthy 30-y-olds versus 69-y-olds.* The tidal flow volume loops for the young adults are shown for a wide range of exercise intensities and over a range of values for $\dot{V}O_2$max of 40–80 mL·kg^{-1}·min^{-1}. Note that expiratory flow limitation in the young only begins to occur at $\dot{V}_E$ ~110–120 L/min and increases in severity at higher ventilations, reaching complete flow limitation at ventilations in excess of 160–180 L/min. In older, healthy subjects significant expiratory flow limitation begins even in moderate exercise at much lower $\dot{V}_E$ than in the young and increases in severity with increasing exercise intensity and ventilatory requirement. Note the increasing end-expiratory lung volume back to and sometimes in excess of resting levels in both age groups commensurate with increasing expiratory flow limitation at high exercise intensities. RV = *residual volume;* TLC = *total lung capacity (Adapted from Johnson et al., 1991a, 1991c).*

outputs substantially higher than those in the older subjects. (The "fitness effect" will be addressed separately in the final section.)

2. **The normal decrease in end-expiratory lung volume (EELV) during exercise is modified substantially in the aged.** Young and old alike show expiratory muscle recruitment and a decrease in end-expiratory lung volume (EELV) at the onset of even mild exercise. As exercise intensity increases beyond the onset of expiratory flow limitation, the older subject tends to show a gradual increase in EELV back toward and even on occa-

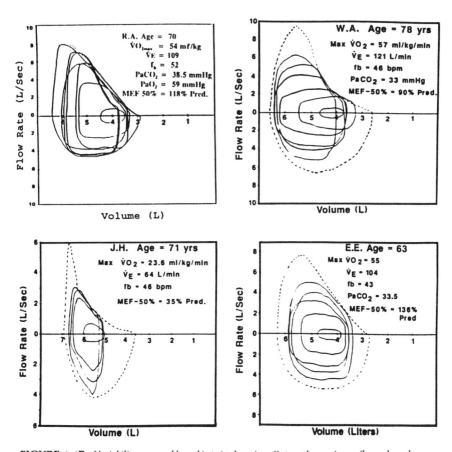

FIGURE 6-6B. *Variability among older subjects in the aging effect on the maximum flow:volume loop; extreme aging effects are exhibited by subject J.H., whereas small effects are shown for subjects E.E. and R.A., with the average age-dependent limitation of maximum flow shown in subject W.A.* Based on the principle of capacity versus demand, note that subjects W.A., R.A., and J.H. reach comparable levels of flow limitation during near-maximal exercise but that subject J.H. achieves this limitation at a much lower ventilatory demand. Subject R.A. was extremely fit. He reached complete limitation to his exercise ventilation during strenuous and maximal exercise and experienced arterial hypoxemia and no hyperventilation. fb = *frequency of breathing; MEF = maximal expiratory flow; Pred. = predicted.*

sion above resting levels. This relative hyperinflation is, of course, necessary in order to find "room" in the flow:volume loop, so that ventilation can increase further with increasing work rate. On the other hand, the absence of a progressive reduction in EELV in older subjects has implications for compromising inspiratory muscle function and for increasing ventilatory work (see below).

3. **Expiratory flow limitation varies greatly among healthy, older individuals.** As with most other aging effects, loss of lung elastic recoil varies greatly among individuals, and this in turn greatly influences the degree of flow limitation incurred during exercise. We provide three examples of healthy, active subjects in Figure 6-6B. Subject W.A. is an extremely fit 78-y-old endurance athlete who shows an average age-related reduction in MEF_{50}. He experiences highly significant flow limitation at a moderate work load, which increases progressively with increasing hyperpnea, and EELV rises to greater than resting values. Contrast this average change due to aging with the two extremes of very little aging effect on flow limitation in a 63-y-old subject (E.E.) and a marked flow limitation seen in a 71-y-old subject (J.H.). Note that subjects W.A. and J.H. reached similar levels of (severe) flow limitation at maximal exercise, but W.A. did so at a greater exercise intensity and minute ventilation.

4. **A greater dead space ventilation with aging requires an increased overall ventilatory response to exercise to maintain normal $\dot{V}_A$ and $PaCO_2$.** Figure 6-7 shows that the dead space volume (V_D) in the healthy aged is about 40–45% of each breath at rest and is consistently greater than the 30–35% V_D:V_T ratios in younger adults. The V_D/V_T ratio falls about equally during exercise in both young and old; therefore, the age difference remains about the same during exercise. The older subjects increase their $\dot{V}_E$ at any given $\dot{V}O_2$ (or $\dot{V}CO_2$) to an extent that elicits the same amount of $\dot{V}_A$ (as in the younger subject) and, thus, alveolar PO_2 and PCO_2 are regulated equally in young and old (see Figure 6-9A). Breathing patterns are also commonly different during exercise, as a healthy aged subject usually shows a higher breathing frequency and a reduced V_T at a given $\dot{V}_E$. This variable reduction in V_T with aging usually occurs in parallel with the reduction in vital capacity. Thus, the aged and the young alike increase V_T during exercise to about 50–60% of vital capacity. The relatively tachypneic breathing pattern in the aged, along with their maldistribution of inspired ventilation, contribute to the increased V_D/V_T.

5. **The aged experience increased work of breathing during exercise.** As shown in Figure 6-8A, the total mechanical work of breathing ($\dot{V}_W$) is increased significantly in the healthy elderly, especially at the moderate work loads. There are two reasons for this. First, the higher overall ventilatory response requires increased pleural pressure development and,

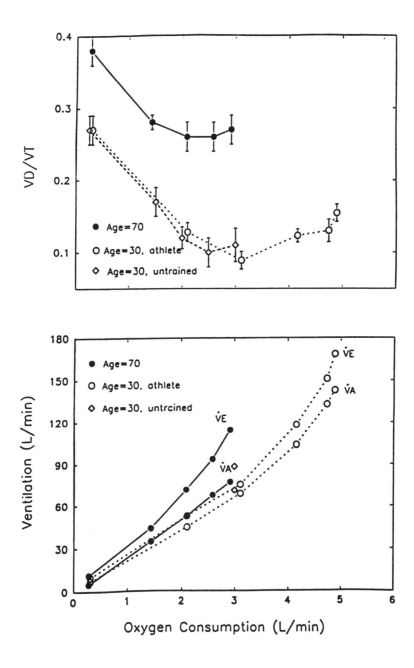

FIGURE 6-7. *Ventilatory responses to exercise in the average healthy 70-y-old (●), untrained 30-y-old (◇)* *and highly trained 30-y-old (○).* Note the higher ratios of dead space to tidal volume in the elderly, their higher overall ventilatory responses ($\dot{V}_E$) to a given exercise intensity, but their comparable levels of alveolar ventilation ($\dot{V}_A$).

therefore, increased ventilatory work. Secondly, factors related to expiratory flow limitation also contribute. First, the higher EELV with increasing exercise displaces a portion of the tidal volume to the upper alinear portion of the pressure:volume relationship, thereby placing a high elastic load on the respiratory muscles; this load must be met by increased pressure development by the inspiratory muscles. This displacement to the upper, stiffer portion of the pressure:volume relationship is reflected in a 30% reduction in dynamic compliance at maximal exercise. Secondly, an increased flow resistance during expiration also requires an increased pressure development by expiratory muscles and increased ventilatory work. Finally, the increased "measured" ventilatory work (V_W) causes increased respiratory muscle $\dot{V}O_2$ ($\dot{V}O_2RM$), but there may also be additional sources of even further increased $\dot{V}O_2RM$. A source of unaccounted-for V_W and $\dot{V}O_2RM$ may be chest-wall distortion accompanying the age-associated limitation in flow and reduction in chest-wall compliance. Shorter inspiratory muscle lengths (at higher EELV) have also been shown to contribute to increased $\dot{V}O_2RM$. The results of these mechanical changes suggest

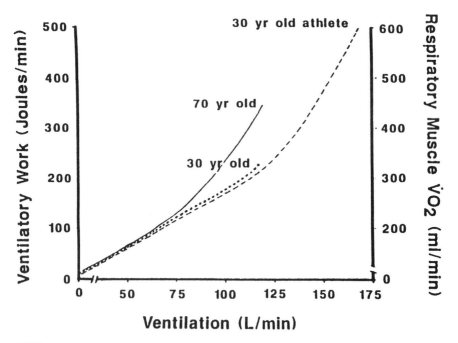

FIGURE 6-8A. *Oxygen cost and work of breathing at various levels of exercise ventilation in the healthy older subject (solid line), in the young trained subject (dashed line), and in the young untrained subject (dotted line).* Note the higher level of ventilatory work and oxygen cost of breathing in the older subject at any given $\dot{V}_E$. The oxygen cost of breathing as a percent of $\dot{V}O_2max$ is 8–10% in the young untrained subject, 13–16% in the young trained subject, and 13–20% in the old trained subject. (Adapted from Johnson & Dempsey, 1991).

that $\dot{V}O_2RM$ at maximal exercise may exceed 10–12% of the total-body $\dot{V}O_2$max in the untrained 70-y-old (at a $\dot{V}_E$ of 75–80 L/min) and may exceed 15% of the total $\dot{V}O_2$max in the highly trained 70-y-old (at a $\dot{V}_E$ of 110 L/min). This $\dot{V}O_2RM$ would be comparable to that measured in the

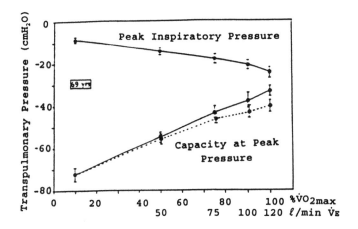

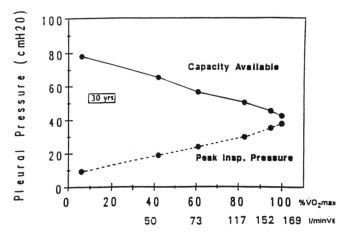

FIGURE 6-8B. *The dynamic capacity for the generation of pleural pressure by the inspiratory muscles (P_{CAP_i}) during exercise at increasing intensities is plotted along with the pressure actually generated during tidal breathing in young adults (30 y) of varying fitness levels and in older highly fit subjects (69 y). Note in both groups at maximal exercise that P_{CAP_i} has decreased (because of increased velocity of shortening and increased end-inspiratory lung volume and, therefore, decreased length of inspiratory muscles) and the pressure generated during tidal breathing has progressively increased. In the young untrained subjects, average inspiratory pressure generated was < 50% of P_{CAP_i} at the normal $\dot{V}O_2$max (43 mL·kg^{-1}·min^{-1}) and maximal $\dot{V}_E$ (~110 L/min) but rose to exceed 85% of P_{CAP_i} in the highly trained at $\dot{V}_E$ > 160 L/min and $\dot{V}O_2$max > 70 mL·kg^{-1}·min^{-1}. The older, fit subjects exceed 80% of P_{CAP_i} at $\dot{V}O_2$max and at maximal $\dot{V}_E$ of only 110 L/min because with exercise they increase ventilatory work much more than do the young, and they decrease P_{CAP_i} more. Adapted from Johnson et al. (1991b, 1991c).*

highly trained athlete at a maximal $\dot{V}_E$ of 170 L/min (Aaron et al., 1992a, 1992b).

6. **The pleural pressure generated by the inspiratory muscles during exercise will be a greater percent of the available (dynamic) capacity for generation of pleural pressure** (P_{CAP_i}) (see Figure 6-8B). Thus, while the younger, untrained subject rarely exceeds 50% of his P_{CAP_i} even at maximal exercise ($\dot{V}_E$ ~110 L/min), the older subject consistently exceeds 50% of inspiratory muscle capacity even at moderate exercise intensities ($\dot{V}_E$ ~70–80 L/min) and exceeds 75% of inspiratory capacity in the fitter, older subject during strenuous to maximal exercise, i.e., when $\dot{V}_E$ is greater than 100 L/min (Johnson et al., 1991b). In many of these subjects, V_E at maximal exercise reaches truly maximal levels, as demonstrated by the failure of added CO_2 to further increase V_E in many of the more highly fit.

7. **Alveolar to arterial gas exchange and pulmonary-vascular hemodynamics probably are only slightly modified by aging.** O_2 and CO_2 exchange during exercise at all intensities undergoes only small modifications with aging; therefore, with a few notable exceptions, arterial blood gas homeostasis stays remarkably constant at all intensities of exercise, even in the most highly fit elderly subjects. These data are summarized in mean and individual subject values in Figure 6-9A and 6-9B. At rest in the healthy older subjects, mean PaO_2 was about 5 mmHg less than in 30-y-olds due to a 5 mmHg widening of A-a DO_2. The A-a DO_2 began to widen beyond 50% $\dot{V}O_2$max to eventually exceed during maximal exercise about 2.5–3 times the values at rest, and as P_AO_2 rose steadily, PaO_2 fell less than 5 mmHg below resting values. Mean $PaCO_2$ also remained normocapnic up to 60–75% $\dot{V}O_2$max and then showed a normal compensatory hyperventilation to 30–35 $PaCO_2$ during strenuous and maximal exercise. We emphasize that there were some exceptions among the subjects studied. PaO_2 was reduced to less than 75 mmHg (87–92% SaO_2) in 4 of 30 subjects and was reduced by about 15 mmHg ($<$ rest) to the 75–78 mmHg range in three others. It is also important to note that younger, healthy subjects (Figure 6-9B) clearly do not show any arterial hypoxemia when $\dot{V}O_2$max is in the range of 35–55 mL·kg^{-1}·min^{-1}; i.e., this occurs only in (some) highly trained younger subjects who have values for $\dot{V}O_2$max greater than 65 mL·kg^{-1}·min^{-1}.

Some recently published studies on arterial blood gases during exercise in older subjects (65–68 y) used healthy trained and untrained subjects, both groups with resting pulmonary function within 20% of the normal age-predicted values (Préfaut et al., 1994). These subjects showed a much more heterogenous response, apparently related to the level of fitness. The untrained older subjects (27.9 ± 1.5 mL·kg^{-1}·min^{-1}) showed—like most of our subjects—a constant PaO_2, a fairly well-regulated $PaCO_2$ (but again no clear hyperventilatory response to maximal exercise), and a

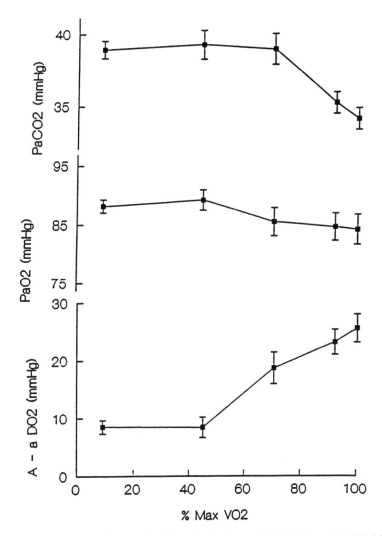

FIGURE 6-9A. *Mean arterial PO_2 and PCO_2 and the alveolar-arterial PO_2 difference (A-a DO2) during incremental progressive exercise in 19 healthy, fit 69-y-olds ($\dot{V}O_2max = 43 \pm 2\ mL\cdot kg^{-1}\cdot min^{-1}$).*

2-3-fold increase in the A-a DO_2 up to maximal exercise; however, all "fit" older subjects showed a progressive decline in PaO_2 throughout exercise to a mean of 70 mmHg, i.e., 25 mmHg less than at rest, at $\dot{V}O_2max$ ($37.8 \pm 2\ mL\cdot kg^{-1}\cdot min^{-1}$). This arterial hypoxemia was due to a combination of a progressive CO_2 retention and the absence of a hyperventilatory response, even at maximal exercise, plus a 3–4-fold increase in A-a DO_2 at maximal exercise. These findings suggest that CO_2 retention and a progressive arterial hypoxemia are readily induced during even mild to moderate exercise with aging, but only in the highly fit older subject. This

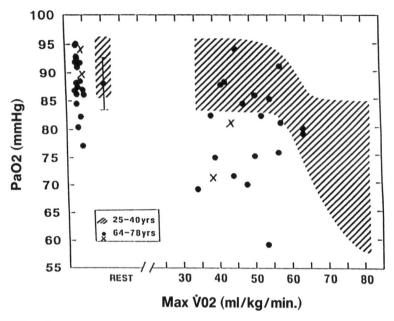

FIGURE 6-9B. *Range of arterial PO_2 during maximal exercise among individual subjects.* The shaded area represents the range of values in young adult subjects of varying $\dot{V}O_2$max. Note the constancy of arterial PO_2 in the young at intense exercise up to a $\dot{V}O_2$max of 60–65 $mL{\cdot}kg^{-1}{\cdot}min^{-1}$, after which the results are highly variable; more than one-third of the young show a significant reduction in arterial PO_2 at maximal exercise. Most of the older, fit subjects (•) show preservation of arterial PO_2 within 10 mm Hg of resting levels, with exceptions in 5 of the subjects who reduced their PaO_2 values to < 75 mm Hg. The mean data of Préfaut et al. (1994) and of Anselme et al. (1994) for their highly-fit master athletes are indicated by **X**.

contrasts markedly with our own study of older subjects who had a wide range of fitness levels ($\dot{V}O_2$max = 26–59 $mL{\cdot}kg^{-1}{\cdot}min^{-1}$) and in whom exercise-induced arterial hypoxemia was very rare, and only occurred in very heavy exercise (Figure 6-9B). Furthermore, $PaCO_2$ occasionally increased slightly in moderate to heavy exercise in our subjects, but a compensatory hyperventilation always occurred during very intense or maximal exercise. The studies do differ in the duration of exercise at each of the progressively increasing exercise intensities used in the test protocol; this might explain why all of the subjects (regardless of age or fitness level) in the study of Préfaut et al. (1994) showed significant CO_2 retention during strenuous and maximal exercise. These same authors published a companion study showing only about one-half of this originally reported reduction in mean arterial PO_2 at maximal exercise in older athletes (Anselme et al., 1994). We recently conducted a 6-y follow-up longitudinal study on a subset of 18 of our subjects as they aged from 66 to 73 y (McClaran et al., 1994); the regulation of SaO_2 and the ventilatory response to all exercise intensities **within** these subjects were very similar to corresponding data from our cross-sectional study (Johnson et al., 1991a, 1991c). On the other hand, these differences in findings—within and between studies—may also reflect the marked variability in the aging effect on lung structure and diffusion surface.

8. **Pulmonary hemodynamics during exercise are altered because of the reduction in pulmonary arteriolar compliance with** healthy aging, so that pulmonary artery pressure (P_{pa}) is increased at any given exercise cardiac output or $\dot{V}O_2$ (Figure 6-10) (Reeves et al., 1989). At maximal exercise, P_{pa} is similar in the older and the younger subjects, but this level of P_{pa} in the older subjects is reached at a substantially lower $\dot{V}O_2$max and $\dot{Q}$max. Pulmonary wedge pressure (P_w) during exercise is also increased with aging, to the extent that during supine exercise P_w can exceed 25 mm Hg at peak work loads.

What, if any, are the consequences of these apparently high pulmonary capillary pressures during strenuous exercise? Some recent data suggest that such high pressures at high Q may: 1) lead to "stress" failure of the blood-gas barrier and; therefore, to increased permeability of the capillary endothelium and 2) cause accumulation of extravascular lung water in the interstitial fluid space (Tsukimoto et al., 1991). Extravascular lung water is not quantifiable in intact humans or animals, but there are some indirect indications of its accumulation under these exercise conditions; these indications include a continued maldistribution of $\dot{V}_A$:Q as

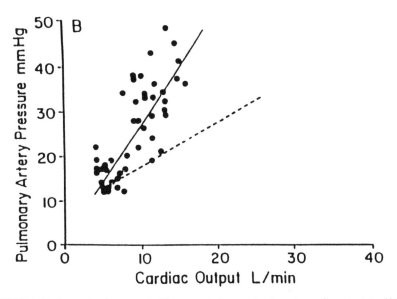

FIGURE 6-10. *Increased pulmonary arterial pressure during exercise at varying cardiac outputs in old (•) versus young subjects (---).* (From Reeves et al., 1989).

measured for a few minutes following heavy exercise in healthy young, fit subjects (Schaffartzik et al., 1992), and increased levels of circulating histamine during heavier exercise in older, fit subjects who develop significant reductions in PaO_2 (Anselme et al., 1994). It was proposed that this increased circulating histamine may be a marker for an inflammatory response to "injury" at the level of the blood-gas barrier (Anselme et al., 1994). On the other hand, in our highly fit subjects we measured lung volume subdivisions, lung closing volume, and diffusion capacity before and within 5 min following maximal exercise of 2–4 min duration and found no consistent change in any of these variables, even in the few subjects who experienced significant arterial hypoxemia at maximal exercise. This evidence bearing on this important issue of fluid accumulation suffers from its reliance on highly indirect, non-specific markers of increased extravascular lung water. However, the available evidence points strongly to the possibility that extremely intense exercise may induce pulmonary edema, which would be a primary explanation for diffusion limitation and perhaps even much of the $\dot{V}_A$:Q maldistribution.

PULMONARY ADAPTATIONS TO CHRONIC EXERCISE

Fitness/Training Effects on the Pulmonary System In The Young Adult

A safe generalization is that, relative to cardiovascular or metabolic links in the oxygen transport chain, the pulmonary system in the young adult undergoes few adaptations to physical training. This generalization is most applicable for the gas exchange function in the lung and to airway mechanics, whereas the respiratory muscles of the chest wall do show some limited adaptability to training.

Sufficient evidence has now accumulated from several animal species and in humans to conclude that physical training is without significant effect on pulmonary gas exchange and that an extraordinary gas exchange capability is not a requisite to superior aerobic performance. This evidence includes the following:

1. Athletic species with both $\dot{V}O_2$max and mitochondrial volume in locomotor muscles 2–3 times that of their nonathletic counterparts of similar body mass (e.g., cow versus horse; dog versus goat) show maximum alveolar-capillary diffusion surface areas that are only 25–50% greater than those of the nonathletic species (Hoppeler et al., 1987).

2. Training effects that are sufficient to increase $\dot{V}O_2$max markedly in young or mature animals (Ross & Thurlbeck, 1992) or in humans at sea level (Reuschlein et al., 1968) or at high altitude (Dempsey et al., 1977) show no significant effects on morphometrically measured diffusion surface or on diffusing capacity of the lung for carbon monoxide (D_LCO).

3. Results from cross-sectional studies of highly trained human athletes are mixed, but the studies of most types of athletes report no significant fitness-related difference in diffusion capacities or A-a DO_2 (at any given $\dot{V}O_2$) (Dempsey et al., 1984, Reuschlein et al., 1968), although some studies of maturing and adult competitive swimmers claim a larger than normal rest and exercise D_LCO (Clanton et al., 1987; Mostyn et al., 1986). These differences seem likely to be due primarily to preselection of these athletes, although some specific effect of long-term swim training is also feasible but as yet unproven in humans.

Mechanical properties of the airways have not been studied in the highly trained animal, and relatively few longitudinal studies of humans are available. In general, lung-volume subdivisions and maximum flow:volume characteristics are no different in the highly trained athlete than in his sedentary counterpart of comparable age, height, and weight (Dempsey et al., 1984; Hagberg et al., 1988b; Reuschlein et al., 1968). Furthermore, even with daily "training" sessions of repeated maximum volitional hyperpneas over many weeks in normal adults (Leith & Bradley, 1976), vital capacity and other lung volume subdivisions remained relatively unchanged. Again, highly trained swimmers may be an exception, as shown by their large TLC, VC, and/or maximum flow:volume loops for a given body size or chest diameter (Armour et al., 1993; Åstrand et al., 1963; Bloomfield et al., 1990; Clanton et al., 1987).

The adaptability of the diaphragm to training has been studied rather extensively in the rat. First, there are some studies (Fregosi & Dempsey, 1986; Metzger & Fitts, 1986) that show no discernible training effects on the diaphragm, despite significant training effects on $\dot{V}O_2max$ and on the aerobic enzymatic capacities of limb locomotor muscles. However, if the training regimen is highly intense and prolonged, a significant training effect on the diaphragm is demonstrable by the increases in succinate dehydrogenase activity, especially in the costal diaphragm (Powers et al., 1992, 1994). In humans there is also evidence of significant effects of chronic running or swimming on respiratory muscle endurance, at least as determined by a prolonged time to "task failure" while breathing at high fixed inspiratory pressures (Clanton et al., 1987; Robinson et al., 1982). The capacity of all inspiratory muscles to generate a high velocity of shortening and maximal (static) pressure across a wide range of muscle lengths was not different in highly trained runners versus untrained, young adults (Johnson et al., 1991c).

Ventilatory function does benefit indirectly from the physical training effects on increasing $\dot{V}O_2max$, namely, the increased aerobic capacity of locomotor muscles and the subsequent reduction in the level of circulating metabolites such as lactate, H+, K+, and norepinephrine. These circulating humoral factors have been implicated as key mediators of the normal hyperventilatory response to heavy exercise. Accordingly, with training of locomotor skeletal muscles, these humoral stimuli are reduced such that for any given intensity of strenuous exercise, $\dot{V}_E$ is considerably reduced and $PaCO_2$ is higher (Casaburi et al., 1987).

It is apparent that there is substantial variation among the different structural and functional capacities of the airways, diffusion surface area, and chest wall musculature in the plasticity of their adaptation to chronic physical training. In most cases the training effect on any aspect of pulmonary structure and function is substantially less than that in the cardiovascular system or in the diffusion surface area or metabolic capacities in locomotor skeletal muscles.

Fitness/Training Effects on the Aging Pulmonary System

Attempts to assess the effects of physical training on the pulmonary system of older adults have relied almost exclusively on cross-sectional data comparisons of older subjects of varying fitness levels. In contrast to the negligible difference in lung volume subdivisions and maximal flow rates when comparisons were made of fit versus less fit younger adults, resting pulmonary function in older fit subjects is clearly different from that in their more sedentary contemporaries. In four such studies using fit subjects whose $\dot{V}O_2max$ levels were 1.5-fold to 2-fold greater than those of less fit subjects, the most consistent differences between subjects in resting pulmonary function were in maximum flow rates, either $FEV_{1.0}$ or MEF_{50}, which were about 20–30% greater in the fit (Table 6-1). (Grimby & Saltin, 1966; Hagberg et al., 1988b; Johnson et al., 1991a). MVV was also usually greater in the fit, whereas vital capacity and total lung capacity were more variable (Hagberg et al., 1988b; Johnson et al., 1993). These older, highly fit subjects still showed expiratory flow rates that were lower and lung closing volumes that were significantly higher than those in younger subjects of any fitness level (Table 6-1).

The more highly fit older subjects also showed lower $\dot{V}_E/\dot{V}O_2$ ratios during submaximal exercise, and these reduced $\dot{V}_E$ values also occurred within older subjects as their $\dot{V}O_2max$ values were increased after 1 y of training (Yerg et al., 1985). Thus, because a given absolute intensity of submaximal exercise represents a lower relative intensity in the trained versus untrained, whether young or old, the trained will exhibit a reduced ventilatory response to the exercise coincident with reduced levels of circulating metabolites.

We do not know if physical training *per se* in these subjects reduces the normal aging effect on lung elastic recoil and resting pulmonary function. The absence of a training effect in the young speaks against this idea, but we do not know if training effects might be different in the aging lung, i.e., might show an interactive effect of aging and training. Our longitudinal study did show substantial declines in MEF_{50} and VC and increases in residual lung volume and lung closing capacity, despite a continued daily

TABLE 6-1. *Lung function at rest: influence of age and fitness*

Variable	Very Fit (70 ± y)	Normally Fit (70 ± y)	Normally or Very Fit (30 y)
Total Lung Capacity (L)	6.80	7.18	6.80
Vital Capacity (L)	4.20	4.26	5.05**
Functional Residual Capacity (L)	3.92	4.24*	3.20**
Maximal Expiratory Flow for 50 s (L/s)	3.41	2.75*	5.26**
Functional Expiratory Volume in 1 s (L)	3.25	2.99*	4.08**
Lung Closing Capacity (L)	3.3	3.3	2.10**
$D_L CO$ (mL·min^{-1}·mm Hg^{-1})	29	27	33**

*$P<0.05$ very fit vs normally fit
**$P<0.05$ young vs old
Mean $\dot{V}O_2$max: **old** very fit = 50 mL·kg^{-1}·min^{-1}, **old** normally fit = 35 mL·kg^{-1}·min^{-1}; **young** very fit = 75 mL·kg^{-1}·min^{-1}; **young** normally fit = 43 mL·kg^{-1}·min^{-1}.

training regimen in highly fit subjects; however, other age-related changes, such as pulmonary diffusion ($D_L CO$) and FRC, did not change further (McClaran et al., 1994). These longitudinal changes in lung function in our highly trained, active subjects paralleled those reported from other longitudinal data obtained in larger numbers of the normal population with identical ages (Ware et al., 1990). So continued habitual activity clearly does **not** protect against an aging effect on lung function. We propose that the enhanced pulmonary function in the highly trained and active elderly subjects observed in cross-sectional studies (see above) reflects an effect of preselection whereby those subjects with more age-resistant pulmonary function and structure stay active longer, probably by choice.

PULMONARY FUNCTION AND HUMAN PERFORMANCE

Pulmonary System Limitations in the Young Adult—Trained And Untrained

In most respects the generalization that the healthy lung and chest wall are "overbuilt" with respect to the demands imposed by even the most extreme exercise intensity is certainly correct. However, there are some important exceptions. First, even in a relatively untrained, young adult whose $\dot{V}O_2$max is less than 50 mL·kg^{-1}·min^{-1}, **diaphragmatic fatigue** does occur when very intense exercise (i.e., greater than 85% $\dot{V}O_2$max) is sustained for 10–20 min to exhaustion (Johnson et al., 1993). This has been documented using bilateral, supramaximal electrical stimulation of the phrenic nerve at 1–20 H$_z$ frequencies before and after such exhaustive exercise. Diaphragmatic force (P_{di}) was reduced 20–50% within 6–8 min following exercise and recovered very slowly over about 1 h following exercise. This so-called low-frequency fatigue of the diaphragm is attributable to both the high level of transdiaphragmatic pressure sustained during the exercise and, just as importantly, the secondary effects of high-intensity exercise of the skeletal muscles, such as extracellular fluid acidosis and the competition between respiratory and locomotor muscles for blood flow (Babcock et al., 1993; Fregosi & Dempsey, 1986).

There are some other "hints" of approaching limits to, or at least inefficient pulmonary system responses in, young untrained subjects at maximal exercise. These include minor limitations to expiratory flow, significant reductions in dynamic compliance of the lung as V_T increases to the relatively flat portion of the pressure:volume relationship (Henke et al., 1988), and the increase in non-uniformity of $\dot{V}_A$:Q distribution coincident with a widening A-a DO$_2$.

Pulmonary system limitations in the young become more evident with greater levels of fitness (e.g., increased $\dot{V}O_2$max and $\dot{V}CO_2$max) because these adaptations allow them to exercise at higher absolute intensities. Given the healthy pulmonary system's relative absence of "plasticity" in response to physical training, it follows that the greater the demand imposed by higher exercise intensities in the well-trained, the closer one approaches the capacity of the unadaptable pulmonary system. The following examples are illustrative of the broad continuum of demand versus capacity in the lung and chest walls among healthy subjects of varying fitness levels.

1. Among the highly fit ($\dot{V}O_2$max > 65 mL·kg^{-1}·min^{-1}), many subjects exhibit values for A-a DO$_2$ greater than 30–40 mm Hg and significant arterial hypoxemia (PaO$_2$ ~ 55–75 mmHg and SaO$_2$ ~ 84–92%) (see Figure 6-9B) (Dempsey et al. 1984, 1990; Johnson et al., 1991c). Prevention of this exercise-induced hypoxemia via small increments in FIO$_2$ was shown to raise $\dot{V}O_2$max while subjects were breathing the oxygen-enriched air; this improvement beyond that of the normal $\dot{V}O_2$max was equivalent to about 1% $\dot{V}O_2$max for every 1% reduction in SaO$_2$ below 92% at maximal exercise (Powers et al., 1989).

2. With increasing $\dot{V}O_2$max, significant expiratory flow limitation occurs progressively with increasing rates of max ventilation. Beginning at about 120–130 L/min $\dot{V}_E$, EELV has a tendency to begin returning toward

resting volumes, and the pressure generated by the inspiratory muscles increases beyond ~ 50% of their capacity (see Figure 6-6A). In many of the highly trained, young endurance athletes, maximal ventilatory capacity was achieved at $\dot{V}O_2$max, and the maximal capacity for pressure generation by the inspiratory muscles was achieved (Johnson et al., 1991c) during tidal breathing.

3. The oxygen cost of ventilation (per L $\dot{V}_E$) rises disproportionately to the increasing $\dot{V}_E$ under conditions of increasing expiratory flow limitations in strenuous exercise to the point where 13–16% of the $\dot{V}O_2$max is required for ventilation in the highly trained at $\dot{V}O_2$max (Aaron et al., 1992b).

4. Significant CO_2 retention (i.e., $PaCO_2$ greater than values at rest) does **not** occur under any circumstances in the healthy lung, although the magnitude of the hyperventilatory response may be constrained in some highly fit subjects under conditions of substantial flow limitation during maximal exercise (Dempsey et al., 1984; Johnson et al., 1991c).

5. The diaphragm **does** show significant increases in aerobic capacity in response to intense and prolonged training; however, this adaptation is not completely protective of the muscle because significant diaphragmatic fatigue is apparent in the highly trained following high-intensity endurance exercise (Babcock et al., 1995). Although the trained and untrained alike do show similar amounts of fatigue following endurance exercise at greater than 85% $\dot{V}O_2$max, the trained athlete can sustain exercise at a higher absolute $\dot{V}_E$ with concomitantly greater diaphragmatic activity. Thus, these data suggest that the training effect on the diaphragm probably just about matched the magnitude of the training effect on other links in the oxygen transport chain that permitted the athlete to achieve a higher $\dot{V}O_2$max.

There is clearly a hierarchy of susceptibility to conditions wherein demand exceeds capacity within the pulmonary system of the young adult. The diaphragm does experience significant fatigue—but clearly not task failure—even in the untrained subject during sustained, heavy exercise. Limitations to alveolar-capillary diffusion resulting in significant arterial hypoxemia is experienced only when $\dot{V}O_2$max is at least 50% greater than normal. Even under these extreme conditions, the effect is not universal among all highly trained individuals. Finally, the ventilatory capacity of the airways and the capacity of the inspiratory muscles to generate pressure are also reached under extraordinary conditions of very high metabolic requirements, but it is likely that these capacities are achieved by **all** highly fit people during maximal exercise.

Finally, it is also important to distinguish between **reaching the limitation** of a specific function of the lung and chest wall and having this function assume the role of a **limiting factor** in exercise performance. As noted earlier, significant diffusion limitation does cause reduced systemic

O_2 transport and will clearly lead to reduced $\dot{V}O_2$max (probably because of a compromised maximal difference between arterial and mixed-venous O_2 content). On the other hand, mechanical limitation to flow does not cause hypoventilation or impaired gas exchange either during progressive exercise to exhaustion or during prolonged intense exercise. There is limited and controversial evidence to date as to whether increased flow limitations and respiratory muscle work or diaphragmatic fatigue will lead to ventilatory limitations during prolonged intense exercise (Gallagher & Younes, 1989).

Pulmonary System Limitations with Healthy Aging in the Trained and Untrained

We have observed in the young adult that the role of the pulmonary system as a limiting factor for maximal oxygen consumption and exercise performance increases as the level of fitness increases and that this occurs because the lung is relatively unadaptable as $\dot{V}O_2$max increases with training. With aging, whether limitations to pulmonary function occur or whether, in turn, pulmonary system limitations to $\dot{V}O_2$max ever occur will depend upon how aging affects the **maximal demands** placed on the system via a changing $\dot{V}O_2$max versus how aging affects structure and function of the lung, airways, and chest wall (i.e., **capacity**). As seen in the examples illustrated below, the variability in the healthy aging process presents various combinations of changing **demand** versus **capacity** of the pulmonary system that may make it more or less susceptible to limitations.

Aging and Limitations in the Untrained, Healthy Subject

First, consider the extreme example of the untrained individual whose $\dot{V}O_2$max decreases normally with aging, for example, from 45 mL·kg^{-1}·min^{-1} at age 30 to 25 mL·kg^{-1}·min^{-1} at age 70, and who has experienced no effects of aging on the lung and chest wall. Clearly in this unlikely event, maintaining the structure of the young lung and chest wall will readily accommodate any demand of the aging, compromised oxygen transport system, so that the pulmonary system would never pose a threat to exercise performance limitation in the aged.

A second scenario in the untrained, aging subject would superimpose a normal aging effect on **both** $\dot{V}O_2$max and on the lung and chest wall capacities. Under this very common condition there would be increased flow limitation with increased ventilatory work, beginning even at submaximal exercise loads; however, in this case the maximum ventilatory requirement at the normal 20-y-old's $\dot{V}O_2$max of 25–30 mL·kg^{-1}·min^{-1} is only about 80 L/min and is clearly achievable within the maximum flow limitations of the normal aging lung. Similarly, the probability of exercise-induced arterial hypoxemia would be negligible because the demands for oxygen transport would again not exceed the capacity for alveolar capillary diffusion, even when reduced by age. So, with respect to pulmonary system limitation, this situation would be much like that in the younger, untrained individual, except for the significant expiratory flow limitation experienced during exercise with aging.

Aging and Limitations in the Fit Subject

An extreme example would be one in which $\dot{V}O_2$max remained > 65 mL·kg^{-1}·min^{-1} as it is in the young, highly fit adult, upon which a normal aging effect on the lung is superimposed. In this case, one would undoubtedly see complete flow and ventilatory limitation and highly significant amounts of exercise-induced arterial hypoxemia even in strenuous but submaximal work. As shown in Figure 6-11, this unlikely case demonstrates that one cannot "fit" the ventilatory and gas exchange demands of the highly conditioned, young adult into the normally aging lung and

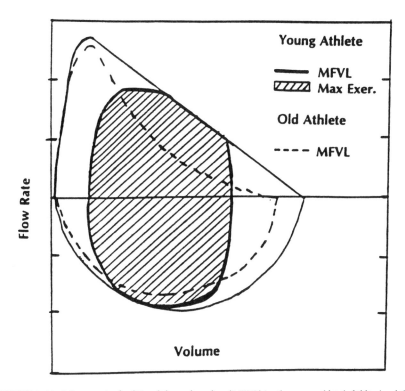

FIGURE 6-11. *Mean maximal volitional flow:volume loop (MFVL) for the young athlete (solid line) and the older athlete (dashed line).* The tidal flow:volume loop during maximal exercise in the young ($\dot{V}O_2$max ~75 mL·kg^{-1}·min^{-1} and maximal $\dot{V}_E$ ~170 L/min) is superimposed on these maximal loops to demonstrate that the airway's capacity for flow and volume in the lung of the 70-y-old athlete ($\dot{V}O_2$max ~43 mL·kg^{-1}·min^{-1} and maximal $\dot{V}_E$ ~115 L/min) is not capable of supporting the ventilatory requirements of the young athlete.

chest wall. While this scenario of an unchanging $\dot{V}O_2$max is very unlikely, there are many highly active, aging subjects in whom $\dot{V}O_2$max does stay relatively high, i.e., not at the level of the young, highly trained, but in the range of 50–60 mL·kg^{-1}·min^{-1}, or two or more times the normal age-related $\dot{V}O_2$max at age 70. The maximal ventilatory response to this maximal metabolic requirement would normally use all of the maximal volitional flow:volume loop, but the ventilatory capacity of the lung and airways of the highly trained, older individual is greater than that of his sedentary, healthy contemporary. Accordingly, a much higher ventilation can be accommodated in the highly fit (versus unfit) 70-y-old before ventilation is truly limited.

Nonetheless, there are some highly-fit, aging subjects whose $\dot{V}O_2$max levels stay sufficiently high and who have experienced sufficiently adverse effects of aging in the lung and airways so that: 1) maximal $\dot{V}_E$ is completely limited at maximal exercise—as demonstrated by the failure of ventilation to increase further when arterial PCO_2 was experimentally increased (via increased $FICO_2$) at maximal exercise (Johnson et al., 1991a, 1991b); and 2) $\dot{V}O_2$max is probably limited (albeit relatively small in most cases) by the widening of the A-a DO_2 and significant arterial hypoxemia, i.e., $SaO_2 < 92\%$ (see Figure 6-9B) in the ~one-fifth of 70-y-olds who are so affected (Powers et al., 1989).

The tendency for limitation in the aging fit pulmonary system at maximal exercise appears to be more likely with flow rate and ventilation than with alveolar to arterial O_2 transport—probably because the normal aging effect is much more prominent on the airways and on lung elastic recoil than on the diffusion surface. An unknown factor with the potential to contribute to exercise limitation is the metabolic and cardiovascular cost of ventilation in highly trained, older subjects working at high ventilatory demand. This might limit exercise performance by having respiratory muscles "stealing" blood flow from locomotor muscles. More assuredly, we would predict, given the much higher pressure development by inspiratory muscles in the older subject during exercise, that diaphragmatic fatigue would be more readily induced during sustained strenuous exercise at less intense work loads than in the younger adult.

It might also be expected that the aging lung would be more susceptible to "failure" in response to the demands of strenuous exercise if additional requirements/limitations are superimposed. For example, exercise-induced hypoxemia would probably be more easily induced at high altitude in the older fit subject—similar to the increased susceptibility of the young, highly trained athlete to experience severe arterial hypoxemia (and limitations of $\dot{V}O_2$max) even at moderate altitudes (Dempsey et al., 1984). Prolonged exercise in the heat causes high breathing frequencies in the young adult; a tachypneic response would add to the already high V_D/V_T in the older subject during similar conditions and may compromise sufficient alveolar ventilation in addition to greatly increasing turbulent flow rate and further increasing airway resistance. Finally, the superimposition of even "mild" chronic airway disease or loss of alveolar surface area on top of already emphysematous-like changes in the normal aging lung would push the older subject to quite severe flow limitation and hypoxemia even in moderately heavy exercise (see Figure 6-6B, Subject J.H.).

DIRECTIONS FOR FUTURE RESEARCH

1. More information is needed regarding the true rate of decline in $\dot{V}O_2$max with aging in men and women, i. e., that due to the direct biological effects of the aging process as opposed to lifestyle and disease factors. The development of new models to isolate the true effects of aging may be needed to effectively pursue this issue.
2. Additional research should investigate the mechanisms underlying the age-related decline in $\dot{V}O_2$max, and the modulatory effects of changes in body composition, disease, and chronic physical activity on these mechanisms. Longitudinal information on the same subjects will be required to answer this question definitively.
3. The mechanisms responsible for the lesser heart rate response and lower stroke volume during submaximal and maximal dynamic exercise with aging need to be identified.
4. The effect of aging on the regulation of blood flow to active skeletal muscle and to the heart during submaximal exercise performed with large muscle groups should be documented. In addition, we need to know if the absolute peak flows to these organs decline with age in proportion to the decline in the peak achievable level of cardiac output.
5. The regulation of blood flow and vascular conductance to areas such as the kidneys and gut during exercise should be studied to ensure that older adults are not subject to excessive vasoconstriction that could result in tissue damage in these regions (Seals, 1993).
6. The possible dissociation of the cardiovascular, metabolic, and thermoregulatory adjustments to prolonged submaximal exercise needs to be investigated to determine if the regulatory signals governing control under these conditions change with age.
7. Because some older adults demonstrate little or no change in $\dot{V}O_2$max levels in response to endurance training, whereas others show marked responsiveness, more insight is needed regarding the factors (e.g., extent of habitual physical activity at baseline, na-

ture of the training stimulus, and genetics) that determine the magnitude of the training-induced increases in $\dot{V}O_2$max levels for individual older adults.

8. The observation that older women do not produce the same left ventricular structural and functional adaptations to endurance exercise training needs to be confirmed; if verified, the mechanisms responsible for this gender specificity should be identified.

9. The interaction among physical training, aging, and hormone replacement therapy on the regulation of arterial blood pressure and other autonomically mediated circulatory adjustments to exercise in postmenopausal women should be characterized.

10. The physiological and nonphysiological reasons underlying the apparent greater rate of decline in endurance exercise performance with advancing age in women versus men need to be identified. Relatedly, the physiological mechanisms responsible for the decline in endurance exercise performance with age in both men and women should be determined.

11. The factors (e.g., nature of the training stimulus) that are important in the improvement of submaximal exercise capacity in older non-athletic adults in response to endurance exercise training need to be determined, along with the exact mechanisms responsible for such improvements.

12. The structural basis for the consistent reduction in lung elastic recoil with the normal aging process needs to be clarified, as do the extent and cause(s) of age-dependent reductions in chest wall compliance.

13. The consistent enhancement of resting pulmonary function in the elderly, highly fit subject is unique in terms of an apparent "training effect." This hypothesis needs in-depth study by means of carefully constructed, large-scale, longitudinal training experiments in the healthy elderly.

14. The reduced compliance of the pulmonary arterioles leads to high pulmonary vascular pressures and resistance at high cardiac outputs in the highly fit elderly. A comprehensive study is needed of the effects of these high pressures on pulmonary edema and on pulmonary gas exchange in the healthy, fit elderly.

15. The increased flow limitation, ventilatory work, and oxygen cost of breathing during exercise in the elderly at all levels of fitness are the most common effects of healthy aging on the response of the pulmonary system to exercise. The role of this increased mechanical cost on exercise performance needs to be determined by the use of imaginative studies employing newer methods of "unloading" the chest wall during prolonged exercise.

SUMMARY AND CONCLUSIONS

1. The $\dot{V}O_2$max levels decrease progressively during adult aging in the general population; the rate of decline is variable and is probably modulated by habitual physical activity, changes in body composition, disease, genetic factors, and, possibly, gender. In humans who engage regularly in vigorous endurance exercise the rate of decrease in $\dot{V}O_2$max with age appears to be ~50% of that exhibited by untrained individuals.

2. A reduction in the maximal achievable cardiac output during exercise, due to declines in maximal heart rate and stroke volume, appears to be the primary mechanism responsible for the decline in $\dot{V}O_2$max with age; a reduction in maximal a-v O_2 D seems to contribute to a lesser extent.

3. There is no compelling evidence that autonomic-circulatory control during submaximal exercise, including the regulation of blood flow to active muscle and the regulation of arterial blood pressure, is altered by the aging process *per se* in humans.

4. During prolonged submaximal exercise performed at the same %$\dot{V}O_2$max in thermoneutral ambient conditions, older adults, despite smaller rises in internal body temperature, demonstrate time-dependent adjustments in whole-body oxygen consumption and cardiovascular function that are similar to those exhibited by younger adults.

5. Some middle-aged and older male and female masters endurance athletes have very high levels of $\dot{V}O_2$max. Previously sedentary middle-aged and older subjects can increase their $\dot{V}O_2$max levels in response to endurance exercise training; there is marked inter-individual variability in the magnitude of response, but the average percent increase with a particular training stimulus appears to be similar in older men and older women.

6. In older men, the increases in $\dot{V}O_2$max with endurance training are primarily caused by increases in maximal, left-ventricular end-diastolic volume, left ventricular systolic function, stroke volume, and cardiac output, with somewhat lesser contributions from increases in maximal a-v O_2 D. Recent findings in older women, however, indicate that the same percent increase in $\dot{V}O_2$max levels with training is solely the result of an increase in maximal a-v O_2 D.

7. In general, older adults experience the same autonomic-cardiovascular adaptations to endurance training as do young adults during rest and submaximal exercise, although older women do not appear to undergo left ventricular changes typically associated with

volume-overload hypertrophy. An exception is the elevation in resting activity of the sympathetic nervous system associated with endurance training, which has not been reported in younger adults.

8. Endurance exercise performance declines progressively after the middle 30s in competitive athletes. In untrained adults, the capacity to perform a particular absolute level of submaximal exercise also declines with age, although the ability to sustain exercise at a particular $\%\dot{V}O_2$max appears to be well preserved. Endurance exercise training can produce marked improvements in submaximal exercise capacity in sedentary older adults.

9. The most consistent aging effects on pulmonary system structure include the loss of lung elastic recoil and a stiffening of the chest wall and pulmonary vasculature.

10. The most common age-dependent changes in the pulmonary system's acute response to exercise are an increased expiratory flow limitation, increased dead space ventilation, and increased ventilatory work and perhaps elevated pulmonary vascular resistance—all of which become obvious during even moderate intensity exercise.

11. Physical training effects on the lung and chest wall are trivial or relatively small in young adults; thus, in the highly fit at a very high $\dot{V}O_2$max, pulmonary gas exchange, pressure generation by inspiratory muscles, and ventilation may often reach limiting values. Furthermore, exercise-induced arterial hypoxemia may become a significant limiting factor to $\dot{V}O_2$max.

12. In contrast to the young adult, older, highly fit, healthy subjects commonly show improved resting lung function—especially greater lung elastic recoil—and, therefore, less flow limitation—than in their less fit contemporaries. Although the cause of the increased pulmonary system capacity (whether it be preselection or a true training effect) is unknown, the increased capacity confers a definite advantage by permitting the fit, older subject to achieve his higher ventilatory requirement at (higher) $\dot{V}O_2$max and $\dot{V}CO_2$.

13. With healthy aging, whether the lung and/or chest wall ever reach their functional limitations during exercise or whether they **cause** exercise performance to be limited, depends on the balance struck between pulmonary system capacity versus demand during the aging process. For example, the demands for ventilation and gas exchange of the highly trained, young adult could not be met by the pulmonary system structure in even the healthiest and fittest 70-y-old. These extremes are approached in some healthy, highly fit, elderly subjects who, having a $\dot{V}O_2$max greater than two times normal, experience significant arterial hypoxemia, complete ventilatory limitation, and an increased effort of breathing

that requires greater than 15% of total $\dot{V}O_2$max. However, these "failures" are extremely rare because the normal aging process appears to affect the capacity of other extra-pulmonary determinants of systemic O_2 transport and utilization at about the same rate as it does those of the lung and chest wall.

ACKNOWLEDGEMENTS

Douglas R. Seals thanks Jennifer Barr for her excellent work on the text of the manuscript, and Kevin Davy, Susan Evans, Mary Jo Reiling, and Edie Stevenson for their development of the figures. His work was supported by grants AG06537 and HL39966 from the National Institutes of Health and by Research Career Development Award AG00423 from the National Institute on Aging. Jerome Dempsey thanks Gundula Birong for her excellent preparation of the manuscript and acknowledges the collaboration of W. Reddan, B. Johnson, S. McClaran, and M. Babcock in the original data collection conducted in the Rankin Laboratory. Many thanks to Ed Coyle for his thoughtful review and to John Sutton for his detailed criticisms and insights. His work was supported by NHLBI and the American Heart Association.

BIBLIOGRAPHY

Aaron, E.A., B.D. Johnson, C.K. Seow, and J.A. Dempsey (1992a). Oxygen cost of exercise hyperpnea: Implications for performance. *J. Appl. Physiol.* 72:1818–1825.

Aaron, E.A., B.D. Johnson, C.K. Seow, and J.A. Dempsey (1992b). The oxygen cost of exercise hyperpnea: Measurement. *J. Appl. Physiol.* 72:1810–1817.

Allen, W.K., D.. Seals, and B.F. Hurley (1985). Lactate threshold and distance-running performance in young and older endurance athletes. *J. Appl. Physiol.* 58:1281–1284.

American Thoracic Society (1991). Lung function testing: Selection of reference values and interpretative strategies. *Am. Rev. Resp. Dis.* 144:1202–1218.

Anselme, F., C. Caillaud, I. Couret, M. Rossi, and C. Préfaut (1994). Histamine and exercise-induced hypoxemia in highly trained athletes. *J. Appl. Physiol.* 76:127–132.

Armour, J., P.M. Donnelly, and P.T.P. Bye (1993). The large lungs of elite swimmers: An increased alveolar number? *Eur. Resp. J.* 6: 237–247.

Åstrand, P.O., L. Engstrom, B.O. Eriksson, P. Karlberg, I. Nylander, B. Saltin, and C. Thoren (1963). Girl swimmers: With special reference to respiratory and circulatory adaptation and gynecological and psychiatric aspects. *Acta. Paediatr. Suppl.* 147:5–71.

Åstrand, P.O., and K. Rodahl (1977). *Textbook of Work Physiology*. New York: McGraw-Hill Book Co.

Babcock, M.A., D. Pegelow, and J.A. Dempsey (1995). Aerobic fitness effects on exercise-induced diaphragm fatigue. *Am. J. Resp. Crit. Care Med.* (Abstract) (In press).

Babcock, M.A., D.F. Pegelow, O. Suman, S.R. McClaran, and J.A. Dempsey (1993). Does the work of the diaphragm alone cause exercise-induced diaphragm fatigue? *Appl. Physiol.* (In press).

Badenhop, D.T., P.A. Cleary, S.F. Schaal, E.L. Fox, and R.L. Bartels (1983). Physiological adjustments to higher- or lower-intensity exercise in elders. *Med. Sci. Sports Exerc.* 15:469–502.

Bader, H. (1983). Importance of the gerontology of elastic arteries in the development of essential hypertension. *Clin. Physiol. Biochem.* 1:36–56.

Belman, M.J., and G.A. Gaesser (1991). Exercise training below and above the lactate threshold in the elderly. *Med. Sci. Sports Exerc.* 23:562–568.

Benestad, A.M. (1965). Trainability of old men. *Acta Med. Scand.* 178:321–327.

Bezucha, G.R., M.C. Lenser, P.G. Hanson, and F.J. Nagle (1982). Comparison of hemodynamic responses to static and dynamic exercise. *J. Appl. Physiol.* 53:1589–1593.

Black, L.F., and R.E. Hyatt (1969). Maximal respiratory pressures: normal values and relationship to age and sex. *Am. Rev. Respir. Dis.* 99:696–702.

Bloomfield, J., B.A. Blansky, and T.R. Ackland (1990). Morphological and physiological growth of competitive swimmers and noncompetitors through adolescence. *Aust. J. Sci. Med. Sport* 22:4–12.

Booth, F.W. (1989). Letter to the editor. *J. Appl. Physiol.* 66:1299.

Bouchard, C., F.T. Dionne, J.A. Simoneau, and M.R. Boulay (1992). Genetics of Aerobic and Anaerobic Performances. In: J.O. Holloszy (ed.) *Exercise and Sport Sciences Reviews*, Vol. 20. Baltimore: Williams & Wilkins, pp. 27–58.

Brandfonbrener, M., M. Landowne, and N.W. Shock (1955). Changes in cardiac output with age. *Circulation* 12:557–566.

Brock, D.B., J.M. Guralnik, and J.A. Brody (1990). Demography and epidemiology of aging in the US. In:

E.L. Schneider and J.W. Rowe (eds.) *Handbook of the Biology of Aging*. San Diego: Academic Press, pp. 3-23.

Brody, J.S., and W.M. Thurlbeck. (1985). Development, growth and aging of the lung. In: A.P. Fishman (ed.) *Handbook of Physiology (Section 3, The Respiratory System, Vol. III, Mechanics of Breathing, Part 1.)* Bethesda: American Physiological Society, pp. 355-386.

Burrows, B., M.G. Cline, R.J. Knudson, L.M. Taussig, and M.D. Lebowitz. (1983). A descriptive analysis of the growth and decline of the FVC and FEV_1. *Chest* 83:717-724.

Buskirk, E.R., and J.L. Hodgson (1987). Age and aerobic power: The rate of change in men and women. *Fed. Proc.* 46:1824-1829.

Carlson, L.A., and B. Pernow (1961). Studies on the peripheral circulation and metabolism in man. I. Oxygen utilization and lactate-pyruvate formation in the legs at rest and during exercise. *Acta Physiol. Scand.* 52:328-342.

Casaburi, R., T.W. Storer, and K. Wasserman (1987). Mediation of reduced ventilatory response to exercise after endurance training. *J. Appl. Physiol.* 63:1533-1538.

Child, J.S., R.J. Barnard, and R.L. Taw (1984). Cardiac hypertrophy and function in master endurance runners and sprinters. *J. Appl. Physiol.* 57:176-181.

Clanton, T.L., G.F. Dixon, J. Drake, and J.E. Gadek (1987). Effects of swim training on lung volumes and inspiratory muscle conditioning. *J. Appl. Physiol.* 62:39-46.

Cleroux, J., C. Giannattasio, G. Bolla, C. Cuspidi, G. Grassi, C. Mazzola, L. Sampieri, G. Seravalle, M. Valsecchi, and G. Mancia (1989). Decreased cardiopulmonary reflexes with aging in normotensive humans. *Am. J. Physiol.* 257:H961-H968.

Coggan, A.R., R.J. Spina, D.S. King, M.A. Rogers, M. Brown, P.M. Nemeth, and J.O. Holloszy (1990). Histochemical and enzymatic characteristics of skeletal muscle in master athletes. *J. Appl. Physiol.* 68:1896-1901.

Coggan, A.R., R.J. Spina, D.S. King, M.A. Rogers, M. Brown, P.M. Nemeth, and J.O. Holloszy (1992). Skeletal muscle adaptations to endurance training in 60- to 70-y-old men and women. *J. Appl. Physiol.* 72:1780-1786.

Conley, D.L., and G.S. Krahenbuhl (1980). Running economy and distance running performance of highly trained athletes. *Med. Sci. Sports Exerc.* 12:357-360.

Cononie, C.C., J.E. Graves, M.L. Pollock, M.I. Phillips, C. Sumners, and J.M. Hagberg (1991). Effect of exercise training on blood pressure in 70-79-y-old men and women. *Med. Sci. Sports Exerc.* 23:505-511.

Convertino, V.. (1991). Blood volume: Its adaption to endurance training. *Med. Sci. Sports Exerc.* 23:1338-1348.

Conway, J., R. Wheller, and R. Sannerstedt (1971). Sympathetic nervous activity during exercise in relation to age. *Cardiovasc. Res.* 5:577-581.

Coyle, E.F., M.K. Henmert, and A.R. Coggan (1986). Effects of detraining on cardiovascular responses to exercise: Role of blood volume. *J. Appl. Physiol.* 60:95-99.

Crapo, R.O. (1993). The Aging Lung. In: D.A. Mahler (ed.) *Pulmonary Disease in the Elderly*, Vol. 63. New York: Marcel Dekker, pp. 1-25

Cunningham, D.A., P.A. Rechnitzer, J.H. Howard, and A.P. Donner (1987). Exercise training of men at retirement a clinical trial. *J. Gerontol.* 42:17-23.

Czernin, J., P. Muller, S. Chan, R. Bruken, G. Porenta, J. Krivokapich, K. Chen, A. Chan, M.E. Phelps, and H.R. Schelbert (1993). Influence of age and hemodynamics on myocardial blood flow and flow reserve. *Circulation* 88:62-69.

Davidson, W.R. Jr., and E.C. Fee (1990). Influence of aging on pulmonary hemodynamics in a population free of coronary artery disease. *Am. J. Cardiol.* 65:1454-1458.

Davy, K.P., and D.R. Seals (1994). Total blood volume in healthy young and older men. *J. Appl. Physiol.* 76:2059-2062.

Davy, K.P., D.G. Johnson, and D.R. Seals (1995). Cardiovascular, plasma, norepinephrine, and thermal adjustments to prolonged exercise in young and older healthy humans. *Clin. Physiol.* (In press).

Dehn, M.M., and R.A. Bruce (1972). Longitudinal variations in maximal oxygen intake with age and activity. *J. Appl. Physiol.* 33:805-807.

De Meersman, R.E. (1993). Heart rate variability and aerobic fitness. *Am. Heart J.* 125:726-731.

Dempsey, J.A., N. Gledhill, W.G. Reddan, H.V. Forster, P.G. Hanson, and A.D. Claremont (1977). Pulmonary adaptation to exercise: Effect of exercise type, duration, chronic hypoxia and physical training. In: P. Milvy (ed.) *The Marathon: Physiological, Medical, Epidemiological, and Psychological Studies. Annals of the New York Academy of Sciences*, Vol. 301. New York: New York Academy of Sciences 301:243-261.

Dempsey, J.A., P.G. Hanson, and K. Henderson (1984). Exercise-induced arterial hypoxemia in healthy humans at sea level. *J. Physiol.* (London) 355:161-175.

Dempsey, J.A., and B.D. Johnson (1992). Demand vs capacity in the healthy pulmonary system. *Schweiz. Z. Sportmed.* 2:55-64.

Dempsey, J.A., S. Powers, and N. Gledhill (1990). Cardiovascular and pulmonary adaptation to physiological activity: Discussion. In: C. Bouchard, R.J. Shephard, T. Stephens, J.R. Sutton, and B.D. McPherson (eds.). *Exercise, Fitness and Health. A Consensus of Current Knowledge*. Champaign, IL: Human Kinetics Publishers, pp. 205-216.

Dempsey, J.A., E.H. Vidruk, and G.A. Mitchell (1985). Pulmonary control systems in exercise: update. *Fed. Proc.* 44:2260–2270.

Denahan, T., J.A. Barney, L.M. Sheldahl, and T.J. Ebert (1993). Lack of changes in cardiac-vagal activity in older males following 12 weeks of aerobic training. *Med. Sci. Sports Exerc.* 25 (Suppl.):S55.

DeVries, H.A. (1970). Physiological effects of an exercise training regime upon men aged 52 to 88. *J. Gerontol.* 25:325–336.

Dill, D.B., S. Robinson, and J.C. Ross (1967). A longitudinal study of 16 champion runners. *J. Sports Med. Phys. Fit.* 7:4–27.

Docherty, J.R. (1990). Cardiovascular responses in ageing: A Review. *Pharm. Rev.* 42:103–125.

Ehrsam, R.E. (1983). Influence of age on pulmonary hemodynamics at rest and during supine exercise. *Clin. Sci.* 65:653–660.

Ehrsam, R.E., A. Perruchoud, M. Oberholzer, F. Burkart, and H. Herzog (1983). Influence of age on pulmonary hemodynamics at rest and during supine exercise. *Clin. Sci.* 65:653–660.

Ehsani, A.A. (1987). Cardiovascular adaptations to exercise training in the elderly. *FASEB J.* 46:1840–1843.

Ehsani, A.A., T. Ogawa, T.R. Miller, R.J. Spina, and S.M. Jilka (1991). Exercise training improves left ventricular systolic function in older men. *Circulation* 83:96–103.

Enright, P.L., R.A. Kronmal, T.A. Manolio, M.B. Shenker, and R.E. Hyatt (1994). Respiratory muscle strength in the elderly. *Am. J. Respir. Crit. Care Med.* 149:430–438.

Esler, M., H. Skews, P. Leonard, G. Jackman, A. Bobik, and P. Korner (1981). Age-dependence of noradrenaline kinetics in normal subjects. *Clin. Sci.* 60:217–219.

Evans, S.L., E.T. Stevenson, H. Keith, and D.R. Seals (1994). Endurance running performance in women: Influence of age in relation to men. *Med. Sci. Sports Exerc.* 26:S137.

Evans, S.L., K.P. Davy, E.T. Stevenson, and D.R. Seals (1995). Physiological determinents of 10-KM performance in highly trained female runners of different ages. *J. Appl. Physiol.* (In press).

Farrell, P.A., J.H. Wilmore, E.F. Coyle, J.E. Billing, and D.L. Costill (1979). Plasma lactate accumulation and distance running performance. *Med. Sci. Sports* 11:338–344.

Fleg, J.L. (1986). Alterations in cardiovascular structure and function with advancing age. *Am. J. Cardiol.* 57:33C–44C.

Fleg, J.L., and E.G. Lakatta (1988). Role of muscle loss in the age-associated reduction in $\dot{V}O_2$max. *J. Appl. Physiol.* 65:1147–1151.

Folkow, B., and A. Svanborg (1993). Physiology of cardiovascular aging. *Physiol. Rev.* 73:725–764.

Forman, D.E., W.J. Manning, R. Hauser, E.V. Gervino, W.J. Evans, and J.Y. Wei (1992). Enhanced left ventricular diastolic filling associated with long-term endurance training. *J. Gerontol.* 47:M56–58.

Foster, V.L., G.J.E. Hume, W.C. Byrnes, A.L. Dickinson, and S.J. Chatfield (1989). Endurance training for elderly women: moderate vs low intensity. *J. Gerontol.* 44:M184–M188.

Fregosi, R., and J.A. Dempsey (1986). The effects of exercise in normoxia and acute hypoxia on respiratory muscle metabolites. *J. Appl. Physiol.* 60:1274–1283.

Fuchi, T., K. Iwaoka, M. Higuchi, and S. Kobayashi (1989). Cardiovascular changes associated with decreased aerobic capacity and aging in long-distance runners. *Eur. J. Appl. Physiol.* 58:884–889.

Gallagher, C.G., and M. Younes (1989). Effect of pressure assist on ventilation and respiratory mechanics in heavy exercise. *J. Appl. Physiol.* 66:1824–1837.

Georges, R., G. Saumon, and A. Louiseau (1978). The relationship of age to pulmonary membrane conductance and capillary blood volume. *Am. Rev. Respir. Dis.* 117:1069–1078.

Gerstenblith, G., E.G. Lakatta, and M.L. Weisfeldt (1976). Age changes in myocardial function and exercise response. *Prog. Cardiovasc. Dis.* XIX:1–21.

Giraud, G.D., M.J. Morton, L.E. Davis, M.S. Paul, and K.L. Thornburg (1993). Estrogen-induced left ventricular chamber enlargement in ewes. *Am. J. Physiol.*, 264:E490–E496.

Goldstein, D.S., C.F. Lake, B. Chernow, M.G. Zeigler, M.D. Coleman, A.A. Taylor, J.R. Mitchell, K.J. Kopin, and H.R. Keiser (1983a). Age-dependence of hypertensive-normotensive differences in plasma norepinephrine. *Hypertension* 5:100–104.

Gosselin, L.E., B.D. Johnson, and G.C. Sieck (1993). Age-related changes in diaphragm muscle contractile properties and myosin heavy chain isoforms. *Am. J. Resp. Care Med.* 150:174–178.

Granath, A., B. Jonsson, and T. Strandell (1964). Circulation in healthy old men, studied by right heart catheterization at rest and during exercise in supine and sitting position. *Acta Med. Scand.* 176:425–446.

Gribbin, B.T., T.G. Pickering, P. Sleight, and R. Peto (1971). Effect of age and high blood pressure on baroreflex sensitivity in man. *Circul. Res.* 29:424–431.

Grimby, G., and B. Saltin (1966). Physiological analysis of physically well-trained middle-aged and older athletes. *Acta Med. Scand.* 179:513–526.

Hagberg, J.M. (1987). Effect of training on the decline of $\dot{V}O_2$max with aging. *FASEB J.* 46:1830–1833.

Hagberg, J.M. (1994). Physical activity, fitness, health, and aging. In: In: C. Bouchard, R.J. Shephard, and T. Stephens (eds). *Physical Activity, Fitness, and Health: International Proceedings and Consensus Statement.* Champaign, IL: Human Kinetics Publishers, pp. 993–1005.

Hagberg, J.M., W.K. Allen, D.R. Seals, B.F. Hurley, A.A. Ehsani, and J.O. Holloszy (1985). A hemodynamic comparison of young and older endurance athlete during exercise. *J. Appl. Physiol.* 58:2041–2046.

Hagberg, J.M., and E.F. Coyle (1983). Physiological determinants of endurance performance as studied in competitive racewalkers. *Med. Sci. Sports Exerc.* 15:287–289.

Hagberg, J.M., J.E. Graves, M. Limacher, D.R. Woods, S.H. Leggett, C. Cononie, J.J. Gruber, and M.L. Pollock (1989). Cardiovascular responses of 70- to 79-y-old men and women to exercise training. *J. Appl. Physiol.* 66:2589–2594.

Hagberg, J.M., D.R. Seals, J.E. Yerg, J. Gavin, R. Gingerich, B. Premachandra, and J.O. Holloszy (1988a). Metabolic responses to exercise in young and older athletes and sedentary men. *J. Appl. Physiol.* 65:900–908.

Hagberg, J.M., J.E. Yerg II, and D.R. Seals (1988b). Pulmonary function in young and older athletes and untrained men. *J. Appl. Physiol.* 65:101–105.

Hanson, J.S., B.S. Tabakin, A.M. Levy, and W. Neede (1968). Long-term physical training and cardiovascular dynamics in middle-aged men. *Circulation* 38:783–799.

Harlan, W.R., A.L. Hull, R.L. Schmouder, J.R. Landis, F.A. Larkin, and F.E. Thompson (1984). High blood pressure in older Americans: The first national health and nutrition examination survey. *Hypertension* 6:802–809.

Heath, G.W., J.M. Hagberg, A.A. Ehsani, and J.O. Holloszy (1981). A physiological comparison of young and older endurance athletes. *J. Appl. Physiol.* 51:634–640.

Henke, K.G., M. Sharratt, D. Pegelow, and J.A. Dempsey (1988). Regulation of end-expiratory lung volume during exercise. *J. Appl. Physiol.* 64:135–146.

Hoeldtke, R.D., and K.M. Cilmi (1985). Effects of aging on catecholamine metabolism. *J. Clin. Endocrinol. Metab.* 60:479–484.

Holloszy, J.O. (1983). Exercise, health, and aging: a need for more information. *Med. Sci. Sports Exerc.* 25:1–5.

Hoppeler, H., S.R. Kayar, H. Claassen, E. Uhlmann, and R.H. Karas (1987). Adaptive variation in the mammalian respiratory system in relation to energetic demand: III. Skeletal muscles: Setting the demand for oxygen. *Resp. Physiol.* 69:27–46.

Hossack, K.F., and R.A. Bruce (1982). Maximal cardiac function in sedentary normal men and women: comparison of age-related changes. *J. Appl. Physiol.* 53:799–804.

Hurley, B.F., D.R. Seals, A.A. Ehsani, L.-J. Cartier, G.P. Dalsky, and J.M. Hagberg (1984). Effects of high intensity strength training on cardiovascular function. *Med. Sci. Sports Exerc.* 16:483–488.

Imai, Y., K. Nagai, M. Sakuma, H. Sakuma, H. Nakatsuka, H. Satoh, N. Minami, M. Munakata, J. Hashimoto, T. Yamagisi, N. Watanabe, T. Yabe, A. Nishiyama, and K. Abe (1993). Ambulatory blood pressure of adults in Ohasama, Japan. *Hypertension* 22:900–912.

Jasperse, J.L., D.R. Seals, and R. Callister (1994). Active forearm blood flow adjustments to handgrip exercise in young and older healthy men. *J. Physiol.* (London) 474:353–360.

Johnson, B.D., M.A. Babcock, O.E. Suman, and J.A. Dempsey (1993). Exercise-induced diaphragmatic fatigue in healthy humans. *J. Physiol.* (London) 460:385–405.

Johnson, B.D., and J.A. Dempsey (1991). Demand vs capacity in the aging pulmonary system. In: J. Holloszy (ed.) *Exercise and Sport Sciences Reviews*, Vol. 19. Baltimore: Williams & Wilkins, pp. 171–210.

Johnson, B.D., W.G. Reddan, D.F. Pegelow, K.C. Seow, and J.A. Dempsey (1991a). Flow limitation and regulation of functional residual capacity during exercise in a fit aging population. *Am. Rev. Resp. Dis.* 143:960–967.

Johnson, B.D., W.G. Reddan, K.C. Seow, and J.A. Dempsey (1991b). Mechanical constraints on exercise hyperpnea in an aging population. *Am. Rev. Resp. Dis.* 143:968–977.

Johnson, B.D., K.W. Saupe, and J.A. Dempsey. (1991c). Mechanical constraints on exercise hyperpnea in endurance athletes. *J. Appl. Physiol.* 72:1818–1825.

Joyner, M.J. (1991). Modeling: Optimal marathon performance on the basis of physiological factors. *J. Appl. Physiol.* 70:683–687.

Joyner, M.J. (1993). Physiological limiting factors and distance running: Influence of gender and age on record performances. In: J.O. Holloszy (ed.) *Exercise and Sport Sciences Reviews*, Vol. 21. Baltimore: Williams & Wilkins, pp. 103–133.

Julius, E.W., A. Amery, L.S. Whitlock, and J. Conway (1967). Influence of age on the hemodynamic response to exercise. *Circulation* 36:220–230.

Kallman, D.A., C.C. Plato, and J.D. Tobin (1990). The role of muscle loss in the age-related decline of grip strength:cross-sectional and longitudinal perspectives. *J. Gerontol.* 54:M82–M88.

Kasch, F.W., J.L. Boyer, S.P. Van Camp, L.S. Verity, and J.P. Wallace (1990). The effect of physical activity and inactivity on aerobic power in older men (a longitudinal study). *Physician Sportsmed.* 18:73–83.

Kohrt, W.M., M.T. Malley, A.R. Coggan, R.J. Spina, T. Ogawa, A.A. Ehsani, R.E. Bourey, W.H. Martin, and J.O. Holloszy (1991). Effects of gender, age, and fitness level on response of $\dot{V}O_2$max to training in 60–71 y olds. *J. Appl. Physiol.* 71:2004–2011.

Kohrt, W.M., R.J. Spina, A.A. Ehsani, P.E. Cryer, and J.O. Holloszy (1993). Effects of age, adiposity, and fitness level on plasma catecholamine responses to standing and exercise. *J. Appl. Physiol.* 75:1828–1835.

Lakatta, E.G. (1993). Cardiovascular regulatory mechanisms in advanced age. *Physiol. Rev.* 73:413–467.

Leith, D.E., and M. Bradley (1976). Ventilatory muscle strength and endurance training. *J. Appl. Physiol.* 41:508–516.

Levy, W.C., M.D. Cerqueira, I.B. Abrass, R.S. Schwartz, and J.R. Stratton (1993). Endurance exercise training augments diastolic filling at rest and during exercise in healthy young and older men. *Circulation* 88:116–126.

Lewis, S.F., W.F. Taylor, R.M. Graham, W.A. Pettinger, J.E. Shutte, and C.G. Blomquist (1983). Cardiovascular responses to exercise as functions of absolute and relative workload. *J. Appl. Physiol.* 54:1314–1323.

Lindbald, L.E. (1977). Influence of age on sensitivity and effector mechanisms of the carotid baroreflex. *Acta Physiol. Scand.* 101:43–49.

Makrides, L., G.J.F. Heigenhauser, and N.L. Jones (1990). High-intensity endurance training in 20- to 30- and 60- to 70-y-old healthy men. *J. Appl. Physiol.* 69:1792–1798.

Marti, B., and H. Howald (1990). Long-term effects of physical training on aerobic capacity: controlled study of former elite athletes. *J. Appl. Physiol.* 69:1451–1459.

Martin III, W.H., W.M. Kohrt, M.T. Malley, E. Korte, and S. Stoltz (1990). Exercise training enhances leg vasodilatory capacity of 65-y-old men and women. *J. Appl. Physiol.* 69:1804–1809.

Martin III, W.H., T. Ogawa, W.M. Kohrt, M.T. Malley, E. Korte, P.S. Keiffer, and K.B. Schechtman (1991). Effects of aging, gender, and physical training on peripheral vascular function. *Circulation* 84:654–664.

McClaran, S.R, M.A. Babcock, D.F. Pegelow, W.G. Reddan, and J.A. Dempsey (1994). Longitudinal study of aging effects on flow limitation during exercise in the healthy elderly adult (abstract). *J. Appl. Physiol.* (In press).

McElvany, G., S. Blackie, N.J. Morrison, P.G. Wilcox, M.S. Fairbarn, and R.L. Pardy (1989). Maximal static respiratory pressures in the normal elderly. *Am. Rev. Respir. Dis.* 139:277–281.

Meredith, C.N., M.J. Zackin, W.R. Frontera, and W.J. Evans (1987). Body composition and aerobic capacity in young and middle-aged endurance-trained men. *Med. Sci. Sports Exerc.* 19:557–563.

Metzger, J.M., and R.H. Fitts (1986). Contractile and biochemical properties of diaphragm: effects of exercise training and fatigue. *J. Appl. Physiol.* 60:1752–1758.

Montoye, H.J. (1984). Age and cardiovascular response to submaximal treadmill exercise in males. *Res. Quart.* 55:85–88.

Montoye, H.J., F.H. Epstein, and M.O. Kjelsberg (1965). The measurement of body fatness. *Am. J. Clin. Nutr.* 16:417–427.

Morlin, C., B.G. Wallin, and B.M. Eriksson (1983). Muscle sympathetic activity and plasma noradrenaline in normotensive and hypertensive man. *Acta Physiol. Scand.* 118:117–121.

Morrow, L.A., O.A. Linares, T.J. Hill, J.A. Sanfield, M.A. Supiano, S.G. Rosens, and J.B. Halter (1987). Age differences in the plasma clearance mechanisms for epinephrine and norepinephrine in humans. *J. Clin. Endocrinol. Metab.* 65:508–511.

Mostyn, J.M., S. Helle, J.B.L. Gee, L.G. Bentivoglio, and D.V. Bates (1986). Pulmonary diffusing capacity of athletes. *J. Appl. Physiol.* 60:1752–1758.

Murray, J.F. (1986). *Aging in the Normal Lung.* 2nd ed. Philadelphia: W.B. Saunders Company, pp. 339–360.

Ng, A.V., R. Callister, D.G. Johnson, and D.R. Seals (1993). Age and gender influence muscle sympathetic nerve activity at rest in healthy humans. *Hypertension* 21:498–503.

Ng, A.V., R. Callister, D.G. Johnson, and D.R. Seals (1994a). Sympathetic neural reactivity to stress does not increase with age in healthy humans. *Am. J. Physiol.* 36:H344–H353.

Ng, A.V., R. Callister, D.G. Johnson, and D.R. Seals (1994b). Endurance exercise training is associated with elevated basal sympathetic nerve activity in healthy older humans. *J. Appl. Physiol.* 77:1366–1374.

Niinimaa, V., and R.J. Shephard (1978). Training and oxygen conductance in the elderly. *J. Gerontol.* 33:354–361.

Ogawa, T., R.J. Spina, W.H. Martin, W.M. Kohrt, K.B. Schechtman, J.O. Holloszy, and A.A. Ehsani (1992). Effects of aging, sex, and physical training on cardiovascular responses to exercise. *Circulation* 86:494–503.

Pines, A., E.Z. Fisman, Y. Levo, M. Averbuch, A. Lidor, Y. Drory, A. Finkelstein, M. Hetman-Peri, M. Moshlowitz, E. Ben-Ari, and D. Ayalon (1991). The effects of hormone replacement therapy in normal postmenopausal women: Measurements of Doppler-derived parameters of aortic flow. *Am. J. Obstet. Gynecol.* 164:806–812.

Poehlman, E.T., A.W. Gardner, and M.I. Goran (1992). Influence of endurance training on energy intake, norepinephrine kinetics, and metabolic rate in older individuals. *Metabolism* 41:941–948.

Poehlman, E.T., and E.S. Horton (1990). Regulation of energy expenditure in aging humans. *Ann. Rev. Nutr.* 10:255–275.

Poehlman, E.T., T. McAuliffe, and E. Danforth Jr. (1990). Effects of age and level of physical activity on plasma norepinephrine kinetics. *Am. J. Physiol.* 258:E256–262.

Pollock, M.L., C. Foster, D. Knapp, J.L. Rod, and D.H. Schmidt (1987). Effect of age and training on aerobic capacity and body composition of master athletes. *J. Appl. Physiol.* 62:725–731.

Port, S., F.R. Cobb, R.E. Coelman, and R.H. Jones (1980). Effect of age on the response of the left ventricular ejection fraction to exercise. *N. Engl. J. Med.* 303:1133–1137.

Poulin, M.J., D.H. Paterson, D. Govindasamy, and D.A. Cunningham (1992). Endurance training of older men: responses to submaximal exercise. *J. Appl. Physiol.* 73:452–457.

Powell, K.E., P.D. Thompson, C.J. Caspersen, and J.S. Kendrick (1987). Physical activity and the incidence of coronary heart disease. *Ann. Rev. Public Health* 8:253-287.

Powers, S.K., D. Criswell, J. Lawler, D. Martin, L.L. Ji, R.A. Herb, and G. Dudley (1994). Regional training-induced alterations in diaphragmatic oxidative and antioxidant enzymes. *Respir. Physiol.* 95:227-237.

Powers, S.K., D. Criswell, F.-K. Lieu, S. Dodd, and H. Silverman (1992). Diaphragmatic fiber type specific adaptation to endurance exercise. *Respir. Physiol.* 89:195-207.

Powers, S.K., J. Lawler, J.A. Dempsey, S. Dodd, and G. Landry (1989). Effects of incomplete pulmonary gas exchange on $\dot{V}O_2$max. *J. Appl. Physiol.* 66:2491-2495.

Préfaut, C., F. Anselme, C. Caillaud, and J. Massé-Biron (1994). Exercise-induced hypoxemia in older athletes. *J. Appl. Physiol.* 76:120-126.

Reeves, J.T., J.A. Dempsey, and R.F. Grover (1989). Pulmonary circulation during exercise. In: E.K. Weir and J.T. Reeves (eds.) *Pulmonary Vascular Physiology and Pathophysiology.* New York: Marcel Dekker, pp. 107-133.

Reuschlein, P.L., W.G. Reddan, J.F. Burpee, J.B.L. Gee, and J. Rankin (1968). The effect of physical training on the pulmonary diffusing capacity during submaximal work. *J. Appl. Physiol.* 24:152-158.

Rivera, A.M., A.E. Pels III, S.P. Sady, M.A. Sady, E.M. Cullinane, and P.D. Thompson (1989). Physiological factors associated with the lower maximal oxygen consumption of master runners. *J. Appl. Physiol.* 66:949-954.

Robinson, S. (1938). Experimental studies of physical fitness in relation to age. *Arbeitsphysiologie* 10:162-323.

Robinson, E.P., and J.M. Kjeldgaard (1982). Improvement in ventilatory muscle function with running. *J. Appl. Physiol.* 52:1400-1406.

Rodeheffer, R.J., G. Gerstenblith, L.C. Becker, J.L. Fleg, M.L. Weisfeldt, and E.G. Lakatta (1984). Exercise cardiac output is maintained with advancing age in healthy human subjects: cardiac dilation and increased stroke volume compensate for a diminished heart rate. *Circulation* 69:203-213.

Rogers, M.A., and W.J. Evans (1993). Changes in skeletal muscle with aging: Effects of exercise training. In: J.O. Holloszy (ed.) *Exercise and Sport Sciences Reviews*, Vol. 21. Baltimore: Williams & Wilkins, pp. 65-102.

Rogers, M.A., J.M. Hagberg, W.H. Martin III, A.A. Ehsani, and J.O. Holloszy (1990). Decline in $\dot{V}O_2$max with aging in master athletes and sedentary men. *J. Appl. Physiol.* 68:2195-2199.

Romanovska, L., J. Ohrastek, and I. Prerovsky (1981). Calf blood flow and vascular resistance during reactive hyperaemia in young athletes and trained middle-aged subjects. *Physiol. Bohemoslov.* 30:275-281.

Ross, K.A., and W.M. Thurlbeck (1992). Lung growth in newborn guinea pigs: Effects of endurance exercise. *Respir. Physiol.* 89:353-364.

Rowe, J.W., and R.L. Kahn (1987). Human aging: usual and successful. *Science* 237:143-149.

Sachs, C., B. Hamberger, and L. Kaijser (1985). Cardiovascular responses and plasma catecholamines in old age. *Clin. Physiol.* 5:553-565.

Saltin, B. (1986). The aging endurance athlete. In: J.R. Sutton and R.M. Brock (eds.) *Sports Medicine for the Mature Athlete.* Indianapolis, In: Benchmark Press, pp. 59-80.

Saltin, B., L.H. Hartley, A. Kilbom, and I. AÅstrand (1969). Physical training in sedentary middle-aged and older men. II. Oxygen uptake, heart rate, and blood lactate concentration at submaximal and maximal exercise. *Scan. J. Clin. Lab. Invest.* 24:323-334.

Schaffartzik, W., D.C. Poole, T. Denon, K. Tsukimoto, M.C. Hogan, J.P. Arocs, D.E. Belmont, and P.D. Wagner (1992). $\dot{V}_A$:Q distribution during heavy exercise and recovery in humans:implications for pulmonary edema. *J. Appl. Physiol.* 72:1657-1667.

Scheuer, J., A. Malhotra, T.F. Schaible, and J. Capasso (1987). Effects of gonadectomy and hormonal replacement on rat hearts. *Circ. Res.* 61:12-19.

Schocken, D.D., J.A. Blumenthal, S. Port, P. Hindle, and E. Coleman (1983). Physical conditioning and left ventricular performance in the elderly: Assessment by radionuclide angiocardiography. *Am. J. Cardiol.* 52:359-364.

Schoenberger, J.A. (1986). Epidemiology of systolic and diastolic systemic blood pressure elevation in the elderly. *Am. J. Cardiol.* 57:45C-51C.

Schulman, S.P., E.G. Lakatta, J.L. Fleg, L. Lakatta, L.C. Becker, and G. Gerstenblith (1992). Age-related decline in left ventricular filling at rest and exercise. *Am. J. Physiol.* 263:H1932-H1938.

Seals, D.R. (1993). Influence of aging on autonomic-circulatory control in humans at rest and during exercise. In: C.V. Gisolfi, D.R. Lamb, and E.R. Nadel (eds.) *Perspectives in Exercise Science and Sports Medicine,* Vol. 6: *Exercise, Heat, and Thermoregulation.* Dubuque: Brown & Benchmark, pp. 257-304.

Seals, D.R., and P.B. Chase (1989). Influence of physical training on heart rate variability and baroreflex circulatory control. *J. Appl. Physiol.* 66:1886-1895.

Seals, D.R., K.P. Davy, M.J. Reiling, and E.T. Stevenson (1994a). Attenuated systolic blood pressure response/METS ratio in endurance trained postmenopausal women. *Med. Sci. Sports Exerc.* 26:S136.

Seals, D.R., J.M. Hagberg, W.K. Allen, B.F. Hurley, G.P. Dalsky, A.A. Ehsani, and J.O. Holloszy (1984a). Glucose tolerance in young and older athletes and sedentary men. *J. Appl. Physiol.* 56:1521-1525.

Seals, D.R., J.M. Hagberg, B.F. Hurley, A.A. Ehsani, and J.O. Holloszy (1984b). Endurance training in older men and women: I. Cardiovascular responses to exercise. *J. Appl. Physiol.* 57:1024-1031.

Seals, D.R., J.M. Hagberg, R.J. Spina, M.A. Rogers, K.B. Schectman, and A.A. Ehsani (1994b). Enhanced left ventricular performance in endurance trained older men. *Circulation* 89:198-205.

Seals, D.R., B.F. Hurley, J.M. Hagberg, J. Schultz, B.J. Linder, L. Natter, and A.A. Ehsani (1985). Effects of training on systolic time intervals at rest and during isometric exercise in men and women 61 to 44 years old. *Am. J. Cardiol.* 55:797–800.

Seals, D.R., J.A. Taylor, A.V. Ng, and M.D. Esler (1994c). Exercise and aging: autonomic control of the circulation. *Med. Sci. Sports Exerc.* 26:568–576.

Spina, R.J., T. Ogawa, W.M. Kohrt, W.M. Martin III, and A.A. Ehsani (1993a). Differences in cardiovascular adaptations to endurance exercise training between older men and women. *J. Appl. Physiol.* 75:849–555.

Spina, R.J., T. Ogawa, W.H. Martin III, A.R. Coggan, J.O. Holloszy, and A.A. Ehsani (1992). Exercise training prevents decline in stroke volume during exercise in young healthy subjects. *J. Appl. Physiol.* 72:2458–2462.

Spina, R.J., T. Ogawa, T.R. Miller, W.M. Kohrt, and A.A. Ehsani (1993b). Effect of exercise training on left ventricular performance in older women free of cardiopulmonary disease. *Am. J. Cardiol.* 71:99–104.

Stevenson, E.T., K.P. Davy, M.J. Reiling, and D.R. Seals (1995). Maximal aerobic capacity and total blood volume in highly trained middle-aged and older female endurance athletes. *J. Appl. Physiol.* 77:1691–1696.

Strandell, T. (1964). Circulatory studies on healthy old men. *Acta Med. Scand.* 175:1–43.

Stratton, J.R., M.D. Cerqueira, R.S. Schwartz, W.C. Levy, R.C. Veith, S.E. Khan, and I.B. Abrass (1992). Differences in cardiovascular responses to isoproterenol in relation to age and exercise training in healthy men. *Circulation* 86:504–512.

Sundlof, G., and B.G. Wallin (1978). Human muscle nerve sympathetic activity at rest. Relationship to blood pressure and age. *J. Physiol.* (London) 274:621–637.

Suominen, H., E. Hiekkinen, H. Liesen, D. Michel, and W. Hollmann (1977). Effects of 8 weeks' endurance training on skeletal muscle metabolism in 56–70-year-old sedentary men. *Eur. J. Appl. Physiol. Occup. Physiol.* 57:176–181.

Takemoto, K.A., L. Bernstein, J.F. Lopez, D. Marshak, S.H. Rahimtoola, and P.A.N. Chandraratna (1992). Abnormalities of diastolic filling of the left ventricle associated with aging are less pronounced in exercise-trained individuals. *Am. Heart J.* 124:143–148.

Taylor, J.A., G.A. Hand, D.G. Johnson, and D.R. Seals (1991). Sympathoadrenal-circulatory regulation during sustained isometric exercise in young and older men. *Am. J. Physiol.* 261:R1061–1069.

Taylor, J.A., G.A. Hand, D.G. Johnson, and D.R. Seals (1992). Augmented forearm vasoconstriction during dynamic exercise in healthy older men. *Circulation* 86:1789–1799.

Thomas, S.G., D.A. Cunningham, P.. Rechnitzer, A.P. Donner, and J.H. Howard (1985). Determinants of the training response in elderly men. *Med. Sci. Sports Exerc.* 17:667–672.

Thurlbeck, W.M. (1991). Morphology of the aging lung. In R.G. Crystal and J.B. West (eds.) *The Lung.* New York: Raven Press, pp. 1743–1748.

Tsukimoto, K., O. Mathieu-Costello, R. Prediletto, A.R. Elliot, and J.B. West (1991). Ultrastructural appearances of pulmonary capillaries at high transmural pressures. *J. Appl. Physiol.* 71:573–582.

Vaitkevicius, P.V., J.L. Fleg, J.H. Engel, F.C. O'Connor, J.G. Wright, L.E. Lakatta, F.C.P. Yin, and E.G. Lakatta (1993). Effects of age and aerobic capacity on arterial stiffness in healthy adults. *Circulation* 88:1456–1462.

Wahren, J., B. Saltin, L. Jorfeldt, and B. Punow (1974). Influence of age on the local circulatory adaptation to leg exercise. *Scan. J. Clin. Lab. Invest.* 33:79–86.

Ware, J.H., D.W. Dockery, T.A. Louis, X. Xu, B.G. Ferris Jr., and F.E. Speizer (1990). Longitudinal and cross-sectional estimates of pulmonary function decline in never-smoking adults. *Am. J. Epidemiol.* 132:685–699.

Warren, B.J., D.C. Nieman, R.G. Dotson, C.H. Adkins, K.A. O'Donnell, B.L. Haddock, and D.E. Butterworth (1993). Cardiorespiratory responses to exercise training in septuagenarian women. *Int. J. Sports Med.* 14:60–65.

Wells, C.L., M.A. Boorman, and D.M. Riggs (1992). Effect of age and menopausal status on cardiorespiratory fitness in masters women runners. *Med. Sci. Sports Exerc.* 24:1147–1154.

Yerg, J.E., D.R. Seals, J.M. Hagberg, and J.O. Holloszy (1985). Effect of endurance exercise training on ventilatory function in older individuals. *J. Appl. Physiol.* 58:791–794.

Yin, F.C., H.A. Spurgeon, G.S. Raizes, H.. Greve, M.L. Weisfeldt, and N.W. Shock (1976). Age associated decrease in chronotropic responses to isoproterenol. *Circulation* 54:161–167.

Younes, M. (1989). Exercise and breathing in health and disease. (Chapter 17, Appendix 4.39). In: M. Kryger (ed.) *Introduction to Respiratory Medicine.* New York: Churchill Livingstone, pp. 331–348.

Younes, M. (1991). Determinants of thoracic excursion during exercise. In: B.J. Whipp and K. Wasserman (eds.) *Pulmonary Physiology and Pathophysiology of Exercise.* (Lung Biology in Health and Disease Series), Vol. 52. New York: Marcel Dekker, pp. 1–67; appendix 4, p. 40.

Ziegler, M.G., C.R. Lake, and I.J. Kopin (1976). Plasma norepinephrine increases with age. *Lancet* 54:1314–1323.

DISCUSSION

BALDWIN: Jerry, how significant is the increase in the oxygen cost of breathing when you compare a young versus old subject at the same absolute level of exercise? Could this be a factor that might contribute to the energy drain during sustained physical activity and adversely affect the endurance performance of the older individual?

DEMPSEY: I think it must be significant. In a young, normally fit person exercising at $\dot{V}O_2$max with a ventilation of 120 L/min, the oxygen cost of breathing is 8–10% of the total body $\dot{V}O_2$. In a 70-y-old, highly fit person with high expiratory-flow limitation and chest wall distortion, the oxygen cost of breathing at that same ventilation was estimated to be 14–16% of the total $\dot{V}O_2$. We were shocked at those differences in ventilatory work. What does the system choose to do with this big load? We thought that what it would do would be to give up. That is, we thought inhibitory afferent feedback from the chest wall (especially via phrenic afferents) would cause the older person to hypoventilate. That didn't happen. They chose to ventilate considerably. Does this affect performance? I don't know for sure. One approach to answer this question would be to have the person exercise and then take the load off the respiratory muscles with a mechanical ventilator.

BALDWIN: Is there some remedial conditioning of alternative muscle groups that can compensate for what you might not normally induce through the training process because of the decline in elasticity of the breathing apparatus?

DEMPSEY: We know the expiratory muscles are highly active in these people, even at mild exercise loads, so I would expect that these muscles become conditioned as expiratory flow limitation occurs. The unfortunate thing is that it won't do any good because the force the expiratory muscles can produce is not the limiting factor to air flow. It is the airway closure that limits expiratory flow rate.

MAUGHAN: Figure 6-1 implies that a decline in maximal oxygen uptake with aging is inevitable. But if a middle-aged population undergoes endurance training, there will be an increase in both $\dot{V}O_2$max and performance. If training begins at a very young age and is progressive, these increases can be expected to continue for many years. If training starts at a very old age, the time available for improvement before the inevitable aging process takes over is going to be much shorter. At what point do you reach a cutoff, and how much improvement may you expect to see in the very old? How many years can they continue to improve?

SEALS: What you can expect is anywhere from no increase to an increase of greater than 50%. An important point is that the inter-individual variability in the magnitude of the increase in $\dot{V}O_2$max in older adults in response to the same endurance training stimulus is remarkable. We really don't understand the basis for this variability. On average, with mild aerobic training you see anywhere from no change to an increase of 10–15%. If they continue to increase the training stimulus up to 70–85% $\dot{V}O_2$max and train 4–5 times a week, over a year's time they will improve $\dot{V}O_2$max about 30%, which is as great or greater than what occurs in a young person.

LAKATTA: There is an important message that becomes somewhat obscured when we emphasize the absence of major changes in overall cardiovascular function with aging. Most of the data produced thus far have dealt with submaximal exercise paradigms, but many are quite convinced of a reduction in maximal cardiovascular reserve based on deficits in heart rate and, in some studies, in stroke volume. Thus, in the cardiovascular system, there can be substantial deficits in the reserve capacity of several of the components, but overall function for submaximal exercise could be preserved. But the issue of the overall reduction in reserve capacity with aging, especially as it relates to diseases that occur later in life, is very important. It gets us to the issue of why we should study aging *per se*. One reason is to be able to understand the interaction of aging and disease processes. *Interaction* is the key word to stress here. First we need to understand disease mechanisms and aging mechanisms separately and then go on to study their interaction. Knowing that there are changes in overall reserve capacity means in healthy older individuals that there are changes in specific regulatory mechanisms that may not be so important by themselves, but are of major importance when the pathophysiological effects of specific diseases enter the picture. At this point, we then see lower thresholds for clinical manifestation of diseases and hence higher prevalence and incidences of these clinical diseases in older individuals. If the emphasis on age-associated changes in cardiovascular function is directed to a continued understanding of mechanisms and how those mechanisms can indeed be shown to affect cardiovascular diseases later in life, preventive therapies can be directed toward attenuating those changes. Perhaps exercise training won't be good enough to prevent some of the age-associated changes, but there are other types of therapies in the offing that run the gamut from other lifestyle changes to pharmacologic agents to gene therapy.

BLOOMFIELD: I was intrigued by the reports that in estrogen-deficient women, resting left ventricular end-diastolic volume does not appear to increase with age as it does with men. There also appears to be a lack of change in peak systolic function of the left ventricle with training in these women. Are there data of this nature on female masters athletes? Secondly, these data suggest some direct effect of estrogen deficiency on the left ventricle function or on cardiac muscle. Do you know of any such mechanism?

SEALS: The echocardiographic data at rest to which you refer actually are the data of Ed Lakatta and he can speak to that issue. The exercise paper in question reported that older men who underwent an endurance exercise training program increased their $\dot{V}O_2$max levels by increasing their maximal cardiac output, which was in turn due to increases in maximal stroke volume. Corollary imaging studies of the left ventricle during supine bicycling exercise showed that the increases in maximal stroke volume measured during treadmill exercise were associated with volume overload hypertrophy of the left ventricle and with an enhancement in left ventricular systolic function. In older women who underwent the same percentage increases in $\dot{V}O_2$max in response to the same endurance training stimulus, the increases in $\dot{V}O_2$max appeared to be due totally to increases in the calculated maximal A-V O_2 difference. There were no increases in treadmill maximal cardiac output. When imaging studies on those women were completed, they confirmed the lack of increases in maximal stroke volume, left ventricular end-diastolic volume, or left ventricular systolic function. In another study, younger women did show increases in maximal cardiac output during treadmill exercise, and these increases were associated with increases in maximal stroke volume. Thus, older women comprise the only group that does not exhibit the classical left-ventricular remodeling and the enhancement of left-ventricular function at peak exercise. The women studied were not on estrogen replacement therapy. There are a few papers in the literature that have reported that chronic estrogen therapy *per se* induces an increase in left ventricular end-diastolic volume. I think this is one of the hypotheses that is going to be hotly studied in the future.

LAKATTA: The Baltimore longitudinal study on aging included about 100 women and 100 men between the ages of 25 y and 85 y who were sedentary and were highly screened to exclude diseases that might impact cardiovascular structure and function. We implemented our study in the sitting position. At rest, older men showed about a 20% average increase in their left ventricular end-diastolic volumes as measured by gated blood-pool scans. We were quite surprised to find that women did not exhibit this increase; rather, their left ventricular end-diastolic volumes at rest did not increase with age. In the supine position, however, some of the age-gender interaction disappears, so part of this effect is a postural effect. The regulation of blood volume and its compartmentalization, in addition to reflex adjustments to posture, may contribute to some of the differences between men and women that account for the age-gender difference in left ventricular end-diastolic volume at rest. During exercise, the left ventricular volume increases from the resting value in both older men and women to a greater extent than in their younger counterparts. The left-ventricular wall thickness that we measured by echocardiography in this subset of the population, as in a larger subset, is the same in both men and women and increases with age between 25 y and 85 y. Similarly, arterial stiffness, as indexed by pulse wave velocity, increases 1.5- to 3-fold in both men and women between these two ages. We are not quite sure about specific, direct estrogen effects on the heart because we don't have enough women on estrogen therapy in our study to specifically answer this question. There is a perimenopausal study in progress now in our Institute on Aging that is primarily looking at bone and other hormonal changes, but cardiac volume will also be measured in this study, so we may derive new information bearing on this issue.

BLOOMFIELD: Dr. Dempsey you have some limited data on older women. Is there any evidence of a gender effect in these pulmonary changes, either in structure or function?

DEMPSEY: Yes. A recent longitudinal study shows that major changes in lung function seem to occur in the 50s and 60s in both genders. These reductions in flow rates and the tendency toward hyperinflation with aging seem to be around 10–13% less marked in the women. I might add that during sleep, there are interesting gender differences, i.e., it is very common in a working population to see a fairly high prevalence of sleep apnea, but the incidence is much lower in women before menopause. After menopause, there is no gender difference.

EICHNER: Are there any data, epidemiologic or otherwise, that forestalling declines in pulmonary function, say by exercise training, wards off pneumonia or bronchitis, or increases the chance of surviving if one contracts bronchitis or pneumonia?

DEMPSEY: First, I don't think exercise training wards off these aging changes. There are cross-sectional data showing that the highly trained 70-y-old has better lung function than his sedentary contemporary, but that idea hasn't held up in longitudinal studies of 18 highly fit active subjects from age 67–73 y. Thus, we must ascribe the disparity in the cross-sectional data to preselection factors, i.e., to a cohort effect, rather than to physical training. The second point is, that what might be a mild respiratory disease in a younger person who quickly gets through it, e.g., reversible airway diseases or asthma, might have more substantial effects in an older person. The healthy, non-smoking, 65-y-old starts off with lung function analogous to that found in mild emphysema, i.e., loss of elastic recall is equivalent to mild emphysema. So, if someone begins with this hyperinflation and susceptibility to airway closure and contracts something like a broncho-constriction or an airway inflammation in addition, it can become extremely serious. As far as ways to prevent this or ameliorate it, physical training doesn't seem to be the answer. The expiratory muscles can be highly trained, but if the airways won't accept the flow, the trained muscles won't help. It may be different for the inspiratory muscles because training may be of some benefit to help the inspiratory muscles handle the substantial work load they are required to produce during exercise in the aged.

EDGERTON: Is a limitation in coughing capacity apparent as one ages, particularly in individuals with acute or chronic deficits in respiratory function?

DEMPSEY: Yes, the cough reflex is something we always want to keep with us; it is very important. It is dependent on a lot of things, including expiratory muscle force, but that is not normally affected much with the normal aging process. However, aging does adversely affect the control of the upper airway, so older people have problems with swallowing, with control of the glottis, and with control of the larynx, all of which can certainly diminish the effectiveness of coughing.

WHITE: The concept of biomarkers in aging is controversial. The use of so-called biomarkers is an attempt to minimize reliance on the chronological index of age. Dr. Dempsey, because ventilation variables lend themselves to measurement, can you identify one or two unambiguous functional indices of aging of this system?

DEMPSEY: My opinion is that loss of lung elastic recoil, as manifested first in expiratory flow limitations upon formed expiration, would be a key indicator of an aging effect on the lung.

WHITE: So, as soon as a change in expiratory flow rate is evident, you would feel that you have evidence of aging of the pulmonary system?

DEMPSEY: Yes. Of course this is in reference to healthy aging. Environmental factors (smoking) and specific congenital diseases can also alter lung elastic recoil, independent of aging.

SUTTON: What about increased airway reactivity? Many athletes have asthma.

DEMPSEY: Agreed. To use changes in expiratory flow rate as an aging biomarker, we would need to consider the effects of bronchoreactivity at any given age. This is not easy to do.

WHITE: Dr. Seals, could you put your finger on one or two functional indices?

SEALS: Maximal oxygen consumption certainly has been kicked around as a possible marker. Maybe Ed Lakatta has a good biomarker for aging of cardiac muscle.

LAKATTA: The whole concept of biomarkers is a very difficult one to cope with because even changes in gene expression that have been identified in cardiac muscle might not be indicative of a true intrinsic aging process. For example, many of the age-associated changes that occur in the regulation of expression of the gene coding for myosin heavy-chain isoforms and for the sarcoplasmic-reticulum pump protein also occur in younger animals under the stress of hypertension. The changes revert when the hypertension is abolished. There are certain phenotypic markers and changes in gene expression that do occur with aging and that could serve as practical reference points for interventions, whether or not we call these biomarkers. With respect to humans, I think the inability of the left ventricle to reduce its volume during systole is the most dramatic difference observed between healthy younger and older individuals. Small improvements in this function can occur in older individuals following chronic endurance training. However this function remains relatively impaired in older athletes when compared to younger sedentary individuals.

KANTER: Jerry, are the mechanical changes that you describe inevitable? I know you've tested masters athletes, but have you tested aged people who have been lifelong athletes? Further, have you seen the paper from Tim Noakes's group in which runners took vitamin C prior to a marathon and displayed diminished upper respiratory tract infection during the week following the race? Do you have any insight on this issue?

DEMPSEY: I didn't even know marathons caused upper respiratory infections! On your first point, the age-associated changes in muscle are not refractory. I am unsure what the true effects of aging are on respiratory muscles in humans. Are the increased airway collapsibility and loss of elastic recoil inevitable? Yes! That's why I think they are pretty good biomarkers of normal aging.

BOUCHARD: I would like to add to previous comments regarding the interaction between regular exercise and disease in older people. We already know that there is considerable heterogeneity in the response to regular exercise, not only in terms of $\dot{V}O_2$max gains or performance improvement, but also in terms of health benefits. There are some people who are physically active but who nonetheless become diabetic or hypertensive or develop coronary heart disease, but many other active people remain free of these clinical manifestations. One explanation for these differences is that people differ in the susceptibility to these diseases and/ or in level of protection derived from regular exercise because of genetic variation at a number of undefined genes. In this regard, the field of nutrition science is ahead of exercise science in the sense that it has begun several years ago to investigate the role of specific genes (e.g., the Apo E, the Apo B, etc.) on the response of plasma lipids and lipoproteins to chronic exposure to high- or low-fat diet, high- or low-cholesterol diet, and other dietary protocols. I suggest that the moment has arrived for us to use similar designs with our own phenotypes and panel of candidate genes. For instance, we know that middle-aged and older men exhibit a mean increase in levels of plasma HDL-cholesterol with regular exercise. However, not all men register an increase. We need to explain this heterogeneity, and I do not believe that we can be successful without taking genetic variation into consideration.

This represents a change in paradigm which, by this way, is experienced by all fields rooted in human biology. The implications are enormous for the research agenda. For instance, instead of assigning subjects at random between control and exercise groups, maybe we need to assign subjects to genotypic groups and test whether the treatment effect differs among genotypes. This approach would be strongly indicated when, for example, a given polymorphism has a substantial effect on the phenotype, such as in the case of the vitamin-D-receptor allelic variation in relation to bone density.

DEMPSEY: I like the idea. But, how specific can we be at this time? What specific markers do we have? If I were trying to discover the cause of variability in the exercise response of left-ventricular ejection function, what phenotypic marker would I use to divide my groups?

BOUCHARD: Of course, it is rather unlikely that ventricular ejection volume variation can be reduced to the effects of one or a few genes.

LAKATTA: I don't think we have a candidate gene but maybe one place to begin to look is at genetic fitness, i.e., focus on those who age successfully and those who age normally and find out which people perform better without doing any regular exercise. Of course, in this regard we would have to devise an instrument to quantify and stratify physical activity within what we now define as the sedentary range. If we can do this, we will take a giant step forward on a lot of the issues raised at this conference. Subsequently, we can perform genetic analyses on those two groups and look for differences in gene type and then try to narrow it down from there.

7

Body Fluid and Temperature Regulation as a Function of Age

W. LARRY KENNEY, Ph.D.

INTRODUCTION

Much of our knowledge about the interactions among age, fluid balance, and the regulation of body temperature during exercise has been gleaned from epidemiological data such as heat wave morbidity and mortality or extrapolated from clinical or institutionalized older populations, or is anecdotal in nature. For those reasons, what is generally accepted as dogma about older[1] men and women exercising in warm environments often has little firm support in the experimental literature. Statements such as "The elderly are less heat tolerant," or "Fluid intake is diminished with aging" are common in exercise science and clinical textbooks, but they concern issues that are far too complex to be simplified into such bromides.

When considering aging and its effect on the regulation of body fluids and body temperature, one must clearly understand the question being posed. Whether the "average" 70-year-old responds differently during sustained activity compared to the "average" 25-year-old is a distinctly different question from "Does aging, independent of concomitant changes in aerobic capacity ($\dot{V}O_2$max), body composition, disease prevalence, etc., result in physiological changes that impact on thermoregulation and fluid balance?" In either case, an important follow-up question for the exercise scientist should be "Are such age-related changes inevitable and irreversible, or are they amenable to intervention?"

A comprehensive review of all aspects of human thermoregulation and body fluid balance is far too broad for treatment in a single chapter. This chapter will focus primarily on the latter two questions posed above. Toward that end, it is important to first examine such issues as morbidity and mortality in older persons during environmental extremes and to consider what constitute "baseline" conditions for older individuals with regard to fluid balance and body temperature; i.e., how different are older versus young men and women in a "normal" resting state? Next, the chapter reviews the impact of age on human physiological responses during exercise in warm environments. Intervention strategies that may affect the ability of older subjects to regulate body fluids and temperature, notably aerobic fitness and heat acclimation, are reviewed. Special attention is given to estrogen deficiency (and supplementation) after menopause—a concomitant of aging in more than half of the population. Finally, responses to exposure to cold are discussed.

Experimental Approaches

Ask the right kind of question-
A question that is worthwhile
And a question that can be
tackled with the tools available
at the time,
For Research is the art of finding
problems that can be solved.

—Otto Warburg and Hans Krebs

There are no comprehensive longitudinal studies of aging and thermoregulation or body fluid balance. Our limited understanding of these topics comes from 1) a few notable longitudinal case study reports (e.g., Robinson et al., 1965), 2) cross-sectional comparisons of older and younger subjects selected randomly or as representative of their respective age groups, and 3) cross-sectional comparisons that attempt to match older and younger subject groups in various ways. The first approach perhaps comes closest to providing a glimpse of true aging changes, yet the results have limited utility because of the few subjects and inattention to inherent limitations in this type of design. The second and third approaches— true cross-sectional comparisons—have merit but study potential age effects rather than aging. Furthermore, it is essential to keep in mind the inherent error introduced into all cross-sectional aging studies by "selective mortality." As pointed out by Epstein (1979), "Subjects over the age of 75 represent . . . biologically superior survivors from a cohort that has experienced at least a 75% mortality."

More germane to this treatise, each of the cross-sectional paradigms above asks a distinctly different question. The second approach typically attempts to answer the question "How does the **average** older adult differ from the **average** younger adult?". The advantage of this approach is that results are more applicable to the general population, e.g., in making health policy decisions involving this rapidly growing group of older individuals. A distinct disadvantage is trying to delineate changes in physiological mechanisms resulting from aging *per se* from those more closely related to other factors that typically change in concert with aging, e.g., $\dot{V}O_2max$, body composition, activity level, ratio of body surface area to body mass, disease presence, socioeconomic influences, etc. If an experiment reports a lower mean sweating rate in a group of 70-year-olds drawn from the general population relative to a group of 30-year-olds, is that deficit due to the 40-y age difference, or does it merely reflect the substantially lower $\dot{V}O_2max$ of an average 70-year-old? This approach is further flawed when exercise is introduced because it is impossible for older and younger subjects who differ in $\dot{V}O_2$max to exercise at the same absolute *and* relative (i.e., %$\dot{V}O_2$max) submaximal intensity.

The third approach, i.e., matching groups of older and younger subjects with respect to as many characteristics as possible, comes closer to answering the question of whether or not age *per se* alters thermoregulatory responses. In such studies, the older adults typically recruited are relatively free of disease and medication, are highly fit, and exercise on a regular basis. Young (20-30-year-old) subjects are then recruited with similar characteristics, most notably $\dot{V}O_2$max, body size, and adiposity, and care is taken to control hydration status and acclimation state. Exercise paradigms can then be designed to impose similar rates of absolute metabolic heat production (a function of the absolute VO_2), while also allowing the older and younger subjects to exercise at similar percentages of $\dot{V}O_2$max (which affect heat loss effector responses). The unstated premise underlying this approach is as follows: If the healthiest, fittest subset of the older population exhibits responses significantly different from their matched younger counterparts, such differences can better be attributed to chronologic age. The results from such studies are directly applicable only to this select subgroup of older men and women and thus may not be true for the older population as a whole; however, it is from this approach that medical and practical concepts can, perhaps, best be derived for older adults.

Recently, a fourth approach has been introduced (Havenith & van Middendorp, 1990; Havenith et al., 1995) in which a large, heterogeneous sample of subjects is tested in a standardized protocol. Dependent variables (e.g., core temperature or heart rate) are then examined for their relative dependence on various physical and physiological variables (including age) using multiple regression analyses. The results of one such study emphasizing aging and heat stress are presented later in the chapter.

EPIDEMIOLOGY

Heat Waves

Epidemiological reports typically use mortality as their criterion measure; thus, data regarding morbidity associated with both heat and cold are generally lacking. High mortality rates among adults over the age of 60 y during climatic heat waves are a ubiquitous phenomenon, yet certification of death as due to excess heat is rare (Oechsli & Buechley, 1970). Because published epidemiological data from heat waves report excess mortality from all causes, few physiological conclusions can be derived; however, the statistics themselves provide some important insights. It is indisputable that the preponderance of hospital presentations and deaths during prolonged hot spells involve men and women over the age of 60 y, and clear evidence exists that this group constitutes the largest at-risk group when exposed to high ambient temperatures.

To cite three examples from the United States, prolonged summer heat waves occurred in 1966 over most of the Midwest, in 1980 in the Midwest and Southern states, and in 1988 over most of the East Coast. Over a 5-d period in St. Louis, Missouri, in 1966, 350 men and women were judged by medical authorities to have died from the effects of heat. Of the 280 cases reviewed by the coroner, 277 were over the age of 60 y (Ellis et al., 1976). Similarly, in the 1980 Memphis, Tennessee, heat wave, there were 483 heat-related hospital presentations (mean age = 69 y) and 83 heat-related deaths (mean age = 70 y) (Applegate et al., 1981). Finally, during the summer of 1988, Allegheny County (Pittsburgh), Pennsylvania, experienced daily high temperatures above 32°C (90°F) for 15 straight days. Over that period, the entire increase in the predicted death rate (107 persons) was fully accounted for by an increased number of deaths of people over the age of 65 (Ramlow & Kuller, 1990) (Figure 7-1). Although most of the dead were women (76%, 57%, and 59% for the three reports cited, respectively), this may simply reflect the larger proportion of women in the older population rather than an age-gender interaction.

From a purely epidemiological standpoint, combined data from St. Louis and Kansas City in 1980 showed that adults over the age of 65 have

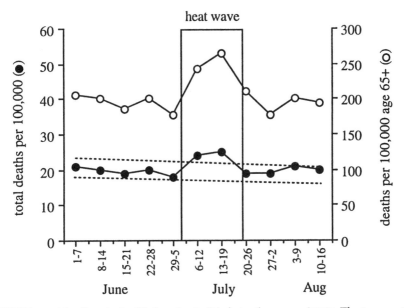

FIGURE 7-1. *Mortality rates for Allegheny County, PA, during the summer of 1988.* The increase in total deaths per 100,000 persons during the heat wave was totally accounted for by the increased death rate of persons over the age of 65 y. The dotted lines illustrate 95% confidence interval for deaths based on the previous 5 y. Redrawn from Ramlow & Kuller (1990).

a 10-fold to 12-fold greater risk of developing heat stroke than do persons under 65 (Jones et al., 1982). An interesting statistical model was developed by Oechsli and Buechley (1970) to examine excess mortality associated with three Los Angeles heat waves. The proportional increase in mortality resulting from high ambient temperatures increased progressively and nonlinearly with both age and temperature. A model that best fit the data incorporated both increasing temperature and advancing age to determine the "age and temperature specific mortality ratio" (Figure 7-2):

$$\text{ATMR} = 90.711 + e^{[-6.577 + 0.034 \cdot \text{age (y)} + 0.077 \cdot \text{temperature (°F)}]}$$

Careful examination of those data shows that 1) the increase in heat-related mortality when peak air temperature stays below 35°C (95°F) is negligible, 2) there are very few heat-related deaths during heat waves in individuals younger than 50, and 3) the risk of an individual dying during

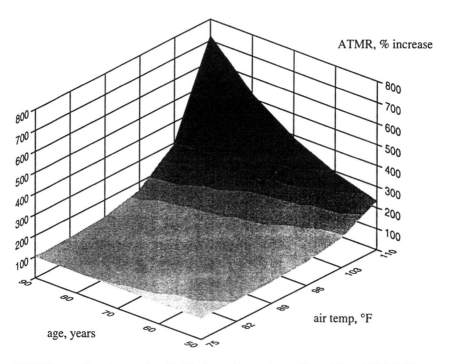

FIGURE 7-2. *Three-dimensional model of the "age and temperature specific mortality ratio" (ATMR) first published by Oechsli & Buechley (1970).* Temperatures are given in °F, as in their original model, and ATMR is expressed as a percentage increase in mortality for a given combination of age and air temperature. The model demonstrates that mortality during heat waves is an exponential function of both age and ambient temperature and that the number of deaths begins to increase significantly at air temperatures above 95°F (35°C) and ages above 50 y.

a heat wave climbs progressively and nonlinearly between the ages of 50 and 90. Further, the single best meteorological predictor of excess mortality is maximal temperature with a 1-d lag, i.e., most deaths occur on the day after the hottest day of a heat wave (Grover, 1938).

However, the impact of socioeconomic status, demography, and other nonphysiological factors on epidemiological heat wave statistics is great. The Centers for Disease Control (CDC) has mapped fatalities due to excessive heat among persons aged 65 and older (Martinez et al., 1989). When such data are mapped, geographical clusters of deaths occur in areas of the United States to an extent not fully explainable by either population density or temperature extremes. These clusters appear in counties that are highly urbanized and (for races other than white) relatively poor. In older populations, alcoholism and the use of tranquilizers and other drugs (Table 7-1) significantly increase the risk of heat stroke (Lomax, 1983). Factors associated with decreased risk include the ability to care for oneself, regular physical activity, and drinking extra liquids (Kilbourne et al., 1982), although the volume of fluids ingested that becomes preventive has not been established. Thus, the interactions of physiological and nonphysiological influences are complex.

Hypothermia

During winter months the mortality rate increases. The increase is more pronounced among older adults (Collins, 1987; Rango, 1984) and is purported to result from an increased incidence of hypothermia and its sequelae (Horvath & Rochelle, 1977). Hypothermia, as used here, refers to abnormally low body core temperatures resulting from cool or cold environmental conditions, as opposed to the common clinical definition of T_c $\leq 35°C$. Published surveys of the mortality risk from hypothermia in the United States between 1970 and 1979 (Rango, 1984) and between 1979 and 1985 (Macey & Schneider, 1993) clearly document increased risk associated with advancing age. Across all ages, exposure-related deaths from hypothermia are highest for nonwhite men and lowest for white women (Rango, 1984). In fact, whereas there is a female bias for risk of death from excessive heat as noted above, there is likewise a strong male bias for deaths from excessive cold (Macey & Schneider, 1993).

As pointed out in a recent review by Young (1991), "Epidemiological analyses of death rates do not provide conclusive evidence for age-related changes in thermoregulatory responses to cold." For instance, hypothermia often results from an alcohol- or drug-related loss of consciousness in cold weather, the incidence of which increases with advanced age (Keatinge, 1986). Also, the notable gender bias mentioned earlier, also seen in laboratory investigations involving passive exposure to cold (Bernstein et al., 1956; Wagner & Horvath, 1985), has been interpreted to imply that

TABLE 7-1. *Drug categories that may induce hyperthermia and/or predispose individuals to heat stroke.* This list is meant to be illustrative, rather than exhaustive. Adapted in part from Lomax (1983).

Drug Category	Potential Effect and Proposed Mechanism
Phenothyazines	Hyperthermia may occur in response to exercise or high ambient temperatures. Risk is increased with longer-acting compounds, e.g., fluphenazine enanthate. Action is primarily by interfering with heat loss mechanisms, rather than actions at the hypothalamic level.
Tricyclic Antidepressants	Hypothermia may occur, especially when combined with other drugs like reserpine, amphetamines, noradrenergic modulators, or cholinomimetic drugs. Hyperpyrexia may occur with overdoses. Main site(s) of actions is unclear.
Opiates	Both opiate use and withdrawal from opiates may cause vasodilation and sweating. Hyperpyrexia has been reported when opiates were given in combination with monoamine oxidase (MAO) inhibitors. Action occurs via blockade of serotonergic pathways (serotonin uptake and metabolism).
Methyldopa	Methyldopa may cause elevations in T_c in hypertensive patients, especially when first taken. Mechanism is thought to beskin vasoconstriction in response to increased circulating sympathomimetic amines.
Amphetamines	Hyperpyrexia and fatal heat stroke are common consequences of acute amphetamine poisoning. Use or abuse in combination with alcohol, MAO inhibitors, barbiturates, and phenothiazines increases this risk. Both central and peripheral actions are important, and exertion and heat waves are often contributing factors.
Antimuscurinic Agents	Belladonna alkaloids induce a rise in T_c which may be significant during exercise at high ambient temperatures. Central and peripheral (suppression of sweating) actions have been noted.
Alcohol and Barbiturates	These drugs cause physiological and behavioral thermoregulatory changes. Alcohol may cause a downward resetting of central thermoceptors and promote dehydration and peripheral vasodilation. In high doses, barbiturates depress all thermoregulatory systems.
Diuretics	Diuretics, having various sites of action, promote varying degrees of water vs. electrolyte loss. Resulting decreases in fluid from both intracellular and extracellular spaces may cause or exacerbate hyperthermia. Effects are exerted both centrally and peripherally.
Adrenergic Antagonists	Actions on control of peripheral (including skin) blood flow have been reported for both α- and β-adrenergic blocking agents.

differences in adiposity and, specifically, in subcutaneous fat thickness and distribution may play a larger role than chronological age. As with heat-related deaths, underlying diseases, medications, and general frailty all contribute to these epidemiological statistics.

BASELINE TEMPERATURE AND
FLUID BALANCE IN OLDER ADULTS

Baseline Body Temperature in Older Adults

It has been reported that baseline body core temperature (T_c) decreases with advancing age and has greater variability in older populations (Howell, 1948; Primrose & Smith, 1982; Salvosa et al., 1971). Such differences in T_c imply either that a lower T_c is defended by differential hypothalamic thermoregulatory mechanisms or, alternately, that older individuals poorly control their heat exchange with the environment and the low T_c is a passive response to environmental temperatures. If such differences do indeed exist, they would have important implications for control of T_c during cold stress, exercise, and other homeostatic challenges.

Rather than being a physiological consequence of aging, the lower T_c of older men and women that is cited in the literature appears to reflect chronic disease and effects of medication. Marion et al. (1991) repeatedly measured the oral and urine temperatures of 93 subjects aged 64–96 who were free from a large number of exclusionary criteria. Those criteria included diseases, low weight, smoking, lack of self-sufficiency, alcohol intake, and medication use. When such factors were excluded, there was no relationship between age and T_c, which averaged 37.0°C $\pm$ 0.45 (s.d.) across all age groups. Nor did the intersubject variability of T_c increase with age, ranging from 36.5–37.6°C for each age group studied (64–72, 73–79, and 80–96 y).

Are Healthy Older Men and Women Chronically Hypohydrated?

Perhaps no area is more replete with anecdotal evidence and facts extrapolated from clinical and institutionalized populations than that of body fluids and aging. For example, in one often cited clinical survey, dehydration (more accurately, hypohydration) was evident in about 25% of nonambulatory geriatric hospital patients (Spangler et al., 1984). In another, a majority of patients over age 65 from six continuing care hospital wards was found to be have elevated serum osmolalities (>296 mOsmol/kg), and a group of 58 patients randomly selected had a mean plasma osmolality of 304 $\pm$ 8 mOsmol/kg at time of hospital admission (O'Neill et al., 1990).[2] When older patients are hospitalized, a common textbook observation, e.g., Agate (1970), is that many cannot or will not spontaneously ask for fluids. Extrapolating such statistics to noninstitutionalized, healthy older men and women may lead to the inaccurate assumption that most older individuals walk around in a frank state of hyperosmolar hypohydration. This does not appear to be the case.

When older subjects report for laboratory studies designed to challenge fluid balance, they are typically in a normal state of hydration (Crowe et al., 1987; Kenney et al., 1990; Phillips et al., 1984a), although a slightly elevated (by 3–6 mOsmols/kg) plasma osmolality is often noted in these older subject groups at "baseline" (Crowe et al., 1987; Faull et al., 1993; Kenney et al., 1990; Mack et al., 1994; Miescher & Fortney, 1989). Such small differences in blood tonicity have led to the conclusion that "healthy, active older [individuals] are hyperosmotic and hypovolemic" (Mack et al., 1994). However, such studies typically require an overnight fast; thus, the "baseline" plasma variables that are reported really reflect a postdehydration state. An overnight fast should more accurately be viewed as a mild dehydration, which selectively renders older subjects slightly hyperosmotic and hypovolemic.

Also, despite the statistics cited above for geriatric hospitals, hypohydration is evident in only about 1% of older patients admitted to community hospitals (Snyder et al., 1987). Even in the hyperosmolar institutionalized patients surveyed by O'Neill et al. (1990) (ages 67–101 y), there was no correlation between age and osmolality. Therefore, it is more plausible that hyperosmolar hypohydration 1) accompanies, or results from, various clinical conditions in older individuals or 2) reflects an age-specific response to mild water deprivation. Both the incidence and the magnitude of chronic hypohydration in the healthy community-dwelling older adult are often overstated.

Spontaneous Fluid Ingestion in Healthy Older Adults

An apparent discrepancy exists in the literature with regard to fluid intake and age. On the surface, it seems difficult to reconcile the above discussion with the fact that laboratory studies typically show a deficient thirst sensation and lower fluid intake when older subjects are challenged by water deprivation or passive heat stress (see below). Do older men and women, on a day-to-day basis, consume less fluid than younger men and women? What dictates spontaneous fluid intake, and do those stimuli change as we age?

Under *ad libitum* conditions, in natural environments, fluid intake has little to do with homeostatic control mechanisms (Phillips et al., 1984b). Neither the amount nor the pattern of fluid intake is regulated physiologically to any great extent; both are governed by the amount and timing of food intake (de Castro, 1988, 1991; Phillips et al., 1984b). Enough fluid is consumed in response to nonregulatory stimuli (i.e., with meals) to maintain adequate fluid balance, and under unstressful conditions the kidney response of older persons is sufficient to maintain this balance. Therefore, afferent physiological signals that arise from a fluid deficit are rarely produced, and physiologically mediated mechanisms are seldom called upon under conditions of normal daily life (de Castro, 1992). This may be especially true for the older adult population, which as a group tends to be sedentary.

When fluids are readily available, independently living healthy older individuals demonstrate daily fluid intakes that are similar to those of younger individuals. In a recent study, 262 adults aged 20–80 were asked to maintain a diary for 7 consecutive days of everything they ate or drank (de Castro, 1992). Data were analyzed for total fluid intake (food water content plus fluids drunk), for water intake in excess of that required for digestion (surplus water), and for fluid ingested as drinks alone. There was no age difference in the overall volume of fluid consumed. Nor was there an age effect for thirst, its relationship to fluid intake, or the amount of fluid ingested relative to the amount of solid food ingested during a meal.[3]

Even when slight reductions of fluid intake have been noted in large surveys of community-dwelling older men and women, their average intake is still well within the normal range (Löwik et al., 1989). In a Dutch survey of 539 apparently healthy, independently living adults aged 65–79 y, daily water intake averaged 2.15 L/d for men and 1.98 L/d for women. Although the nonalcoholic beverage intake of the 75–79-year-old group was significantly lower than that of younger subjects, even the lowest daily intake reported (1.87 L/d) was well within what the authors considered the normal range of 1.6–2.4 L/d. However, it is important to realize, as pointed out by Rolls (1989), that if older individuals do not feel well or if access to palatable fluids is in any way restricted, problems may develop.

AGE AND RESPONSE TO DEHYDRATION

Mild Fluid Deprivation

There is sound evidence that older subjects have more difficulty defending their fluid balance in response to mild dehydration caused by water deprivation than do younger people. Thus, problems related to fluid balance in older men and women may only become apparent when homeostasis is challenged. In this population even seemingly mild stresses, such as the fluid restriction imposed prior to surgery or laboratory procedures in hospital settings, may create a disturbance in fluid balance that is difficult to self-correct (Leaf, 1984). The disturbed fluid and electrolyte homeostasis in older individuals has been linked to both altered renal function and deficiencies in thirst mechanisms. Responses to the dehydration induced by exercise and thermal stresses will be discussed separately.

Renal Fluid Conservation. The effects of aging on kidney function have been extensively reviewed (e.g., Epstein, 1979; Levi & Rowe, 1992). Progressive changes in both the structure and function of the kidney are evident beginning roughly at age 40 (Lindeman & Goldman, 1986). Blood vessels, glomeruli, tubules, and interstitium all seem to be targets for aging effects. Perhaps most importantly, though, a loss of functioning nephrons requires the surviving nephron pool to handle an increased solute and fluid load. Most age-related disturbances in renal fluid handling can be traced to this increased load per functional nephron (Lindeman & Goldman, 1986).

The normal renal response of young people to water deprivation is a marked decrease in urine flow, a moderate increase in urine osmolality, and a significant decrease in free-water clearance. It has long been recognized that the aged kidney is less responsive to water deprivation. Age differences in renal fluid conservation have been noted after 9 h (Faull et al., 1993), 12 h (Rowe et al., 1976), and 29 h (Lindeman et al., 1960) of fluid deprivation. After an overnight fast of 9 h, 58–74-year olds had a significantly lower mean urine osmolality (508 versus 842 mOsmols/kg) and higher plasma osmolality (294 versus 291 mOsmols/kg) and free-water clearance (-0.35 vs -0.95 mL/min) than a group of 18–45-year-old controls (Faull et al., 1993). In response to 12 h of fluid deprivation, a similar group of older subjects was less able than young or middle-aged subjects to significantly alter urine flow rate, urine osmolality, or osmolar clearance (Rowe et al., 1976).

This decreased ability of the kidneys of older adults to concentrate urine and thus minimize free-water clearance after water deprivation appears to be an intrarenal defect occurring at the nephron level. While this relative inability has often been attributed to the concomitant decrease in glomerular filtration rate (GFR) with aging, this belief is not universally held. Rowe et al. (1976) found no relationship between GFR and urine osmolality after the 12-h water deprivation, suggesting that although the lower GFR probably contributes to the increased excretion of free water in older subjects, the cause is more complex. Other contributing factors may include increases in medullary blood flow, decreases in countercurrent exchange efficiency (Rowe et al., 1976), and defects in solute transport from the tubular lumen to the medullary interstitium (Epstein, 1979).

Most investigations into the response of plasma vasopressin concentrations [AVP] (hormonal antidiuresis) of older subjects to fluid deprivation have shown older subjects to have the same or greater [AVP] than do younger controls before and after 24 h of water deprivation (Phillips et al., 1984a). A reduced renal responsiveness to circulating AVP has been proposed. However, a more recent study found just the opposite. After an overnight fast, older men had significantly higher plasma osmolalities than did younger men (294 vs 291 mOsmols/kg), yet plasma [AVP] was significantly lower (0.5 vs 2.3 pmol/L) (Faull et al., 1993). Such AVP levels in the older men would not be expected to achieve urine osmolalities greater than 400 mOsmols/kg. Because those subjects had urine osmolalities of >500 mOsmols/kg, this concentration was most likely caused by mechanisms other than those involving [AVP].

When low doses of AVP are infused in men and women over the age of 65, they respond normally (Lindeman et al., 1966); however, when higher doses are infused, maximum urine osmolality is significantly diminished (Miller & Shock, 1953).

Thirst. Under normal conditions, increased thirst and fluid intake defend against any threats to fluid homeostasis that may result from altered free-water clearance by the kidneys. Therefore, although an inadequate renal response to mild water deprivation may play a role in any fluid volume depletion occurring in older persons, reduced thirst is probably more important (Phillips et al., 1993). *Ad libitum* fluid intake can be directly measured, but thirst is typically assessed using visual-analog scales involving questions such as, "How thirsty do you feel now?". Care should be taken to ensure that older subjects interpret such scales and rate their thirst sensations in a manner similar to younger subjects.

After a 24-h period of restricted water intake that caused an equal weight loss in older and younger subjects, a group of healthy men 67–75 years old were less thirsty and replaced less of the fluid deficit over the next 2 h than did young controls (Figure 7-3A) (Phillips et al., 1984a). This initial finding of reduced thirst with advancing age has since been confirmed (Crowe et al., 1987; Mack et al., 1994; Phillips et al., 1991a) using various paradigms for inducing thirst and/or a water deficit. For example, Crowe et al. (1987) found that after young subjects ingested 20 mL/kg water loads, thirst was suppressed for 1–2 h and then increased progressively over the following 5–6 h, whether they were initially depleted or not. Conversely, water-replete older men (mean age = 72 y) showed no alteration in their thirst ratings over the entire 7 h following the water loads, despite clear indications that osmotic thirst stimulis had occurred. Such reduced thirst in older individuals seems to be due to a lower thirst sensitivity to hypertonicity because the thirst response of older men to a hypertonic infusion of saline without volume depletion is likewise blunted (Figure 7-3B) (Phillips et al., 1991a).

Voluntary fluid intake after dehydration is also influenced by non-thirst factors such as fluid availability and palatability. While thirst and intake are separate entities, they seem to be affected in parallel by age, and increasing the availability or palatability of fluids does not increase water deprivation-induced fluid intake in older men and women (Phillips et al., 1993). After two separate bouts of dehydration (fluid deprivation plus a dry diet), healthy older men were offered either water (or mineral water) or a variety of palatable beverages, including cola and orange juice (Phillips et al., 1991b). Orange juice was consumed in larger volumes on single occasions, suggesting a higher palatability, yet over 2 h there was no difference in fluid consumption between trials or beverages. Although these results imply that palatability alone is insufficient to overcome the reduced thirst, the tonicity of the fluid consumed may be important in the time course (Gisolfi et al., 1992) and effectiveness of rehydration (Phillips et al., 1993).

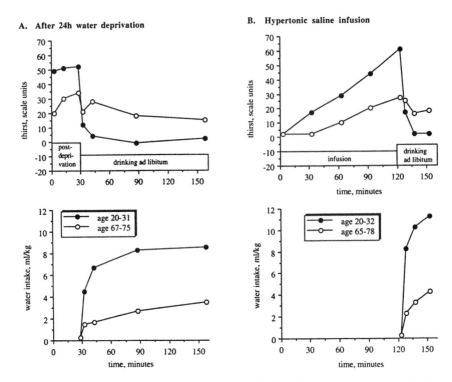

FIGURE 7-3. *Thirst perception and fluid intake of young and older subjects in response to two perturbations, 24 h of water deprivation (A) and venous infusion of hypertonic (5%) saline (B).* In each case, the thirst ratings and hydration response of the elderly group were blunted, compared to the young group. Redrawn from data published in Phillips et al. (1984a; panel A data) and Phillips et al. (1991a; panel B data).

Heat Exposure and Exercise

Like fluid deprivation, passive exposure to hot environments for prolonged periods and exercise in warm conditions also cause a hyperosmolar hypohydration. As with fluid deprivation, older men and women often respond with altered renal and thirst responses to these challenges to fluid homeostasis. Miescher & Fortney (1989) studied the thirst and rehydration responses of five older (61–67 y) and six younger (21–29 y) men during a 4-h resting exposure at 45°C, 25% rh. Only during the final hour were subjects allowed to drink water *ad libitum*. The older men responded with greater increases in rectal temperatures during the exposure, despite similar losses of body weight (~1.5%), suggesting similar sweating rates. During the rehydration phase, older men consumed similar volumes of water, with both groups replacing about half the fluid deficit. Men who drank both the greatest and the least amounts were in the older group;

because the sample size was so small, further conclusions are difficult to draw. However, the older men had a lower thirst rating despite chronically higher plasma osmolalities.

Recently, Mack et al. (1994) reexamined the question of osmotic control of thirst and free-water clearance in healthy older (>65) and younger (<28) men. In order to promote a greater degree of dehydration (~2.5% of body weight), the subjects exercised on a cycle ergometer in a hot (36°C) dry environment for 105 min. A 3-h rehydration period followed. During dehydration, the plasma osmolality threshold for increased thirst was elevated in the older men. During rehydration, less fluid was consumed by the older subjects; however, the relationship between fluid intake and thirst was unchanged (Figure 7-4). In addition, there was an attenuated renal response in the older subjects, i.e., production of a less concentrated urine during dehydration and a less dilute urine during rehydration.

Potential Contributing Factors

Drug Effects. The increased use of prescription medication compounds the deficient responses of older persons to mild dehydration (Levi & Rowe, 1992). Most sedatives and mild tranquilizers affect both thirst and the synthesis and release of AVP. Likewise, lithium and demeclocycline inhibit the action of AVP at the renal tubules. Finally, the use of osmotic diuretics for such conditions as hypertension or congestive heart failure needs to be carefully monitored to prevent hypohydration.

Fitness and Lifestyle Influences. While changes in thirst and renal function in response to dehydration seem to occur in healthy, medically screened older adults, the influence of low cardiorespiratory fitness and/or sedentary lifestyle has not been examined to any great extent. The group of 98 subjects studied by Rowe et al. (1976) included "active community-dwelling volunteers" who were rigorously screened for the presence of any diseases that could influence renal function, but their activity levels were not described.

The previously mentioned group of older subjects studied by Mack et al. (1994) reveals an unintended result. Subjects presented at the laboratory for that study after an overnight fast, at which time they demonstrated lower urine flows, higher urine osmolalities, and lower free-water clearances than did young controls. If one looks at the overnight fast not as a control period but as a perturbation similar to that imposed by Faull et al. (1993), the older men showed greater, rather than attenuated, responses. These men were described as "healthy, active" volunteers, although their average $\dot{V}O_2max$ of 21.7 mL·kg^{-1}·min^{-1} suggests that they were not highly fit. Although the authors concluded that the relative hypohydration of this group was chronic, a plausible alternate conclusion

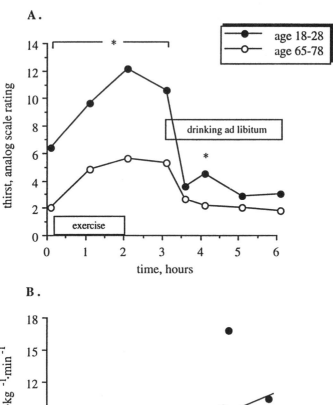

FIGURE 7-4. *(A) Subjective thirst ratings of young and older men during and after 105 min of exercise (60% $\dot{V}O_2 max$) in a warm (36°C) environment. The combination of exercise and high ambient temperature caused a 2.2–2.5% reduction in body weight in each group. (B) The relationship between the rate of fluid intake during the initial 30 min of rehydration after exercise and peak subjective thirst rating was unaffected by age.* Redrawn from Mack et al. (1994). An asterisk denotes a significant age-related difference (P<0.05).

might be that these older subjects responded more appropriately than did the young controls with respect to renal function (but not thirst!) after mild water deprivation.

When we tested groups of young (20–30-year-old) and middle-aged (49–60-year-old) men matched for $\dot{V}O_2$max and body composition, many, but not all, of the aforementioned age-associated differences disappeared. In one study (Kenney et al., 1990), responses to a 24-h fluid deprivation stimulus followed by an exercise-heat challenge were examined. All of these middle-aged men were highly fit, regular aerobic exercisers. In this case, there were no age differences in plasma osmolality, plasma electrolyte concentration, or urine osmolality before or after the 24-h deprivation period or after the heat test (48°C; 90 min rest, 30 min exercise, 60 min recovery with *ad libitum* water ingestion). Nor were there any differences in urine output or water consumption.

On the other hand, in a more recent study using similarly matched subject groups, we found a distinct failure of older (67 ± 1 y) men to concentrate their urine during a more prolonged exercise bout lasting 90 min (Bell et al., 1994). Urine osmolality and free-water clearance did not change in the older men because of their inability to reduce urine flow rate. It is not surprising, perhaps, that a greater challenge to homeostasis is needed for age-related sequelae to appear in fit older individuals.

AGE AND RESPONSE TO EXERCISE IN WARM ENVIRONMENTS

Dynamic exercise presents a multitude of challenges to the interactive regulatory processes that maintain homeostasis. Performance of the exercise in a warm environment adds significantly to those challenges. Delivery of oxygen to active muscle involves a local decrease in vascular resistance occurring primarily through locally mediated vasodilator mechanisms. This peripheral vasodilation in turn creates a challenge to blood flow delivery that is met by both increases in cardiac output (central mechanisms) and adjustments in vascular resistance in nonactive tissues (peripheral mechanisms). The mechanisms by which these challenges are met create another series of regulatory problems, including difficulties in regulation of blood pressure and core temperature. Despite the seeming immensity of these challenges to homeostasis, *in vivo* regulation is usually accomplished with a remarkably high degree of precision. The following section asks the question "How does chronologic age influence the various homeostatic mechanisms by which the body responds to dynamic exercise in the heat?".

Control of Skin Blood Flow

Humans respond physiologically to heat stress through two effector mechanisms: by dramatically increasing skin blood flow (SkBF) and by the production and subsequent evaporation of eccrine sweat. The former determines the rate at which heat is convected from the body core to the skin, whereas the latter accounts for the majority of the dissipation of that heat to the environment. Various aspects of the control of SkBF during exercise have been recently reviewed (Johnson, 1992; Kenney & Johnson, 1992). During exercise SkBF over most of the body is determined by a competition between vasoconstrictor and vasodilator influences. In fact, there is dual efferent neural control of SkBF—a noradrenergic vasoconstrictor system common to all regional circulations and a sympathetic vasodilator system. Although the precise mechanisms through which this latter system functions are not clearly understood, it is of major importance in the control of SkBF during exercise. Activation of this system can fully dilate cutaneous arterioles, increasing whole-body SkBF to levels approaching 8 L/min (Rowell, 1974).

The influence of age on control of SkBF may best be discussed within the context of the pattern of SkBF control during prolonged upright exercise. Under such conditions, particularly in warm environments, T_c does not usually reach an equilibrium but continues to increase. The competition between the skin and working muscle for a limited cardiac output is formidable. As soon as a characteristic threshold is surpassed, the increase in T_c is accompanied by a parallel steep rise in SkBF. However, SkBF does not increase without limit, and an attenuated rate of increase occurs above a T_c of about 38°C, such that an apparent upper limit to SkBF is reached (Brengelmann et al., 1977; Kenney et al., 1991, 1994; Nadel et al., 1979). If SkBF is plotted as a function of T_c during exercise, three distinct phases—threshold, steep rise, and attenuated rise—are seen.

Is chronologic age associated with an altered SkBF response during exercise in a hot environment? And if so, by what mechanism(s) does age exert this effect? In a series of studies (Kenney, 1988; Kenney & Anderson, 1988; Kenney et al., 1990, 1991; Tankersley et al., 1991), we compared the SkBF responses of older fit ($\dot{V}O_2$max = 45–50 mL·kg^{-1}·min^{-1}) healthy men and women aged 50–75 with a sample of 20–30-year-old subjects with similar physical and physiological characteristics. Contrary to earlier reports (e.g., Hellon & Lind, 1958), older individuals typically respond to exercise with less skin vasodilation than that exhibited by their younger counterparts. Although exercise intensity and ambient conditions differed among the studies, there was a consistent effect of age on the SkBF:T_c relationship, which is shown in Figure 7-5.

The threshold T_c for increasing SkBF is unchanged by age, but the slope of the relationship is decreased. A reasonable interpretation of this systematic change would be that age affects SkBF peripherally rather than centrally (i.e., at the hypothalamus) (after Nadel et al., 1971).

As in Figure 7-5, changes in forearm blood flow (FBF) measured with strain gauges have traditionally been used to assess changes in SkBF. Because the underlying assumptions for using FBF to assess SkBF have not been proven for older individuals, we reexamined temperature data from

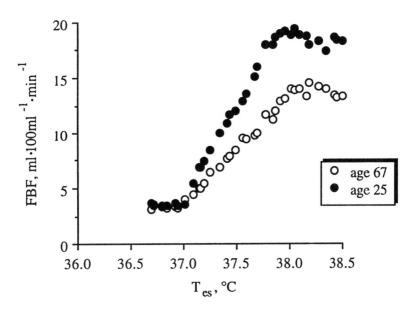

FIGURE 7-5. *Representative data from one young and one older subject tested by Kenney (1988).* Although there was no difference in the esophageal temperature (T_{es}) threshold for increased forearm blood flow (FBF), the slope of the response was consistently attenuated in the older subjects, as was the maximal FBF achieved.

the studies cited above, this time estimating whole-body SkBF from heat balance measurements (Kenney & Havenith, 1991). The estimated SkBFs for the respective older groups ranged from 24–40% lower than those for their matched young counterparts. It is obvious from these data that older men and women increase SkBF to a significantly smaller degree during combined exercise and heat stress than do younger men. Although the mean SkBF response across a group of older subjects is lower than that for a fitness-matched group of young subjects, the range of responses within the older group is typically larger. In our subject samples, a few men over the age of 65 exhibited fairly high levels of SkBF; however, several others had severe limitations to increasing SkBF during a heat challenge, rarely exceeding a FBF of 10–12 mL·100 mL^{-1}·min^{-1}. (FBF for young subjects under similar conditions is typically 20–25 mL·100 mL^{-1}·min^{-1}.)

As discussed above, evidence (e.g., Phillips et al., 1984a) has suggested that aging is accompanied by changes in both thirst and renal function that ultimately lead to a state of hyperosmolar hypohydration. Because hypovolemia and hypertonicity of the blood can each cause a reduced SkBF (Fortney et al., 1981, 1984; Nadel et al., 1980), we manipulated fluid intake to determine if hypohydration and age were independent factors controlling SkBF during a heat challenge (Kenney et al., 1990). Eighteen hours of water deprivation induced a hyperosmolar hypohydration in each group similar to that reported for free-living older subjects (Miescher & Fortney, 1989). Regardless of hydration state, FBF was lower during exercise in the heat in the older subjects. The effects of age were independent from those of the induced hypohydration, suggesting that the age effects on SkBF are not artifactual hydration effects.

An alternate hypothesis might be that an increased sympathetic (noradrenergic) vasoconstrictor tone may limit heat-induced skin vasodilation in older individuals. Vasoconstrictor tone in humans is mediated through α-noradrenergic sympathetic pathways. If older individuals have an exaggerated α-noradrenergic vasoconstriction that limits dilation, blocking the constrictor system should lead to a "normalization" of their SkBF response, i.e., it should become more like that of younger individuals. When we systemically blocked α-receptors with the selective α_1-antagonist prazosin, there was no selective effect of the drug on the SkBF response of older men (Kenney et al., 1991).

Because structural changes that are independent of aerobic fitness occur in aging skin, the most plausible explanation for the lower skin vasodilation with age is that structural changes within the cutaneous vessels limit the extent of vasodilation. The magnitude of maximal vasodilation that can be elicited by prolonged local heating of the forearm appears to be diminished in older men (Rooke et al., 1994), an effect that appears to decline fairly linearly between the ages of 20 and 80 y (Martin & Kenney, unpublished data).

Cardiac Output and Its Distribution

Cardiac Output and Age. Whether or not exercise cardiac output ($\dot{Q}$) declines with age is extremely controversial, and there is abundant evidence for both opinions in the literature. This topic is confounded by differences in exercise intensity (relative versus absolute), subject screening for underlying diseases, subject fitness level and training status, and the method used to measure $\dot{Q}$. During submaximal exercise, $\dot{Q}$ has been reported to be lower (McElvaney et al., 1989; Ogawa et al., 1992; Strandel, 1964), similar (Fleg, 1986; Hagberg et al., 1985), and even higher (Becklake et al., 1965; Kanstrup & Ekblom, 1978) in older subjects than in young subjects.

A unifying hypothesis may lie in the reported mechanisms that account for age-related differences (or nondifferences in some cases) in $\dot{Q}$ with advanced age. Gerstenblith, Lakatta, and their colleagues have suggested that during exercise, the mechanisms through which older subjects achieve high cardiac outputs shift from dependence on catecholamine-mediated increases in heart rate and inotropy to greater reliance on the Frank-Starling mechanism (Gerstenblith et al., 1987; Lakatta, 1986; Schulman et al., 1992). Left ventricular diastolic filling declines with age, with older men showing lower peak filling rates at rest, at 50% $\dot{V}O_2$max, and at maximal exercise intensities (Schulman et al., 1992). This decline is not secondary to a lower $\dot{V}O_2$max but rather is related to a decrease in β-adrenergic responsiveness (Schulman et al., 1992). Under conditions in which venous return and ventricular filling would be expected to be compromised, one might expect that older subjects would be less able to compensate for lower filling rates by sympathetic means. This would explain why lower stroke volumes and cardiac outputs are seen in older men 1) during upright, but not supine, exercise (Fagard & Staessen, 1991) and 2) when skin venous pooling is augmented by the imposition of an additional heat stress (Kenney, 1988).

In addition, some data suggest that age-related changes in Q may be gender-specific (Hossack & Bruce, 1982; Spina et al., 1993). Only one study has reported exercise Q in both older and younger individuals during exercise in a warm environment (Kenney, 1988). Older (55–68 y) and younger (19–30 y) men (n = 4) and women (n = 8), matched for $\dot{V}O_2$max, exercised at a low intensity (40% $\dot{V}O_2$max) at 37°C ambient temperature. The 55–68-year-old subjects had significantly lower Qs than did younger subjects, even though they were exercising at the same absolute workload and percentage of $\dot{V}O_2$max. When we recently repeated those measures on a group of male subjects (unpublished data), those age differences in Q disappeared. The women in the 1988 study were all postmenopausal, and none was taking estrogen replacement therapy. The possibility that the lack of cyclic estrogen influences may influence cardiac function deserves attention in future studies.

Regional Blood Flow. Although increasing cardiac output helps meet the dual demand for increased blood flow to working muscle and to the skin, there is a limited ability for cardiac output to increase as central filling pressure falls. An additional circulatory adjustment during dynamic exercise in the heat is the sympathetically mediated redistribution of blood flow away from visceral organs, such as the liver and kidneys, to augment perfusion of skin and active muscle vascular beds (Figure 7-6). Diversion of blood from these two regions allows for a redistribution of 800 mL/min or more to the skin circulation (Rowell, 1974, 1986).

We recently compared the renal blood flow (RBF) responses of 60–70-year-old and 20–30-year-old men before, during, and after a bout of exercise in a warm (30°C) environment (Kenney & Zappe, 1994). To better determine the effects of chronological age (i.e., to minimize the effects of confounding variables), the distinct age groups were matched with respect to body size, adiposity, and $\dot{V}O_2$max. Baseline data were collected for a full day, and exercise tests were performed twice, on the first and fourth days of a heat acclimation protocol.

Baseline RBF was 21% lower for the 60–70-year-old group (753 ± 116 mL/min versus 959 ± 104 mL/min) (Figure 7-7). Such age-associated reductions in RBF at rest are well documented (Davies & Shock, 1950;

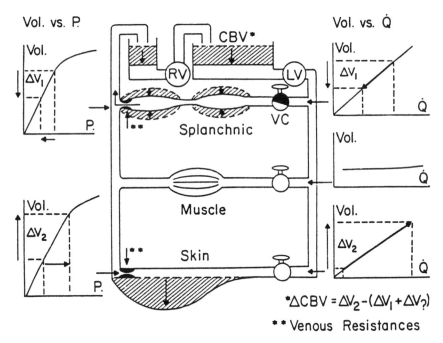

Vol. vs. P

CBV*

Vol. vs. Q̇

Splanchnic

Muscle

Skin

VC

RV   LV

*ΔCBV = ΔV₂-(ΔV₁+ΔV?)

$$^*\Delta CBV = \Delta V_2 - (\Delta V_1 + \Delta V_?)$$

** Venous Resistances

FIGURE 7-6. *Schematic illustration of how the cardiovascular system compensates for the high skin blood flows that accompany exercise in hot environments.* Blood flow increases to both active muscle and skin vaculature. Splanchnic and skin circulations are highly compliant, as shown in the plots of volume (Vol.) versus pressure (P.) on the left, whereas muscle beds are relatively non-compliant due to mechanical influences. The panels on the right show the relationships between volume (Vol.) and flow (Q̇). Skin vasodilation reduces the blood volume available for right ventricular (RV) filling, and central venous pressure falls. Left ventricular (LV) output can be maintained only by depleting the preventricular sump (CBV). Partial compensation is achieved by vasoconstriction (VC) of renal (not shown) and splanchnic beds. From Rowell (1983) with permission.

Watkin & Shock, 1955). During exercise at 50% $\dot{V}O_2$max, RBF decreased to a significantly greater extent in the 20–30-year-old group on each exercise day, decreasing by 508 and 365 mL/min during exercise on days 1 and 4 (reductions of 45% and 36%, respectively). For the 60–70-year-old subjects, the RBF decreases were only 98 (12%) and 83 (12%) mL/min on each of the two days. During recovery, RBF increased in the younger men but decreased below exercise levels in the older men (Figure 7-7). In both groups, the recovery RBF (averaged over 150 min) remained significantly below pre-exercise values (P<0.05).

There was no significant effect of age on plasma norepinephrine concentration ([NE]) at any time, although the mean [NE] of the older group during exercise was 20–25% lower than that of the young men during exercise. When the reduction in RBF was plotted against surrogate measures of sympathetic activity (HR or [NE]), data from both groups fell

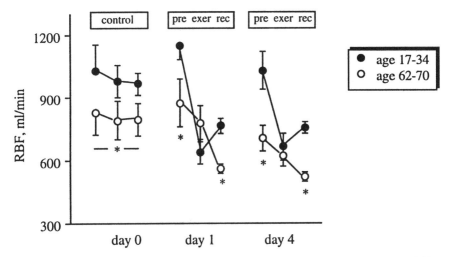

FIGURE 7-7. *Renal blood flow (measured by para-aminohippurate clearance) of young (filled circles) and older (open circles) men (n = 6 per group) on a control day (no exercise, day 0), and on the first and fourth days of exercise in a warm environment.* On each day, data collected at several time points were pooled to reflect average values before exercise (pre), over 90 min of exercise at 50% $\dot{V}O_2$max (exer), and through 2.5 h of recovery (rec). Bars represent 1 SEM. An asterisk denotes a significant age difference (P<0.05).

along a single line, suggesting that sympathetic control of RBF is not altered by age. Rather, the lesser redistribution of blood flow from the kidneys results merely from the age difference in resting RBF "reserve." During sustained exercise, the ability to redistribute 350–500 mL/min of flow to the skin is a relatively small contribution (Zambraski, 1990), yet coupled with splanchnic vasoconstriction (Rowell et al., 1965), approximately 1 L·min^{-1} of cardiac output may be redistributed. This may be of important consequence for older patients with left ventricular dysfunction and thus a limited ability to increase cardiac output.

Unpublished data from our laboratory show that control of splanchnic blood flow (SBF, measured by indocyanine green dilution) during exercise is not altered by age at low workloads provided that the older subjects have high $\dot{V}O_2$max levels. Unlike the kidneys, however, there is no age difference in resting SBF. Age differences in the redistribution of splanchnic blood flow are deserving of further study.

Sweat Gland Function

More so than any other species, humans rely to a large degree on the ability to activate eccrine sweat glands and the subsequent ability of those glands to produce and secrete sweat onto the skin surface in order to regulate body temperature under heat stress conditions. Because myriad factors affect whole-body sweating and evaporative rates in humans, a basic question to be considered is whether or not aging alters the eccrine gland response to a standardized stimulus. Isolated eccrine glands can be excised and stimulated in vitro (e.g., Sato & Sato, 1983), or cholinergic analogs such as methylcholine (MCh) or pilocarpine can be injected intradermally or induced via iontophoresis.

There is a large interindividual variability in the sweat gland responses to such sudorific stimuli; however, some clear effects of aging are evident. Local sweating rates are lower in older subjects for a given pharmacological stimulus, an effect that can be attributed to a smaller sweat output per activated gland (Ellis et al., 1976; Kenney & Fowler, 1988; Sato & Timm, 1988; Silver et al., 1964). The density of active eccrine glands is unaffected by age. The same pattern, i.e., similar active gland densities but lower gland outputs, has also been shown for heat-activated sweat glands during exercise in dry heat (Anderson & Kenney, 1987).

When do these changes occur? Sato (1993) has stated, "Aging has very little effect on the pharmacologically induced maximal sweat rate until the 60s, but glandular function gradually declines in the 70s and 80s." This seems to be an oversimplification for several reasons. In the subjects tested by Ellis et al. (1976), there was a distinct age difference in MCh-induced sweating. (These subjects were drawn at random from a hospitalized population.) However, the authors noted that in the older subjects who exhibited higher sweat outputs, ". . . the texture and appearance of the skin . . . appeared more youthful and elastic and less wrinkled to the naked eye than of those whose sweat response was poor or absent." Thus, local skin aging, perhaps as a result of lifetime exposure to ultraviolet radiation, may play a role.

We injected various concentrations of MCh intradermally in three age groups of fit, heat-acclimated men (aged 22–24 y, 33–40 y, and 58–67 y) (Kenney & Fowler, 1988). Their respective mean sweat gland productions at each concentration are shown in Figure 7-8. Although only the oldest and youngest group responses differed significantly, it is interesting that the 33–40-year-old group exhibited sweat outputs that were intermediate in each case, suggesting perhaps a continuous decline throughout adulthood. These data also strongly suggest that this decrement is not a function of a decreased $\dot{V}O_2$max or differing body size or composition, as subject groups were matched for these characteristics and were rigorously heat acclimated.

Failure to take into account heat acclimation, whether natural or artificial, can lead to erroneous conclusions. For example, one study reported that old and young men matched for $\dot{V}O_2$max had similar sweating rates in response to pilocarpine iontophoresis; however, these results were confounded by comparing an older group of men who were actively training (4 h of vigorous exercise per week for the previous 23 y!) with a young sedentary group (Buono et al., 1991). Sweat glands can even undergo "lo-

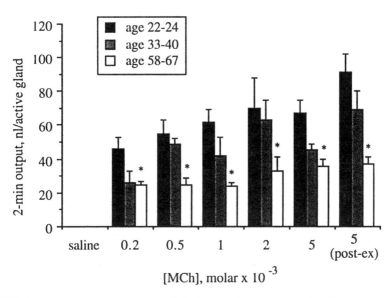

FIGURE 7-8. *Mean sweat output per activated gland, measured 2 min after intradermal injection of various concentrations of acetyl-β-methylcholine chloride (MCh) in three age groups of fit, heat-acclimated men (n = 5 per group).* Bars represent 1 SEM. While only the oldest and youngest group responses differed significantly, the 33–40-year-old group exhibited sweat outputs that were intermediate at each concentration of MCh, suggesting a continuous decline throughout adulthood. Redrawn from Kenney & Fowler (1988).

cal training" by repeatedly immersing the skin in hot water. When such a protocol is performed, older individuals increase local sweat production, but to a lesser degree than do young men and women (Ogawa & Ohnishi, 1989).

There is good evidence that there are regional differences in sweat gland function between older and younger persons. Foster et al. (1976) demonstrated that forehead and limb sweating was more reduced by age than was trunk sweating in response to MCh injection. The same was true during passive heating (legs and feet in a warm water bath while sitting at 35°C), i.e., an age difference was noted on the thighs, but not on the back (Inoue et al., 1991). In each case, gland output was lower in older men at peripheral sites, but not at central locations. A logical hypothesis may be that glandular function declines in a peripheral-to-central direction as skin ages.

Sweating Responses

The age-related deficit in drug- or heat-activated sweat gland function described above does not necessarily translate into lower local or whole-body sweating rates during heating or exercise. Sweating rate depends not only on physiological factors but also on environmental influ-

TABLE 7-2. *Results of studies examining the effects of age on sweating responses, 1956–1994.* ↓ implies a significantly lower response in older subjects; NS implies no significant age-related difference.

Reference	T_a, rh	$\dot{V}O_2$max similar?	Accli- mated?	Rest or Exercise	Sweating Rate	Sweating Onset	Sweating Slope
Anderson & Kenney, 1987	48°, 15%	Y	Y	E(40%)	↓	-	-
Armstrong & Kenney, 1993	46°, 11%	Y	both	R	↓peak	NS	NS
Cable & Green, 1990	22°, 50%	N	N	E/R	↓	-	-
Crowe & Moore, 1973	30°[1]	N	N	R	-	↓	-
Drinkwater & Horvath, 1979	35°, 60%	N	N	E (35%)	↓	-	-
	48°, 10%				↓	-	-
Drinkwater et al., 1982	40°, 40%	N	N	R	NS	NS	NS
Fennell & Moore, 1973	27°[1]	N	N	R	-	-	-
Hellon & Lind, 1956	38°, 60%	N	N	R	NS	↓	NS
Hellon et al., 1956	38°, 55%	N	N	E/R	NS[2]	-	-
Inoue et al., 1991	35°[3]	N	N	R	NS	↓	-
		N	Y		↓	↓	-
Kenney, 1988	37°, 60%	Y	N	E (40%)	NS	-	-
Kenney & Anderson, 1988	37°, 60%	Y	Y	E (40%)	NS	-	-
Kenney et al., 1990	48°, 15%	Y	N	E (43%)	NS	-	-
Lind et al., 1970	various	N	N	E/R	NS[2]	-	-
Mack et al., 1994	36°, 30%	N	N	E (60%)	NS	-	-
Miescher & Fortney, 1989	45°, 25%	N	N	R	NS	-	-
Pandolf et al., 1988	49°, 20%	Y	both	E (45%)	NS	NS	NS
Robinson et al., 1965[4]	40°, 20%	N	both	E	↓	-	-
Sagawa et al.,1988	40°, 40%	N	N	R	NS	NS	-
Shoenfeld et al., 1978	90°, 4%	N	N	R	↓	-	-
Smolander et al., 1990	30°, 80%	Y	N	E (30%)	NS	NS	NS
	40°, 20%				NS	-	↓
Tankersley et al., 1991	30°, 55%	N	N	E (68%)	↓	NS	↓
		Y	N		NS	NS	NS
Wagner et al. , 1972	49°, 15%	N	both	E	↓	-	-
Yousef et al., 1984	desert	N	N	E (40%)	NS	-	-

[1] plus hand in hot water bath
[2] ↓ during work, ↑ during rest
[3] plus legs in hot water bath
[4] longitudinal comparison of 4 men

ences. Table 7-2 provides summary data from 24 published studies over the past 39 y that compared sweating rates and/or local sweating characteristics in young and older subjects. Most studies reported no significant age-related difference in sweating. In many of the studies that did report significantly lower sweating responses, two conclusions may be drawn: 1) as is the case with skin blood flow, $\dot{V}O_2$max and heat acclimation are more important in determining sweating rate than is age, and 2) peak sweating rates may be lower in older men and women, although very large interindividual variability exists. Such potential differences may be masked by environmental influences, among other factors.

Heat Storage and Body Temperature

Contradictions in the literature about whether or not older subjects are relatively less "heat tolerant" than young subjects can for the most part be easily resolved by controlling for differences in $\dot{V}O_2$max. Older literature demonstrated a decreased work-heat tolerance (greater physiological strain) in older men and women (Drinkwater & Horvath, 1979; Hellon et al., 1956; Hellon & Lind, 1956; Wagner et al., 1972). This conclusion is still valid for the general population of older men and women, whose lower $\dot{V}O_2$max on average predetermines that a given absolute work intensity comprises a greater percentage of their maximal capacities. However, when old and young subjects are matched for $\dot{V}O_2$max and can, therefore, exercise at the same absolute and relative intensities, there are seldom differences in either T_c or calculated heat storage (Kenney, 1988; Kenney et al., 1990, 1991; Pandolf et al., 1988; Tankersley et al., 1991). The one exception to this conclusion from our laboratory was also the only study in which women comprised the sample of subjects tested (Kenney & Anderson, 1988). A group of postmenopausal women (52–62 y) not taking estrogen was matched for $\dot{V}O_2$max with younger women and exercised without fluid replacement at 35–40% $\dot{V}O_2$max in both a warm humid environment (37°C, 60% rh) and a hot dry environment (48°C, 15% rh). In each environment, the older women responded with greater rates of rise in core temperature during exercise.

Havenith and colleagues have applied a novel approach to determine the relative influences of various individual characteristics on heat strain. Rather than matching subject groups that differ in only one characteristic (such as age), this methodology involves testing a large number of heterogeneous subjects and using multiple regression analyses to determine the influence of various individual characteristics on a dependent response of interest (Havenith & van Middendorp, 1990). We applied this methodology to determine the relative influences of several independent variables, i.e., age, adiposity, and $\dot{V}O_2$max, on the dependent variables, rectal temperature (T_{re}) and heat storage (S), during 1 h of low-intensity (60 W), steady-state, cycle exercise in a warm (35°C) environment (Havenith et al., 1995). Fifty-six subjects, aged 20–73, were selected; there was no correlation between age and $\dot{V}O_2$max in this group, but there were large ranges of values in both age and $\dot{V}O_2$max. Final T_{re} and S were both significantly correlated with $\dot{V}O_2$max. After inclusion of the $\dot{V}O_2$max effect into the prediction models, neither age nor adiposity had a significant influence. We concluded that when natural variation in physical fitness is introduced in a test population, the age effect appears to be relatively negligible.

Thus, despite clear influences of age on the control of sweat gland function and SkBF, it is debatable whether or not age-related differences (which tend to be peripheral in nature) have much importance with regard to the control of body temperature during exercise. The impact of hypovolemia on thermoregulation may provide a close analogy. During exercise in a hypovolemic state, T_c increases; therefore, the core-to-skin temperature gradient increases. Because overall core-to-skin heat transfer is a product of: 1) SkBF, 2) this gradient, and 3) the specific heat of the blood, the lower SkBF under such conditions is offset by the larger thermal gradient. In hypovolemic subjects, a 30% lower maximal SkBF creates a difference in heat transfer of less than 10% (Nadel, 1986). It is, therefore, interesting to also note that the relatively lower SkBF levels in the fit, healthy, older subjects mentioned above do not typically translate into greater heat storage or poorer heat tolerance. In the case of SkBF, the maintenance of lower mean skin temperatures by older subjects facilitates a similar rate of convective heat transfer from core-to-skin because the thermal gradient is larger (Kenney & Havenith, 1993).

Control of Plasma Volume

Resting plasma volume (PV) is not fixed for an individual but rather is influenced by a variety of factors, including body size, lean body mass, chronic diseases, physical activity and trained state, heat acclimation, and hydration status. Therefore, it is not surprising that there is disagreement in the literature as to whether older men and women have similar or lower plasma volumes than do younger persons of the same gender. Three recent studies have used the Evan's blue dye-dilution technique to measure PV in older and younger men. In an unmatched but healthy active group of men, Mack et al. (1994) saw significantly lower plasma volumes in subjects older than 65 y (43 ± 2 mL/kg) versus those younger than 30 y (48 ± 3 mL/kg). When Davy and Seals (1994) matched men in their 60s with men in their 20s on the basis of regular daily physical activity, a similar difference was noted (50 ± 2 versus 39 ± 2 mL/kg). A requirement for inclusion in that study was that subjects be physically untrained. When Bell (1993) matched older and younger subjects for $\dot{V}O_2$max rather than for activity, such differences disappeared, and older subjects actually had slightly but nonsignificantly higher plasma volumes (48 ± 2 versus 43 ± 3 mL/kg). Standardizing for lean body mass rather than body weight does not account for the differences among studies, although the loss of lean body mass which typically accompanies aging certainly strongly influences PV. It is proposed that, like many other factors affecting thermoregulation, PV is probably only secondarily influenced by age and is more strongly influenced by physical activity and $\dot{V}O_2$max.

During exercise, fluid is shifted from the vascular space into the extravascular compartment. The magnitude of this translocation is determined by Frank-Starling forces (primarily hydrostatic and oncotic pressure gradients), which are, in turn, a function of exercise intensity, ambient conditions, posture, and other factors associated with dynamic exercise (Harrison, 1985). A greater loss of plasma volume is associated with greater increases in T_c, a relative tachycardia, and hypotension during exercise in hot environments.

Some authors have also suggested in recent years that control of plasma volume may be more labile in older exercising subjects. However, a thorough review of the data in this area makes it difficult to support the contention that age is associated with greater losses of plasma volume (ΔPV) during exercise. That is not to say that this may not be true for a given set of conditions, because significantly greater shifts of fluid out of the vascular compartment in older subjects have been noted. Rather, those findings simply are not universal. Miescher & Fortney (1989) saw larger protein and fluid losses in older versus younger men during 3 h of passive heating, losses that took longer to restore when drinking was initiated. Mack et al. (1994), on the other hand, noted no age difference in ΔPV during prolonged exercise in the heat. Results from our own studies have been mixed. In one set of studies, we noted that older women demonstrated significantly larger ΔPV during exercise in warm humid, but not in hot dry, conditions (Kenney & Anderson, 1988). In another, age was associated with a larger loss of PV when subjects were well hydrated, but the age difference disappeared if the same men were hypohydrated (Kenney et al., 1990).

At present, no conclusions can be drawn about control of intravascular fluid volume during exercise with aging. More systematic investigations, perhaps focusing on age differences in intravascular protein (Kenney et al., 1990) and protein translocation, are necessary before a clear hypothesis can be stated.

EXERCISE TRAINING AND HEAT ACCLIMATION IN OLDER ADULTS

The distinct effects of endurance exercise training versus heat acclimation on the control of body temperature and body fluid balance have not been completely studied, even in young subjects. Part of this problem stems from the difficulty in separating the two. The attainment of a fully acclimated state necessitates performance of exercise in a warm environment. Passive exposure, as in a sauna or steam room, conveys some, but not all, of the benefits of repeated exercise in the heat. Conversely, exercise training involves the regular elevation of body temperature and sweating, which serves to partially acclimate the individual even if exercise is performed in a cool environment.[4] There is a dearth of exercise training studies in the literature involving men and women over the age of 65 or 70, and fewer yet that have examined the control of body temperature and fluids before and after a training regimen.

Exercise Training Effects on Thermoregulation

Regular exercise training appears to positively alter thermoregulatory effector (SkBF and sweating) responses to exercise in the heat. Roberts et al. (1977) trained eight young subjects 1 h/d for 10 d at 75% $\dot{V}O_2$max to examine the effects of such an acute training regimen on both sweating and SkBF. Training, which increased $\dot{V}O_2$max by 12%, resulted in a higher local sweating rate on the chest and a higher SkBF at a given T_c because training lowered the thresholds for the onset of sweating and skin vasodilation. The slope of the relationship between chest sweating rate and T_c was only slightly increased with training and that for SkBF versus T_c was unaffected. As reviewed above, age appears to adversely affect SkBF and, to a lesser degree, sweating during exercise in the heat. Because of the lack of good exercise training studies performed with older subjects, one might pose the question "Can older subjects who maintain a high $\dot{V}O_2$max via regular exercise offset these decrements in SkBF and sweating?".

Tankersley et al. (1991) addressed this question by recruiting three groups of subjects who differed in age and $\dot{V}O_2$max in the following way. A group of 13 older (O) men (58–74 y) was recruited, seven of whom were senior athletes with high values for $\dot{V}O_2$max relative to their age group (HO). Each of the remaining six older subjects had a normal $\dot{V}O_2$max for his age (NO). Also tested were seven young men (Y) who were well matched with the HO for $\dot{V}O_2$max and well matched with the NO for training status, i.e., active but not trained. Each subject performed a 20-min exercise bout at 65–70% $\dot{V}O_2$max in a warm (30°C) environment. Results are shown in Figure 7-9. Although significant differences in FBF and sweating rate (SR) were noted between only the Y and NO groups, the HO group demonstrated responses that were intermediate, somewhat lower than those of the Y but higher than those of the NO. It follows from these data that regular exercise training in older subjects may help offset the age-related decline in heat loss function.

Although no true longitudinal training studies have been conducted with subjects past the age of 65, the aforementioned work by Havenith et al. (1995) supports the conclusions of Tankersley et al. (1991). Inclusion of $\dot{V}O_2$max into regression models eliminated age as a significant predictor of core temperature. On the other hand, FBF and forearm vascular conductance (FVC = FBF standardized for mean arterial pressure) were significantly related to both age (y) and $\dot{V}O_2$max (mL·kg^{-1}·min^{-1}), according to the following equations:

FBF $= 8.4 - 0.17$ age $+ 0.35 \ \dot{V}O_2$max, and
FVC $= 7.7 - 0.3$ age $+ 0.5 \ \dot{V}O_2$max.

Weight loss due to sweating was a function of fitness-related variables only.

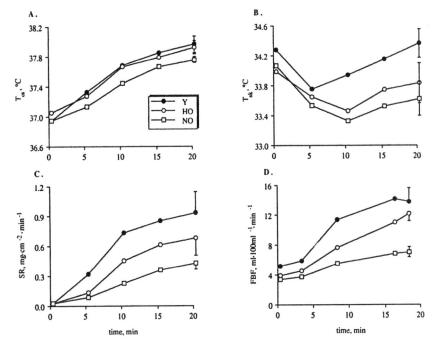

FIGURE 7-9. *Esophageal temperature (A), mean skin temperature (B), chest sweating rate (C), and forearm blood flow (D) responses of three groups of subjects who differed in age and $\dot{V}O_2max$.* The high-fit older (HO) group consisted of seven senior athletes with high $\dot{V}O_2max$ levels relative to their ages, whereas the normally fit older (NO) subjects had normal $\dot{V}O_2max$ levels for their ages. The young men (Y) were well matched with the HO for $\dot{V}O_2max$ and well matched with the NO for training status, i.e., active but not trained. Each subject performed a 20-min exercise bout at 65–70% $\dot{V}O_2max$ in a warm (30°C) environment. Significant differences in FBF and SR were noted only between the Y and NO groups; the HO group demonstrated responses that were intermediate. Each data point is the group mean ± *SEM*. Redrawn from Tankersley et al. (1991).

Heat Acclimation and Age

In the 1960s, Robinson et al. (1965) published a more or less longitudinal account of the ability to acclimatize to the heat. Four men aged 44–60 "acclimatized about as well" during repeated work at 40°C, 25% rh as they had 21 y earlier. Yousef et al. (1984) and Pandolf et al. (1988) each confirmed the ability of middle-aged men to acclimate to repeated exercise-heat exposures. In the latter study, middle-aged men (mean age = 46 y) actually responded with less strain than men aged 21 y during the first several exposures, an advantage apparently conferred by their greater weekly aerobic activity (subjects were matched for $\dot{V}O_2max$). This advantage was negated by the heat acclimation because the younger men had similar responses after the initial few days.

Early studies involving young subjects (e.g., Hellon & Lind, 1958) and the effects of heat acclimation reported lower SkBF after acclimation. However, these lower blood flows were apparently the result of lower core and skin temperatures for a given exercise intensity. Similar to training-induced adaptations, heat acclimation leads to a higher SkBF for a given T_c via a threshold change (Hessemer et al., 1986; Roberts et al., 1977) in young subjects. Furthermore, this adaptation can occur without any increase in $\dot{V}O_2$max (Roberts et al., 1977). Because an acute hypervolemia fails to significantly alter SkBF (Nadel et al., 1980), this increased SkBF may be independent of the expansion of blood volume that accompanies both exercise training and heat acclimation (as noted by Fortney et al., 1981), but the exact mechanism is unknown.

We recently published data that show that heat acclimation confers similar effects on SkBF and local sweating in young and older men during 90 min of passive heating (60 min progressive increase in air temperature from 28°C to 46°C, followed by sustained heating at 46°C for 30 min) (Armstrong & Kenney, 1993). After a 9-d active heat acclimation period, both older (61 ± 1 y) and younger (26 ± 2 y) men demonstrated similar reductions in baseline rectal and mean body temperatures. There was, in both age groups, a greater effector response at a given T_c, resulting from a threshold shift. Although acclimation increased sweating rate in both groups, the older men had significantly lower sweating rates on the chest before and after acclimation.

THE POSTMENOPAUSAL WOMAN

No chapter on the physiology of aging would be complete without mention of menopause, a concomitant of the aging process that occurs in more than half the population. Because thermoregulatory function and body fluid balance are both altered by menstrual cycle phase, it is not surprising that the cessation of regular hormonal cycling causes sometimes profound effects on the control of body temperature and fluids. There is a vast literature dealing with the causes, physiology, and treatment of vasomotor ("hot flashes") and sudomotor ("night sweats") instability during menopause. Although these symptoms reflect a thermoregulatory manifestation secondary to this change in hormonal control, little is known about changes in baseline temperature regulation or in thermoregulatory control during exercise in perimenopausal and postmenopausal women.

Estrogen Replacement Therapy

The effects of therapeutic estrogen replacement therapy (ERT) on thermoregulation have not been systematically examined. In young eumenorrheic women, an elevated progesterone concentration has been implicated in the post-ovulatory rise in body temperature, but potential roles for estrogens in thermoregulation have been ignored for the most part. Exogenous estrogen (17β-estradiol, E_2) administration causes the conservation of water and electrolytes in women (Aitken et al., 1974; Blahd et al., 1974), resulting in a significant hemodilution and expansion of plasma volume (Whitten & Bradbury, 1951). Although E_2 increases the firing rates of warm-sensitive neurons in the preoptic anterior hypothalamus in rats (Silva & Boulant, 1986), which should stimulate heat loss responses, no similar evidence exists in humans.

We tested a small group of postmenopausal women before and after 14–23 d of ERT (Tankersley et al., 1992). The daily dosage of E_2 administered was sufficient to significantly increase plasma E_2 concentrations without affecting progesterone levels. Core temperature was consistently ~0.5°C lower after ERT, both at rest under well-controlled conditions and during exercise in a warm environment. There was no change in resting or exercise $\dot{V}O_2$, but FBF and local sweating were higher at any given T_c (Figure 7-10). Furthermore, exercise heart rate was significantly lower after ERT, the probable consequence of an isotonic hemodilution. Thus, both thermoregulatory and cardiovascular strain experienced during heat and exercise stress seem to be reduced by acute ERT. Whether these are transient effects or whether continued ERT maintains these advantages is currently under investigation.

In light of the foregoing discussion, it is interesting to revisit the fact that we have seen age-related differences in thermoregulatory responses in only one study in which older and younger subjects are matched for $\dot{V}O_2$max. The older subjects in that study (Kenney & Anderson, 1988)— eight 52–62-year-old postmenopausal women—were not given ERT.

AGE AND RESPONSE TO COLD ENVIRONMENTS

Compared to the relatively voluminous literature on age and heat stress, there have been few studies on the effect of age on physiological responses to cold. In general, reports contending that older men and women demonstrate a relative inability to maintain their body temperatures when exposed to cold conditions (Collins et al., 1977; Fox et al., 1973; Horvath & Rochelle, 1977; Lybarger & Kilbourne, 1985; Yousef & Golding, 1989) far exceed those that have shown no age effect (Bernstein et al., 1956; Wagner & Horvath, 1985). However, it has been suggested that age may be a secondary factor in determining tolerance to cold.

There is a notable gender difference in laboratory investigations involving passive exposure to cold. Older women are often able to maintain body temperatures as well as younger women—and better so than older men—during cold exposure (Bernstein et al., 1956; Wagner & Horvath, 1985). These results have been interpreted to imply that differences in body size and adiposity (specifically, subcutaneous fat thickness and dis-

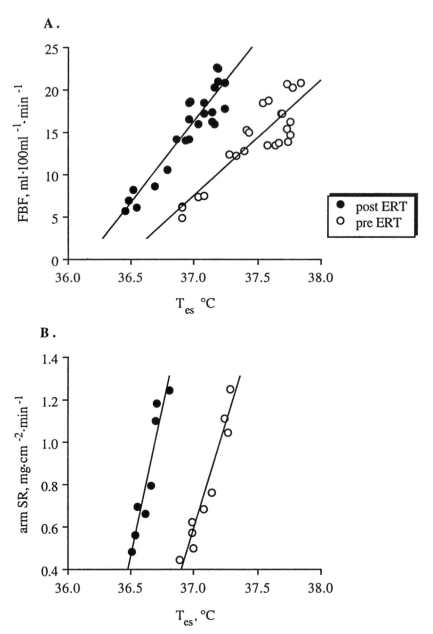

FIGURE 7-10. *The effects of acute estrogen replacement therapy (ERT) on control of (A) forearm blood flow and (B) arm sweating rate.* Data from one representative woman are shown from an exercise test (cycle exercise at 40% VO$_2$max, 25°C ambient temperature) performed before and 23 d after beginning ERT. ERT shifted the esophageal temperature (T$_{es}$) threshold for both effector responses to a lower core temperature without affecting the slope of the response. Redrawn from Tankersley et al. (1992).

tribution) may play a larger role than does chronological age in determining core temperature responses to cold. In one of the few studies to match subject groups for surface area-to-mass ratio, Wagner et al. (1974) saw no age difference in the rectal temperature response of men who sat for 30 min at 17°C. No body composition data were reported in that study; however, two studies comparing older and younger women support the aforementioned interpretation. Bernstein et al. (1956) reported no age difference in the rectal temperature response to 3 h of rest in a cool (17°C) room. A later study (Wagner & Horvath, 1985) reported that older women (average age of 61 y) were able to maintain T_c during 2 h at 10°C, whereas the T_c of 21-year-old women dropped slightly. In both of these studies, the older women had higher percentages of body fat and smaller surface area-to-mass ratios than did the young women.

On the other hand, recent evidence shows that aerobic fitness has little effect on the T_c drop at rest and during low-intensity exercise in the cold (Falk et al., 1994). In that study, neither age nor $\dot{V}O_2max$ had an effect on thermal comfort or cold sensation at 5°C. However, T_{re} dropped faster in 55–70-year-old men than in men in their 20s, regardless of $\dot{V}O_2max$.

DIRECTIONS FOR FUTURE RESEARCH

Many questions are yet to be answered regarding the regulation of body fluids and temperature in older adults. Some have been noted throughout this chapter, and a select few important areas will be highlighted here.

1. First and foremost, issues of aging in women need to be addressed more directly and comprehensively. Changes in thermoregulatory function and fluid balance related to aging must be separated from those associated with menopause, as defined by the loss of cyclic hormonal function, because the latter may be amenable to intervention. With respect to hormonal replacement therapy, direct effects of estrogen supplements versus combination therapies (estrogen + progestins) on thermoregulation have not been examined. The underlying mechanisms through which hormonal actions are exerted also have not been investigated.

2. Skin is the locus of the two primary effectors of heat loss, i.e., cutaneous arterioles and eccrine sweat glands. Aging of skin is inevitable, yet the rate of structural and functional age-related changes varies greatly. The role of ultraviolet light and other environmental influences should be addressed in concert with aging studies. New and better methods are needed to quantify such changes and effects.

3. Better longitudinal training studies should be designed to examine the potential impact of various modes of exercise training on acute and long-term thermoregulation and control of body fluids.
4. Similarly, mechanisms that underlie heat acclimation may well change as we age. The ability to expand plasma volume with either endurance training or heat acclimation involves plasma protein translocation and/or synthesis, and we know little at this time about the effects of age on those mechanisms.
5. Finally, there are complex interactive effects of age and aerobic fitness on thirst sensitivity and renal function. These interactions have not been explored, yet they serve as the underlying data on which fluid replacement issues in older men and women will ultimately be determined.

SUMMARY

Epidemiological evidence of increased mortality among older men and women from hyperthermia and hypothermia should **not** be interpreted as implying that aging *per se* confers an intolerance to environmental extremes. Furthermore, healthy independently living older men and women demonstrate daily fluid intakes well within the normal range and easily maintain adequate fluid homeostasis. However, there are age-related changes in both thirst and renal function that become evident and important under stressful conditions (dehydration, continuous exposure to hot weather) or when illness or incapacity increase water loss or prevent easy access to palatable fluids.

With respect to exercise in warm environments, few studies have attempted to delineate the effects of chronologic age from related factors such as differences in $\dot{V}O_2$max, habitual activity, and body composition in determining thermoregulatory and body fluid responses. When the effects of chronic diseases and sedentary lifestyle are kept to a minimum, heat tolerance appears to be minimally compromised by age. $\dot{V}O_2$max is more important than age in predicting body temperature during exertion, although peripheral physiological mechanisms (control of skin blood flow and sweating) associated with heat dissipation are clearly altered as the skin ages. Dehydration effects may be magnified in older individuals, and rehydration may be compromised by age-related differences in thirst sensitivity and renal function.

The efficacy of various interventions (aerobic training, acclimation, etc.) in improving thermoregulatory responses of older individuals has not been adequately studied. Older men and women are capable of acclimating to hot conditions, but the time course of physiological changes underlying acclimation with age is unexplored. Another intervention that holds promise is estrogen replacement therapy in postmenopausal women.

Estrogen replacement therapy acutely affects temperature regulation and control of body fluids in a positive direction, but the chronic effects are not known.

Tolerance to cold exposure under resting conditions may be less dependent on age and aerobic fitness than on body composition. Studies of older and younger subjects exercising in cold environments are lacking altogether, including important studies into the possible preventive effects of regular physical activity on physiological responses to cold stress.

FOOTNOTES

[1]Where possible, as when citing specific data from the literature, age ranges are provided in lieu of arbitrary descriptors such as "elderly," "old age," very old," etc. When specific ages or ranges are not available, the comparative "older" will be used to differentiate a cross-sectional difference between adults over the age of 60 and those younger than 30.

[2]Various clinical definitions exist with respect to "normal" serum osmolality. For the purpose of simplicity, a working definition of 275-295 mOsmols/kg is suggested here.

[3]There were two factors that did show a clear age-related effect in this study. The first was the type of fluid ingested. Older subjects drank less alcohol and more coffee and tea; young subjects drank significantly more sugared soda and diet soda. The second difference was in the timing of spontaneous drinking. Older subjects drank fluids earlier in the day, but drinking declined markedly in the evening. Notable in this diurnal pattern was the lack of any relationship with thirst. Rather, such a pattern has been attributed to a conscious attempt to avoid the need to micturate during the night.

[4]An interesting distinction between training effects and those associated with sweating was made by Hessemer et al. (1986). These authors showed that inhibiting sweating during exercise by blowing cool air over the skin ("sweatless training") eliminated the training effect on sweating threshold previously reported by Roberts et al. (1977).

ACKNOWLEDGEMENTS

The work performed in the author's laboratory was funded by NIH Grant AG07004, The Pennsylvania State University Gerontology Center, and an NIH Biomedical Research Support Grant. The technical support and medical assistance of the Noll Physiological Research Center faculty, staff, and graduate students are thankfully acknowledged. The scientific contributions to this area of study by former graduate students Clarke G. Tankersley and Dion H. Zappe are duly and gratefully noted, as are the editorial comments of William J. Evans, Barbara J. Rolls, and Susan M. Puhl.

BIBLIOGRAPHY

Agate, J. (1970). *The Practice of Geriatrics*. London: Heinemann.

Aitken, J.M., R. Lindsay, and D.M. Hart (1974). The redistribution of body sodium in women on long-term oestrogen therapy. *Clin. Sci. Mol. Med.* 47:179-187.

Anderson, R.K., and W.L. Kenney (1987). Effect of age on heat-activated sweat gland density and flow during exercise in dry heat. *J. Appl. Physiol.* 63:1089-1094.

Applegate, W.B., L. Runyan, M.L. Brasfield, C. Williams, C. Konigsberg, and C. Fouche (1981). Analysis of the 1990 heat wave in Memphis. *J. Am. Geriatr. Soc.* 29:37-342.

Armstrong, C.G., and W.L. Kenney (1993). Effects of age and acclimation on responses to passive heat exposure. *J. Appl. Physiol.* 75:2162-2167.

Becklake, M.R., H. Frank, G.R. Dagenais, G.L. Ostiguy, and C.A. Guzman (1965). Influence of age and sex on exercise cardiac output. *J. Appl. Physiol.* 20:938-947.

Bell, G.W. (1993). Effect of age on the control of plasma volume during exercise and heat acclimation. Unpublished M.S. Thesis, The Pennsylvania State University.

Bell, G.W., D.H. Zappe, R.F. Wideman, and W.L. Kenney (1994). Inability of healthy older men to concentrate urine during prolonged exercise. *FASEB J.* 8:A588 (abstract).

Bernstein, L.M., L.C. Johnston, R. Ryan, T. Inouye, and F.K. Hick (1956). Body composition as related to heat regulation in women. *J. Appl. Physiol.* 9:241-256.

Blahd, W.H., M.A. Lederer, and E.T. Tyler (1974). Effect of oral contraceptives on body water and electrolytes. *J. Reprod. Med.* 13:223–225.

Brengelmann, G.L., J.M. Johnson, L. Hermansen, and L.B. Rowell (1977). Altered control of skin blood flow during exercise at high internal temperatures. *J. Appl. Physiol.: Respirat. Environ. Exerc. Physiol.* 43:790–794.

Buono, M.J., B.K. McKenzie, and F.W. Kasch (1991). Effects of ageing and physical training on the peripheral sweat production of the human eccrine sweat gland. *Age & Ageing* 20:439–441.

Cable, N.T., and N.T. Green (1990). The influence of bicycle exercise, with or without hand immersion in cold water, on forearm sweating in young and middle-aged women. *Exper. Physiol.* 75:505–514.

Collins, K.J. (1987). Effects of cold on old people. *Br. J. Hosp. Med.* 38:506–514.

Collins, K.J., C. Dore, A.N. Exton-Smith, R.H. Fox, I.C. Macdonald, and P.M. Woodward (1977). Accidental hypothermia and impaired temperature homeostasis in the elderly. *Br. Med. J.* 1:353–356.

Crowe, J.P., and R.E. Moore (1973). Physiological and behavioral responses of aged men to passive heating. *J. Physiol. (London)* 236:43P.

Crowe, M.J., M.L. Forsling, B.J. Rolls, P.A. Phillips, J.G.G. Ledingham, and R.F. Smith (1987). Altered water excretion in healthy elderly men. *Age and Ageing* 16:285–293.

Davies, D.F., and N.W. Shock (1950). Age changes in glomerular filtration rate, effective renal plasma flow and tubular excretory capacity in adult males. *J. Clin. Invest.* 29:496–507.

Davy, K.P., and D.R. Seals (1994). Total blood volume in healthy young and older men. *J. Appl. Physiol.* 76:2059–2062.

de Castro, J.M. (1988). A microregulatory analysis of spontaneous fluid intake by humans: evidence that the amount of fluid ingestion and its timing is governed by feeding. *Physiol. Behav.* 43:705–714.

de Castro, J.M. (1991). The relationship of spontaneous macronutrient and sodium intake with fluid ingestion and thirst in humans. *Physiol. Behav.* 49:513–519.

de Castro, J.M. (1992). Age-related changes in natural spontaneous fluid ingestion and thirst in humans. *J. Gerontol.* 47:P321–P330.

Drinkwater, B.L., and S.M. Horvath (1979). Heat tolerance in aging. *Med. Sci. Sports Exerc.* 11:49–55.

Drinkwater, B.L., J.F. Bedi, A.B. Louks, S. Roche, and S.M. Horvath (1982). Sweating sensitivity and capacity of women in relation to age. *J. Appl. Physiol.* 53:671–676.

Ellis, F.P., A.N. Exton-Smith, K.G. Foster, and J.S. Weiner (1976). Eccrine sweating and mortality during heat waves in very young and very old persons. *Israel J. Med. Sci.* 12:815–817.

Epstein, M. (1979). Effects of aging on the kidney. *Fed. Proc.* 38:168–172.

Fagard, R., and J. Staessen (1991). Relation of cardiac output at rest and during exercise in essential hypertension. *Am. J. Cardiol.* 67:585–589.

Falk, B., O. Bar-Or, J. Smolander, and G. Frost (1994). Response to rest and exercise in the cold: effects of age and aerobic fitness. *J. Appl. Physiol.* 76:72–78.

Faull, C.M., C. Holmes, and P.H. Baylis (1993). Water balance in elderly people: is there a deficiency of vasopressin? *Age and Ageing* 22:114–120.

Fennell, W.H., and R.E. Moore (1973). Responses of aged men to passive heating. *J. Physiol. (London)* 231:118P.

Fleg, J.L. (1986). Alterations in cardiovascular structure and function with advancing age. *Am. J. Cardiol.* 57:33C–44C.

Fortney, S.M., E.R. Nadel, C.B. Wenger, and J.R. Bove (1981). Effect of acute alterations of blood volume on circulatory performance in humans. *J. Appl. Physiol.: Respirat. Environ. Exerc. Physiol.* 50:292–298.

Fortney, S.M., C.B. Wenger, J.R. Bove, and E.R. Nadel (1984). Effect of hyperosmolality on control of blood flow and sweating. *J. Appl. Physiol.: Respirat. Environ. Exerc. Physiol.* 57:1688–1695.

Foster, K.G., F.P. Ellis, C. Dore, A.N. Exton-Smith, and J.S. Weiner (1976). Sweat responses in the aged. *Age and Ageing* 5:91–101.

Fox, R.H., R. MacGibbon, L. Davies, and P.M. Woodward (1973). Problem of the old and the cold. *Br. Med. J.* 1:21–24.

Gerstenblith, G., D.G. Renlund, and E.G. Lakatta (1987). Cardiovascular response to exercise in younger and older men. *Fed. Proc.* 46:1834–1839.

Gisolfi, C.V., R.W. Summers, H.P. Schedl, and T.L. Bleiler (1992). Intestinal water absorption from select carbohydrate solutions in humans. *J. Appl. Physiol.* 73:2142–2150.

Grover, M. (1938). Mortality during periods of excessive temperature. *Pub. Health Rep.* 53:1122–1143.

Hagberg, J.M., W.K. Allen, D.R. Seals, B.F. Hurley, A.A. Ehsani, and J.O. Holloszy (1985). A hemodynamic comparison of young and older endurance athletes during exercise. *J. Appl. Physiol.* 58:2041–2046.

Harrison, M.F. (1985). Effects of thermal stress and exercise on blood volume in humans. *Physiol. Rev.* 65:149–209.

Havenith, G., Y. Inoue, V. Luttikholt, and W.L. Kenney (1995). Age predicts cardiovascular, but not thermoregulatory responses to humid heat stress. *Eur. J. Appl. Physiol.* 70:88–96.

Havenith, G., and H. van Middendorp (1990). The relative influence of physical fitness, acclimation state, anthropometric measures and gender on individual reactions to heat stress. *Eur. J. Appl. Physiol.* 61:419–427.

Hellon, R.F., and A.R. Lind (1956). Observations on the activity of sweat glands with special reference to the influence of ageing. *J. Physiol. (London)* 133:132–144.

Hellon, R.F., and A.R. Lind (1958). The influence of age on peripheral vasodilation in a hot environment. *J. Physiol. (London)* 141:262–272.

Hellon, R.F., A.R. Lind, and J.S. Weiner (1956). The physiological reactions of men of two age groups to a hot environment. *J. Physiol. (London)* 133:118P–131P.

Hessemer, V., A. Zeh, and K. Bruck (1986). Effects of passive heat adaptation and moderate sweatless conditioning on responses to heat and cold. *Eur. J. Appl. Physiol.* 55:281–289.

Horvath, S.M., and R.D. Rochelle (1977). Hypothermia in the aged. *Environ. Health Perspect.* 20:127–130.

Hossack, K.F., and R.A. Bruce (1982). Maximal cardiac function in sedentary normal men and women: comparison of age-related changes. *J. Appl. Physiol.* 53:799–804.

Howell, T.H. (1948). Normal temperature in old age. *Lancet* i:517–518.

Inoue, Y., M. Nakao, T. Araki, and H. Murakami (1991). Regional differences in the sweating responses of older and younger men. *J. Appl. Physiol.* 71:2453–2459.

Johnson, J.M. (1992). Exercise and the cutaneous circulation. In: J.O. Holloszy (ed.) *Exerc. and Sport Sci. Reviews.* Baltimore: Williams and Wilkins, pp. 59–97.

Jones, S.T., A.P. Liang, E.M. Kilbourne, M.R. Griffin, P.A. Patracia, S.G. Fite Wassilak, R.J. Mullan, R.F. Herrick, H.D. Donnell, K. Choi, and S.B. Thacker (1982). Morbidity and mortality associated with the July 1980 heat wave in St. Louis and Kansas City, MO. *J. Am. Med. Assoc.* 247:3327–3331.

Kanstrup, I.-L., and B. Ekblom (1978). Influence of age and physical activity on central hemodynamics and lung function in active adults. *J. Appl. Physiol.* 45:709–717.

Keatinge, W. (1986). Medical problems of cold weather. *J. Royal Coll. Physic. (London)* 20:283–287.

Kenney, W.L. (1988). Control of heat-induced vasodilation in relation to age. *Eur. J. Appl. Physiol.* 57:120–125.

Kenney, W.L., and R.K. Anderson (1988). Responses of older and younger women to exercise in dry and humid heat without fluid replacement. *Med. Sci. Sports Exerc.* 20:155–160.

Kenney, W.L., and S.R. Fowler (1988). Methylcholine activated eccrine sweat gland density and output as a function of age. *J. Appl. Physiol.* 65:1082–1088.

Kenney, W.L., and G. Havenith (1991). Aging, skin blood flow, and heat tolerance. In: *Proc. Int. Conf. Human-Environ. Systems,* Tokyo, Japan, pp. 87–90.

Kenney, W.L., and G. Havenith (1993). Heat stress and age: skin blood flow and body temperature. *J. Therm. Biol.* 18:341–344.

Kenney, W.L., and J.M. Johnson (1992). Control of skin blood flow during exercise. *Med. Sci. Sports Exerc.* 24:303–312.

Kenney, W.L., C.G. Tankersley, D.L. Newswanger, D.E. Hyde, and S.M. Puhl (1990). Age and hypohydration independently influence the peripheral vascular response to heat stress. *J. Appl. Physiol.* 68:1902–1908.

Kenney, W.L., C.G. Tankersley, D.L. Newswanger, and S.M. Puhl (1991). Alpha-1 adrenergic blockade does not alter control of skin blood flow during exercise. *Am. J. Physiol. (Heart Circ. Physiol.)* 260:H855–H861.

Kenney, W.L., and D.H. Zappe (1994). Effect of age on renal blood flow during exercise. *Aging Clin. Exp. Res.* 6:293–302.

Kenney, W.L., D.H. Zappe, C.G. Tankersley, and J.A. Derr (1994). Effect of systemic yohimbine on the control of skin blood flow during local heating and dynamic exercise. *Am. J. Physiol.* 266:H371–H376.

Kilbourne, E.M., K. Choi, T.S. Jines, and S.B. Thacker (1982). Risk factors for heat stroke: a case control study. *J. Am. Med. Assoc.* 247:3332–3336.

Lakatta, E.G. (1986). Hemodynamic adaptations to stress with advancing age. *Acta Med. Scand.* suppl. 711:39–52.

Leaf, A. (1984). Dehydration in the elderly. *N. Engl. J. Med.* 311:791–792.

Levi, M., and J.W. Rowe (1992). Renal function and dysfunction in aging. In: D.W. Seldin and G. Giebisch (eds.) *The Kidney: Physiology and Pathophysiology.* New York: Raven Press, pp. 3433–3456.

Lind, A.R., P.W. Humphreys, K.J. Collins, K. Foster, and K.F. Sweetland (1970). Influence of age and daily duration of exposure on responses of men to work in heat. *J. Appl. Physiol.* 28:50–56.

Lindeman, R.D., and R. Goldman (1986). Anatomic and physiologic age changes in the kidney. *Exp. Gerontol.* 21:379–406.

Lindeman, R.D., T.D. Lee, M.J. Yiengst, and N.W. Shock (1966). Influence of age, renal disease, hypertension, diuretics, and calcium on the antidiuretic response to suboptimal infusions of vasopressin. *J. Lab. Clin. Med.* 68:206–223.

Lindeman, R.D., H.C. Van Buren, and L.G. Raisz (1960). Osmolar renal concentrating ability in healthy young men and hospitalized patients without renal disease. *N. Engl. J. Med.* 262:1306–1314.

Lomax, P. (1983) Drug-induced changes in the thermoregulatory system. In: M. Khogali and J.R.S. Hales (eds.) *Heat Stroke and Temperature Regulation.* Sydney: Academic Press, pp. 197–212.

Löwik, M.R.H., S. Westenbrink, K.F.A.M. Hulshof, C. Kistemaker, and R.J.J. Hermus (1989). Nutrition and aging: dietary intake of apparently healthy elderly. *J. Am. Coll. Nutr.* 8:347–356.

Lybarger, J.A., and E.M. Kilbourne (1985). Hyperthermia and hypothermia in the elderly: an epidemiology review. In: B.B. Davis and W.G. Wood (eds.) *Homeostatic Function and Aging.* New York: Raven Press, pp. 149–156.

Macey, S.M., and D.F. Schneider (1993). Deaths from excessive heat and excessive cold among the elderly. *Gerontologist* 33:497–500.

Mack, G.W., C.A. Weseman, G.W. Langhans, H. Scherzer, C.M. Gillen, and E.R. Nadel (1994). Body fluid in dehydrated healthy older men: thirst and renal osmoregulation. *J. Appl. Physiol.* 76:1615–1623, 1994.

Marion, G.S., K.P. McGann, and D.L. Camp (1991). Core body temperature in the elderly and factors which influence its measurement. *Gerontology* 37:225–232.

Martinez, B.F., J.L. Annest, E.M. Kilbourne, M.L. Kirk, K.J. Lui, and S.M. Smith (1989). Geographic distribution of heat-related deaths among elderly persons. *J. Am. Med. Soc.* 262:2246–2250.

McElvaney, G.N., S.P. Blackie, N.J. Morrison, M.S. Fairbarn, P.G. Wilcox, and R.L. Pardy (1989). Cardiac output at rest and in exercise in elderly subjects. *Med. Sci. Sports Exerc.* 21:293–298.

Miescher, E., and S.M. Fortney (1989). Responses to dehydration and rehydration during heat exposure in young and older men. *Am. J. Physiol. (Regulatory Integrative Comp. Physiol.)* 257:R1050–R1056.

Miller, J.H., and N.W. Shock (1953). Age differences in the renal tubular response to antidiuretic hormone. *J. Gerontol.* 8:446–450.

Nadel, E.R. (1986). Non-thermal influences on the control of skin blood flow have minimal effects on heat transfer during exercise. *The Yale J. Biol. Med.* 59:321–327.

Nadel, E.R., E. Cafarelli, M.F. Roberts, and C.B. Wenger (1979). Circulatory regulation during exercise in different ambient temperatures. *J. Appl. Physiol.* 46:430–437.

Nadel, E.R., S.M. Fortney, and C.B. Wenger (1980). Effect of hydration state on circulatory and thermal regulations. *J. Appl. Physiol.* 49:715–721.

Nadel, E.R., J.W. Mitchell, B. Saltin, and J.A.J. Stolwijk (1971). Peripheral modifications to the central drive for sweating. *J. Appl. Physiol.* 31:828–833.

Oechsli, F.W., and R.W. Buechley (1970). Excess mortality associated with three Los Angeles September hot spells. *Environ. Res.* 3:277–284.

Ogawa, T., and N. Ohnishi (1989). Trainability of sweat glands in the aged. In: M.K. Yousef (ed.) *Milestones in Environmental Physiology.* The Hague: SPB Academic Publishing, pp. 63–71 .

Ogawa, T., R.J. Spina, W.H. Martin, W.M. Kohrt, K.B. Schechtman, J.O. Holloszy, and A.A. Ehsani (1992). Effects of aging, sex, and physical training on cardiovascular responses to exercise. *Circulation* 86:494–503.

O'Neill, P.A., E.B. Faragher, I. Davies, R. Wears, K.A. McLean, and D.S. Fairweather (1990). Reduced survival with increasing plasma osmolality in elderly continuing care patients. *Age and Ageing* 19:68–71.

Pandolf, K.B., B.S. Cadarette, M.N. Sawka, A.J. Young, R.P. Francesconi, and R.R. Gonzalez (1988). Thermoregulatory responses of middle-aged and young men during dry-heat acclimation. *J. Appl. Physiol.* 65:65–71.

Phillips, P.A., M. Bretherton, C.I. Johnston, and L. Gray (1991a). Reduced osmotic thirst in healthy elderly men. *Am. J. Physiol.* 261:R166–R171.

Phillips, P.A., C.I. Johnston, and L. Gray (1991b). Thirst and fluid intake in the elderly. In: D.J. Ramsay and D.A. Booth (eds.) *Thirst: Physiological and Psychological Aspects.* London: Springer-Verlag, pp. 403–411.

Phillips, P.A., C.I. Johnston, and L. Gray (1993). Disturbed fluid and electrolyte homeostasis following dehydration in elderly people. *Age and Ageing* 22:26–33.

Phillips, P.A., B.J. Rolls, M.L. Ledingham, M.L. Forsling, J.J. Morton, M.J. Crowe, and L. Wollner (1984a). Reduced thirst after water deprivation in healthy elderly men. *N. Engl. J. Med.* 311:753–759.

Phillips, P.A., B.J. Rolls, M.L. Ledingham, and J.J. Morton (1984b). Body fluid changes, thirst and drinking in man during free access to water. *Physiol. Behav.* 33:357–363.

Primrose, W.R., and L.R.N. Smith (1982). Oral and environmental temperatures in a Scottish urban geriatric population. *J. Clin. Exp.Gerontol.* 42:151–165.

Ramlow, J.M., and J.H. Kuller (1990). Effects of the summer heat wave of 1988 on daily mortality in Allegheny County, PA. *Publ. Health Rep.* 105:283–289.

Rango, N. (1984). Exposure-related hypothermia mortality in the United States, 1970-79. *Am. J. Publ. Health* 74:1159–1160.

Roberts, M.F., C.B. Wenger, J.A.J. Stolwijk, and E.R. Nadel (1977). Skin blood flow and sweating changes following exercise training and heat acclimation. *J. Appl. Physiol.* 43:133–137.

Robinson, S., H.S. Belding, F.C. Consolazio, S.M. Horvath, and E.S. Turrell (1965). Acclimatization of older men to work in the heat. *J. Appl. Physiol.* 20:583–586.

Rolls, B.J. (1989). Regulation of food and fluid intake in the elderly. *Ann. NY Acad. Sci.* 561:217–225.

Rooke, G.A., M.V. Savage, and G.L. Brengelmann (1994). Maximal skin blood flow is decreased in elderly men. *J. Appl. Physiol.* 77:11–14.

Rowe, J.W., N.W. Shock, and R.A. DeFronzo (1976). The influence of age on the renal response to water deprivation in man. *Nephron* 17:270–278.

Rowell, L.B. (1974). Human cardiovascular adjustments to exercise and thermal stress. *Physiol. Rev.* 54:75–159.

Rowell, L.B. (1983). Cardiovascular aspects of human thermoregulation. *Circ. Res.* 52:367–379.

Rowell, L.B. (1986). *Human Circulation: Regulation During Physical Stress.* New York: Oxford University Press.

Rowell, L.B., J.R. Blackmon, R.H. Martin, J.A. Mazzerella, and R.A. Bruce (1965). Hepatic clearance of indocyanine green in man under thermal and exercise stresses. *J. Appl. Physiol.* 20:384–394.

Sagawa, S., K. Shiraki, M.K. Yousef, and K. Miki (1988). Sweating and cardiovascular responses of aged men to heat exposure. *J. Gerontol.* 43:M1–M8.

Salvosa, C.B., P.R. Payne, and E.F. Wheeler (1971). Environmental conditions and body temperatures of elderly women living alone or in local authority homes. *Br. Med. J.* ii:656–659.

Sato, K. (1993). The mechanism of eccrine sweat secretion. In: C.V. Gisolfi, D.R. Lamb, and E.R. Nadel (eds.) *Perspectives in Exercise Science and Sports Medicine, Vol. 6: Exercise, Heat, and Thermoregulation.* Dubuque: Brown & Benchmark, pp. 85–118.

Sato, K., and F. Sato (1983). Individual variation in structure and function of human eccrine sweat gland. *Am. J. Physiol.* 245:R203–R208.

Sato, K., and D. Timm (1988). Effect of aging on pharmacological sweating in man. In: A.M. Klingman and Y. Takase (eds.), *Cutaneous Aging.* Tokyo: University of Tokyo Press, pp. 127–134.

Schulman, S.P., E.G. Lakatta, J.L. Fleg, L. Lakatta, L.C. Becker, and G. Gerstenblith (1992). Age-related decline in left ventricular filling at rest and exercise. *Am. J. Physiol.* 263:H1932–H1938.

Shoenfeld, Y., R. Udassin, Y. Shapiro, A. Ohri, and E. Sohar (1978). Age and sex differences in response to short exposure to extreme dry heat. *J. Appl. Physiol.* 44:1–4.

Silva, N.L., and J.A. Boulant (1986). Effects of testosterone, estradiol, and temperature on neurons in preoptic tissue slices. *Am. J. Physiol.* 250:R625–R632.

Silver, A., W. Montagna, and I. Karaean (1964). Age and sex differences in spontaneous, adrenergic, and cholinergic human sweating. *J. Invest. Dermatol.* 43:255–256.

Smolander, J., O. Korhonen, and R. Ilmarinen (1990). Responses of young and older men during prolonged exercise in dry and humid heat. *Eur. J. Appl. Physiol.* 61:413–418.

Snyder, M.A., D.W. Feigal, and A.L. Arieff (1987). Hypernatraemia in elderly patients: a heterogenous, morbid and iatrogenic entity. *Ann. Intern.Med.* 107:309–319.

Spangler, P.F., T.R. Risley, and D.D. Bilyew (1984). The management of dehydration and incontinence in non-ambulatory geriatric patients. *J. Appl. Behav. Anal.* 17:397–401.

Spina, R.J., T. Ogawa, W.M. Kohrt, W.H. Martin, J.O. Holloszy, and A.A. Ehsani (1993). Differences in cardiovascular adaptations to endurance exercise training between older men and women. *J. Appl. Physiol.* 75:849–855.

Strandel, T. (1964). Circulatory studies on healthy older men. *Acta Med. Scand.* 175 (suppl. 414):1–44.

Tankersley, C.G., D.J. Mikita, W.C. Nicholas, and W.L. Kenney (1992). Estrogen replacement in middle-aged women: thermoregulatory, cardiovascular, and body fluid responses to exercise in the heat. *J. Appl. Physiol.* 73:1238–1245.

Tankersley, C.G., J. Smolander, W.L. Kenney, and S.M. Fortney (1991). Sweating and skin blood flow during exercise: effects of age and maximal oxygen uptake. *J. Appl. Physiol.* 71:236–242.

Wagner, J.A., and S.M. Horvath (1985). Influences of age and gender on human thermoregulatory responses to cold exposures. *J. Appl. Physiol.* 58:180–186.

Wagner, J.A., S. Robinson, and R.P. Marino (1974). Age and temperature regulation of humans in neutral and cold environments. *J. Appl. Physiol.* 37:562–565.

Wagner, J.A., S. Robinson, S.P. Tzankoff, and R.P. Marino (1972). Heat tolerance and acclimatization to work in the heat in relation to age. *J. Appl. Physiol.* 33:616–622.

Watkin, D.M., and N.W. Shock (1955). Agewise standards for CIN, CPAH, and TmPAH in adult males. *J. Clin. Invest.* 34:969.

Whitten, C.L., and J.T. Bradbury (1951). Hemodilution as a result of estrogen therapy. Estrogenic effects in the human female. *Proc. Soc. Exp. Biol. Med.* 78:626–629.

Young, A.J. (1991). Effects of aging on human cold tolerance. *Exp. Aging Res.* 17:205–213.

Yousef, M.K., D.B. Dill, T.F. Vitez, S.D. Hillyard, and A.S. Goldman (1984). Thermoregulatory responses to desert heat: age, race and sex. *J. Gerontol.* 39:406–414.

Yousef, M.K., and L.A. Golding (1989). Thermal homeostasis and aging. In: M.K. Yousef (ed.) *Milestones in Environmental Physiology.* The Hague: SPB Academic Publ., pp. 53–61.

Zambraski, E.J. (1990). Renal regulation of fluid homeostasis during exercise. In: C.V. Gisolfi and D.R. Lamb (eds.) *Prospectives in Exercise Science and Sports Medicine, Vol. 3: Fluid Homeostasis During Exercise.* Carmel, IN: Cooper Publishing Group, pp. 247–280.

DISCUSSION

BAR-OR: You have compared epidemiologic data and claims with the laboratory-based evidence and have managed to dispel some myths and fads regarding the responses of aged people to warm or cool environments. It is particularly important that you have included some information about possible interactions between temperature regulation and medications, a topic of major relevance to this population. With respect to future research, my own shopping list of unresolved issues includes some methodological aspects. First, we need to know how best to equate subjects who differ in age. Should they be equated for absolute maximal $\dot{V}O_2$, for $\dot{V}O_2$ max/kg, for level of habitual activity, for state of health, or for adiposity? Regarding the latter, it is important to consider not only subcutaneous fat thickness, but also the total fat mass because fat has considerably lower specific heat than any other tissue, which has implications to the rate of body cooling and heating. A second unresolved methodological issue is how to equate the metabolic heat stress (i.e., exercise intensity) among various age groups tested in the laboratory. Third, there is a lack of good research on the interactions among age, temperature regulation, fluid balance, and medications. Finally, from a public health as well as a theoretical point of view, we must find ways of enhancing the thirst of older people to increase their fluid intake during heat stress.

KENNEY: I agree with those points.

MORA: We need to seriously consider the deterioration of neural circuits in the brain that control the physiological systems that decline with age. The same could be said regarding temperature regulation. For instance, we now know that a degeneration of the catecholamine systems and possibly other neurotransmitter systems in the hypothalamus occurs with age and that this phenomenon influences the morphology and functioning of organs such as the skin, kidney, sweat glands, etc., that respond to temperature challenges. In your opinion what is the importance of a degeneration of the neurochemical systems in the brain that control body temperature relative to the importance of degeneration or dysfunction of the peripheral mechanisms?

KENNEY: Through age 85 or 90, in presumably healthy adults, we see little evidence of central nervous system deterioration that impacts directly on body temperature regulation. As I mentioned, if one eliminates confounding effects such as low body weights, medication effects, alcohol intake, etc., baseline body temperature (from measures of urine temperature upon awakening in the morning) among the elderly is very similar to that of younger individuals. When we look at fluid deprivation, exercise, or passive heating as perturbations, the predominance of the differences that we see in healthy older versus younger subjects are, in my opinion, more the result of peripheral age-related changes. The body turns on appropriate effector mechanisms at the same core and skin temperatures; however, subsequent to turning on thermoregulatory systems, the rate of change of the systems per given increase in body temperature is attenuated.

MORA: In animals, I agree that there are few central differences in temperature control at various ages when one examines thermoregulation in a basal state or at a neutral ambient temperature. The problem starts when aged animals are challenged by putting them in an extremely hot or cold environment. **TIPTON:** It is hard for me to believe that there are no age-induced changes in the hypothalamus that affect thermoregulation.

KENNEY: I certainly do not want to imply such a notion unequivocally based on the available human data. I think there are clearly changes in synaptic function and efferent outflow that occur in the aging brain. It's also fairly clear that there are effects on the brain of both estrogen supplementation and lack of cycling estrogen that change central thermoregulatory effector functions.

TIPTON: Dr. Sato and others suggest that the eccrine sweat gland changes structurally with training and exposure to heat. Are these changes true for the elderly?

KENNEY: Dr. Sato has elegantly shown that sweat output per sweat gland is primarily a function of sweat gland size, which changes both chronically and acutely. With respect to adaptability, Drs. Ogawa and Ohnishi had older (61–73 y) and younger (19–29 y) subjects put their forearms in hot water baths for 30 min/d, day after day, to locally "train" sweat glands. While both younger and older subjects demonstrated an increase in forearm sweating (presumably output per gland), the increase was about 50% smaller in the older subjects. Dr. Sato commented at a previous GSSI meeting that he doesn't think sweat-gland function changes much below the age of 70, but I would disagree. We see a fairly linear decline from age 40 through 85 in the volume of sweat per gland in response to pharmacological stimulation with sudorific agents such as methylcholine (Kenney & Fowler, 1988).

BALDWIN: The renin-angiotensin-aldosterone system is pivotal for both fluid retention and fluid intake. We also know that aged individuals tend to be more hypertensive. Is there an alteration in this system with aging?

KENNEY: We haven't looked directly at the renin side of the axis. We often see markedly lower concentrations of circulating aldosterone during exercise in older subjects. I believe Dr. Nadel's group has likewise seen age differences in plasma aldosterone. Tankersley et al. (1992) demonstrated an aldosterone-lowering effect of estrogen replacement therapy in postmenopausal women. In neither case does a change in plasma aldosterone affect sweat electrolytes. I think this area really hasn't been examined sufficiently.

Because of the way we design our experiments and because we use very fit, healthy, older individuals, we don't see either differences in control of blood pressure or the magnitude of blood pressure change during thermal challenges that might be secondary to aging.

NADEL: Similar to sweat glands, the response of the kidney to aldosterone is appropriate in older people. It seems that the system is responding in an appropriate way, even though aldosterone levels are slightly altered.

Mack et al. (1994) showed that older people tended to have a slightly higher plasma osmolality at baseline and even after drinking 400 mL of water, so it appears that in these older people there was an upward adjustment in the point about which they regulated their plasma osmolality.

KENNEY: We need to be careful about how we control experiments that involve hydration and aging. Faull et al. (1993) recently demonstrated that as little as 8–9 h of overnight fasting was a substantial fluid deprivation stimulus for older subjects. When we design laboratory experiments, it's typical to have older and younger subjects show up at the lab early in the morning after an 8–12 h fast. We must be careful that we are not changing what we consider to be a control condition into something that is actually a mild fluid deprivation stimulus. When older subjects show up at the lab for such experiments, they tend to have plasma osmolalities 3–6 mOsmols/kg higher than those of younger subjects. This may not represent a true baseline, but rather a differential response to an overnight fast.

NADEL: Larry has made a very good point. Older people tend to have a slightly different fluid distribution space than younger people. When arriving in the lab, we always give our subjects a water challenge and allow them to respond to that over the following hour so that they are well hydrated prior to study. Even after a water challenge, our older people still were regulating about a higher plasma osmolality. I agree that we should standardize our methods of testing to reduce variability due to factors such as activity, adiposity, hydration, and others.

KENNEY: The issue of plasma volume illustrates that point nicely as well. If older and younger subjects are drawn randomly from the population, there is a significantly lower baseline plasma volume (PV) in older men and women, regardless of whether you standardize PV to total body weight or to lean body mass. In the Davy and Seals (1994) study, subjects were matched on the basis of regular physical activity, and there was still a significantly lower plasma volume in the older subjects. Conversely, when we match our subjects on the basis of $\dot{V}O_2$max, this PV difference disappears. This is a clear illustration that investigators must be very careful about what questions they are asking. No one method of designing cross-sectional age experiments gets at all of the pertinent issues.

MAUGHAN: The death rates during cold waves among the elderly seem to rise according to the distance from the equator, which indicates that this seasonal mortality rhythm is related to the ambient temperature. Is this effect caused by age-related differences in ability to detect a change in temperature and to respond accordingly?

KENNEY: Epidemiological data from anywhere in the world show that death rates go up in the winter versus the summer months—whether in Hawaii or Alaska. So it's not purely a cold-temperature effect. However, as you said, as one moves further from the equator, this winter "excess mortality" increases. My feeling is that age *per se* does not directly cause people to be less cold-tolerant or to have a higher incidence of deaths from hypothermia. However, differences in body composition, body size, surface area-to-mass ratio, and the use of most medications influence that response to cold. Cold tolerance is different from heat tolerance in that a high $\dot{V}O_2$max is not protective, as recently shown by Falk et al. (1994). Older men had a more rapid drop in core temperature at rest and during low-intensity exercise at 5°C. In the older subjects, there was no protective effect of having a higher $\dot{V}O_2$max on this response. In my opinion, other factors, in particular, fat beneath the skin and throughout the body, body size, etc., play a greater role than age *per se*.

BAR-OR: Furthermore, even though the older and younger men were also matched for skinfold thickness, the thermoregulatory difference still existed in favor of the younger men.

KANTER: In light of the fact that left-ventricular function declines with age and that as one ages there is more of a reliance on the Frank-Starling mechanism for enhancing stroke volume, coupled with the fact that skin-blood flow decreases with age, it is of particular importance for the elderly to be able to maintain blood volume. Assuming that the elderly can more or less maintain a blood volume similar to that of younger individuals, do you have any insights into what types of diet or beverage exercising elderly persons might consume to insure that they better maintain blood volume? One obvious thing that you can suggest is sodium to help maintain blood volume, but that raises the issue of hypertension and sodium intake.

KENNEY: With respect to the reported relative inability of older exercising subjects to maintain volume in the intravascular space, I think it's less an issue of electrolytes than of differences in intravascular proteins. These proteins, primarily albumin, maintain the high colloidal (oncotic) intravascular pressure which holds fluid inside that space. We often see lower circulating protein concentrations and total protein and albumin contents in even very fit, healthy, exercising subjects. This may in some way relate to an inability to keep fluid in the vascular space during thermal and exercise challenges. The relative magnitude of plasma volume losses during exercise versus passive heat exposure is situational. Miescher and Fortney (1989) showed that older subjects lose much greater portions of their plasma volumes than do younger subjects during 3 h of rest in a hot dry environment without fluid replacement. We have seen this difference in comparing older and younger women exercising in warm and humid, but not in hot and dry environments.

Hypertension unrelated to age limits the ability of the skin to vasodilate. In terms of the trade-off between increasing sodium intake to maintain plasma volume and the detrimental effects of high sodium intakes on blood pressure in sodium-sensitive individuals, I think the amount of sodium needed to support maintenance of intravascular volume and to aid in release of fluid from the gut into that space is fairly small when you look at it terms of the overall daily salt intake of the average American.

KANTER: If an aged person were to increase sodium intake during exercise, what would that do to taste perception, and would it encourage greater fluid intake?

KENNEY: I am unaware of any data on that topic.

WHITE: Are there credible data, or do you have an opinion, on any adjustments in beverage composition that would enhance fluid replacement in old persons? It strikes me there are three possibilities: 1) enhance the magnitude or rate of fluid absorbed, 2) provide more benefits per unit volume, or 3) enhance the thirst sensation so more is consumed once one starts drinking.

KENNEY: I haven't seen any data on enhancing absorption of fluid and keeping it in the intravascular space, so I couldn't even begin to speculate. With respect to what the elderly prefer to drink and would drink more of, there was a very nice paper by Flavia Meyer in Dr. Bar-Or's lab showing that children have a clear taste preference for grape as opposed to orange or cherry or other flavors. Several studies have looked at issues of palatability in older men and women by comparing intake of orange juice versus tea versus sodas versus water, etc., but within one fixed set of electrolyte and carbohydrate constraints, I don't think taste preference issues of the elderly have been addressed adequately.

DAVIS: What do you think is (are) the mechanism(s) of thirst decline in the elderly? A better understanding of the mechanisms might help us with decisions about what seems to be one of the more important aspects of impaired thermoregulation in older person.

KENNEY: I think it's an age-related difference in the total integrated response. It probably reflects changes in brain function and brain processing. The primary stimulus for thirst is hypertonicity as reflected by changes in serum osmolality. There are tremendous effects of changes in cerebrospinal fluid osmolality on hypothalamic function and effector function. It's a complex integrative problem that nobody yet has addressed in its entirety.

NADEL: Hypovolemia is a secondary drive for thirst. We repeated the Phillips study involving hypertonic saline infusion in older and younger people. Increased plasma osmolality increases the thirst drive, but the increased plasma volume decreases the same drive using this protocol. The differences between younger and older people disappear. So there may be some subtleties concerning which of the sensory systems declines with aging. It shouldn't be surprising that the thirst sense is dulled with aging; other sensory-processing pathways decline with aging as well. The sense of smell decreases dramatically with aging, as do the senses of taste, hearing, and vision.

WHITE: Do you have data to resolve the question of whether the age-related difference in sweat output per gland is a difference in rate, in magnitude, or both?

KENNEY: It's a difference in both rate and magnitude.

SEALS: Is there clear evidence that older people have an impaired ability to regulate internal body temperature during exercise in warm ambient conditions?

KENNEY: While our paradigm of matching older and younger subjects for $\dot{V}O_2$max is far from perfect, it is probably the best way to answer that specific question. When we ask individuals in their 70s and those in their 20s who are of the same gender, equally heat acclimated, etc., to exercise at the same absolute *and* relative intensity, we almost never see differences in the rate of rise in body core temperature, as measured in the esophagus at heart level. As an aside, I think we need to be careful in interpreting aging studies that use rectal temperature as the criterion measure of core temperature because of possible age-associated differences in blood-flow distribution. I think there is a clear dichotomy in the literature between conclusions based on rectal temperature versus esophageal and sometimes even tympanic temperature as the criterion measure of body-core temperature.

BAR-OR: There is one more factor that we have to take into consideration when discussing relative versus absolute metabolic heat load, and this is body size. We have been taking for granted for decades that a given submaximal $\dot{V}O_2$/kg represents the same relative metabolic heat stress among people. But this may not be so when people differ in body size (both body mass and skin surface area). Based on scaling logic, one should not merely divide by body weight when people differ markedly in their size.

COYLE: In your 1988 paper you showed that when older and younger men and women exercised at the same absolute $\dot{V}O_2$, which also happens to be the same percent of $\dot{V}O_2$max because the old are better trained, that the older subjects have a significantly lower cardiac output. Of course with that design, you can't control the state of training. Is cardiac output an important effector for heat loss in dissipating the heat to the skin?

KENNEY: I would not categorize cardiac output as a true effector response for heat loss, but it is the primary system subserving the increase in skin blood flow that allows convection of heat from the muscle to the skin where it can be dissipated. An additional but uncompleted phase of that study is to take sedentary groups of both ages and put them through a structured endurance training program. After the training program, we are retesting them at both the same relative and the same absolute intensities used before training. I think we *will* have a better picture of true training effects, but we don't have those data yet.

8

The Relationship Between Nutrition and Exercise in Older Adults

JEFFREY B. BLUMBERG, Ph.D.

MOHSEN MEYDANI, D.V.M., Ph.D.

INTRODUCTION

Biology and Chronology in Age-Related Changes

Our early modern concepts about the aging process were shaped by the work of Shock (1983) at the National Institute on Aging. He and his colleagues described apparently progressive, age-related declines in several physiological variables, e.g., basal metabolic rate, renal plasma flow, and maximal breathing capacity, as well as changes in body composition, such as the loss of lean body mass. It was thought that these changes were underlying factors in the growing prevalence of chronic diseases such as cancer and osteoporosis among the elderly. Thus, the progressive loss of fitness and independence in older adults was believed to result from the combination of the aging process itself and associated chronic degenerative conditions. Regardless of the actual etiology, this real increase in disability common to the elderly translates directly into the diminished strength and mobility necessary to engage in activities of daily living. Katz et al. (1983) have calculated that of those individuals who reach age 65, only the first half of their remaining life spans will be active and independent.

It is only now becoming clear that many of the physiologic changes in older people previously attributed exclusively to aging and chronic disease are due significantly to lifestyle factors such as diet and physical inactivity (Table 8-1). Indeed, it has been estimated that the leading causes of death in the United States, including heart disease, cancer, stroke, accidents, and pulmonary disease, are largely due to environmental determinants of aging. Bortz (1982) has noted that many of the progressive declines in physiologic function observed after age 30, e.g., losses in cardiac output, muscle size and strength, glucose clearance rate, bone mineral content, and maximal oxygen consumption, also occur rapidly in healthy young adults during immobilization. Thus, Bortz (1982, 1989) has suggested

TABLE 8-1. *Characteristics associated with aging, disuse syndromes, and exercise.* ↓ = decrease; ↑ = increase; - = no change.

Characteristic	Aging	Disuse	Exercise
Metabolic Variables			
Basal metabolic rate	↓	↓	↑/-
Glucose tolerance	↓	↓	↑
Muscle glycogen	↓	↓	↑
Insulin responsiveness	-/↓	↓	--
Calcium balance	↓	↓	↑
LDL cholesterol	↑	↑	--
Body Composition Variables			
Lean body mass	↓	↓	↑
Fat mass	↑	↑/↓	↓
Bone mass	↓	↓	↑/-
Total body water	↓	↓	↑/-

that at least a portion of the changes that are commonly attributed to aging are in reality caused by disuse and, as such, are subject to correction.

The indication that chronology can be separated from biology by modifying diet/nutritional status and physical activity has broad implications for both public health policy and clinical therapeutics. Importantly, a dynamic interrelationship exists between these factors, i.e., in older people nutrition influences the ability to undertake and benefit from exercise, and physical activity modifies nutrient requirements and nutritional status (Figure 8-1) (Evans & Meredith, 1989).

The major determinants of muscular weakness in old age appear to be senescent musculoskeletal changes, concomitant chronic disease(s) and associated drug therapies, disuse atrophy, and undernutrition (Fiatarone & Evans, 1993). The complexity of the interactions among these contributing factors makes it difficult to elucidate the pathogenesis of muscle dysfunction in the elderly. For example, an increasingly sedentary lifestyle among older people is nearly universal in industrialized countries, so the separation of genetic aging from disuse atrophy is not readily accomplished. Nonetheless, changes in muscle usually attributed to aging include decreases in the quantity of contractile elements and in metabolic capacities. With an entire adulthood characterized by inactivity, disuse may serve to enhance true age-related losses of endurance, strength, and flexibility, leading to further inactivity and disuse. The effects of age and disuse may in turn exacerbate subclinical disorders such as intraabdominal obesity, glucose intolerance, osteopenia, hypertension, and dyslipemia. These problems, together with the drugs used to treat them (e.g., diuretics that deplete tissue electrolytes, and corticorsteroids with their catabolic effects), may further limit activity in a vicious downhill spiral. The poor nutritional status of older adults and the prevalence of protein-calorie malnutrition, especially among institutionalized elderly, contribute directly to impairments in muscle morphology, physiology, and function.

Despite the difficulty in identifying the precise contribution of each of these determinants to muscle dysfunction with age, there are apparent

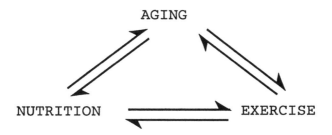

FIGURE 8-1. *Schematic diagram of interactions among aging, nutrition, and exercise*

benefits of dietary and exercise interventions addressing the overlapping impact of disuse atrophy, malnutrition, drug-induced nutrient deficiencies, and disease. Evidence that diet and nutritional status can impact upon risk for chronic disease (National Research Council, 1989a) and that increased physical activity prolongs average life span supports this concept (Blair et al., 1989; Paffenbarger et al., 1986; Pekkanen et al., 1987).

Physical Fitness and Exercise Among the Elderly

Clinical studies of diet and physical fitness have focused primarily on younger adults. While many of the concepts developed in this population are applicable to the elderly, it is important to appreciate the substantial heterogeneity in age and fitness that characterizes this group. In the United States, people over 65 y constitute about 12% of the total population, with those between 65–74, 75–84, and >85 y equaling about 62%, 29%, and 9% of the older population, respectively. The prevalence of disability increases progressively with advancing age such that the inability to perform four basic activities of daily living (eating, toileting, walking, and transferring) affects 10% of those aged 65–74, 20% of those 75–84, and 40% of those >85 y (Federal Council on Aging, 1981; Manton & Soldo, 1985). In the Framingham Study, 5% of men and 10% of women aged 65–74 y and 12% of men and 30% of women aged 75–84 y were unable to walk 800 m; 15% of men and 45% of women aged 65–74 y and 28% of men and 65% of women aged 75–84 y were unable to lift 4.5 kg (Jette & Branch, 1981).

Williamson et al. (1964), charting the principal disabilities in an elderly English community, found that the average individual had 3.3 disabilities, with 65% of the population exhibiting vision and hearing losses, 45% musculoskeletal impairments, 27% cognitive disability, 20% cardiac insufficiency, and 20% urinary dysfunction. The leading causes of disability in U.S. men and women have been characterized as arthritis and rheumatism (32% and 16%, respectively), heart conditions (22% and 25%), hypertension (11% and 6%), visual impairment (9% and 8%), diabetes (6% and 6%), impairment of lower extremities and hips (6% and 4%), and impairments of back and spine (4% and 3%) (National Council for Health Statistics, 1979).

Geographic and occupational factors partly determine the levels of physical activity and fitness in older individuals; e.g., farmers and other people in rural areas tend to have greater aerobic capacities than those living in urban settings (Bailey et al., 1974). However, the aging process itself appears to be associated with a reduction in voluntary activity in both laboratory animals (Mondon et al., 1985) and in man. While declines in activity and fitness in developed countries occur soon after adolescence, even among highly active Masai men $\dot{V}O_2$max declines to 40 mL·kg^{-1}·min^{-1}

after age 51 from an average rate of 58 mL·kg^{-1}·min^{-1} measured in younger men (Mann et al., 1965).

As described above, the complex interplay among normal aging, disease, and disuse makes it difficult to readily ascribe specific determinants to the loss of physical fitness and function. Beyond the factors of aging, disease, and disuse, preconceived societal notions about aging may predispose individuals to greatly reduced expectations with regard to physical performance. Such preconceptions may promote inactivity in women at an even earlier age than in men (Blair et al., 1989). In a survey of Californians 50–64 y, only 2% of women and 8% of men reported regular vigorous exercise during the previous year (Sallis et al., 1985). Paffenbarger et al. (1986) reported that among Harvard graduates of all ages not more than 20% spent more than 2 h/wk playing sports. These figures illustrate Americans' sedentary existence and, together with typical dietary patterns, explain why as many as 20% and 40% of middle-aged and older men and women, respectively, are classified as obese; some subsets of the populations show even higher rates, e.g., 61% of black women aged 45–54 y are identified as overweight (National Council for Health Statistics, 1987). Obesity itself can subsequently discourage exercise because of the extra imposition of effort required for breathing and moving (Whipp & Davis, 1984). In addition, illness and fear of injury also contribute to sedentary behaviors in older adults (Wagner et al., 1992).

NUTRITIONAL STATUS IN OLDER ADULTS

Nutritional status surveys of older adults consistently show only a low-to-moderate prevalence of frank nutrient deficiencies but a substantial risk for other deficiencies based upon nutrient intakes below Recommended Dietary Allowances (RDA) (National Research Council, 1989b). Risk for deficiencies of vitamins A and D, thiamin, riboflavin, and folic acid, in addition to calcium and zinc are most commonly reported (Russell & Suter, 1993; Zheng & Rosenberg, 1989). It is important to note that use of the current RDAs as standards for evaluation do not account for evidence suggesting an age-related increase in the requirement for several nutrients, nor do they suggest optimal intakes relevant to caloric expenditure, health promotion, or reduction of risk from chronic disease (Blumberg, 1991). Many of the impairments in muscle function observed in malnourished patients closely resemble those found with aging although they are readily reversible upon renourishment as noted by Russell et al. (1983) in their treatment of patients with anorexia nervosa.

The efficacy of nutritional interventions on muscle dysfunction in geriatric patients with chronic undernutrition remains to be demonstrated. While limited information is available concerning the role of minerals such as magnesium and zinc in exercise and aging, more data have been published concerning vitamins.

Vitamins

Muscle function can be impaired by frank and subclinical vitamin deficiencies, which are common among the elderly. The status of thiamin, niacin, and riboflavin, because of their association with energy metabolism, are particularly relevant to the performance of exercise and heavy physical activity (Belko et al., 1983; Sauberlich et al., 1979). Vitamin D may play a role in the myopathy of aging (Sorensen et al., 1979). As noted below, vitamin E and perhaps other dietary antioxidants appear to play an important role in the protection of muscle damage induced by eccentric exercise, particularly in older adults.

Thiamin. Thiamin as thiamin pyrophosphate is a coenzyme required for the oxidative decarboxylation of α-keto acids and for the activity of transketolase in the pentose phosphate pathway. There is a wide variability of reported low thiamin intake (0–47%) and low biochemical indices of thiamine status (0–15%) in older adults (Russell & Suter, 1993). Because older persons have lower energy intakes, the RDA for vitamin B1 for those 51+ y is reduced relative to the RDA for young adults by 20% and 9% to 1.2 and 1.0 mg for men and women, respectively. However, some surveys report that a third of the elderly still consume substantially less than the recommended 0.5 mg/1000 kcal.

Race and economic status are strongly associated with thiamin intake as well as niacin and riboflavin intake; the lowest intakes are found among black, elderly males with incomes below the poverty level. Although Knippel et al. (1986) found that thiamin supplementation at 900 mg/d for 3 d increased the anaerobic threshold in trained cyclists during maximal cycle ergometry, no studies relating thiamin status to performance measures have been conducted in older adults.

Niacin. Niacin functions as a component of two coenzymes, nicotinamide adenine dinucleotide (NAD) and nicotinamide adenine dinucleotide phosphate (NADP), necessary for glycolysis, fatty acid metabolism, and tissue respiration. Niacin intakes of less than two-thirds the RDA range from 0–53% of surveyed elderly, depending on race and income (Gray et al., 1983). The 1989 RDA for older men and women was reduced 21% and 13% from that of younger adult males and females, respectively, to 15 and 13 mg of niacin equivalents, respectively. Mean niacin intakes decrease with advancing age even among apparently healthy, independent older populations (Sahyoun, 1992). The prevalence of abnormal N-methylnicotinamide excretion in urine increases with age and sickness and has been reported in 1–50% of heterogeneous elderly populations. In young adults niacin prevents the rise in plasma free-fatty acids during exercise, and at high intakes niacin appears to be associated with no change in performance but greater fatigue (Bergstrom et al., 1969). Pernow and Saltin (1971) found that providing niacin supplements to glycogen-depleted subjects decreased their endurance; comparable data in older adults are not available.

Riboflavin. Riboflavin functions primarily as a component of two flavin coenzymes, flavin mononucleotide (FMN) and flavin adenine dinucleotide (FAD), that catalyze many oxidation-reduction reactions. The RDA of riboflavin for those 51+ y is reduced 18% and 8% for men and women, respectively, from that of younger adults. There is a wide spectrum of riboflavin intakes among the elderly, with 0–36% of elderly subjects reported to have intakes below two-thirds the RDA of 1.4 and 1.2 mg for men and women, respectively (Alexander et al., 1984). A tendency toward lower mean erythrocyte glutathione reductase activity coefficients (EGR-AC) which occurs with age, independent of riboflavin intake and gender. This may indicate lower metabolic requirements for riboflavin in the aged, due to lower energy and protein intakes or other age-related changes in the absorption and/or metabolism of the vitamin (Garry et al., 1982). Using EGR-AC as an index of riboflavin nutriture, 0–28% of healthy elderly have been found deficient, with a greater prevalence noted among geriatric patients. Based on a graded repletion study conducted in Guatemala with healthy older people, Boisvert and Russell (1993) concluded that the dietary requirement for older adults is the same as that for younger people and, therefore, should not have been reduced. Moreover, Winters et al. (1992) showed that exercise training of women aged 50–67 y resulted in an increased ERG-AC and decreased urinary riboflavin excretion (indicators of riboflavin depletion) when riboflavin intake was held at the 1989 RDA value. Thus, the RDA for riboflavin in older adults contains little margin for error and should be raised to the amounts recommended for younger adults aged 25–50 y (i.e., 1.7 and 1.3 mg for men and women, respectively).

Vitamin D. Vitamin D is essential for the proper formation of the skeleton and for mineral homeostasis but has also been implicated in skeletal muscle function via the existence of 1,25-dihydroxyvitamin D_3 receptors (Simpson et al., 1985). Further, vitamin D appears important in the regulation of ATP and phosphate concentrations and calcium metabolism in the sarcoplasmic reticulum and mitochondria of muscle (Boland, 1986). As summarized by Krall et al. (1989), the mean vitamin D dietary intake among free-living elderly in North America and in Europe is about 2.5 μg/d and rarely exceeds the RDA for older adults of 5.0 μg/d. Increasing vitamin D intakes to 10 μg/d through supplementation is still not adequate in many elderly to bring plasma 25-hydroxyvitamin D concentrations into acceptable normal ranges (Gloth et al., 1991). Because of age-related impairments in vitamin D synthesis in skin and metabolism, Russell and Suter (1993) have indicated that the present RDA for vitamin D is too low to maintain steady serum parathyroid hormone concentrations and bone health. Supplements of vitamin D administered to school children revealed no effect on measures of submaximal performance (Berven, 1963); no studies have directly examined the influence of vitamin D status on exercise capacity in older adults.

Vitamin E. The most widely accepted biological function of vitamin E is related to its role as a free-radical scavenger preventing the chain reaction of lipid peroxidation events. However, beyond this direct antioxidant action, vitamin E also serves to stabilize membranes, regulate membrane fluidity, affect nucleic acid metabolism, regulate protein synthesis, and modulate xenobiotic biotransformation (Meydani, 1987). Recent studies have demonstrated that vitamin E also serves to modulate protein kinase C activity, the arachidonic acid cascade, and immune function. The RDA for vitamin E for adult men and women is 10 and 8 mg α-tocopherol equivalents, respectively. (Vitamin E is a mixture of tocopherols; α-tocopherol is often used as a marker for vitamin E activity.) Deficiencies of vitamin E are rarely present without other signs of malnutrition. Murphy et al. (1990) analyzed the second U.S. National Health and Nutrition Examination Survey (NHANES II) and reported daily mean vitamin E intake in men and women at 9.6 and 7.0 mg, respectively; daily median intakes were 7.3 and 5.4 mg, respectively. Vitamin E intakes declined steadily with age such that men and women older than 65 y were consuming a significantly lower daily mean of 8–3 and 6.6 mg, respectively; daily median intakes were 6.0 and 4.9 mg, respectively.

The α-tocopherol concentration in blood better reflects vitamin E status than does dietary intake. Serum α-tocopherol levels increase with age, at least into the seventh decade, in association with its carrier lipoprotein and in relation to liver stores of vitamin E (Blumberg, 1987). Meydani and Blumberg (1992) examined the Boston Nutritional Status survey and reported mean plasma α-tocopherol in men aged 60–90+ y was 27 μmol/L; when stratified by age, mean plasma vitamin E decreased from 32 to 21 μmol/L. A similar pattern was observed in women, with a mean plasma vitamin E of 31 μmol/L and a declining trend from 32 to 26 μmol/L between 60 and 90+ y.

Vitamin E has long been postulated to benefit physical performance based largely on findings from tocopherol-deficient animals, e.g., increased urinary excretion of creatine and phosphate, increased oxidation of polyunsaturated fatty acids, decreased ATP production, and increased levels of lactate and pyruvate, leading to a form of muscular dystrophy (Shephard, 1983). While most studies on vitamin E in sports have failed to demonstrate significant ergogenic effects, clinical trials have shown that α-tocopherol supplementation reduces exercise-induced lipid peroxidation (Dillard et al., 1978; Goldfarb et al., 1989). In addition, Simon-Schnass and Pabst (1988) found that vitamin E supplementation at 400 mg/d prevented the loss in anaerobic threshold seen in mountain climbers at high altitudes, and Sumida et al. (1989) reported that 300 mg α-tocopherol/d for 4 wk lowered the increases in serum markers of cell-membrane damage (malondialdehyde, β-glucuronidase, mitochondrial glutamic-oxaloacetic transaminase) seen after exhaustive exercise on a bicycle ergometer.

Although the evidence cited above is based on studies of young adults, vitamin E may provide particular protection against exercise-induced oxidative injury in older adults (Meydani et al., 1993). (See later discussion on acute-phase immune responses.) The potential for antioxidant protection against free-radical pathology generated during exercise, while promising but not unequivocally proven, has led some investigators to recommend vitamin E supplements for athletes (Packer et al., 1993; Shephard, 1984).

The increased production of reactive oxygen species associated with exercise has given rise to the hypothesis that antioxidant nutrients in addition to vitamin E may play a protective role, if not necessarily an ergogenic one, during strenuous physical activity (Table 8-2). For example, although most studies of exercise after vitamin C (ascorbic acid) supplementation show little or no beneficial action, under certain conditions of dose and duration, Bramich and McNaughton (1987) found that ascorbic acid increased muscle strength and reduced $\dot{V}O_2$max. Furthermore, high-dose combinations of vitamins C and E and β-carotene have been found effective in reducing measures of lipid peroxidation such as serum malondialdehyde and exhaled pentane (Singh, 1992). In addition, Dragan et al. (1990) administered 150 μg/d selenium for 2 wk in a crossover study to Romanian elite swimmers and reported that the treatment reduced levels of serum lipid peroxides and increased concentrations of serum glutathione. With the exception of vitamin E, the use of antioxidant nutrients singly or in combination has not been tested in older adults engaged in exercise programs.

Protein

Dietary protein provides about 10–20% of total energy intake in both young and older adults, despite the smaller energy intake characteristic of the latter group (Munro, 1964). While a number of reports have identified

---

TABLE 8-2. *Potential sources of reactive oxygen species generated during exercise*

- Antioxidant nutrient depletion
- Arachidonic acid metabolism
- Catecholamine oxidation
- Inhalation of pro-oxidant environmental pollutants
- Release of iron and heme protein
- Mechanical damage to skeletal muscle
- Increased electron transport in mitochondria
- Phagocyte recruitment/activation
- Tissue ischemia/reperfusion

protein-calorie malnutrition as a major problem among the elderly, this status appears almost exclusive to elderly individuals afflicted with diseases associated with wasting. From the Boston Nutritional Status Survey of 686 free-living older adults, Sahyoun (1992) and McGandy et al. (1986) reported median absolute protein intakes of 78 and 62 g in men and women, respectively; these values are higher than the RDA of 63 and 50 g for men and women, respectively, and equivalent to 17% of total calorie intake. However, biochemical markers for protein status generally decline with advancing age from 60–69 y to 90+ y. For example, Munro (1992) reported age-related declines in plasma albumin (from 42 to 37 g/L in men and 42 to 36 g/L in women), serum transferrin (from 3.00 to 2.66 g/L in men and 2.97 to 2.51 g/L in women), serum total protein (from 70 to 68 g/L in men and 69 to 66 g/L in women), and serum transthyretin (from 5.5 to 3.7 μmol/L in men and 5.0 to 4.2 μmol/L in women). Age-related increases were noted in blood urea nitrogen (from 6.8 to 8.5 mmol/L in men and 6.0 to 8.5 mmol/L in women), serum creatinine (from 76 to 95 μmol/L in women), and serum ceruloplasmin (from 322 to 363 mg/L in men). Recently, Campbell et al. (1994b) completed a nitrogen balance study in elderly subjects and recalculated results from three previous studies of protein requirements in older adults using the same balance formula. They estimated the dietary protein requirement of healthy older men and women to be 0.91 ± 0.043 g$\cdot$kg$^{-1}\cdot$d^{-1}. This value is higher than the current RDA of 0.8 g$\cdot$kg$^{-1}\cdot$d^{-1} and is considerably greater than the 0.6 g$\cdot$kg$^{-1}\cdot$d^{-1} established by the 1985 joint FDA/WHO/UNU Expert Consultation. Campbell et al. (1994b) concluded that a safe protein allowance for the elderly requires an intake of 1.0–1.25 g$\cdot$kg$^{-1}\cdot$d^{-1} from a diet containing high-quality protein.

Energy

Energy and macronutrient intakes decrease with aging (Elahi et al., 1983; McGandy et al., 1966). Sahyoun (1992) assessed dietary energy consumption in the Boston Nutritional Status Survey and reported median intakes of 1852 and 1468 kcal in free-living men and women, respectively. The lowest intakes were found among the 90+ y subjects, who reported mean intakes of 1357 and 1020 kcal in men and women, respectively. As noted in other surveys of older adults, these values are substantially below the RDA for older adults (2300 and 1900 kcal for men and women, respectively). When energy was calculated per unit of body weight, median values for men and women were similar (25 and 23 kcal/kg, respectively) but, again, lower than recommended intakes of 30 kcal/kg. Of course, estimation of total daily energy intakes based on food record data has serious limitations. Direct measurement of total daily energy expenditure using doubly-labeled water now provides a more accurate estimate of daily energy needs of the elderly. However, as is the case with many other nutrients, the dietary energy needs of older adults are being reevaluated.

Changing energy requirements with age are not only affected by the energy needed for physical activity but also by the changes in resting metabolic rate. Prately et al. (1994) reported that resting metabolic rates in older men increase significantly as a result of resistance training. Similarly, Campbell et al. (1994a) found that weight maintenance during 12 wk of resistance training by older adults is associated with increased caloric requirements. Roberts et al. (1992) suggested that the current RDA for energy intake in elderly men may not only significantly underestimate usual energy requirements but, further, that the low levels of energy expenditure implied by the RDA may favor increases in body fat mass.

Most of the studies concerning the relationship between physical activity and food intake have ignored older individuals (Poehlman, 1992). In one of the few reports available, Goran and Poehlman (1992) monitored 11 elderly subjects and found that endurance training increased mean maximal oxygen consumption by 9% and resting metabolic rate by 11%. However, there was no significant change in total energy intake during 10 d of training with light exercise because of a compensatory decline in ordinary physical activity between training sessions. But when these subjects engaged in moderately intense exercise training, mean spontaneous energy intake increased by 17%. These authors also reported that relative macronutrient intake did not change during the study, suggesting that endurance training does not selectively influence macronutrient intake in older adults.

Moderate exercise training is not usually associated with improvements in nutrient intake or dietary quality in sedentary, mildly obese women (Nieman et al., 1989, 1990). Butterworth et al. (1993) engaged 12 women aged 67–85 y in 12 wk of moderate exercise training (30–40 min of fast walking 5 times/wk) but found no significant changes in means for body weight or nutrient intake, despite an improved aerobic capacity. However, relative to a group of sedentary older women, the trained subjects had higher mean energy and nutrient intakes, especially when expressed on a weight-adjusted basis (e.g., 5 g versus 3 g carbohydrate/kg). When exercise training becomes strenuous, an increase in energy and nutrient intake can be expected (Blair et al., 1985).

BODY COMPOSITION CHANGES WITH AGING

Lean Body Mass

Aging is associated with changes in body composition such that between 25 and 75 y the lipid compartment expands from 14% to 38% of the total body weight, while total body water (mainly extracellular water) and lean body mass decline. The loss of muscle mass is reflected by creatinine excretion rates of about 2000 mg/h at age 20 to 1000 mg/h at age 90 (Tzankoff & Norris, 1978). Direct regional assessment of the cross-sectional area of skeletal muscle by computed tomography indicates that muscle can account for 90% of the area in active young men but only 30% in frail elderly women (Fiatarone et al., 1991). This decline in lean body mass, termed sarcopenia, is accelerated after menopause and at advanced ages (Rosenberg, 1989). Sarcopenia is associated with an increase in intramuscular fat (Borkan et al., 1983).

Cohn et al. (1980) observed that loss of skeletal muscle may be related to the reduction in bone density seen in the elderly. Differentiating muscle and non-muscle mass via assessment of total body potassium and nitrogen, they determined that skeletal muscle loses protein with advancing age, whereas protein in non-muscle tissue is maintained. Flynn et al. (1989) suggested that there may also be a gender difference in the rate of body composition changes with age because the most rapid loss of total body potassium occurs between 41–60 y in men but only after 60 y in women.

The impact of the age-related changes in lean body mass on nutritional status and physical fitness are substantial. Because basal metabolism strongly reflects the lean, metabolizing component of body mass, energy requirements may be diminished by about 100 kcal per decade after age 45 (Tzankoff & Norris, 1977). As energy intake is reduced with age due to a lower basal metabolic rate (and a more sedentary lifestyle), it becomes increasingly difficult for an older person to satisfy his or her micronutrient requirements through diet alone. The functional significance of this change is also substantial, as preservation of the fat-free compartment is highly predictive of muscle function and mobility in the very old (Fiatarone et al., 1991).

Frontera et al. (1991) examined the isokinetic strength of the elbow and knee extensors and flexors in healthy older adults and observed that strength was 16–27% lower in those 65–78 y than in those 45–54 y. When strength was adjusted for fat-free mass or muscle mass, the age-related differences were not significant (except for knee extensors). When strength was expressed per kilogram of muscle mass, gender differences were smaller or absent. This study indicates that muscle mass is the major determinant of the age- and gender-related differences in muscle strength independent of muscle location (upper versus lower extremities) and function (extension versus flexion). Thus, if muscle mass can be preserved into old age, it would be reasonable to expect that muscle strength could also be preserved. Although the reduction in muscle mass with age appears to account for the quantitative loss of strength, qualitative changes in maximal force production may result from decrements in neural recruitment capacity (Bruce et al., 1989). Fiatarone et al. (1990) reported that resistance training can restore some muscle mass and strength even in the very old who have lost substantial amounts of both; the observation that inadequate intakes of vitamin D, magnesium, calcium, and zinc intakes are associated with sarcopenia suggest that appropriate nutritional intervention may be synergistic with the resistance training.

The impact of sarcopenia extends beyond its contribution to weakness, risk of falls, and inability to perform activities of daily living. The importance of muscle mass to the maintenance of basal metabolic rate and physical activity implicate sarcopenia as a risk factor in many of the leading chronic diseases common to older adults including Type II diabetes, coronary artery disease, and hypertension.

Bone

Peak bone mass is achieved at about age 23. The two types of skeletal tissue, cortical and trabecular bone, behave differently in response to aging. In cortical bone, which accounts for three-fourths of the weight of the skeleton, there is an age-related reduction in thickness and an increase in porosity. Progressive cortical thinning occurs mainly by removal of bone from the inner (endosteal) surface and results from increased bone resorption which is not entirely compensated by an increase in bone formation. Trabecular bone loss occurs as a result of thinning of normal trabeculae and of destruction of entire trabeculae. This latter mechanism accounts for two-thirds of trabecular bone loss and leads to a change in the network arrangement (Parfitt, 1987). As it appears that lost trabeculae cannot be replaced, prevention of bone loss is of key importance.

The major determinants of bone volume include genetics and the status of sex hormones, calcium and vitamin D nutriture, and exercise. As comprehensively reviewed by Bloomfield (1995), there is strong evidence that physical activity with reasonable loading and weight bearing by the skeleton will postpone osteoporosis. This stimulatory effect of physical loading and weight bearing on the density and stability of the skeleton seems to last over most of the life span, not only during childhood and adolescence (Suominen et al., 1984). However, exercise and high dietary calcium may preferentially alter bone density at different skeletal sites. For example, Nelson et al. (1991) found that 1 y of brisk walking for 4 d/wk by postmenopausal women arrested the age-associated loss of trabecular bone from spine. They found no additional benefit when the walking exercise was combined with increased milk consumption, although increased dietary calcium had an independent effect on femoral bone density. Age-associated decreases in the efficiency of calcium absorption and the synthesis of vitamin D in skin, in combination with typical low dietary intakes of these nutrients, especially in older adults, significantly jeopardize the maintenance of bone density with aging. In addition, exercise may increase bone density via an influence on hormonal status, as suggested by the results of Nelson et al. (1988), who found that the level of

1,25-dihydroxyvitamin D in active women was higher than that in sedentary women, although their 25-hydroxyvitamin D levels were similar; thus, exercise may enhance the conversion of vitamin D to its biologically active form to increase calcium absorption and bone density.

Adipose Tissue

While lean body mass decreases with age, the amount of body fat generally increases until the eighth decade, after which it decreases again (Noppa et al., 1979; Novak, 1972). In a cross-sectional comparison of 514 people who ranged in age from 29 y to 96 y, Silver et al. (1993) found that the percentages of body fat as measured by bioelectrical impedance did not increase significantly after the age of 40 y, particularly between 40–84 y. It appears that an increase of body weight, rather than a true age-related increase in a percentage of body fat, is the principal basis for the increase of body fat in the elderly. This contention is supported by the data of Silver et al. (1993) who found in a nursing home population that fat comprised 18% of body mass in those 65–74 y, 15% in those 75–84, and 18% in those over 85 y. However, greater proportions of body fat were observed by Durenberg et al. (1988), who used skinfold measurements and regression equations to assess body composition in subjects who ranged in age from 60 y to 83 y; they reported values of 28% and 39% fat in men and women, respectively. However, it has been noted that use of biological impedance and skinfold measurements to assess body fat in elderly people may not be especially accurate because the predictive equations in these methods were derived mostly from young healthy individuals. Bjorntorp (1991) reported that in the average lean man and woman, fat constitutes about 15% and 25% of body weight, respectively. In contrast, male and female endurance athletes have only about 7–15% of their body weights as fat.

Deposition of fat is characterized by its topographical distribution, generally classified as: 1) no particular concentration of fat in a given area; 2) subcutaneous deposition in the trunk, particularly in the abdominal area, called android or male-type fat deposition; 3) intraabdominal fat, called abdominal visceral obesity when it is in excess; or 4) gluteofemoral fat deposition or gynoid type, which is observed primarily in females (Campaigne, 1990). With advancing age, fat is redistributed from subcutaneous to the intraabdominal compartments (Borkan et al., 1983). Central or android distribution of fat both in young and middle-aged individuals is a strong predictor of obesity-related metabolic abnormalities, including hyperlipidemia, glucose intolerance, hypertension, stroke, coronary heart disease, and mortality (Schwartz et al., 1991). There are metabolic differences between adipocytes from various regions; e.g., gynoid body fat is less closely associated with metabolic abnormalities than is android type (Bjorntorp, 1988). Intraabdominal fat measured by computed tomography in 15 healthy 60–82 y men was two-fold greater than that of young men aged 24–31 (Schwartz et al., 1991); following 6 mo of an endurance training program, the central intraabdominal fat in these elderly subjects was reduced by more than 20%. Aerobic exercise training preferentially mobilizes fat from central fat depots in both males and females (Despres, 1991; Despres et al., 1988, 1991). However, loss of intraabdominal fat in women is expected only when weight loss is substantial.

While catecholamine-mediated lipolysis is reduced in aged fat cells (Lonnqvist et al., 1990), exercise training in elderly subjects is still capable of stimulating this process to some extent. With exercise, fat is mobilized from adipose tissue in response to stimulation of an intracellular lipase by catecholamines (Arner, 1988). The fatty acids resulting from hydrolysis of triglycerides are transported in loose combination with plasma albumin to muscle, where they are released, absorbed, and oxidized. Glycerol is not used directly as a substrate but undergoes gluconeogenesis in the liver to restock liver glycogen stores which, in turn, provide glucose as a fuel for muscle metabolism (Bjorntorp, 1991). Therefore, older individuals with a more central distribution of adiposity can benefit from endurance training, which increases the capacity of skeletal muscle to use fat as an energy source and thereby reduces central fat depots and associated risks of android fat distribution.

AGE-ASSOCIATED CHANGES IN ACUTE-PHASE IMMUNE RESPONSES FOLLOWING ECCENTRIC EXERCISE

Exercise increases oxidative metabolism and produces reactive oxygen species. These changes appear to play a key role in altering the fatty acid composition of cell membranes; the permeability of those membranes, resulting in leakage of enzymes; and the release of chemotactic factors, all of which elicit metabolic events that lead to muscle fiber degradation and the subsequent repair processes. Strenuous and exhaustive exercise as well as unaccustomed exercise induce oxidative damage and muscle injury (Evans & Cannon, 1991; Packer, 1984). Damage to sarcomeres at the Z-band level, followed by movement of fluids into the muscle cells, is the characteristic of muscle damage described by Warhol et al. (1985) in postrace muscle biopsies taken from marathon runners. Biopsies taken 8–12 wk after the race showed the presence of central nuclei and satellite cells and an indication of a regeneration process. Similar damage is also observed in muscle fiber architecture following eccentric exercise, i.e., running down a slope, lowering a heavy barbell, and other types of exercise that require force production as muscles lengthen. This type of exercise is most likely to cause delayed-onset muscle damage (Friden et al., 1983) and accompanying muscle soreness (Asmussen, 1956).

Exercise-induced damage to muscle fibers stimulates a wide range of defensive reactions known as the acute-phase immune response, similar to that produced by the immune system against infection. The acute-phase response stimulated by muscle injury promotes clearance of damaged tissue and promotes the repair and regeneration process (Kampschmidt, 1981). Inflammatory cells infiltrating at the site of muscle damage are one of the sources of reactive oxygen species generated by a bout of exercise.

Evans and Cannon (1991) indicated that the early manifestations of the acute-phase response after exercise are similar to the response seen with infection and are mediated through activation of complement, possibly via release of fragments from damaged muscle. This activation is followed by an increase in circulating neutrophils and by their infiltration at the site of muscle damage; neutrophils may be drawn by specific chemoattractants such as C5a. The magnitude of increase in circulating neutrophils following continuous exercise for several hours is dependent on the duration and intensity of exercise. Furthermore, a greater increase of neutrophils has been reported following eccentric exercise than after concentric exercise (Smith et al., 1989).

Evidence suggests that neutrophils are activated following exercise to phagocytize tissue debris and to release cytotoxic factors such as elastase, lysozyme, and reactive oxygen species. Reactive oxygen species can also be produced via a transient localized interruption of blood flow to a group of muscle fibers, resulting in ischemia-reperfusion injury. Interruption of blood flow can occur through an increase of intramuscular pressure or blockage of circulation by an accumulation of large numbers of neutrophils in the microcirculation. The cytotoxic factors can affect the surrounding tissue and degrade the basement membrane of the microvasculature and thus promote further leukocyte infiltration (Meydani & Evans, 1993).

Neutrophils have a relatively short half-life within tissue of 1–2 d (Bainton, 1988). Neutrophil accumulation and subsequent release of cytotoxic factors lead to infiltration and accumulation of monocytes at the site of injury; the monocytes are then transformed into macrophages. Substantial accumulation of monocytes in skeletal muscle is found after the completion of marathon races (Round et al., 1987). These cells are activated, phagocytize cell debris, and they secrete cytotoxic factors and peroxidative cytokines such as interleukin (IL)-1 and tumor necrosis factor-α (TNFα) (Cannon et al., 1990, 1991). Cannon et al. (1989) have presented immunohistochemical evidence for the presence of IL-1 in muscle biopsies taken from vastus lateralis muscle up to 5 d following downhill running. These cytokines promote protein breakdown at the site of the injury and increase hepatic synthesis of proteins, including antioxidant enzymes.

The antioxidant response of older adults to strenuous types of exercise appears to be diminished relative to that of young individuals (Meredith et al., 1989a). Following a single bout of high-intensity eccentric exercise, previously sedentary old men showed a prolonged increase in the rate of muscle protein breakdown, evidenced by an increase in the ratio of 3-methylhistidine/creatinine in the urine; this ratio peaked 10 d after the exercise bout (Evans et al., 1986). In addition, an increase in circulating interleukin-1 was observed 3 h after the exercise in these old men. Endurance-trained old men performing the same exercise did not display increases in interleukin-1; however, the concentrations of interleukin-1 in their plasma samples that were obtained before exercise were significantly higher than those in untrained subjects.

Zerba et al. (1990) observed that muscle from senescent mice is more susceptible to injury and is damaged more severely by eccentric contractions than is muscle from young and adult mice; further, a lower maximal isotonic force was noted in the older animals. No differences were observed in the degree of injury between young and adult mice, suggesting that muscle susceptibility to injury increases in the late stages of the life span. Pretreatment of old mice with polyethylene-glycol-superoxide dismutase (PEG-SOD) provided immediate protection against injury (Zerba et al., 1990), indicating that, in addition to the effect of mechanical strain, oxidative damage contributes to the initial injury during the eccentric contraction. Thus, although the activity of antioxidant enzymes in muscle may increase with age, the ability of these enzymes to protect against oxidative injury may be inadequate to meet demands under conditions of oxidative stress (Oliver et al., 1987).

Eccentric exercise-induced muscle damage can last for up to 6 wk (Byrnes et al., 1985). Ultrastructural examination of muscle biopsy samples reveals significantly greater amounts of muscle damage in older men performing 45 min of high-intensity eccentric exercise compared to the damage seen in young men performing the exercise at a similar intensity (Manfredi et al., 1991). Old skeletal muscle appears to be more susceptible to eccentric exercise-induced injury, in part because older men are typically less active and fit (Meredith et al., 1989a). Skeletal muscle in older individuals may also contain muscle fibers that are more susceptible to injury (Armstrong et al., 1983).

To a certain extent, muscle damage seen in older subjects may also be due to the accumulation of oxidized forms of proteins (Oliver et al., 1987). Rates of lipid peroxidation as well as antioxidant enzyme activities in skeletal muscle increase with advancing age (Oliver et al., 1987). However, the age-related accumulation of oxidized proteins in muscle suggests there is a relatively greater increase in pro-oxidant reactions than in antioxidant defenses. This imbalance may contribute to the reduced ability of the elderly to mount an acute-phase response to muscle damage. Cannon et al. (1990) observed greatly attenuated neutrophil accumulation and plasma creatine kinase elevation in untrained older men (>55 y) when compared to young men (<30 y) during the 24 h period following 45 min of downhill running; vitamin E supplementation significantly increased the postexercise rise in circulating neutrophils and creatine kinase activity in the older subjects to levels comparable to those of the younger men. At the time of peak concentrations in the plasma, creatine kinase activity was significantly correlated with superoxide release from neutrophils. The association of this circulating enzyme that has leaked from muscle with neutrophil mobilization and function supports the concept that neutrophils are involved in the delayed increase in muscle membrane permeability after damaging exercise. Further, increases in superoxide production by circulating neutrophils and endotoxin-induced production of interleukin-1 and TNFα by neutrophils *ex-vivo* was attenuated when subjects were supplemented with vitamin E (Cannon et al., 1990, 1991). These data indicate that vitamin E supplementation may affect the rate of repair of skeletal muscle following muscle damage and that these effects may be more pronounced in older subjects. The alterations observed in fatty acid composition, vitamin E, and lipid-conjugated dienes in muscle and elevations in urinary lipid peroxides after the eccentric exercise were consistent with the concept that vitamin E provides protection against exercise-induced oxidative injury (Meydani et al., 1993). Several potential mechanisms of action of vitamin E and other antioxidant nutrients have been proposed with regard to their ability to modulate immune responses during exercise (Table 8-3) (Cannon & Blumberg, 1994).

CHANGES IN PROTEIN REQUIREMENTS FOR ACTIVE OLDER ADULTS

The requirements of the elderly for individual essential amino acids and for total protein are uncertain because the available data are limited and often contradictory. However, the effects of a variety of biological, environmental, and social factors impacting upon the elderly generally suggest that their protein needs are higher than those of young adults. Based upon these factors, tentative recommendations have been offered that protein requirements for older adults should be higher than those currently provided by international authorities (Young, 1990).

TABLE 8-3. *Potential mechanisms underlying modulation of immune responses during exercise by antioxidant nutrients*

- Neutralization of immunosuppressive reactive oxidants
- Inhibition of protein kinase C and NADPH-oxidase activation
- Modulation of intracellular cyclic nucleotides
- Synthesis of immunoregulatory prostaglandins
- Protection of 5·lipoxygenase
- Regulation of cytokine production
- Antagonism of histamine-induced immunosuppression

Decreased physical activity, a lower intake of energy and protein, and reduced protein turnover with advancing age lead to a substantial loss of body protein and reduced muscle mass in the elderly. In studies of 959 sedentary men, Tzankoff and Norris (1977) demonstrated a substantial decline in 24-h creatinine excretion with each decade of life after the age of 20–30 y. Investigating 200 healthy men and women 45–78 y old, Evans (1992) indicated that muscle mass is the major determinant of age- and sex-related differences in strength and physical capacity in the elderly. Therefore, exercise training and adequate protein intake may preserve muscle mass in the elderly and help to prevent the age-associated decline in metabolic rate and loss of muscle mass due to protein degradation.

As previously noted, many age-related changes in muscle metabolism and function appear due more to disuse than than to age *per se* (Evans, 1993; Fiatarone & Evans, 1993). Disuse of muscle leads to a disproportionate loss of contractile proteins; atrophy of muscle fibers; a decreased capacity of muscle to effectively utilize fatty acids, glucose, and pyruvate; and an increased risk of glucose intolerance. Maintenance or resumption of physical activity in older individuals may reverse the decrease in energy intake, promote protein synthesis, and improve nutritional status. These changes may result from exercise itself and/or from nonspecific activity apart from exercise, such as changes in appetite regulation, food consumption, and the thermic effect of feeding.

In one investigation of the influence of activity on body composition and metabolic rate, Meredith et al. (1987) studied 12 men aged 22–59 y who had been habitually active for at least 2 y and found no age-related difference in muscle mass. They also determined that mean basal metabolic rate was the same for younger and older subjects, despite the fact that the average energy requirement of the older subjects was 17% lower and their average aerobic capacity was 15% lower per unit of body weight. The older subjects performed less physical activity per week compared to the younger subjects, and energy intake and aerobic capacity were associated with the amount of physical activity performed per week. Thus, the declining muscle mass, physical capacity, and increase of body fat that often are observed within this age range are primarily due to decreased physical activity rather than to aging *per se* (Meredith et al., 1987).

Even though protein ordinarily provides only a minor source of energy for muscle function, protein requirements appear to increase with exercise training in both young and older adults. For example, Gontzea et al. (1974, 1975) examined young but sedentary adults fed 1.0-1.5 g protein·kg^{-1}·d^{-1} and found that nitrogen balance became negative with the onset of a cycle ergometer exercise program for 4 d. Also, Tarnopolsky et al. (1988) calculated greater protein requirements for young bodybuilders and endurance-trained men relative to sedentary controls by extrapolating from nitrogen balances obtained with protein intakes of 1.7-2.7 g·kg^{-1}·d^{-1}.

Furthermore, Frontera et al. (1988) found that after 12 wk of progressive, high-intensity, strength training of healthy men aged 60–72 y, the strength of knee extensors and flexors increased, along with the total volume of the thigh musculature. A similar improvement in muscle size and strength has been reported in very old (86–96 y) institutionalized subjects who participated in a high-intensity, progressive-resistance training program (Fiatarone et al., 1990). Finally, Meredith et al. (1988) found that supplementing elderly volunteers with a daily protein/energy supplement increased the size and mass of their mid-thigh muscles more than those of non-supplemented controls after 12 wk of resistance training; however, the gain in strength was similar in both groups.

Age-associated declines in muscle mass and strength occur to a lesser extent in physically active than in sedentary individuals (Fiatarone & Evans, 1993). Despite a reduced muscle mass with aging, habitual physical activity increases protein turnover and protein requirements in the elderly. Following a single bout of eccentric exercise, Fielding et al. (1991) found that older untrained men produced increases in whole-body protein turnover similar to those seen in younger untrained men. However, the older men had an exaggerated proteolytic response, and the protein loss was principally derived from myofibrillar proteolysis (postexercise excretion of urinary 3-methylhistidine was 37% higher than in young men).

Meredith et al. (1989b) have estimated that 0.98 g·kg^{-1}·d^{-1} of good quality protein intake is necessary to maintain nitrogen balance in a well-trained middle-aged man; further, they suggested that 1.38 g·kg^{-1}·d^{-1}, more than the present RDA, will assure a safety margin in regularly active, middle-aged individuals. Studies indicate that there is a higher dietary protein need at the initiation of training, when there is a dramatic change in muscle metabolism. In world-class bodybuilders, protein constitutes 20% of total energy (Manore et al., 1993). It appears that protein requirement remains somewhat elevated as long as training continues (Evans, 1993).

Nitrogen balance studies indicate that the dietary protein needs of subjects engaging in habitual endurance exercise activities are greater than the current RDA of 0.8 g·kg^{-1}·d^{-1} and average 0.94 g·kg^{-1}·d^{-1}. However, using ^{15}N-glycine as a tracer and estimating 3-methylhistidine excretion, Meredith et al. (1989b) found that protein needs of physically active men were not greater than those of sedentary men. If the protein requirement is expressed as a percent of the total energy intake, only 7% of that energy must be derived from protein. Therefore, habitually active people may not require supplementary protein if their diets are similar to those of typical Americans, who consume 12–15% of their total energy as protein. However, particular attention should be given to the protein needs of those elderly individuals who attempt to lose weight by exercising and restricting their dietary energy intakes.

Rudman and Feiler (1989) and others have documented a 20–65% prevalence of protein-calorie malnutrition among institutionalized elderly. Protein-calorie malnutrition has been documented as an important cause of muscle dysfunction, including selective fiber atrophy and disorganization of myofibrils. Decreases in oxidative enzyme capacity and glycogen content of muscle as well as electrolyte imbalances in association with increased water content are characteristic of this condition (Heymsfield et al., 1982). Functional impairments observed in patients with protein-calorie malnutrition include decreased strength, abnormal force/frequency ratios, and prolonged relaxation time (Jeejeebhoy, 1986).

NUTRITION, EXERCISE, AND COMMON GERIATRIC DISORDERS

The etiology of chronic disorders in older adults is multifactorial and includes interacting elements of genetics and environment. In the absence of any current practical application of preventive genetics, the primary interventions to compress morbidity in the elderly remain pharmacotherapy and/or alteration of lifestyle factors such as diet, exercise, and smoking behaviors. The evidence of a beneficial effect of diet modification and exercise on reducing the risk of osteoporosis is quite strong (Bloomfield, 1995), whereas available information on the effect of exercise on inflammatory diseases such as arthritis and on the vulnerability of older active people to infectious diseases is limited.

Insulin Resistance, Glucose Intolerance, and Type II Diabetes

Aging is associated with inactivity, increased adiposity, and a central distribution of fat, interrelated factors that are also associated with insulin resistance and glucose intolerance. Relative body weight is consistently linked to the prevalence of diabetes mellitus, and the prevention or treatment of obesity through caloric restriction is a critical component in the management of diabetes. Limited and sometimes contradictory studies have implicated a potentially beneficial role of soluble dietary fiber, antioxidant vitamins, and chromium in the primary and/or secondary prevention of diabetes. In addition to nutritional considerations, it is noteworthy that even in older adults whose glucose tolerance is within normal standards for younger people, blood glucose and insulin levels tend to be higher following an oral glucose challenge (Gumbiner et al., 1989). Thus, the degree to which diet and/or aging, *per se*, is responsible for the deterioration in glucose regulation is not clear.

The mechanisms by which exercise improves insulin sensitivity in young adults appear, in part, to be related to increases in the number and/or activity of glucose-transporter proteins and subsequent enhancement of glucose uptake by skeletal muscle. Glycogen synthase activity probably is increased with training, resulting in more glycogen synthesis and non-oxidative disposal of glucose; however, these changes appear rather short-lived and mostly disappear within a few days of the discontinuation of regular exercise (Horton, 1986). Kirwan et al. (1993) tested the effects of a vigorous endurance exercise program in healthy 60–70 y old men and women and reported significantly lower plasma insulin concentrations during induced hyperglycemia after the training. Insulin action appeared improved by the exercise (i.e., glucose disposal rate was unchanged despite the blunted insulin response) to levels typical of young adults. Hughes et al. (1993) found that regularly performed aerobic exercise with no change in body composition had a significant chronic effect by increasing glucose tolerance, peripheral insulin action, and GLUT-4 protein in older men and women with impaired glucose tolerance; this effect was independent of the intensity of the exercise.

Although physical activity is already recommended by physicians to patients with Type II diabetes because exercise presumably increases tissue sensitivity to insulin, it is less clear whether or not exercise is effective in preventing this disease. However, Helmrich et al. (1991) prospectively examined patterns of physical activity and other personal characteristics in almost 6000 male college alumni and reported that leisure time physical activity expressed in kilocalories expended per week was inversely related to the development of non-insulin-dependent diabetes mellitus; for each 500 kcal increment in energy expenditure from 500 to 3500 kcal, the age-adjusted risk for diabetes was reduced by 6%. The protective effect of physical activity was noted to be the greatest in those persons at highest risk, i.e., with obesity, hypertension, and/or family history of diabetes.

Dyslipidemia

Dyslipidemia is common in older adults and appears related to diet and inactivity, but other factors are also involved. These include: obesity; diabetes mellitus; pharmacotherapy with thiazide diuretics, beta-adrenergic blockers, glucocorticoids, and other drugs; and diseases of the thyroid, kidney, and liver. High levels of physical activity are associated in cross-sectional studies of young and middle-aged individuals with less-atherogenic lipoprotein profiles, including reduced concentrations of plasma triglycerides (TG) and very-low-density lipoproteins (VLDL), and elevated concentrations of high-density lipoprotein cholesterol (HDL-C), HDL_2-C, and apolipoprotein A-I (Cook et al., 1986; Haskell, 1986). The mechanisms for exercise-related improvements in dyslipidemia are unclear but may involve lipoprotein lipase-induced enhancement of VLDL-TG and subsequent production of HDL particles, increased lecithin-cholesterol acyl-transferase activity, and/or reduced hepatic clearance of HDL particles due to inhibition of hepatic TG lipase activity.

Although some studies indicate that in older men the total cholesterol and LDL-C levels are more related to body fatness than to physical training, Tamai et al. (1988) have shown that HDL-C is higher and total cholesterol/HDL-C is lower in trained elderly men even after correcting for fatness. Studies by Coon et al. (1989) and Houmard et al. (1991) both suggest that HDL-C in healthy older men is more closely related to fitness, percent body fat, and fat distribution than to age. However, prospective studies indicate no beneficial effect of low-intensity endurance training on the lipoprotein profiles of older adults. Pavlou et al. (1989) and Schwartz et al. (1991) have shown that in older adults, as in younger individuals, high-intensity training decreases TG and increases HDL-C but does not change total or LDL cholesterol.

Hypertension

Drug treatment of hypertension in the elderly is effective in reducing the risk of stroke and atherosclerotic cardiovascular disease. However, the adverse responses to antihypertensive therapy suggest a need to more closely examine the efficacy of nonpharmacologic regimens, including low-sodium diets, endurance exercise, and weight loss, especially in patients with mild to moderate hypertension. Strong and consistent correlations between body mass and blood pressure and between obesity and hypertension have been reported in virtually every epidemiologic study of these relationships. Other than caloric intake, the strongest body of evidence for an effect of nutrients on hypertension concerns the high intake of sodium and/or the low intake of potassium (Intersalt Cooperative Research Group, 1988), although some evidence also indicates that low intake of calcium is a risk factor for hypertension (McCarron & Morris, 1985). Examination of the relationships among other dietary factors, including alcohol, protein, fiber, and ratio of polyunsaturated to saturated fat, has yielded weak and inconsistent results.

Cross-sectional and cohort studies generally reveal modestly lower systolic and diastolic blood pressures (about 5–10 mm Hg) in physically active people, but the magnitude of difference depends upon the type and intensity of exercise and the position in which the blood pressure was measured. Paffenberger et al. (1983) and Blair et al. (1984) measured leisure time activity and $\dot{V}O_2$max values, respectively, in large, prospective cohort studies and concluded that increased fitness is protective against the development of hypertension. The effect was independent of age, obesity, and family history. However, in their analysis of a 20-y follow-up study of middle-aged Finnish men, Pekkanen et al. (1987) could not support such a conclusion. Seals et al. (1984) and Stratton et al. (1992) conducted intervention trials with intensive endurance training in older individuals but detected no significant decrement in resting blood pressure. In contrast, Hagberg et al. (1989) showed a training-related decrease in blood pressure responses to acute submaximal exercise in hypertensive patients aged 60–69 y. Thus, some studies suggest that habitual activity and physical fitness may improve the control of hypertension, but the lack of consistency among reports, perhaps due to differences in the populations studied, and the absence of a clear mechanism of action make specific recommendations for the elderly difficult.

Cancer

The evidence supporting the role of diet in the prevention of cancer has been deemed strong enough to warrant recommendations designed to reduce the risks of developing certain forms of the disease, particularly cancers of the breast and colon (National Research Council, 1989a). Such measures include increased daily consumption of fruits (2–4 servings); vegetables (3–5 servings), particularly those rich in antioxidant vitamins C and E and β-carotene; and whole-grain cereal products. In addition, reducing total fat intake to no more than 30% of total calories and minimizing intake of alcohol and salt-cured, salt-pickled, and smoked foods are part of the consensus on chemopreventive diets.

There is a growing body of strongly suggestive epidemiologic evidence that physical activity is associated with decreased overall cancer mortality and decreased incidence of specific types of cancer (Shephard, 1990). Although the magnitude of risk reduction is small, almost 20 studies have observed that physical activity is inversely associated with colorectal cancer; more limited evidence indicates a similar inverse relationship between physical activity and the incidence of breast cancer and cancers of the reproductive system in women (Sternfeld, 1992). Several potential biological bases for these relationships have been proposed; in the case of colon cancer, these include exercise-induced increases in gastrointestinal motility, and for breast and reproductive system cancers, proposed mechanisms include alteration of sex hormone status directly via action on the pituitary gland or indirectly via a reduction of fat stores. Further, moderate exercise may serve to promote greater antioxidant enzyme activity or immune responsiveness with a subsequent beneficial impact on cancer risk.

Atherosclerotic Cardiovascular Diseases

Atherosclerotic cardiovascular diseases, including coronary heart disease (CHD), peripheral arterial disease (PAD), and stroke, make up the largest group of vascular diseases in the United States and have the greatest effect on morbidity and mortality. Rates of and population risk for CHD are most strongly related to the average serum cholesterol level (or, more specifically, to the average LDL-C or LDL-C/HDL-C ratio). The mean serum cholesterol level in turn is significantly determined by dietary factors, particularly saturated fatty acids (such as palmitic and myristic acids), cholesterol, and perhaps hydrogenated (trans-) polyunsaturated fatty acids. A growing body of evidence implicates other dietary factors in the reduction of CHD risk, including moderate intakes of alcohol and more generous consumption of soluble fiber, n-3/n-6 polyunsaturated fatty acids, and monounsaturated fatty acids. Recently, an inverse correlation between CHD and the status of beta carotene and the antioxidant vitamins C and E has been observed in experimental and epidemiological studies (Enstrom et al., 1992; Rimm et al., 1993; Stampfer et al., 1993). The biological basis for this effect appears to be related to a reduction in the oxidative modification of LDL-C and the subsequent transformation of monocytes to foam cells (Steinberg et al., 1989). There is also evidence suggesting that a poor status of folic acid, vitamin B12, and/or vitamin B6 may be associated with CHD via the subsequent elevation of homocysteine, an independent risk factor for CHD (Stampfer et al., 1992). Peripheral arterial disease and stroke appear to be influenced by the same dietary risk factors as CHD, but the importance of these risk factors appears smaller relative to other determinants, such as smoking and diabetes for PAD, and hypertension for stroke.

Several early cohort and case-control studies first established the relationship between physical activity and CHD. Paffenbarger & Hale (1975) examined this relationship in longshoremen and reported that CHD mortality was higher for workers with lower levels of work-related activity when compared with those engaged in more vigorous work. Morris et al. (1980) determined correlations between leisure time activity and initial CHD in a large cohort of civil servants and found those who did not participate in vigorous leisure time activities had higher risks of both fatal and non-fatal CHD events. Paffenbarger et al. (1978) found that the risk of a first heart attack was higher in college alumni with low levels of contemporary leisure time physical activity than in those who were more active; further, this risk was lower for those who engaged in strenuous sports play than in more casual activities at any given level of energy expenditure. Siscovick et al. (1982) observed that among persons who habitually engaged in low levels of vigorous activity, the overall risk of primary cardiac arrest was increased relative to those who were more vigorous during their leisure time activities. Garcia-Palmieri et al. (1982) and Salonen et al. (1982) have reported similar results from studies in Puerto Rico and Finland, respectively. Generally, the magnitude of the relative risk between the low- and high-activity groups is about 2.0 after adjusting for potential confounding factors such as age, smoking, obesity, hypertension, and family history.

DIRECTIONS FOR FUTURE RESEARCH

Our understanding of the relationship between nutrition and physical fitness in older adults has grown sufficiently for us to recognize that in combination they possess the ability to slow or reverse several age-associated signs and symptoms such as loss of muscle mass and the subsequent decrease in strength and mobility. Continuing advances in this area are providing the basis for an integrated approach to the treatment of frailty as well as to the prevention and management of many chronic diseases common among the elderly. However, enough is not known about different types of exercise regimens and the associated changes in nutrient requirements optimal to such programs to accurately prescribe an individualized approach targeted at a specific disorder.

Epidemiological studies provide substantial evidence linking vigorously active lifestyles with reduced risk for several chronic diseases. However, there is a serious need for prospective and long-term trials that directly evaluate the combined effect of endurance training and nutritional intervention in older (not just middle-aged) and very old people and that assess appropriate clinical and disease endpoints. Dietary modification in these studies should include not only caloric restriction and weight loss, but also a significant improvement in protein and micronutrient status. During the aging process there appears to be an untoward change in the balance between antioxidant defenses in skeletal muscle and vulnerability to injury from oxidative stress induced by exercise. While still largely unexplored, the available evidence suggests that older adults engaged in exercise training and physically active lifestyles may benefit from nutritional interventions that enhance antioxidant status.

There is a need for new prospective trials to focus on the specific characteristics of the most efficacious exercise training (type, duration, intensity, and frequency) and its application to specific groups by age, sex, race, and risk or severity of disease. These studies should also include other relevant variables, e.g., body mass index, fat distribution, and immune responsiveness, that will be useful in determining which other physiological characteristics predict the most favorable outcomes for dietary and exercise programs.

There is remarkably little information available about strength training and its potential efficacy in reducing the risk of or managing chronic conditions. Despite the evidence demonstrating the benefits of progressive resistance training on muscle mass and strength, studies are lacking that focus on prevention and treatment of chronic disease and the qualitative and quantitative differences such interventions may present relative to (or in combination with) endurance exercise. Attention should also be directed to the differential benefits of exercise programs, e.g., the action on microvascular versus macrovascular injury in diabetes and on stroke versus coronary artery disease in atherosclerotic diseases.

The role of exercise and diet in the prevention and treatment of inflammatory diseases such as arthritis as well as infectious diseases common among elderly are not well studied, although it is reasonable to speculate about potential benefits of exercise and diet interventions. The apparent inverse relationship between exercise and cancer risk must be more fully examined, e.g., through case-control investigations, before the suggestive evidence now available can be translated into recommendations.

Despite the recognition of lack of exercise as a major public health concern, there has been little systematic assessment of the health risks of exercise in older people. Older people can be predisposed to injury due to their health status, difficulties with balance and/or gait, and greater vulnerability to environmental extremes in temperature (Table 8-4) (Fiatarone & Evans, 1990). Little information is available on the relationships among nutritional status; the type, intensity, and duration of vigorous exercise; and the risk of untoward cardiovascular events in older people. Studies are also needed to assess the potential risk for both immediate and delayed episodes of exercise-induced hypoglycemia in diabetes and the association of these events with dietary patterns.

SUMMARY

Many diseases and disabilities associated with advancing age are also associated also with age-related changes in diet and physical activity. Increasingly, evidence is forthcoming that many of these diseases and disabilities are more closely linked to the changes in diet and activity than they are to age *per se*. Older people often consume less than the Recommended Dietary Allowances (RDA)(which may already be inadequate) for thiamin, niacin, riboflavin, vitamin D, and vitamin E, and there is reason to suspect that these low vitamin intakes may contribute to disability and disease. Evidence is accumulating that dietary supplementation with vitamin E and other antioxidant compounds may provide protection against cellular damage caused by oxidant stress, including the oxidant stress induced by exercise.

Muscle disuse and insufficient ingestion of dietary protein and total dietary energy contributes to a loss of lean tissue in the elderly and to musculoskeletal frailty common in this age group. Rather than needing less protein in their later years, it now appears that older people may ac-

TABLE 8-4. *Potential risks of exercise in older adults*

Metabolic/Nutritional	Cardiovascular	Musculoskeletal
Dehydration	Arrhythmia	Falls
Heat stroke	Cardiac arrest	Fractures
Hyperglycemia	Claudication	Hernia
Hypoglycemia	Hypertension	Ligament injury
Hypothermia	Hypotension	Muscle soreness
Nutrient deficiencies	Infarction	Soft tissue ulceration
Pharmacokinetic changes	Ischemia Syncope	Synovitis

tually require a greater intake of dietary protein than indicated by the RDA. Coupled with an increased emphasis on strength training, it seems likely that increased dietary protein could lead to a better maintenance of lean body mass and to a reduced incidence of falls and other consequences of frailty in older individuals.

The immune systems of older people may be impaired relative to those of young people in the ability to respond to the oxidative stress and resultant tissue damage associated with strenuous exercise. Old muscle is apparently more susceptible to damage induced by eccentric muscle actions, but vitamin E supplementation may attenuate these adverse effects of exercise.

Although studies on older populations are sparse, there is some reason to suggest that there may be a potentially positive effect of combining dietary modification with exercise training to reduce the risk of osteoporosis, Type II diabetes, coronary artery disease, hypertension, and perhaps some types of cancer. Much more research on all of these topics is required before definitive recommendations can be made for diet and exercise in older persons.

BIBLIOGRAPHY

Alexander, M., G. Emanuel, J.T. Pinto, and R.S. Rivlin (1984). Relation of riboflavin nutriture in healthy elderly to intake of calcium and vitamin supplements: evidence against riboflavin supplementation. *Am. J. Clin. Nutr.* 39:540–546.

Armstrong, R.B., R.W. Ogilvie, and J.A. Schwane (1983). Eccentric exercise-induced injury to rat skeletal muscle. *J. Appl. Physiol.* 54:80–93.

Arner, P. (1988). Control of lipolysis and its relevance to development of obesity in man. *Diabetes Metab. Rev.* 4:507–515.

Asmussen, E. (1956). Observations on experimental muscular soreness. *Acta Rheum. Scand.* 2:109–116.

Bailey, D.A., R.J. Shephard, R.L. Mirwald, and G.A. MacBride (1974). Current levels of Canadian cardiorespiratory fitness. *Can. Med. Assoc. J.* 111:25–30.

Bainton, D.F. (1988). Phagocytic cells: Developmental biology of neutrophils and eosinophils. In: J.I. Gallin, I.M. Goldstein, and R. Snyderman (eds.) *Inflammation: Basic Principles and Clinical Correlates.* New York: Raven Press, pp. 265–280.

Belko, A.Z., E. Obarzanek, H.J. Kalkwarf, M.A. Rotter, S. Bogusz, D. Miller, J.D. Haas, and D.A. Roe (1983). Effects of exercise on riboflavin requirements of young women. *Am. J. Clin. Nutr.* 37:509–517.

Bergstrom, J., E. Hultman, L. Jorfeldt, B. Pernow, and J. Wahren (1969). Effect of nicotinic acid on physical working capacity and on metabolism of muscle glycogen in man. *J. Appl. Physiol.* 26:170–176.

Berven, H. (1963). The physical working capacity of healthy children. Seasonal variation and effect of ultraviolet radiation and vitamin D supply. *Acta Pediatr.* 148 (Suppl.):1–4.

Bjorntorp, P. (1988). The associations between obesity, adipose tissue distribution and disease. *Acta Med. Scand. Suppl.* 723:121–134.

Bjorntorp, P. (1991). Importance of fat as a support nutrient for energy: metabolism of athletes. *J. Sports Sci.* 9:71–76.

Blair, S.N., N.N. Goodyear, L.W. Gibbons, and K.H. Cooper (1984). Physical fitness and incidence of hypertension in healthy normotensive men and women. *JAMA* 252:487–453.

Blair, S.N., D.R. Jacobs, and K.E. Powell (1985). Relationships between exercise or physical activity and other health behaviors. *Public Health Rep.* 100:172–180.

Blair, S.N., H.W. Kohl, and R.S. Paffenberger (1989). Physical fitness and all-cause mortality: A prospective study of healthy men and women. *JAMA* 262:2395–2399.

Bloomfield, S. (1995). Bone, ligaments and tendons. In: C.V. Gisolfi, E.R. Nadel, and D.R. Lamb (eds.) *Perspectives in Exercise Science and Sports Medicine, Vol. 8: Exercise in Older Adults.* Carmel, IN: Cooper Publishing Group, pp 175–235.

Blumberg, J.B. (1991). Considerations of the recommended dietary allowances for older adults. *Clin. Appl. Nutr.* 1:9–18.

Blumberg, J.B. (1987). Vitamin E requirements during aging. In: O. Hayaishi and M. Mino (eds.) *Clinical and Nutritional Aspects of Vitamin E.* Amsterdam: Elsevier Science, pp. 53–61.

Boisvert, W.A., and R.M. Russell (1993). Riboflavin requirement of healthy elderly humans and its relationship to micronutrient composition of the diet. *J. Nutr.* 123:915–925.

Boland, R. (1986). Role of vitamin D in skeletal muscle function. *Endocr. Rev.* 7:434–448.

Borkan, G.A., D.E. Hults, S.G. Gerzof, A.H. Robbins, and C.K. Silbert (1983). Age changes in body composition revealed by computed tomography. *J. Gerontol.* 38:673–677.

Bortz, W.M. (1982). Disuse and aging. *JAMA* 248:1203–1208.

Bortz, W.M. (1989). Redefining human aging. *J. Am. Geriatr. Soc.* 37:1092–1095.

Bramich, K., and L. McNaughton (1987). The effects of two levels of ascorbic acid on muscular endurance, muscular strength and on $\dot{V}O_2max$. *Int. Clin. Nutr. Rev.* 7:5–10.

Bruce, S., D. Newton, and R. Woledge (1989). Effect of age on voluntary force and cross-sectional area of human adductor poilicis muscle. *Q. J. Exp. Physiol.* 74:359–362.

Butterworth, D.E., D.C. Nieman, and B.J. Warren (1993). Exercise training and nutrient intake in elderly women. *J. Am. Diet. Assoc.* 93:653–657.

Byrnes, W.C., P.M. Clarkson, J.S. White, S.S. Hsieh, P.N. Frykman, and R.J. Maughan (1985). Delayed onset muscle soreness following repeated bouts of downhill running. *J. Appl. Physiol.* 59:710–715.

Campaigne, B.N. (1990). Body fat distribution in females: metabolic consequences and implications for weight loss. *Med. Sci. Sports Exerc.* 22:291–297.

Campbell, W.W., M.C. Crim, V.R. Young, and W.J. Evans (1994a). Increased energy requirements and changes in body composition with resistance training in older adults. *Am. J. Clin. Nutr.* 60:167–175.

Campbell, W.W., M.C. Crim, G.E. Dallal, V.R. Young, and W.J. Evans (1994b). Increased protein requirements in elderly people: new data and retrospective reassessments. *Am. J. Clin. Nutr.* 60:501–509.

Cannon, J.G., and J.B. Blumberg (1994). Acute phase immune responses in exercise. In: C.K. Sen, L. Packer, and O. Hnninen (eds.) *Exercise and Oxygen Toxicity.* Amsterdam: Elsevier Science Publishers, pp. 447–462.

Cannon, J.G., R.A. Fielding, M.A. Fiatarone, S.F. Orencole, C.A. Dinarello, and W.J. Evans (1989). Interleukin-1β in human skeletal muscle following exercise. *Am. J. Physiol.* 257:R451–455.

Cannon, J.G., S.N. Meydani, R.A. Fielding, M.A. Fiatarone, M. Meydani, M. Farhangmehr, S.F. Orencole, J.B. Blumberg, and W.J. Evans (1991). Acute phase response in exercise. II. Associations between vitamin E, cytokines, and muscle proteolysis. *Am. J. Physiol.* 260: R1235–R1240.

Cannon, J.G., S.F. Orencole, R.A. Fielding, M. Meydani, S.N. Meydani, M.A. Fiatarone, J.B. Blumberg, and W.J. Evans (1990). The acute phase response in exercise I: The interaction of age and vitamin E on neutrophils and muscle enzyme release. *Am. J. Physiol.* 259: R1214–R1219.

Cohn, S.H., D. Vartsky, S. Yasurura, A. Savitsky, I. Zanazi, A. Vaswani, and K.J. Ellis (1980). Compartmental body composition based on total body potassium and calcium. *Am. J. Physiol.* 239:E524–E530.

Cook, T.C., R.E. Laporte, R.A. Washburn, N.D. Traven, G.W. Slemenda, and K.F. Metz (1986). Chronic low level physical activity as a determinant of high density lipoprotein cholesterol and subfractions. *Med. Sci. Sports Exerc.* 18:653–657.

Coon, P.J., E.R. Bleecker, D.T. Drinkwater, D.A. Meyers, and A.P. Goldberg (1989). Effects of body composition and exercise capacity on glucose tolerance, insulin and lipoprotein lipids in healthy older men: A cross-sectional and longitudinal intervention study. *Metab. Clin. Exp.* 38:1201–1206.

Despres, J.P. (1991). Obesity, regional adipose tissue distribution and metabolism: effect of exercise. In: D.R. Romsos, J. Himms-Hagen, and M. Suzuki (eds.) *Obesity: Dietary Factors and Control.* Tokyo: Japan Scientific Society Press and Karger, pp. 251–259.

Despres, J.P., M.C. Pouliot, S. Moorjani, A. Nadeau, A. Tremblay, P.J. Lupien, G. Theriault, and C. Vouchard (1991). Loss of abdominal fat and metabolic response to exercise training in obese women. *Am. J. Physiol.* 261:E159–E167.

Despres, J.P., A. Tremblay, A. Nadeau, and C. Bouchard (1988). Physical training and changes in regional adipose tissue distribution. *Acta Med. Scand.* 723:205–212.

Dillard, C.J., R.E. Litov, W.M. Savin, E.E. Dumelin, and A.L. Tappel (1978). Effects of exercise, vitamin E and ozone on pulmonary function and lipid peroxidation. *J. Appl. Physiol.* 45:927–932.

Dragan I., V. Dinu, M. Mohora, and E. Cristea (1990). Studies regarding the antioxidant effects of selenium on top swimmers. *Rev. Rouman. Physiol.* 27:15–20.

Durenberg, P., K. van der Kooy, T. Hulshof and P. Evers (1988). Body mass index as a measure of body fatness in the elderly. *Eur. J. Clin. Nutr.* 43:231–236.

Elahi, V.K., D. Elahi, R. Andres, J.D. Tobin, M.G. Butler, and A.H. Norris (1983). A longitudinal study of nutritional intake in men. *J. Gerontol.* 38:162–180.

Enstrom, J.E., L.E. Kanim, and M.A. Klein (1992). Vitamin C intake and mortality among a sample of the United States Population. *Epidemiology* 3:194–202.

Evans, W.J. (1993). Exercise and protein metabolism. In: A.P. Simploulos and K.N. Pavlou (eds.) *Nutrition and Fitness for Athletes.* Basel: Karger, pp. 21–23.

Evans, W.J. (1992). Exercise, nutrition, and aging. *J. Nutr.* 122:796–801.

Evans, W.J., and J.G. Cannon (1991). The metabolic effects of exercise-induced muscle damage. In: J.O. Holloszy (ed.) *Exerc. Sport Sci. Rev.* Baltimore: Williams & Wilkins, pp. 99–126.

Evans, W.J., and C.N. Meredith (1989). Exercise and nutrition in the elderly. In: H.N. Munro and D.E. Danford (eds.) *Nutrition, Aging, and the Elderly*. New York: Plenum Press, pp. 89–126.

Evans, W.J., C.N. Meredith, J.G. Cannon, D.A. Dinarello, W.R. Frontera, V.A. Hughes, B.H. Jones, and H.G. Knuttgen (1986). Metabolic changes following eccentric exercise in trained and untrained men. *J. Appl. Physiol.* 61:1864–1868.

Federal Council on Aging (1981). The need for long-term care: a chartbook of the Federal Council on the Aging. In: U.S.G.P. Office (ed.) Washington, D.C.: pp. OHDS 81-20704.

Fiatarone, M.A., and W.J. Evans (1993). The etiology and reversibility of muscle dysfunction in the aged. *J. Gerontol.* 48:77–83.

Fiatarone, M.A., and W.J. Evans (1990). Exercise in the oldest old. *Top. Geriatr. Rehabil.* 2:63–77.

Fiatarone, M.A., E.C. Marks, N.D. Ryan, C.N. Meredith, L.A. Lipsitz, and W.J. Evans (1990). High-intensity strength training in nonagenarians. *JAMA* 263:3029–3034.

Fiatarone, M.A., E.F. O'Neill, N. Ryan, L. Joseph, S.B. Roberts, J.J. Kehayias, L.A. Lipsitz, and W.J. Evans (1991). Body composition and muscle function in the very old. *Med. Sci. Sports Exerc.* 23:S20.

Fielding, R.A., C.A. Meredith, K.P. O'Reilly, W.R. Frontera, J.G. Cannon, and W.J. Evans (1991). Enhanced protein breakdown following eccentric exercise in young and old men. *J. Appl. Physiol.* 71:674–679.

Flynn, M.A., G.B. Nolph, A.S. Baker, W.M. Martin, and G. Krause (1989). Total body potassium in aging humans: a longitudinal study. *Am. J. Clin. Nutr.* 50:713–717.

Friden, J., J. Seger, M. Sjostrom, and B. Ekblom (1983). Adaptive response in human skeletal muscle subjected to prolonged eccentric exercise. *Int. J. Sports Med.* 4:177–183.

Frontera, W.R., V.A. Hughes, K.J. Lutz, and W.J. Evans (1991). A cross-sectional study of muscle strength and mass in 45- to 78-yr-old men and women. *J. Appl. Physiol.* 71:644–650.

Frontera, W.R., C.N. Meredith, K.P. O'Reilly, H.G. Knuttgen, and W.J. Evans (1988). Strength conditioning in older men: Skeletal muscle hypertrophy and improved function. *J. Appl. Physiol.* 64:1038–1044.

Garcia-Palmieri, M.R., R.J. Costas, M. Cruz-Vidal, P.D. Sarlie, and R.J. Havlik (1982). Increased physical activity: a protective factor against heart attacks in Puerto Rico. *Am. J. Cardiol.* 50:749–755.

Garry, P.J., J.S. Goodwin, and W.C. Hunt (1982). Nutritional status in a healthy elderly population: riboflavin. *Am. J. Clin. Nutr.* 36:902–909.

Gloth, F.M., J.D. Tobin, S.S. Sherman, and B.W. Hollis (1991). Is the recommended daily allowance for vitamin D too low for homebound elderly? *J. Am. Geriatr. Soc.* 39:137–141.

Goldfarb, A.H., M.K. Todd, B.T. Boyer, H.M. Alessio, and R.G. Cutler (1989). Effect of vitamin E on lipid peroxidation at 80% VO_2max. *Med. Sci. Sports Exer.* 21:S16–20.

Gontzea, I., P. Sutzescu, and S. Dumitrache (1975). The influence of adaptation to physical effort on nitrogen balance in man. *Nutr. Rep. Int.* 11:231–236.

Gontzea, I., P. Sutzescu, and S. Dumitrache (1974). The influence of muscle activity on nitrogen balance and the need for protein. *Nutr. Rep. Int.* 10:35–43.

Goran, M.I., and E.T. Poehlman (1992). Endurance training does not enhance total energy expenditure in healthy elderly persons. *Am. J. Physiol.* 263:E950–E957.

Gray, G.E., A. Paganinin-Hill, and R.K. Ross (1983). Dietary intake and nutrient supplement use in a Southern California retirement community. *Am. J. Clin. Nutr.* 38:122–128.

Gumbiner, B., K.S. Polonsky, W.F. Beltz, P. Wallace, G. Brechtel, and R.I. Fink (1989). Effects of aging on insulin secretion. *Diabetes* 38:1549–1456.

Hagberg, J.M., S.J. Montain, W.H. Martin, and A.A. Shsam (1989). Effect of exercise training in 60- to 69-year old persons with essential hypertension. *Am. J. Cardiol.* 64:348–352.

Haskell, W.L. (1986). The influence of exercise training on plasma lipids and lipoproteins in health and disease. *Acta Med. Scand. Suppl.* 711:25–37.

Helmrich, S.P., D.R. Ragland, R.W. Leung, and R.S. Paffenbarger (1991). Physical activity and reduced occurrence of non-insulin-dependent diabetes mellitus. *N. Engl. J. Med.* 325:147–152.

Hermansen, L., E. Hultman, and B. Saltin (1967). Muscle glycogen during prolonged severe exercise. *Acta Physiol. Scand.* 71:129–139.

Heymsfield, S., V. Stevens, R. Noel, C. McManus, J. Smith, and D. Nixon (1982). Biochemical composition of muscle in normal and semi-starved human subjects: relevance to anthropometric measurements. *Am. J. Clin. Nutr.* 36:131–142.

Holloszy, J.O., and E.F. Coyle (1984). Adaptation of skeletal muscle to endurance exercise and their metabolic consequences. *J. Appl. Physiol.* 56:831–838.

Horton, E.S. (1986). Exercise and physical training: effects on insulin sensitivity and glucose metabolism. *Diabetes Metab. Rev.* 2:1–17.

Houmard, J.A., W.S. Wheeler, M.R. McCammon, D. Holbert, R.G. Israel, and H.A. Barakat (1991). Effects of fitness level and regional distribution of fat on carbohydrate metabolism and plasma lipids in middle- to older-aged men. *Metab. Clin. Exp.* 40:714–719.

Hughes V.A., M.A. Fiatarone, R.A. Fielding, B.B. Kahn, C.M. Ferrara, P. Shepherd, E.C. Fisher, R.R. Wolfe, D. Elahi, and W. Evans (1993). Exercise increases muscle GLUT-4 levels and insulin action in subjects with impaired glucose tolerance. *Am. J. Physiol.* 264:E855–E862.

Hultman, E. (1967). Physiological role of muscle glycogen in man, with special reference to exercise. *Circ. Res.* 20 (supp. 1): I99–I112.

Intersalt Cooperative Research Group (1988). Intersalt: An international study of electrolyte excretion and blood pressure. Results for 24 hour urinary sodium and potassium excretion. *Br. Med. J.* 297:319–328.

Jeejeebhoy, K.N. (1986). Muscle function and nutrition. *Gut* 27:25–39.

Jette, A.M., and L.G. Branch (1981). The Framingham disability study: II. Physical disability among the aging. *Am. J. Public Health* 71:1211–1216.

Kampschmidt, R. (1981). Leukocytic endogenous mediator/endogenous pyrogen. In: P. Canonico, M. Powanda (ed.) *The Physiologic and Metabolic Responses of the Host.* Amsterdam: Elsevier/North Holland, pp. 55–74.

Katz, S., L.G. Branch, M.H. Branson, J.A. Papsidero, J.C. Beck, and D.S. Greer (1983). Active life expectancy. *N. Engl. J. Med.* 309:1218–1224.

Kirwan, J.P., W.M. Kohrt, D.M. Wojta, R.E. Bourey, and J.O. Holloszy (1993). Endurance exercise training reduces glucose-stimulated insulin levels in 60- to 70-year old men and women. *J. Gerontology Med. Sci.* 48:M84–M90.

Knippel, M., L. Mauri, R. Belluschi, G. Bana, C. Galli, G.L. Pusterla, M. Spreafico, and E. Troina (1986). The action of thiamin on the production of lactic acid in cyclists. *Med. Sport* 39:11–15.

Krall, E.A., N. Sahyoun, S. Tannenbaum, G.E. Dallal, and B. Dawson-Hughes (1989). Effect of vitamin D intake on season variations in parathyroid hormone secretion in postmenopausal women. *N. Engl. J. Med.* 321:1777–1783.

Lonnqvist, F., B. Nyberg, H. Wahrenberg, and P. Arner (1990). Catecholamine-induced lipolysis in adipose tissue of the elderly. *J. Clin. Invest.* 85:1614–1621.

Manfredi, T.G., R.A. Fielding, K.P. O'Reilly, C.N. Meredith, H.Y. Lee, and W.J. Evans (1991). Serum creatin kinase activity and exercise-induced muscle damage in older men. *Med. Sci. Sports Exerc.* 23:1028–1034.

Mann, G.V., R.D. Shaffer, and A. Rich (1965). Physical fitness and immunity to heart disease in Masai. *Lancet* 2:1308–1310.

Manore, M.M., J. Thompson, and M. Risso (1993). Diet and exercise strategies of world-class body builder. *Int. J. Sport Nutr.* 3:76–86.

Manton, K.G., and B.J. Soldo (1985). Dynamics of health changes in the oldest old: new perspectives and evidence. *Milbank Mem. Fund Q.* 63:206–285.

McCarron, D.A., and C.D. Morris (1985). Blood pressure response to oral calcium in persons with mild to moderate hypertension. A randomized, double-blind, placebo-controlled, crossover trial. *Ann. Intern. Med.* 103:825–831.

McGandy, R.B., C.H. Barrows, M. Spanias, A. Meredith, J.L. Stone, and A.H. Norris (1966). Nutrient intakes and energy expenditure in men of different ages. *J. Gerontol.* 21:581–587.

McGandy, R.B., R.M. Russell, S. Hartz, R.A. Jacob, S. Tannenbaum, H. Peters, N. Sahyoun, and C.L. Otradovec (1986). Nutritional status survey of healthy noninstitutionalized elderly: Energy and nutrient intakes from three-day diet records and nutrient supplements. *Nutr. Res.* 6:785–798.

Meredith, C.N., W.R. Frontera, and W.J. Evans (1988). Effect of diet on body composition changes during strength training in elderly men. *Am. J. Clin. Nutr.* 47:767.

Meredith, C.N., W.R. Frontera, E.C. Fusher, V.A. Hughes, J.C. Herland, J. Edwards, and W.J. Evans (1989a). Peripheral effects of endurance training in young and old subjects. *J. Appl. Physiol.* 66:2844–2849.

Meredith, C.N., M.J. Zackin, W.R. Frontera, and W.J. Evans (1987). Body composition and aerobic capacity in young middle-age endurance-trained men. *Med. Sci. Sports Exerc.* 19:557–563.

Meredith, C.N., M.J. Zackin, W.R. Frontera, and W.J. Evans (1989b). Dietary protein requirements and body protein metabolism in endurance-trained men. *J. Appl. Physiol.* 66:2850–2856.

Meydani, M. (1987). Dietary effects of detoxification processes. In: J.N. Hathcock (ed.) *Nutritional Toxicology.* Florida: Academic Press, pp. 1–39.

Meydani, M., and J.B. Blumberg (1992). Vitamin E. In: S.C. Hartz, R. Russell and I.H. Rosenberg (eds.) *Nutrition in the Elderly—The Boston Nutritional Status Survey.* London: Smith-Gordon & Company, pp. 103–110.

Meydani, M., and W.J. Evans (1993). Free radicals, exercise, and aging. In: B.P. Yu (ed.) *Free Radicals in Aging.* Boca Raton: CRC Press, pp. 184–199.

Meydani, M., W.J. Evans, G. Handleman, L. Biddle, R.A. Fielding, S.N. Meydani, J. Burrill, M.A. Fiatarone, J.B. Blumberg, and J.G. Cannon (1993). Protective effect of vitamin E on exercised induced oxidative damage in young and older adults. *Am. J. Physiol.* 264:R992–R998.

Mondon, C.E., C.B. Dolkas, C. Sims, and G. Reaven (1985). Spontaneous running activity in male rats: effect of age. *J. Appl. Physiol.* 58:1553–1557.

Morris, J.N., M.G. Everitt, R. Pollard, S.P. Chave, and A.M. Semmece (1980). Vigorous exercise in leisure-time: protection against coronary heart disease. *Lancet* 2:1207–1210.

Munro, H.N. (1964). An introduction to nutritional aspects of protein metabolism. In: H.N. Munro and J.B. Allison (eds.) *Mammalian Protein Metabolism.* New York: Academic Press, pp. 3–39.

NUTRITION AND EXERCISE **383**

Munro, H.N. (1992). Protein. In: S.C. Hartz, R. Russell, and I.H. Rosenberg (eds.) *Nutrition in the Elderly: The Boston Nutritional Status Survey.* London, U.K.: Smith-Gordon & Co., pp. 75–85.

Murphy, S.P., A.F. Subar, and G. Block (1990). Vitamin E intakes and sources in the United States. *Am. J. Clin. Nutr.* 52:361–367.

National Council for Health Statistics (1987). Anthropometric reference data and prevalence of overweight. United States 1976–1980. *National Health Survey,* series 11, no. 238: DHHS publication no. (PHS) 87–1688. Hyattsville, MD: National Center for Health Statistics.

National Council for Health Statistics (1979). *National Center for Health Services Research: Health United States:* DHEW publication [PHS] 79–1232. Hyattsville, MD:National Center for Health Statistics.

National Research Council (1989a). *Diet and Health: Implication for Reducing Chronic Disease Risk.* Committee on Diet and Health, Food and Nutrition Board Commission on Life Sciences: National Academy Press, Washington, D.C.

National Research Council (1989b). *Recommended Dietary Allowances.* Subcommittee on the Tenth Edition of the RDAs. Food and Nutrition Board, Commission on Life Sciences. Washington, D.C.: National Academy Press.

Nelson, M.E., F.A. Dilmanian, G.E. Dallal, and W.J. Evans (1991). A one-year walking program and increased dietary calcium in postmenopausal women: Effects on bone. *Am. J. Clin. Nutr.* 53:1304–1311.

Nelson, M.E., C.N. Meredith, B. Dawson-Hughes, and W.J. Evans (1988). Hormone and bone mineral status in endurance-trained and sedentary postmenopausal women. *J. Clin. Endocrinol. Metab.* 64:927–933.

Nieman, D.C., J.V. Butler, L.M. Pollet, S.J. Dietrich, and R.D. Lutz (1989). Nutrient intake of marathon runners. *J. Am. Diet. Assoc.* 89:1273–1278.

Nieman, D.C., L.M. Onash, and J.W. Lee (1990). The effect of moderate exercise training on nutrient intake in mildly obese women. *J. Am. Diet. Assoc.* 90:1557–1562.

Noppa, H., M. Anderson, C. Bengtsson, A. Bruce, and B. Isaksson (1979). Body composition in middle aged women with special reference to the correlation between body fat mass and anthropometric data. *Am. J. Clin. Nutr.* 32:438–443.

Novak, L.P. (1972). Aging, total body potassium, fat free mass and cell mass in males and females between ages 18 and 85 years. *J. Geront.* 27:438–443.

Oliver, C.N., B. Ahn, E.J. Moerman, S. Goldstein, and E. Stadtman (1987). Age-related changes in oxidized proteins. *J. Biol. Chem.* 262:5488–5491.

Packer, L. (1984). Vitamin E, physical exercise, and tissue damage in animals. *Med. Biol.* 62:105–109.

Packer, L., A.Z. Reznick, I. Simon-Schnass, and S.V. Landvik (1993). Significance of vitamin E for the athlete. In: L. Packer and J. Fuchs (eds.) *Vitamin E in Health and Disease.* New York: Marcel Dekker, Inc., pp. 465–471.

Paffenbarger, R.S., and W.E. Hale (1975). Work activity and coronary heart mortality. *N. Engl. J. Med.* 292:545–550.

Paffenbarger, R.S., R.T. Hyde, A.L. Wing, and C.C. Hsieh (1986). Physical activity, all-cause mortality, and longevity of college alumni. *N. Engl. J. Med.* 314:605–613.

Paffenbarger, R.S., A.L. Wine, and R.T. Hyde (1978). Physical activity as an index of heart attack risk in college alumni. *Am. J. Epidemiol.* 108:161–175.

Paffenberger, R.S., A.L. Wing, R.T. Hyde, and D.L. Jung (1983). Physical activity and incidence of hypertension in college alumni. *Am. J. Epidemiol.* 117:245–251.

Parfitt, A.M. (1987). Bone remodeling and bone loss: Understanding the pathophysiology of osteoporosis. *Clin. Obstet. Gynecol.* 30:789–793.

Pavlou, C.N., S. Krey, and W.P. Steffee (1989). Exercise as an adjunct to weight loss and maintenance in moderately obese subjects. *Am. J. Clin. Nutr.* 49:1115–1118.

Pekkanen, J., B. Marti, A. Nissinen, and J. Tuomilehto (1987). Reduction of premature mortality by high physical activity: A 20 year follow-up of middle-aged Finnish men. *Lancet* 1:1473–1479.

Pernow, B., and B. Saltin (1971). Availability of substrates and capacity for prolonged heavy exercise in man. *J Appl. Physiol.* 31:416–418.

Poehlman, E.T. (1992). Energy expenditure and requirements in aging humans. *J. Nutr.* 122:2057–2065.

Pratley, R., B. Nicklas, M. Rubin, J. Miller, A. Smith, M. Smith, B. Hurley, and A. Goldberg (1994). Strength training increases resting metabolic rate and norepinephrine levels in healthy 50- to 65-yr-old-men. *J. Appl. Physiol.* 76:133–137.

Rimm, E.B., M.J. Stampfer, A. Ascherio, E. Giovannucci, G.A. Colditz, and W.C. Willett (1993). Vitamin E consumption and the risk of coronary heart disease in men. *N. Engl. J. Med.* 328:1450–1456.

Roberts, S.B., V.R. Young, P. Fuss, M.B. Heyman, M. Fiatarone, G.E. Dallal, J. Cortiella, and W.J. Evans (1992). What are the dietary energy needs of elderly adults? *Int. J. Obes.* 16:969–976.

Rosenberg, I.H. (1989). Summary comments: Epidemiological and methodological problems in determining nutritional status of older persons. *Am. J. Clin. Nutr.* 50:1231–1233.

Round, J.M., D.A. Johnes, and G. Cambridge (1987). Cellular infiltrates in human skeletal muscle: exercise induced damage as a model for inflammatory muscle disease? *J. Neurol. Sci.* 82:1–11.

Rudman, D., and A. Feiler (1989). Protein-calorie undernutrition in the nursing home. *J. Am. Geriatr. Soc.* 37:173–183.

Russell, D., P. Prendergast, D. Darby, P. Garfinkel, J. Whitwell, and N.K. Jeejeebhoy (1983). A comparison between muscle function and body composition in anorexia nervosa: the effect of refeeding. *Am. J. Clin. Nutr.* 38:229–237.

Russell, R.M., and P.M. Suter (1993). Vitamin requirements of the elderly: An update. *Am. J. Clin. Nutr.* 58:4–14.

Sahyoun, N. (1992). Nutrient intake by the NSS elderly population. In: S. Hartz, I.H. Rosenberg, and R.M. Russell (eds.) *Nutrition in the Elderly: The Boston Nutritional Status Survey.* London, U.K.: Smith-Gordon & Co., pp. 31–44.

Sallis, J.F., W.L. Haskell, P.D. Wood, and S.P. Fortman (1985). Physical activity assessment methodology in the Five City project. *Am. J. Epidemiol.* 121:96–106.

Salonen, J.T., P. Puska, and J. Tuomilehto (1982). Physical activity and risk of myocardial infarction, cerebral stroke and death: a longitudinal study in Eastern Finland. *Am. J. Epidemiol.* 115:526–537.

Sauberlich, H.E., Y.F. Herman, C.O. Stevens, and R.H. Herman (1979). Thiamin requirement of the adult human. *Am. J. Clin. Nutr.* 32:2237–2248.

Schwartz, R.S., W.P. Shuman, V. Larson, K.C. Cain, G.W. Fellingham, J.C. Beard, S.E. Kahn, J.R. Stratton, M.D. Cerqueira, and I.B. Abrass (1991). The effect of intensive endurance exercise training on body fat distribution in young and old men. *Metabolism* 40:545–554.

Seals, D.R., J.M. Hagberg, B.E. Hurley, A.A. Ehsanim, and J.O. Holloszy (1984). Endurance training in older men and women: I. Cardiovascular responses to exercise. *J. Appl. Physiol.* 57:1024–1030.

Shephard, R.J. (1984). Athletic performance and urban air pollution. *Can. Med. Assoc. J.* 131:105–107.

Shephard, R.J. (1990). Physical activity and cancer. *Int. J. Sports Med.* 11:413–420.

Shephard, R.J. (1983). Vitamin E and athletic performance. *J. Sports Med.* 23:461–468.

Shock, N.W. (1983). Aging of physiological systems. *J. Chronic Dis.* 36:137–142.

Silver, A.J., C.P. Guillen, M.J. Kahl, and J.E. Morley (1993). Effect of aging on body fat. *J. Am. Geriatr. Soc.* 41:211–213.

Simon-Schnass, I., and H. Pabst (1988). Influence of vitamin E on physical performance. *Int. J. Vitam. Nutr. Res.* 58:49–53.

Simpson, R.U., G.A. Thomas, and A.J. Arnold (1985). Identification of 1,25-dihydroxyvitamin D3 receptors in muscle. *J. Biol. Chem.* 260:8882–8891.

Singh, V.N. (1992). A current perspective on nutrition and exercise. *J. Nutr.* 122:60–765.

Siscovick, D.S., N.S. Weiss, A.P. Hallstrom, T.S. Invi, and D.R. Peterson (1982). Physical activity and primary cardiac arrest. *JAMA* 248:3113–3117.

Smith, L.L., M. McCammon, S. Smith, M. Chamness, R.G. Israel, and K.F. O'Brien (1989). White blood cell response to uphill walking and downhill jogging at similar metabolic loads. *Eur. J. Appl. Physiol.* 58:833–837.

Sorensen, O.H., B.I. Lund, B. Saltin, B.J. Lund, R.B. Andersen, L. Hjorth, F. Melsen, and L. Mosekilde (1979). Myopathy in bone loss of ageing: Improvement by treatment with 1 alpha-hydroxycholecalciferol and calcium. *Clin. Sci.* 56:157–161.

Stampfer, M.J., C.H. Hennekens, J.E. Manson, G.A. Colditz, B. Rosner, and W.C. Willett (1993). Vitamin E consumption and the risk of coronary disease in women. *N. Engl. J. Med.* 328:1444–1449.

Stampfer, M.J., R. Malinow, W.C. Willett, L.M. Newcomer, B. Upson, D. Ullmann, P.V. Tishler, and C.H. Hennekens (1992). A prospective study of plasma homocyst(e)ine and risk of myocardial infarction in US physicians. *JAMA* 268:877–881.

Steinberg, D., S. Parthasarathy, T.E. Carew, J.C. Khoo, and J.L. Witztum (1989). Beyond cholesterol: modifications of low-density lipoprotein that increase its atherogenicity. *N. Engl. J. Med.* 320:915–924.

Sternfeld, B. (1992). Cancer and the protective effect of physical activity: The epidemiological evidence. *Med. Sci. Sports Exerc.* 24:1195–1209.

Stratton, J.R., M.D. Cerqueira, R.S. Schwartz, W.C. Levy, R.C. Veith, S.E. Kahn, and I.B. Abrass (1992). Differences in cardiovascular responses to isoproterenol in relation to age and exercise training in healthy men. *Circulation* 86:504–512.

Suominen, H., E. Heikkinen, P. Vainio, and T. Lahtinen (1984). Mineral density of calcaneus in men at different ages: A population study with special reference to lifestyle factors. *Age Ageing* 13:273–277.

Sumida, S., K. Tanaka, H. Kitao, and F. Nakadomo (1989). Exercise-induced lipid peroxidation and leakage of enzyme before and after vitamin E supplementation. *Int. J. Biochem.* 21:835–838.

Tamai, T., T. Nakai, H. Takai, R. Fujiwara, S. Miyabo, M. Higuchi, and S. Kobayashi (1988). The effects of physical exercise on plasma lipoprotein and apolipoprotein metabolism in elderly men. *J. Gerontol.* 43:M75–M80.

Tarnopolsky, M.A., J.D. MacDougall, and S.A. Atkinson (1988). Influence of protein intake and training status on nitrogen balance and lean body mass. *J. Appl. Physiol.* 64:187–193.

Tzankoff, S.P., and A.H. Norris (1977). Effect of muscle mass decrease on age-related basal metabolic rate changes. *J. Appl. Physiol.* 43:100–110.

Tzankoff, S.P., and A.H. Norris (1978). Longitudinal changes in basal metabolism in man. *J. Appl. Physiol.* 45:536–539.

Wagner, E.H., A.Z. LaCroix, D.M. Buchner, and E.B. Larson (1992). Effects of physical activity on health status in older adults: I. Observational studies. *Ann. Rev. Public Health* 13:451–468.

Warhol, M.J., A.J. Siegel, W.J. Evans, and L.M. Silverman (1985). Skeletal muscle injury and repair in marathon runners after competition. *Am. J. Pathol.* 118:331–339.

Whipp, B.J., and J.A. Davis (1984). The ventiltory stress of exercise in obesity. *Am. Rev. Respir. Dis.* 129:S90–S92.

Williamson, J., I.H. Stokoe, and S. Gray (1964). Old people at home: their unreported needs. *Lancet* 1:1117–1120.

Winters, L.R.T., J.S. Yoon, H.J. Kalkwarf, J.C. Davies, M.G. Berkowitz, J. Haas, and D.A. Roe (1992). Riboflavin requirements and exercise adaptation in older women. *Am. J. Clin. Nutr.* 56:526–532.

Young, V. (1990). Amino acids and protein in relation to the nutrition of elderly people. *Age Ageing* 19:510–524.

Zerba, E., T.E. Komorowski, and J.A. Faulkner (1990). Free radical injury to skeletal muscles of young, adult, and old mice. *Am. J. Physiol.* 258:C429–C435.

Zheng, J.J., and I.H. Rosenberg (1989). What is the nutritional status of the elderly? *Geriatrics* 44:57–64.

DISCUSSION

EVANS: There is a potential impairment in the way older people adjust to changes in energy intake. With Sue Roberts we overfed and underfed young and old people. After the overfeeding or underfeeding for two weeks, young people become hypophagic or hyperphagic, respectively, i.e., they accommodate quite easily. Old people don't do that; when they are overfed, they stay fat for a long time, and, more importantly, when they are underfed, their body weights remain low for a long time. We know about an impaired thirst mechanisms in old people, and we are now beginning to realize that they also have impaired appetite mechanisms.

BLUMBERG: Hopefully, some of those studies will help reinforce the fact that changes in the capacity for adaptation with age, for example in the efficiency of nutrient absorption and metabolism, can have a dramatic impact on nutritional requirements in older people. Add these so-called "age-related" changes in nutritional requirements to the impact of exercise and its influence on dietary requirements, and you can see the potential for further exacerbating the problem of inadequate nutritional status in the elderly.

The RDA for riboflavin is reduced for people over 51 y based on the assumption that because older people are less active, they require less energy and thus less riboflavin. However, recent studies suggest that riboflavin is really not directly linked to energy requirements but is closely associated with protein intakes due to the formation and storage of flavoproteins. Thus, riboflavin requirements not only do not decrease with age in older people, they actually increase significantly, perhaps in association with protein requirements, and, as demonstrated by Laura Winters's group (1992) at Cornell University, riboflavin requirements increase in association with vigorous exercise. I think this situation illustrates the fact that contrary to earlier thinking and in contrast to the RDA, the requirements for several micronutrients not only do not decrease but actually increase with age. This, of course, presents us with a major problem of determining how best to induce older adults to consume these greater amounts of vitamins and minerals when their total energy and food intake is low. If we succeed in motivating older people to exercise, without marked changes in the dietary pattern, the gap between their real intakes as well as the RDA and their true requirement to maintain physiologic function may increase further.

There is a very dynamic interrelationship between diet and exercise. If you wish to achieve a maximal benefit from exercise, then you will have to ensure an optimal intake of essential nutrients. It is interesting to note the complete lack of benefit observed with a nutritional supplement in the FICSIT study by Maria Fiatarone (*N. Engl. J. Med.*, 330:1769, 1994) conducted at Tufts University. However, in this important study, while the strength training intervention was individually calibrated and quite aggressive at 80% of the one-repetition maximum, the nutritional intervention was very conservative in supplying only 33% of the RDA for the micronutrients and was provided in identical fashion to everyone. Given the fact that the RDAs for many nutrients are inadequate to the needs of older people, especially those engaged in exercise programs, and given that the nutritional intervention was not based upon the actual nutritional status of the subjects, the lack of benefit is not surprising. The mean caloric intake of about 1450 kcal/d of these very old nursing home residents underscores their undoubtedly low nutritional status at the beginning of the study. It is imperative that we initiate research that focuses on optimizing nutritional status to determine whether some synergy can be demonstrated with the exercise.

EVANS: We thought that resistance training might actually increase protein requirements, but because resistance training is so profoundly anabolic, we see an almost immediate drop in nitrogen excretion. So in fact, protein requirements are significantly reduced if protein requirement is defined as that amount of protein needed to maintain nitrogen balance. These results have positive implications in renal patients, for example, who have to subsist on very low dietary protein intakes. If they eat a bit more protein while they engage in a program of resistance training, they can probably reduce their nitrogen excretion and enhance their muscle mass. That is one of the hypotheses we will be testing next year.

BLUMBERG: I would like point out that the study by Wayne Campbell et al. (1994a) at Tufts University demonstrated a 15% increase in energy requirements in older men and women after 12 wk of upper- and lower-body resistance training. He also employed two different protein intakes (0.8 or 1.6 $g \cdot kg^{-1} \cdot d^{-1}$) but was unable to show any difference between these two diets with regard to strength performance.

EVANS: But the difference was almost significant ($P < 0.08$).

BLUMBERG: Then perhaps there is some suggestion of an effect on strength with changing protein intakes.

MAUGHAN: The gain in body fat sometimes seems to be an inevitable consequence of aging, but for some, that is obviously not true. To what extent is the typical age-associated fat gain due to changes in activity or to changes in other factors?

BLUMBERG: It is quite difficult to attribute the magnitude of changes in body composition seen as people grow older to a function of primary or secondary aging processes. It appears relatively clear in this case that genetics, diet, and physical activity play a role, with the environmental factors being quite important. It is instructive to note that even lean young people who stay moderately active throughout life still present with small increases in body fat, although nothing like we see with sedentary people eating typical American diets.

MAUGHAN: Obviously, if one increases physical activity, one can increase total energy intake and therefore increase the intake of all the nutrients. But that causes some potential problems if the exercise increases the nutrient requirements in excess of the increase in intake that is stimulated. To what extent can we rely on an increase in activity rather than dietary fortification to meet those needs?

BLUMBERG: We need to promote both exercise and increased nutrient density for older people. If people increase their energy expenditure in physical activity, they will increase their nutrient intake, although we do not know to what extent. However, we must be careful not to assume that just because physically active people will eat more, that they will eat more healthfully. They could simply meet their increased energy requirements through high-fat, nutrient-poor diets. Thus, we must continue to promote healthy dietary patterns in conjunction with exercise. While this may theoretically be a successful strategy for apparently healthy, community-based, older people, there remains a major obstacle with the institutionalized, frail elderly who, even if engaged in an exercise program, may consume too little food to provide all their micronutrient requirements. Some of the preliminary work by Sue Roberts at Tufts University which suggests that older people may not be able to fully adapt their energy intakes after underfeeding or overfeeding may have implications with regard to their changing energy requirements with exercise. We do not know that older people who increase their physical activity will automatically and adequately increase their energy and micronutrient intakes.

MAUGHAN: That's my concern. With young people, the message is simple: if you exercise more, you will eat more and get your nutrient requirements. But with the elderly, we may need to say that if you exercise more, you not only will have to eat more, but you will also need some supplements.

BLUMBERG: While we do not have the data which unequivocally demonstrate that nutrient supplementation is always necessary for active older people, I believe that there are many situations where it represents part of a rational solution for dealing with the risk of nutritional deficiencies common to much of this population.

REAVEN: What is the scientific basis for prescribing low-fat, high-carbohydrate diets for older individuals?

BLUMBERG: The fact is that there is very little direct scientific evidence available to support the application of these dietary recommendations to older people. The recommendations have been extrapolated from studies, primarily epidemiological studies, conducted in young and middle-aged people. These investigations associated low-fat and high-fiber diets rich in fruits and vegetables with a reduced risk of heart disease, hypertension, Type II diabetes, and some forms of cancer. However, these recommendations have never been tested through prospective clinical trials. Nor has it been demonstrated that older people can readily achieve the dietary patterns or amounts of food intake suggested by these guidelines.

REAVEN: I would like to go one step further and raise the possibility that low-fat, high-carbohydrate diets may be counterproductive in older individuals. First of all, if you are concerned about energy intake being too low in this age group, restricting fat and recommending high fiber diets is unlikely to increase the intake of food. Secondly, a significant problem, as you have shown, is that older individuals often become more sedentary and less physically active, changes that will make them more insulin resistant, hyperinsulinemic, and with higher triglyceride and lower HDL-cholesterol levels. All of these responses to a low-fat, high-carbohydrate diet will increase risk of coronary heart disease. When patients with diabetes are admitted to a nursing home, they are immediately put on a "diabetic diet," usually low in fat and high in carbohydrate. We have compared such "diabetic diets" with what they eat when they freely choose. When compared to the diabetic diets, the diets they self-selected resulted in a similar level of LDL cholesterol and unchanged glycemic control; the patients were happier, and they actually had a slight increase in weight. I think it is important before we begin recommending diets that we ask ourselves why we are doing it, and what are the associated benefits and risks.

BLUMBERG: I agree that this is an extraordinarily important point. However, it represents a significant challenge to change what now represents a consensus about healthy diets for all Americans over the age of two years. The Dietary Guidelines for Americans represent the recommendation of a joint committee of the Department of Health and Human Services and the U.S. Department of Agriculture. It is important that we determine through new studies whether these guidelines represent what is really optimal for older people, what magnitude of benefit might be obtained by adhering to them, and whether they can be realistically achieved.

REAVEN: I may add that the American Diabetes Association has finally changed their dietary recommendations. They now recommend that intake of saturated fat should be decreased, but no longer stipulate that it should be replaced with carbohydrate.

BLUMBERG: It will be very interesting to assess the impact of the new

ADA report about appropriate diets for diabetics. The recommended changes substantially alter the way clinicians have instructed their patients for many years. Everyone has accepted the old recommendations as conventional wisdom. I wonder how long it will take to turn around the thinking about these new dietary guidelines?

EVANS: We published a paper showing that exercise had the expected effects of improving insulin sensitivity and glucose tolerance, but when the subjects were required to consume a high-carbohydrate, low-fat diet and to exercise strenuously for 12 wk, nobody improved. In fact, the diet completely obliterated the effects of the exercise.

EDDY: Gerald, are you recommending a diet with 40% of the energy derived from fat?

REAVEN: There are now abundant data, both in patients with Type II diabetes and in non-diabetic subjects with syndromes associated with resistance to insulin action, that they would be better off on a diet in which saturated fat is replaced with monounsaturated and polyunsaturated fat. Such diets are as effective as low-fat, high-carbohydrate diets in terms of lowering LDL cholesterol, but do not raise concentrations of glucose, insulin, and triglycerides, or lower HDL-cholesterol levels.

MAUGHAN: Dr. Blumberg, I would like to re-emphasize your point about the RDA as it applies to individuals. Are we agreed that just because 20–50% of the population have vitamin intakes below the RDA, that doesn't necessarily mean that some individuals in the population are failing to consume enough vitamins to meet their individual requirements?

BLUMBERG: Absolutely. It is important to keep in mind that the each RDA represents a population-based value. Given the tremendous heterogeneity present in the population, especially the older segment, it is possible that intakes at or even below the RDA for a specific vitamin may be adequate to meet the needs of some particular individual. Nonetheless, it is useful to keep in mind the many factors in older people that may contribute to increasing the need for vitamins; these factors include the presence of chronic diseases, use of medications, prevalence of gastric atrophy, and exercise programs.

KANTER: The only antioxidant nutrient that you stressed was vitamin E. You said very little, if anything, about vitamin C, beta-carotene, or any of the minerals (copper, zinc, magnesium, selenium, iron) involved in antioxidant enzyme production. Is there any information on the role played by these nutrients in older persons?

BLUMBERG: My emphasis on vitamin E is based upon what is available in the literature. Vitamin E has been an understandably popular focus of attention due to its role as an effective, chain-breaking antioxidant in membranes. While it would be reasonable to postulate a similarly important role for beta-carotene, another lipid-soluble antioxidant, I am not aware of any studies the relationship between exercise and any of the carotenoids. In fact, the entire relationship between antioxidant defenses and physical activity deserves substantially more attention because of the increase in oxidative stress associated with exercise.

Interestingly, exercise itself can enhance some antioxidant defenses via induction of antioxidant enzymes such as superoxide dismutase. This adaptation might suggest that there is no corresponding increase in the need for dietary antioxidants. While some of our data suggests that this might be the case for younger people, it is not true for older people engaged in strenuous exercise. Older adults are more vulnerable to any pro-oxidant challenge, including exercise, and appear unable to fully defend themselves against toxicity from reactive oxygen species through increased production of antioxidant enzymes. Thus, they may possess much higher requirements for dietary antioxidants like vitamins C and E and beta-carotene to maintain physiologic function and minimize free-radical-induced injury.

KANTER: Is it fair to say that if antioxidant enzyme levels increase, the requirements for minerals such as selenium, copper, zinc, and manganese would increase as well?

BLUMBERG: Yes, that is a fair assumption because we recognize the essentiality of these minerals by their roles as cofactors in enzymes. Examples are copper, manganese, and zinc in superoxide dismutase, selenium in glutathione peroxidase, and iron in catalase. Importantly, intakes of zinc below 66% of the RDA are very common among older people.

DAVIS: The release of oxygen radicals is an important aspect of the normal function of immune cells such as neutrophils, monocytes, and macrophages. You have suggested that vitamin E as an antioxidant might impair that function. In addition, you reported that vitamin E decreased the response of important cytokines that are released by these cells; these include interleukin-1, interleukin-6, and tumor-necrosis factor that are necessary for proper tissue repair following damage as well as for defense against infections and cancer. Therefore, I wonder if this effect of vitamin E should be considered as positive or negative.

BLUMBERG: Before beginning our vitamin E studies, we recognized that dampening peroxide tone through vitamin E intervention might not be beneficial because events like the respiratory burst from neutrophils are essential to muscle repair and remodeling. However, we found that vitamin E actually enhanced all the acute-phase immune responses, including neutrophil concentrations and respiratory activity. Previous studies in cell culture have demonstrated that vitamin E possesses chemotaxic properties for immune cells. Based in part on our observation of a positive correlation between superoxide release and plasma creatine kinase levels, we hypothesized that vitamin E may be protecting the neutrophil membrane from auto-oxidation and thus increasing the cell's effectiveness in clearing damaged tissue and enhancing muscle repair. We also found that vitamin E reduced the exercise-induced stimulation of cyto-kine production, at least interleukin-1 and interleukin-6. These cytokines may play a role in muscle remodeling after exercise. However, it is impor-tant to note that while we observed less production of these pro-inflam-matory mediators, they were still present. It seems unlikely that any antioxidant nutrient intervention would be able to entirely obliterate cytokine production. It would be worthwhile testing whether parameters of the acute-phase immune response, such as production of cytokines or creatine kinase, may serve as a marker for the ability of muscle to respond to a particular exercise intervention and whether modulation of dietary vitamin E may influence the change in a beneficial fashion.

EICHNER: Creatine kinase activity was higher in older runners after downhill running, despite vitamin E supplements, as I understand it. Yet, I believe other investigators have shown no change or lower activities of creatine kinase after vitamin E supplementation. Do supplements of vit-amin E decrease or increase muscle damage in older exercisers? Or is creatine kinase activity not a valid marker of muscle damage?

EVANS: Plasma creatine kinase activity is not a good indicator of muscle damage. In our opinion, CK release is more of an indication of the on-going process of repair than it is of damage.

TIPTON: You seem to be more convinced about the disuse hypothesis of aging than you are about the free-radical hypothesis of aging. I am per-suaded that there is something to the free-radical theory and am biased in favor of the concept of an antioxidant cocktail for older individuals and more emphasis on micronutrients than on calories.

BLUMBERG: It is interesting to note the apparent paradox between the disuse hypothesis and the free-radical hypothesis of aging. Inactivity would appear to spare the body from some oxidative stress, whereas exercise clearly increases oxidative metabolism and the generation of free-radical species. Nonetheless, there is compelling data regarding both the accumulation of injury and the increased susceptibility to free-radical attack with age. The ability of dietary antioxidants to counter the oxida-tive modification of LDL-cholesterol, the UV-photooxidation of the crys-talline lens, and the oxidative damage to nucleic acids suggests a value for increased intakes of antioxidants to reduce the risk of heart disease, cataracts, and cancer, respectively. We also recognize the dynamic inter-relationship between the antioxidant nutrients and enzymes, so it is rea-sonable to postulate a greater efficacy from a "cocktail" than from any single antioxidant compound. However, with regard to combination anti-oxidant formulations, and especially their impact on exercise, there is little evidence available and none in older adults.

EDGERTON: I am curious about the definition of deficiency states for nutrients in older people. The current standards are based on young people, so is it possible that these standards don't apply to older individuals?

BLUMBERG: Yes, the RDA standard for people over 51 y is essentially an extrapolation from data obtained in younger people. Inadequate consumption or risk for deficiency are frequently but arbitrarily defined as intakes below 75% or 67% of the RDAs. The 1989 RDAs include data published in the mid-1980s from studies conducted in older populations. These studies indicate greater requirements for several vitamins, including B6, B12, D, riboflavin, and folic acid. More importantly, the criteria employed in developing the RDAs lack the sensitivity to detect subtle nutrition-sensitive alterations in metabolism during the aging process and they place little weight on the risk factors for chronic diseases common among the elderly. Further, the RDAs ignore the impact of physical activity on nutrient requirements beyond an assumption about normal habits of sedentary Americans.

For middle-aged and older adults, it seems to me more appropriate to consider other criteria, such as the preservation of physiologic function and body composition. Levels of intake should be identified that are associated with the maintenance (or restoration) of immune responses, blood pressure, bone density, and other functions responsive to diet. Moreover, results of epidemiologic studies that reveal risk reductions for chronic disease through associations between specific nutrient intakes and conditions such as cancer, heart disease, and osteoporosis should also be considered in formulating recommended intakes.

BALDWIN: You suggested that resistance training in the elderly increases energy expenditure and energy requirement. Does this mean that there is an increase in the resting metabolic rate and also the need for energy intake? If so, this is somewhat surprising to me.

BLUMBERG: The study by Wayne Campbell et al. (1994a) found that combined upper- and lower-body resistance training for 12 wk was associated with an mean increase of 15% in energy intake required for body weight maintenance. They found that fat mass decreased and fat-free mass increased in these weight-stable subjects, with the change in fat-free mass representing total body water, but not either protein plus mineral mass or body cell mass. Thus, the exercise was associated with an apparent increase in resting metabolic rate due to an increase in the metabolic activity of lean tissue and not an increase in the amount of lean tissue mass.

BALDWIN: But if they maintained their body weights while they lost fat, they must have gained muscle.

EVANS: We saw an increase in body-water content, but not a significant increase in muscle mass. It may be that our techniques were not sensitive enough to pick up small changes in muscle mass that occurred in just 12 wk. But there was a significant increase in resting metabolic rate that we think was attributed to increased protein turnover, which we detected with turnover studies.

BALDWIN: If adult rats accustomed to an *ad libitum* mixed diet containing 40% of energy as carbohydrate, 40% as fat, and 20% as protein are shifted to a diet that contains only 2% protein but more fat and carbohydrate, they consume more calories but undergo a marked loss of body mass that is reflected in the loss of muscle, in spite of the fact that they consume more energy. In fact, their loss of body mass exactly mimics what we see when we restrict caloric intake by 50%. There is something about the protein in the diet that has a tremendous impact, and I think we need to pay more attention to it, particularly in aged populations.

BOUCHARD: The issue of exercise and resting metabolic rate is one which has been studied extensively in the obesity research community. The bulk of the evidence is in the opposite direction from that described by Dr. Evans, i.e., most studies find no effect of exercise training on resting metabolic rate. The only circumstances in which an effect is found are 1) when the resting metabolic rate is measured the day after the last exercise bout, and that effect is thought to be simply a carryover effect of the previous session because it disappears by 48 h; or 2) when caloric intake is increased relative to the increased energy expenditure of the exercise program, which is an effect of the caloric intake and not of the exercise *per se*.

HASKELL: Claude, are those all endurance training studies? Bill Evans was talking about resistance training; do you think there is any difference?

BOUCHARD: Three modalities have been used, endurance, high-intensity exercise, and resistance training; the same trends have been observed for all modalities.

WILLIAMS: Should we be recommending nutritional supplements to older persons who are serious sport competitors?

BLUMBERG: I do not want to over-promise the benefits of such supplementation. Clearly, nutritional deficiencies are associated with impairment in work performance. However, there is very little evidence to suggest that providing the required or optimal amount of any micronutrient will improve maximal performance. Most of the studies conducted to date do not show that one can jump higher, run farther, or swim faster after taking a nutrient supplement. However, recent studies do suggest that providing optimal levels of more vitamins may be associated with a reduction in the degree of tissue injury resulting from exercise and improvements in the rate of muscle repair. It is not yet clear whether this situation translates in a direct and practical application to training regimens for athletes or sports activities for "week-end warriors," although it does suggest a real benefit.

9

Insulin Resistance and Aging:
Modulation by Obesity and Physical Activity

Gerald M. Reaven, M.D.

INTRODUCTION

There is a general agreement that glucose tolerance decreases with age, and states of glucose intolerance are much more common in the elderly. For example, the prevalence of impaired glucose tolerance (IGT) and non-insulin-dependent diabetes (NIDDM) combined was 11.2% for all adults ages 20–74 y, but 27%, almost a threefold increase, for those aged 65–74 y (Harris et al., 1987). These figures emphasize the enormous clinical and public health consequences of this age-related deterioration of glucose tolerance as the proportion of the population over the age of 65 increases (Kane et al., 1981). In light of these data, understanding the nature of this age-related decline in glucose tolerance becomes of paramount importance. More specifically, it becomes crucial to distinguish between the inevitable consequences of aging on glucose tolerance, as differentiated from the deleterious impact of a number of age-related variables on glucose homeostasis in older individuals. For example, as individuals get older, they often become heavier, are less physically active, have chronic diseases, and are more often taking medication for various diseases. All of these variables can have untoward effects on glucose homeostasis. The practical importance of this distinction is self-evident; the greater the role played by age-related variables in the glucose intolerance of aging, the more successful will be interventions aimed at preventing the adverse consequences of this phenomenon.

The goal of this chapter is to review the changes in glucose tolerance that occur with aging and to evaluate the degree to which they are secondary to age-associated changes—primarily obesity and physical inactivity. Because glucose tolerance is ultimately a manifestation of the interplay between insulin secretion and insulin action, it is necessary to review data on the effects of age on these processes and to show how these effects can be modulated by age-related variables. In particular, evidence will be presented demonstrating that the decrease that occurs with aging in the ability of insulin to stimulate glucose uptake is most closely related to age-associated changes in obesity and physical activity and is, therefore, the defect most amenable to intervention.

GLUCOSE INTOLERANCE AND AGING: STATEMENT OF PROBLEM AND MEDICAL IMPLICATIONS

It is estimated that the 98% of the diabetes present in those over 45 y of age is non-insulin-dependent (Harris, 1985). Data from the 1984 to 1986 National Health Interview Survey indicate that about 1 in 10 adults aged 65 and older have NIDDM (U.S. Department of Health and Human Services: Current Estimates from the National Health Interview Survey: United States, 1986). This may in fact be an underestimate because it is based on self-report, and a previous population survey that validated patient history with oral glucose tolerance tests showed that there are an approximately equal number of undiagnosed diabetics (Harris et al., 1987).

Patients with diabetes are at risk for a number of other health problems in addition to the morbidity and mortality associated directly with diabetes. These include: a) large vessel (macrovascular) disease leading to coronary heart disease (CHD), skin ulcers, and amputations; b) small vessel (microvascular) disease that results in kidney disease and blindness; c) neuropathy that causes pain and numbness in the extremities, as well as abnormalities in blood pressure and heart rate; and d) an increased susceptibility to infection. The total economic burden of NIDDM, including health care expenditures and lost productivity due to disability and premature mortality, was estimated at approximately $19.8 billion in 1986, of which approximately half was attributable to persons over 65 years of age who had diabetes (Huse et al., 1989).

Although the impact of NIDDM is important, the health-related implications of the decrease in glucose tolerance that occurs with aging are not confined to an increased prevalence of diabetes. As mentioned previously, the glucose intolerance of aging is associated with a decrease in the ability of insulin to stimulate tissue glucose uptake. If the endocrine pancreas can respond to this defect by increasing insulin secretion, glucose tolerance can be maintained and NIDDM prevented. On the other hand, this state of insulin resistance and compensatory hyperinsulinemia is not benign, and it is now clear (Laws & Reaven, 1993; Reaven, 1988) that a series of abnormalities associated with these defects increases the risk of CHD. This issue will also be discussed in detail in a subsequent section, but at this juncture it suffices to simply indicate that the negative effects of the age-associated development of resistance to insulin-mediated glucose uptake are not limited to increasing the prevalence of NIDDM.

EFFECT OF AGE ON GLUCOSE TOLERANCE

Animal Data

It would not be appropriate in the context of this chapter to review all of the published data of the effect of age on glucose tolerance in animals. However, a few comments on results of studies performed in rats (the species most often studied) may be useful.

Perhaps the most complete study of the effect of age on glucose tolerance in rats was that of Klimas (1968), who performed oral glucose tolerance tests (700 mg/kg) on 20 rats each at 1, 3, 6, 10, 14, 18, 26, 30, and 34 mo of age. Deterioration of oral glucose tolerance was noted to occur within the first 6 mo, but there were no further changes as rats lived to 34 mo. The changes that did occur in the first 6 mo were quantitatively modest, and the data suggested that there may have been no real decline in glucose tolerance beyond 3 mo of age.

The protocol utilized in this excellent study introduces a technical problem that occurs when attempts to assess the effect of age on glucose tolerance in the rat are confounded by the fact that adult rats get heavier as they get older. Should the glucose challenge given to a 2-year-old, 1000-g rat be four times greater than that given to a 2-month-old, 250-g rat? This adjustment must be questioned in view of the fact that most of the difference in weight between the two different-aged rats is due to adipose tissue, and adipose tissue consumes relatively little glucose (Moody et al., 1970). The importance of the issue can be seen in Figure 9-1, which compares plasma glucose responses of two groups of rats given oral glucose in standard doses and then in doses normalized to the animals' weights (Bracho-Romero & Reaven, 1977). When 1.8 g/kg of glucose was given, plasma glucose concentrations were somewhat higher in the 12-week-old, 400-g rats than in the 6-week-old, 150-g rats (Figure 9-1A). However, when the oral glucose was given as a standard dose of 270 mg, the plasma glucose response was actually lower in the older rats. Thus, the effect of age on glucose tolerance depended upon the experimental protocol used.

Unfortunately, there is no accepted "right way" to deal with this dilemma. In an effort to avoid the problem, as experimental rats grew from 3–9 mo of age, we fed them a diet that was less calorically dense than conventional rat chow (Bracho-Romero & Reaven, 1977). By preventing substantial weight gain in rats beyond the age of 3 mo, it was possible to compare oral glucose tolerance in rats of similar weight, but of different ages. As indicated in Figure 9-2, the plasma glucose concentrations were somewhat higher in the 9-month-old than in the 3-month-old rats of similar weight. It should also be noted that the plasma insulin responses of the older rats were also higher at every time point. These data suggest that glucose tolerance deteriorates with age to a modest degree in the rat. Because this was associated with higher insulin levels, the decrease in glucose tolerance was most likely due to an age-related decline in insulin-stimulated glucose uptake.

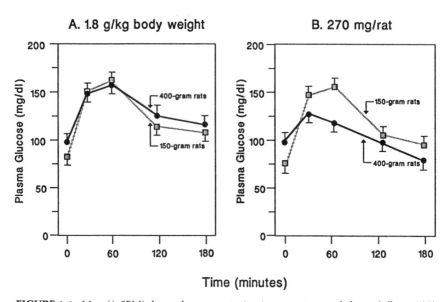

FIGURE 9-1. *Mean (± SEM) plasma glucose concentrations in response to an oral glucose challenge of (A) 1.8 g/kg body weight or of (B) 270 mg per rat in rats weighing either 150 or 400 g. Adapted from J. Am. Geriatr. Soc. 25:299-302, 1977, with permission.*

Human Data

There is considerable evidence that plasma glucose concentrations increase with age. For example, based upon an extensive review of available literature, Davidson (1979) estimated that the plasma glucose concentration 120 min after an oral glucose load increases from 1–11 mg/dL per decade, whereas Andres (1971), using a similar approach, developed a nomogram indicating that the plasma glucose level 120 min after oral glucose increased approximately 10 mg/dL per decade. However, it must be emphasized that these generalizations were derived to a significant extent from investigations that had not controlled for age-associated changes in degree of adiposity, level of physical activity, and general state of health, all of which we now recognize as profoundly affecting glucose tolerance. These confounding factors have been addressed in more recent studies, and a somewhat different picture of the relationship between age and glucose tolerance has evolved.

For example, Maneatis and colleagues (1982) measured plasma glucose response to a 75-g oral glucose load, the standard glucose load recommended by the National Diabetes Data Group (1979), in 206 physically

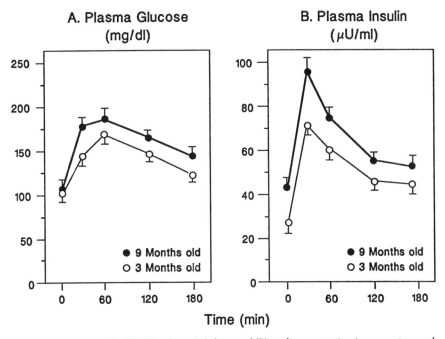

FIGURE 9-2. *Means (± SEM) for plasma (A) glucose and (B) insulin concentrations in response to an oral glucose challenge of 1.8 g/kg body weight in 3-month-old and 9-month-old rats of similar weight.* Adapted from *J. Am. Geriatr. Soc.* 25:299-302, 1977, with permission.

active and generally healthy 47- to 90-year-old residents of a retirement community—127 women and 79 men. For the men, there was no significant correlation between age and response to oral glucose, but for the women, there was a modest correlation ($r = 0.26$ $P<0.01$) that was attenuated, but still persisted, even after adjustment for obesity and level of physical activity ($r = 0.22$, $P<0.025$). This study was the first to propose that deterioration of glucose tolerance with age is relatively modest in magnitude, and not necessarily an inevitable consequence of aging.

A similar conclusion can be drawn from a subsequent report by Zavaroni et al. (1986). These authors studied 732 factory workers in Parma, Italy, aged 22–73 y, and found modest positive correlations between glucose response to a 75-g oral glucose challenge and age in both men ($r = 0.27$, $P<0.001$) and women ($r = 0.16$, $P<0.005$). Percent of ideal body weight, leisure time physical activity, and use of diabetogenic drugs also correlated with glucose response, however. When the effect of these variables was taken into account, the magnitude of the relationship between age and plasma glucose was reduced, and age accounted for only about 6% of the variance in glucose response in the men and 1% in the women. These results provide further evidence that aging *per se* plays a relatively minor role in the deterioration of glucose tolerance that occurs with age.

Additional support for the view that glucose intolerance is not an inevitable consequence of aging can be found in the report by Wang et al. (1989). They studied a population of male office workers and laborers, each group divided into two age groups: 20–40 y and 40–69 y. The four groups, young laborers, young office workers, older laborers, and older office workers, were similar in degree of obesity as estimated by body mass index. Incremental plasma glucose responses to an oral glucose challenge were lowest in the younger laborers and highest in the older office workers. The glucose responses were higher in both older groups compared with the younger groups, but the increase with age when young and old office workers were compared was much greater than the increase with age in laborers. In fact, there was no statistically significant decline in glucose tolerance with age in the laborers, and the plasma glucose response was significantly lower in older laborers than in older office workers. This study again demonstrates that glucose tolerance can deteriorate with age, but it is clear that the degree to which this occurs can be modified dramatically by level of habitual physical activity.

However, the most informative study as to the relative effect of age *per se*, as differentiated from the impact of age-related variables such as obesity and level of activity on glucose tolerance, is the recent report from Shimokata and colleagues (1991). They studied 743 healthy men and women from 17–92 years of age, having excluded subjects who either had diseases or were taking medications known to affect glucose tolerance.

Volunteers were divided into three age groups: 17–39 y, 40–59 y, and 60–92 y. When differences in degree of obesity, fat distribution, and fitness ($\dot{V}O_2$max) were taken into account, the means for plasma glucose concentration 120 min after oral glucose were similar in the two younger groups, and an increase in the mean 2-h plasma glucose level was limited to the group aged 60–92 y. However, even in this instance, it is possible that the decline in glucose tolerance in the older group might not be caused by age *per se*. It is now recognized that individuals can differ not only in their overall degrees of obesity but also in body fat distribution (Bouchard et al., 1993). Furthermore, there is considerable evidence that the metabolic impact of adipose tissue can also vary as a function of regional distribution (Bouchard et al., 1993). Perhaps of greatest relevance at this juncture is the observation that the degree of abdominal obesity, as estimated by the ratio of waist-to-hip girth (WHR), was a significant predictor of the development of NIDDM (Ohlson et al., 1985). Because visceral fat in the abdominal region increases with age (Borkan et al., 1983), it is possible that the decrease in glucose tolerance described by Shimokata et al. (1991) in the 60–92 age group was due to a greater degree of visceral abdominal obesity in the oldest age group.

Based on the foregoing analysis, it seems justified to conclude that there is not a progressive and inevitable deterioration of glucose tolerance with age. Furthermore, previous estimates of the untoward effects of age on glucose tolerance have been confounded by not taking into consideration the impact of important age-related variables, i.e., obesity and physical inactivity. When this is done, the effect of age is greatly attenuated, and it is possible that age *per se* may have little or no adverse effect on glucose tolerance. Finally, it must be emphasized that most studies have used the plasma glucose concentration following a 75-g oral glucose challenge as the measure of glucose tolerance. Although this is the standard way to diagnose diabetes (National Diabetes Data Group, 1979), it should be emphasized that it overestimates the magnitude of glucose intolerance that occurs with age. For example, the data for two age groups depicted in Figure 9-3 contrast the mean plasma glucose concentrations for 180 min after an acute challenge with 75 g of glucose with those concentrations from 8:00 a.m. to 4:00 p.m. in response to conventional meals (Fraze et al., 1987). It can be seen from the data in the left panel (9-3A) that the group aged 60 y and older had significantly higher plasma glucose concentrations 60 and 120 min after the acute glucose load. The results in the right panel (9-3B) compare day-long glucose concentrations in response to identical test meals in the two age groups, and it is obvious that the difference between the younger and older individuals was markedly diminished. Indeed, the total integrated glucose response from 8:00 a.m. to 4:00 p.m. of the older group was increased by only 8%. These studies were performed

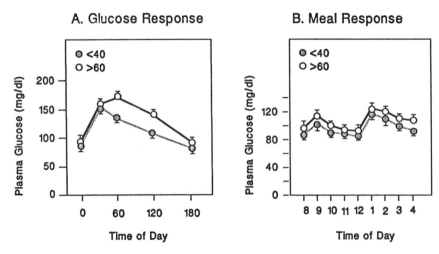

A. Glucose Response

B. Meal Response

FIGURE 9-3. *Mean (± SEM) plasma glucose concentrations in response to (A) a 75-g oral glucose challenge or (B) before and after breakfast (20% of total daily energy intake) and lunch (40% of total daily energy intake) in individuals <40 years old (●---●) and >60 years old (○—○).* Adapted from J. Am. Geriatr. Soc. 35:224-228, 1987, with permission.

in healthy, non-obese individuals, and the results emphasize the fact that day-long plasma glucose concentrations in these older subjects were comparable to the values in the younger subjects.

EFFECT OF AGE ON INSULIN RESISTANCE AND INSULIN SECRETION

As described previously, there is abundant evidence that glucose tolerance decreases with age. Irrespective of the relative importance of aging versus age-associated variables in this phenomenon, the loss of glucose homeostasis must be secondary to defects in insulin action and/or insulin secretion. This section will review relevant data concerning the changes in insulin action and insulin secretion that occur with aging and will evaluate the relative importance of age, as contrasted to age-related variables, in these events.

Animal Data

In order to understand the effect of age on the endocrine pancreas, it is necessary to distinguish between maximal insulin secretion per pancreas and maximal insulin secretion per pancreatic β-cell. As rats grow older, fatter, and less active, the total pancreas increases in weight, with an increase in both the size and number of islets of Langerhans; hence β-cell mass increases with age (Curry et al., 1984; Reaven & Reaven, 1981; Reaven et al., 1979, 1983a, 1983b, 1987). The magnitude of these changes can be modified by differences in strain and gender of rats. For example, the increase in pancreatic insulin secretory mass is greater in Sprague-Dawley than in Fischer 344 rats (Curry et al., 1984; Reaven & Reaven, 1981; Reaven et al., 1979) and is also accentuated in males as compared to female rats (Reaven et al., 1987). Furthermore, the age-associated increase in pancreatic insulin secretory mass can be attenuated (Reaven & Reaven, 1981; Reaven et al., 1983a, 1983b) by preventing obesity (decreasing caloric intake), changing diet composition (high sucrose intake), or by increasing the level of habitual physical activity (rats living in exercise wheel cages). However, in all of these instances, and irrespective of total β-cell mass, insulin secretion per β-cell declines progressively with age. This change is independent of strain of rat (Curry et al., 1984), gender (Reaven et al., 1987) and environmental manipulation (Reaven & Reaven, 1981; Reaven et al., 1983a, 1983b), and it appears to be an inevitable consequence of aging.

Thus, the pancreatic hyperplasia that occurs with aging in rats seems to represent an effort of the organism to compensate for the decrease in insulin secretion per β-cell, and the observed increase in the mass of insulin secretory cells is highly correlated with the amount of insulin secretion necessary to prevent deterioration of glucose homeostasis as rats age. For example, as will be discussed in detail subsequently, the ability of insulin to stimulate glucose disposal is decreased by obesity, and an older and fatter rat has a larger insulin secretory mass than a leaner rat of the same age (Curry et al., 1984; Reaven & Reaven, 1981; Reaven et al., 1979, 1983a, 1983b, 1987). Thus, although the decrease in maximal insulin secretion *per β-cell* is similar in the two groups of older rats, maximal glucose-stimulated insulin secretion by the pancreas will be greater in the older, and fatter, rats.

Because maximal total insulin response to a glucose challenge is preserved in rats as they mature, while glucose tolerance tends to deteriorate, there must be a defect in insulin action in older rats. Narimiya et al. (1984) measured this directly. In rats of three different ages, endogenous insulin secretion was inhibited, and insulin was infused to achieve the same steady-state degree of physiological hyperinsulinemia (SSPI) in each animal. The same amount of dextrose was also continuously infused in each rat. The resulting steady-state plasma glucose concentration (SSPG) provided a measure of the ability of equal concentrations of insulin to stimulate glucose disposal in animals of different ages. The results of this study are illustrated in Figure 9-4. It can be seen that the SSPI concentrations were similar in the three groups (9-4A). Despite this, the SSPG concentrations (9-4B) increased almost fourfold as rats grew from 1.5 to 4 months of age. Thus, there was a dramatic decrease in the ability of insulin to stimulate glucose disposal over this 2.5 mo period. On the other hand, there was essentially no change in SSPG concentrations as rats aged from 4 to 12 months of age. It should be noted that weight more than doubled between 1.5 and 4 months of age. However, from 4 to 12 mo, despite the longer aging interval, there was little change in SSPG and a much smaller change in weight. This evidence suggests that the increase in SSPG occurred early in the maturation process, presumably due to the weight gain. The fact that values for SSPG did not increase from 4 to 12 months of age suggests that the aging process had little, if any, effect on insulin action. These *in vivo* observations have been confirmed by studies in which the ability of insulin to stimulate glucose uptake was quantified in perfused hindlimbs of rats of different ages (Goodman et al., 1983; Narimiya et al., 1984). The results of these experiments also demonstrated that a dramatic decline in insulin action occurred as rats matured, with little change being seen from 4 months to 2 years of age.

To further examine the relative effects of weight gain versus maturation, Santos et al. (1989) studied three groups of rats. One grew without any intervention until 5 months of age. Another group was fed an energy-restricted diet so the rats did not gain weight as they grew older. A third group was placed in exercise wheel cages and allowed to exercise and eat *ad libitum*. This group also did not gain weight with aging. Insulin action, assessed by the steady-state plasma glucose concentration as previously described (Figure 9-4), was significantly lower in the two groups of leaner rats. This shows that weight maintenance, accomplished either by restriction of energy intake or by exercise training, can attenuate the insulin resistance associated with the maturation process in rats.

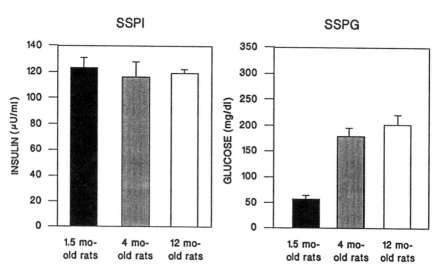

FIGURE 9-4. *Mean (± SEM) steady-state plasma insulin (SSPI) and glucose (SSPG) concentrations in 1.5-, 4-, and 12-month-old rats.* Adapted from *Am. J. Physiol.* 246 Endocrinol. Metab. 9:E397–E404, 1984, with permission.

The data presented so far provide a coherent hypothesis concerning the effect of age on insulin secretion, insulin action, and glucose tolerance in rats. A decrease in maximal glucose-stimulated insulin release per pancreatic β-cell appears to be an inevitable consequence of aging, whereas a decrease in insulin-stimulated glucose uptake is primarily due to the obesity and physical inactivity that accompany aging. If rats remain lean and physically active as they age, significant increases in insulin resistance do not develop, the pancreatic islets are able to secrete enough insulin to maintain normal glucose homeostasis despite decreases in insulin secretory capacity per β-cell, and relatively little evidence of β-cell hyperlasia is seen. The more obese and sedentary rats become as they grow older, the greater the resistance to insulin-stimulated glucose uptake; in this situation, increasingly greater quantities of insulin must be secreted to maintain normal glucose tolerance, thereby accentuating the need for β-cell hyperplasia. If the need for insulin exceeds the capacity of the pancreas to secrete it, glucose homeostasis will be lost. However, in the case of the rats, there seems to be no limit in the degree of β-cell hyperplasia that can occur, and spontaneous hyperglycemia does not develop.

Human Data

As in rats, absolute concentrations of plasma insulin in humans tend to stay the same or rise with age (Reaven & Reaven, 1985). If glucose tolerance declines with age, and insulin concentrations do not, the simplest conclusion is that the ability of insulin to stimulate glucose disposal must decrease with age. Over the last several years a good deal of evidence has been published in support of this generalization (DeFronzo, 1979; Fink et al., 1983, 1986; Reaven et al., 1989a; Rowe et al., 1983). Before continuing the discussion of the relationship between aging and insulin action, it is necessary to emphasize that just because circulating plasma insulin concentrations in older healthy subjects are similar to or greater than those in younger individuals, it does not follow that insulin secretory function is unaffected by age. The importance of this distinction will become apparent when the relationship between age and NIDDM is addressed.

Rather than review the evidence that aging is associated with resistance to insulin-mediated glucose uptake, a conclusion that is widely accepted, it seems more useful to focus on three aspects of this problem that may be controversial. The first issue relates to whether or not the development of insulin resistance is progressive with aging. Although this is often suggested to be the case (DeFronzo, 1979; Fink et al., 1983; Rowe et al., 1983), the results of hyperinsulinemic, euglycemic clamp studies shown in Figure 9-5 indicate that this issue may be more complicated. These data depict the ability of similar steady-state plasma concentrations of infused exogenous insulin to promote glucose uptake in a group of healthy, nondiabetic volunteers, divided into three age groups: 21–34, 35–54, and >55 years of age. As can be seen in Figure 9-5A, the average insulin-stimulated glucose uptake (metabolic clearance rate) values for the two younger age groups were equal, whereas the values for those >55 years of age were decreased by approximately 25% on average. Essentially similar data have been published by Fink and colleagues (1986), suggesting that the defect in insulin action may not be progressive with aging, but manifested only in the older population. It can be seen from Figure 9-5B that this age-related decline in glucose disposal occurred despite the presence of higher steady-state plasma insulin concentrations in those >55 years of age. These data are of particular interest in light of the previously discussed evidence of Shimokota and colleagues (1991) that, when the effect of differences in obesity and $\dot{V}O_2$max are taken into consideration, only healthy individuals above the age of 60 show a decline in glucose tolerance.

The values for glucose uptake shown in Figure 9-5 are often assumed to represent a specific increase in the ability of insulin to stimulate glucose uptake. In fact, this is not the case, and what is actually being measured is a combination of glucose uptake in the basal state plus the increment in glucose uptake due to the action of insulin. Thus, even if it is assumed that glucose uptake is decreased on the average in individuals >60 years of age, it is not clear if the age-related defect involves basal glucose uptake, insulin-stimulated glucose uptake, or both. In that context, data from our research group (Reaven et al., 1989a) and that of Pacini et al. (1988) have attempted to make that distinction. The results of the two

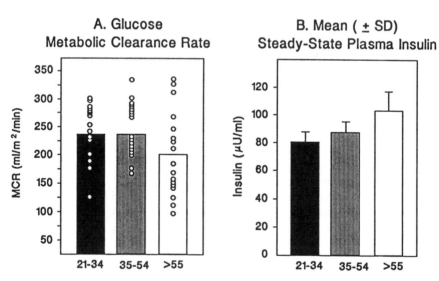

FIGURE 9-5. *Mean glucose metabolic clearance rates (A) and steady-state plasma insulin concentrations (B) during hyperinsulinemic, euglycemic clamp studies in 14 subjects aged 21–34, 17 subjects 35–54, and 17 subjects more than 55 years of age. Individual data are shown as open circles.* Adapted from *J. Am. Geriatr. Soc.* 37:735–740, 1989, with permission.

studies are quite comparable, both demonstrating that the degree of insulin resistance present in healthy, older individuals was relatively modest in magnitude, and could be seen both at basal insulin levels and during periods of physiological hyperinsulinemia.

If it is assumed that there is a decrease of modest magnitude in glucose uptake under basal condition and in response to insulin in individuals over the age of 60, it is necessary to evaluate the relative roles of aging, as distinct from age-related variables, in this change. Perhaps the best way to begin this analysis is to focus on the individual data seen in Figure 9-5A. It can be seen that the degree of variability in values for glucose uptake in normal humans was essentially doubled in subjects 55 years of age or older. There are several possible explanations for these findings. For example, older individuals tend to be relatively more obese (Novak, 1972), and obesity is a factor well known to increase resistance to insulin-stimulated glucose uptake (Olefsky et al., 1974a; Rabinowitz & Zierler, 1962). Although efforts have been made to control for body weight in recent studies, more subtle changes in body composition associated with aging might help explain the increased variability in insulin action. Because it appears that insulin sensitivity is directly related to muscle mass and inversely proportional to adiposity (Yki-Järvinen & Koivisto, 1983), the relative decrease in muscle mass (and increase in adiposity) that tends to occur in older individuals might be responsible for the age-related decline in basal and insulin-stimulated glucose uptake. For example, as discussed previously, age is also associated with an increase in visceral abdominal obesity (Borkan et al., 1983), and there is evidence (Park et al., 1991) that this change is associated with a decrease in insulin-mediated glucose disposal. This issue has been recently addressed by Boden et al. (1993), who compared insulin-mediated glucose uptake in healthy older and younger individuals, and also measured body composition and insulin-stimulated blood flow to the leg. The results demonstrated that data for body fat and glucose uptake in both elderly and younger subjects were highly correlated in a negative fashion. In contrast, glucose uptake did not vary as a function of age. These data provide further support for the view that a decline in insulin-mediated glucose uptake is not an inevitable consequence of aging.

Finally, it has been shown that maximal aerobic capacity, a reflection of level of habitual physical activity, is directly correlated to insulin-mediated glucose uptake (Rosenthal et al., 1983). In general, individuals tend to become more sedentary as they age, and differences in level of physical activity could also contribute to the variability of results noted in studies of insulin action. Given these data, it is obvious that the healthier, leaner, and more physically active the older individuals being studied, the more difficult it will be to document any reduction in insulin action. Support for this generalization can be found in the results of Hollenbeck et al. (1985), who studied 20 non-obese men over 60 years of age—13 who were healthy but not engaged in a regular exercise program, and seven who exercised for at least 45 min, 3 or more times per wk. All had normal glucose tolerance. Although body mass index (BMI) was the same in the two groups, the sedentary group had significantly more body fat. Maximal aerobic power ($\dot{V}O_2$max) was significantly higher in the group of subjects who exercised regularly. Insulin-mediated glucose uptake as measured by the insulin clamp technique was significantly higher in the exercising group, and there was a strong correlation ($r = 0.74$ $P<0.001$) between $\dot{V}O_2$max and *in vivo* insulin action, independent of BMI and percent body fat.

In summary, there is considerable evidence that glucose disposal decreases with age. However, because plasma insulin concentrations do not decline with age, serious disruptions of glucose homeostasis can be prevented despite this defect. Although controversies remain, certain generalizations as to the relationship between age and glucose disposal seem to be justified. Specifically, glucose uptake does not seem to decline progressively with age in healthy, non-obese, and active individuals. It is impossible to exclude the possibility that in some persons glucose disposal may begin to fall off after the age of 60, but even in these individuals the change is relatively modest in magnitude. Finally, it is apparent that increases in degree of adiposity and decreases in level of habitual physical activity account for most, if not all, of the loss of glucose tolerance with aging.

CLINICAL IMPLICATIONS OF AGE-RELATED INSULIN RESISTANCE

Non-Insulin-Dependent Diabetes

The data showing that the glucose intolerance of aging can be significantly modulated by changes in degree of adiposity and physical activity provides unambiguous evidence as to why increasing activity and decreasing obesity should be key elements of community health strategists. On the other hand, the fact that resistance to insulin-mediated glucose disposal can be prevented to a substantial degree if older subjects remain healthy, non-obese, and physically active does not negate the relationship between this defect, when it is present, and the development of NIDDM in older subjects. There is general agreement that resistance to insulin-stimulated glucose disposal by muscle can be demonstrated in the vast majority of patients with NIDDM (Donner, 1985; Ginsberg et al., 1975; Reaven, 1983). A similar defect in muscle insulin action has also been consistently seen (Reaven, 1983; Shen et al., 1970) in patients with impaired glucose tolerance (IGT). Of great interest is the observation that the magnitude of insulin resistance is relatively similar in patients with IGT or NIDDM (Reaven et al., 1989b). Consequently, it seems reasonable to conclude that resistance to insulin-mediated muscle glucose uptake is present in the great majority of individuals with glucose intolerance, but that this defect, by itself, can account neither for the development of significant hyperglycemia in patients with NIDDM nor for the severity of fasting hyperglycemia in these individuals.

Insulin resistance can also be demonstrated in a significant number of individuals with normal glucose tolerance, and the ability of these individuals to maintain glucose homeostasis appears to be due to their capacity to sustain a state of chronic hyperinsulinemia (Hollenbeck & Reaven, 1987). By inference, it seems most likely that NIDDM with significant fasting hyperglycemia will develop only when insulin-resistant subjects are not capable of secreting enough insulin to compensate for the defect in cellular insulin action. This possibility has received considerable experimental support from both cross-sectional and longitudinal studies (Haffner et al., 1990; Reaven & Miller, 1968; Saad et al., 1989; Sicree et al., 1987; Warram et al., 1990; Zimmet et al., 1978), and there is considerable evidence that patients with NIDDM and significant hyperglycemia are characterized by the combination of muscle resistance to insulin-mediated glucose uptake and an insulin secretory response of insufficient magnitude to overcome the abnormality in insulin action.

Given this background, a reasonable hypothesis to account for the increased prevalence of NIDDM in older individuals is that they are unable to compensate for the insulin resistance associated with aging by increasing insulin secretion to the requisite degree. At first, this notion might seem to be at odds with the fact that absolute concentrations of plasma insulin do not appear to be lower in older, as compared to younger individuals (Reaven & Reaven, 1985). Perhaps the implication of these findings can best be understood by inspection of the data (Fraze et al., 1987) in Figure 9-6A. These measurements show the responses of plasma insulin concentrations to meals between 8:00 a.m. and 4:00 p.m. in individuals aged less than 40 y and greater than 60 y; the plasma glucose responses to these same meals can be seen in Figure 9-3B. Inspection of the results in Figures 9-3B and 9-6A indicates that the day-long plasma insulin concentrations in the older group (Figure 9-6A) were not high enough to prevent some increase in the day-long plasma glucose responses of those in the over 60 years group (Figure 9-3B). The simplest interpretation of these data is that the older group is more insulin resistant and cannot increase the insulin secretory response to the degree necessary to prevent the modest increase in plasma glucose response seen in Figure 9-3B. However, as the data in Figure 9-6B show, the day-long insulin concentrations in the group over 60 y can prevent any increase in plasma free-fatty acid (FFA) concentrations. Thus, although the pancreatic insulin secretory responses in these older subjects were insufficient to prevent increases in ambient glucose concentrations (Figure 9-3B), the changes in glucose were minor in magnitude, and plasma FFA concentrations did not

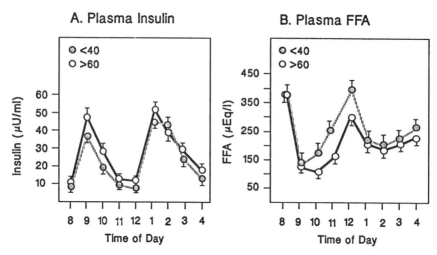

FIGURE 9-6. *Mean (± SEM) plasma insulin (A) and FFA (B) concentrations before and after breakfast (20% of total daily energy intake) and lunch (40% of total daily energy intake) in individuals <40 years old (●---●) and >60 years old (○—○). Adapted from J. Am. Geriatr. Soc. 35:224–228, 1987, with permission.*

increase. (The importance of secreting enough insulin to maintain normal FFA concentrations will be discussed later in this section.)

If it is accepted that NIDDM and significant hyperglycemia develop when insulin-resistant subjects cannot maintain a state of hyperinsulinemia, the increased prevalence of NIDDM in older subjects can be understood only if we know why they are less able to maintain the requisite state of compensatory hyperinsulinemia. Although this question cannot be answered definitively, consideration of the effect of age on pancreatic function in the rat provides one possible explanation. As discussed previously, both glucose and insulin concentrations in plasma of the rat tend to increase with age (Bracho-Romero & Reaven, 1977), whereas maximal glucose-stimulated insulin release *per β-cell* declines with age (Curry et al., 1984; Reaven & Reaven, 1981; Reaven et al., 1979, 1983a, 1983b, 1987). As discussed previously, the individual β-cell in the aged rat functions less effectively, but the rat compensates by increasing its β-cell mass, thereby maintaining the degree of insulin secretion required to prevent any significant decline in glucose tolerance.

Unfortunately, because insulin secretory capacity per β-cell mass in human beings has not been determined experimentally, we do not know whether insulin secretion per β-cell declines with increasing age, as in the rat. However, some evidence suggests that islet-cell hyperplasia can occur in human beings as a function of obesity or aging, or both (Maclean & Ogilvie, 1955). Therefore, for the purposes of this discussion, we will postulate that the age-related decline in insulin secretory capacity per β-cell described in the rat also occurs also to some degree in human beings. If this formulation is accepted, the greater prevalence of NIDDM among the elderly should not be surprising. In the first place, the increase in body weight and decrease in physical activity that is often associated with growing older will serve only to accentuate the genetic defect in insulin-stimulated glucose disposal that characterizes patients with NIDDM. As a result, the need to secrete increasingly greater quantities of insulin to maintain glucose homeostasis will tend to increase with age. Assuming that this is accompanied by an inevitable decline in glucose-stimulated insulin release *per β-cell*, it becomes more difficult for the pancreas to compensate to this increased demand. Given this situation, the likelihood that NIDDM will develop increases substantially.

It should be emphasized that only relatively small decrements in plasma insulin concentrations are associated with the development of significant hyperglycemia in patients with NIDDM (Fraze et al., 1985). In this context, insulin resistance at the level of the adipose tissue appears to offer a reasonable explanation for why the loss of insulin secretory function with aging can be so powerful. Specifically, adipose tissue is very insulin-sensitive, and plasma free-fatty acid (FFA) concentrations are half-maximally suppressed at a plasma insulin concentration of ~20 mU/mL (Swislocki et al., 1987). Thus, small changes in plasma insulin concentration can have profound effects on plasma FFA concentration. It has also been shown that ambient plasma FFA concentrations are higher than normal in patients with NIDDM, i.e., their adipose tissue is also insulin-resistant (Fraze et al., 1985; Golay et al., 1987; Swislocki et al., 1987). Furthermore, the greater the increase in plasma FFA concentrations, the higher the plasma glucose concentrations (Golay et al., 1987).

It is apparent from the data in Figure 9-6B that plasma FFA levels can be maintained normally in older subjects as long as their ambient insulin concentrations are also normal (Figure 9-6A). On the other hand, the degree of insulin resistance in these subjects was relatively mild, attested to by the fact that their day-long plasma glucose concentrations were only modestly elevated (Figure 9-3B). Thus, if these older individuals had been genetically more insulin resistant or fatter or less active, their inability to increase their insulin secretory response above the "normal" level would have led to an increase in plasma FFA concentrations, a marked accentuation in ambient plasma glucose concentrations, and the development of frank NIDDM.

Coronary Heart Disease

In the preceding section an effort has been made to relate age-related changes in insulin action and insulin secretion to the increased prevalence of NIDDM that occurs with aging. Although this is a major health concern, the adverse effect of age-related variables on insulin action is not confined to the development of NIDDM. Although compensatory hyper-insulinemia can overcome the resistance to insulin-mediated glucose that is commonly seen in older individuals (DeFronzo, 1979; Fink et al., 1983, 1986; Reaven et al., 1989b; Rowe et al., 1983), this victory is not without cost. There is a large body of evidence linking insulin resistance and compensatory hyperinsulinemia to a cluster of abnormalities that increase risk of CHD. This concept, introduced in 1988 and designated as Syndrome X (Reaven, 1988), has received considerable experimental support since then (Ferrannini et al., 1991; Haffner et al., 1990; Landin et al., 1990), and the number of abnormalities associated with insulin resistance, compensatory hyperinsulinemia, and CHD has grown substantially (Laws & Reaven, 1993).

Because insulin resistance and compensatory hyperinsulinemia play a central role in regulation of lipoprotein metabolism (Reaven, 1988; Reaven & Chen, 1988), the dyslipidemia associated with these changes provides an explanation for a link between insulin metabolism and CHD. Resistance to insulin-mediated glucose disposal and compensatory hyperinsulinemia correlate strongly with secretion rate of very low-density lipoprotein (VLDL)-triglyceride (TG) and with plasma TG concentration in both hypertriglyceridemic and normotriglyceridemic individuals (Garg et al., 1988; Olefsky et al., 1974a; Reaven et al., 1967; Tobey et al., 1981). Experimental manipulations that modify insulin action and/or plasma insulin concentrations lead to predictable changes in VLDL-TG secretion rates and plasma TG concentrations. For example, weight loss is associated with increases in insulin-mediated glucose uptake and a decrease in plasma insulin concentration, hepatic VLDL-TG secretion, and plasma TG concentration (Olefsky et al., 1974b). In contrast, ingestion of a high-carbo-hydrate diet leads to day-long parallel increases in plasma concentrations of insulin and TG (Farquhar et al., 1966).

Once plasma VLDL-TG pool-size increases, associated abnormalities of plasma lipoprotein metabolism develop. The best established of these is low concentration of high-density lipoprotein (HDL)-cholesterol (Zava-roni et al., 1985). When insulin-mediated glucose uptake is quantified in normal volunteers, the subset of subjects that is most insulin resistant has the highest concentrations of insulin and TG and the lowest concentrations of HDL-cholesterol (Laws & Reaven, 1992). The associations of insulin resistance with plasma TG and HDL-cholesterol concentrations are independent of obesity, either general or abdominal, and level of habitual activity as estimated by maximal oxygen consumption (Laws & Reaven, 1992).

In addition to a low HDL-cholesterol, hypertriglyceridemia is associated with two other important changes in lipoprotein metabolism that increase the risk of CHD, i.e., small, dense LDL-particles (Austin et al., 1988) and the accentuation of postprandial lipemia (Patsch et al., 1992).

Whether or not these changes are directly due to insulin resistance and compensatory hyperinsulinemia, or simply secondary to the hypertriglyceridemia that develops in subjects who are insulin resistant and hyperinsulinemic, is not clear. However, among 100 normal subjects we studied, those with small, dense LDL particles were relatively insulin resistant, glucose intolerant, hyperinsulinemic, hypertensive, and hypertriglyceridemic, and had lower HDL-cholesterol concentrations (Reaven et al., 1993).

The lipid abnormalities related to insulin resistance and compensatory hyperinsulinemia are known to increase the risk of CHD. The strong association of low plasma concentrations of HDL-cholesterol to CHD risk has been shown in numerous studies (Assmann & Schulte, 1992; Castelli et al., 1977; Manninen et al., 1992; Miller & Miller, 1975). In contrast, controversy continues as to whether or not hypertriglyceridemia is an "independent" risk factor for CHD (Austin, 1991; Criqui et al., 1993; Hulley et al., 1980; Reaven, 1993). Although a high plasma TG concentration and CHD are strongly correlated in univariate analysis, the relationship between hypertriglyceridemia and CHD often loses statistical significance in multivariate analyses when variations in plasma HDL-cholesterol and glucose are taken into consideration (Austin, 1991; Criqui et al., 1993; Hulley et al., 1980; Reaven, 1993). However, as previously emphasized, plasma glucose, insulin, TG, and HDL-cholesterol concentrations are themselves highly correlated. The problems with performing multivariate analysis to ascertain which of a series of variables is "independently" related to CHD, when the measures are themselves highly correlated, have recently been emphasized (Austin, 1991). Furthermore, recent reports examining the contributions of HDL-cholesterol and TG concentrations to risk for CHD showed the highest risk in men with low HDL-cholesterol and high TG concentrations (Assmann & Schulte, 1992; Manninen et al., 1992). Similarly, in the initial report demonstrating the increased risk for CHD associated with small, dense LDL-particles, it is notable that subjects with this lipoprotein abnormality had relatively low HDL-cholesterol and high TG concentrations (Austin et al., 1988), again demonstrating the presence of a cluster of metabolic abnormalities.

Insulin resistance and compensatory hyperinsulinemia also appear to be associated with changes that accentuate thrombosis formation by increasing coagulation and inhibiting fibrinolytic processes (Juhan-Vague et al., 1991, 1993; Landin et al., 1990; Potter van Loon et al., 1993). For example, concentration of plasminogen activator-inhibitor-1 (PAI-1) is associated with myocardial infarction, and PAI-1 levels are also highly correlated with insulin and triglyceride concentrations and with insulin resistance (Juhan-Vague et al., 1991, 1993; Landin et al., 1990; Potter van Loon et al., 1993). Because insulin resistance, hyperinsulinemia, and hypertriglyceridemia are themselves highly correlated (Garg et al., 1988; Olefsky et al.,

1974a; Reaven, 1988; Reaven et al., 1967; Tobey et al., 1981), it is not clear which of these changes is most important in regulation of PAI-1 levels. However, these observations provide further support for the role played by insulin resistance and hyperinsulinemia in the pathogenesis of CHD.

There is also evidence that insulin resistance and compensatory hyperinsulinemia play a role in the etiology and clinical course of a substantial portion of patients with high blood pressure. Specifically, patients with high blood pressure, as a group, are resistant to insulin-mediated glucose uptake and hyperinsulinemic when compared to a closely matched population with normal blood pressure (Reaven, 1988, 1991). These abnormalities persist despite successful drug treatment of hypertension and can be seen in both obese and nonobese individuals (Reaven, 1988, 1991). Furthermore, abnormalities of insulin metabolism can be discerned in normotensive, first-degree relatives of patients with high blood pressure (Facchini et al., 1992; Ferrari et al., 1991) but not in patients with secondary forms of hypertension (Shamiss et al., 1992). The fact that insulin resistance and hyperinsulinemia can be demonstrated in patients at risk for the development of hypertension further supports the view that these abnormalities may play a role in regulation of blood pressure.

On the other hand, two major arguments have been advanced against the view that insulin resistance and hyperinsulinemia are involved in blood pressure regulation. Acute hyperinsulinemia in human beings leads to vasodilation, and blood pressure does not increase (Anderson & Mark, 1993). In addition, blood pressure does not change when insulin is infused into dogs for periods of up to two weeks (Hall et al., 1990). However, blood pressure does increase when rats are infused with insulin (Brands et al., 1991). Furthermore, blood pressure falls when insulin dose is decreased in obese, hypertensive patients with NIDDM (Tedde et al., 1989) and increases when insulin treatment is initiated in patients with NIDDM who are poorly controlled on oral agents (Randeree et al., 1992).

Secondly, it has been argued that a relationship between insulin level and blood pressure cannot always be seen in population studies. For example, it has been reported that blood pressure and insulin concentration are significantly correlated in Caucasians, but in neither Afro-Americans nor Pima Indians (Saad et al., 1991). On the other hand, hypertensive Afro-Americans are insulin resistant and hyperinsulinemic when compared to Afro-Americans with normal blood pressure (Falkner et al., 1990, 1993), raising questions as to the significance of the lack of a relationship between blood pressure and insulin described in Afro-Americans in epidemiological studies.

Evidence that insulin resistance and compensatory hyperinsulinemia play a role in the clinical course of patients with high blood pressure is even more convincing. In the first place, these subjects tend to be glucose intolerant, and there is certainly evidence that this abnormality would increase their risk of CHD (Reaven, 1988, 1991; Vaccaro et al., 1992). In addition, hypertriglyceridemia is commonly seen in patients with essential hypertension and in their first-degree relatives (Facchini et al., 1992; Ferrari et al., 1991; Reaven, 1988, 1991). The association between insulin resistance and compensatory hyperinsulinemia in the development of hypertriglyceridemia, as well as the relationship between an increase in plasma TG concentration and CHD, have already been discussed. Further bolstering the link between abnormal insulin metabolism, high blood pressure, and CHD is the recent observation that patients with high blood pressure and EKG evidence of CHD were insulin resistant and hyperinsulinemic when compared to a matched group of patients with high blood pressure who did not demonstrate ischemic EKG changes (Sheu et al., 1992). In light of these considerations, there appears to be ample evidence that the development of CHD in patients with hypertension may be secondary to the defects in insulin metabolism that exist in these subjects.

There is now abundant evidence that insulin resistance, compensatory hyperinsulinemia, dyslipidemia, hypertension, and defects in hemostatic function cluster in individuals (Facchini et al., 1992; Ferrannini et al., 1991; Ferrari et al., 1991; Haffner et al., 1990; Juhan-Vague et al., 1993; Landin et al., 1990; Laws & Reaven, 1993; Reaven, 1988, 1991). As stated previously, this cluster of abnormalities was proposed to represent a previously undescribed syndrome (Syndrome X), with resistance to insulin-mediated glucose disposal as the basic abnormality. Figure 9-7 summarizes the current status of Syndrome X. It is proposed that individual variations in the degree of insulin resistance are secondary to both genetic and environmental influences. For example, obesity, *per se*, can lead to a decrease in insulin-mediated glucose uptake, whereas weight loss in obese individuals is associated with enhanced *in vivo* insulin action (Olefsky et al., 1974b). However, obesity is not the only environmental change that can modulate insulin resistance, and level of habitual physical activity seems to be as potent as obesity in this regard (Bogardus et al., 1985; Rosenthal et al., 1983). Furthermore, it is also known that exercise training can enhance insulin sensitivity, lower plasma TG and insulin levels, lower blood pressure, and increase HDL-cholesterol concentrations (Krotkiewski et al., 1979; Schwartz 1987). However, the fact that obesity and habitual activity can modify the presentation of Syndrome X does not mean that Syndrome X is determined solely by these environmental variables. For example, in non-diabetic volunteers of European and Native American backgrounds, less than 50% of the total variance in insulin-stimulated glucose uptake could be attributed to the combined effects of differences in age, maximal oxygen consumption, and obesity (Bogardus et al., 1985). Age had relatively little effect, and the relative impact of differences in maximal oxygen consumption was at least as great as that due to variations in body weight. Furthermore, when obese and non-obese individuals are matched for degree of hyperinsulinemia, the phenotypic manifestations of Syndrome X are present to a similar degree (Zavaroni et al., 1994).

All of the clinical features of Syndrome X can develop independently of obesity, sedentary activity, and so on; consequently, some of the terms used to describe Syndrome X, i.e., "the deadly quartet" (Kaplan, 1989) or the "GHO Syndrome" (glucose intolerance, hypertension, and obesity) (Modan et al., 1985), are misleading. These terms imply that obesity is an essential attribute of the system complex being described. This conclusion is not meant to denigrate the impact of variations in weight and level of physical activity on resistance to insulin-mediated glucose disposal, and there is no question that all of the manifestations of Syndrome X will be accentuated when individuals become heavier and/or less active. On the other hand, it is necessary to emphasize that insulin resistance, and the consequent manifestations of this defect, are not dependent upon obesity or a sedentary lifestyle.

This section provides a summary of the evidence that resistance to insulin-mediated glucose disposal predisposes individuals to develop a cluster of associated abnormalities that increase the risk of CHD, as outlined in Figure 9-7. Irrespective of the relative importance of nature and nurture in regulation of insulin-mediated glucose disposal, the physiological response to a decrease in this function is that the pancreatic β-cells will

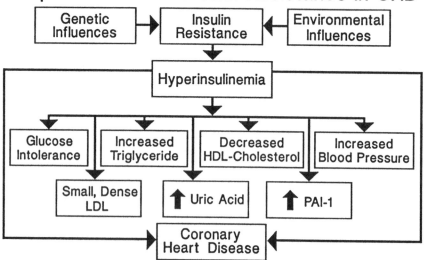

Proposed Role for Insulin Resistance in CHD

FIGURE 9-7. *Diagramatic representation of the sequence of events postulated to stem from resistance to insulin-mediated glucose disposal and to make up the current version of Syndrome X.*

secrete more insulin to compensate for this defect. If this state of compensatory hyperinsulinemia cannot be maintained, glucose intolerance will develop. If the pancreas can compensate, the resultant state of compensatory hyperinsulinemia will put subjects at risk to develop all of the abnormalities outlined in Figure 9-7. These observations serve to further emphasize the adverse health-related impact of the insulin resistance that develops with aging. Thus, whether to prevent NIDDM or CHD, efforts to maintain normal insulin action as individuals age are of paramount importance.

PREVENTION OF AGE-RELATED INSULIN RESISTANCE

The discussion to this point has on repeated occasions emphasized the fact that both the resistance to insulin-mediated glucose disposal and the glucose intolerance associated with aging are due, in large part, to the increase in adiposity and decrease in physical activity that often occur as individuals grow older. As a corollary, remaining lean and physically active should minimize to a substantial degree the insulin resistance associated with aging and, by inference, decrease the likelihood of developing detrimental consequences. Unfortunately, there are no long-term prospective studies that definitively address this issue, but there are cross-sectional observations that provide considerable support for this point of view.

In the case of obesity, weight loss will enhance insulin-mediated glucose uptake, improve glucose tolerance, lower circulating concentrations of insulin and TG, and decrease blood pressure (Olefsky et al., 1974b; Reisin et al., 1978). Furthermore, weight loss in older patients with NIDDM will greatly improve glycemic control (Reaven et al., 1985). Indeed, the beneficial impact of weight loss on insulin resistance and its associated cluster of untoward events is so well appreciated that it has attained the realm of the conventional clinical practice of medicine.

Based upon studies in both Pima Indians and individuals of European descent, it is quite likely that variations in degree of aerobic fitness are as powerful as the degree of obesity in modulation of insulin-mediated glucose uptake (Bogardus et al., 1985). Despite these data, modulation of physical activity as a way of improving insulin sensitivity is rarely awarded the attention given to control of obesity.

Discussions of the health-related implications of level of physical activity usually focus on exercise training programs. However, it must be appreciated that there is a significant direct relationship between $\dot{V}O_2max$ and insulin-mediated glucose uptake in the population at large (Rosenthal et al., 1983). Furthermore, as described previously, when older laborers were compared to similarly aged office workers, glucose tolerance was significantly better in the laborers (Wang et al., 1989). Perhaps the most clinically relevant finding in this context was that of Frisch et al. (1986), who studied the effect of having participated in college athletics on the subsequent development of diabetes in women up to 70 years of age. More than 5000 living college alumnae were divided into two groups— former college athletes and nonathletes. The former college athletes tended to be leaner and more physically active throughout life. Nonathletes had 3.4 times the risk of developing diabetes, compared with the athletes. These data highlight the fact that when the problem of glucose intolerance and NIDDM in older individuals is addressed, emphasis on physical activity should not be made at the time individuals enter the geriatric age group, but at considerably younger ages and, optimally, throughout the life span.

Additional support for this notion can be derived from the results of three epidemiologic studies that evaluated the impact of leisure time activity on the development of NIDDM (Helmrich et al., 1991; Manson et al., 1991, 1992). Although details of the three studies varied somewhat, the conclusions were quite similar in that they all demonstrated a significant reduction in incidence of NIDDM in individuals who exercised as compared to those who did not. Common to all three studies was the fact that the beneficial effects of exercise were independent of differences in family history of diabetes or degree of obesity. In two of the studies (Helmrich et al., 1991; Manson et al., 1992) there was evidence that the more frequent and/or intense the exercise, the greater the reduction in risk of developing NIDDM. Finally, in the study by Helmrich et al. (1991), the protective benefit was especially evident in those at increased risk of NIDDM, i.e., those with a family history of NIDDM or a high body mass index.

A much smaller case-controlled study, but one that provides data comparing the relative effects of obesity and physical activity, was that of Seals and associates (1984), who compared oral glucose tolerance in five groups. There were three groups of older men (14 older, endurance-trained masters athletes; 12 older, untrained men; 9 older, lean, untrained men) and two groups of younger men (15 young, endurance-trained athletes and 15 young, untrained men). Both the younger and older athletes were leaner than the corresponding groups of untrained men. Total glucose responses to an oral glucose challenge (summations of the glucose levels at all the time points) were lower in young and old athletes and in young, untrained men than in the two groups of untrained, older men. In fact, the glucose response to the oral glucose was as low in the masters athletes as in the young athletes, illustrating that in these vigorously exercising individuals there was no age-associated decline in glucose tolerance. It is also of note that of the two variables, leanness and physical fitness, the latter appeared to be a more powerful determinant of glucose response, given that the older athletes had markedly better responses than the older, lean, physically inactive men. Insulin levels were also measured and were found to be significantly lower in the athletes, older and younger. These data strongly suggest that the effect of exercise training was to enhance insulin-mediated glucose disposal, a conclusion consistent with the previously discussed results of Hollenbeck et al. (1985), who directly evaluated the effect of chronic exercise on glucose disposal in older subjects. Parenthetically, Seals et al. (1984) commented upon the difficulty of recruiting lean, inactive older men for their study, indicating that physical activity is an important component in permitting individuals to remain lean as they age.

The studies described above have emphasized how important the level of physical activity can be in preventing the development of NIDDM, presumably by modulation of the changes in insulin action and glucose tolerance that are associated with aging. These results should be not surprising in view of the abundant evidence that insulin-mediated glucose uptake is increased in response to exercise training programs (Lampman et al., 1985; Reaven & Reaven, 1985; Rodnick et al., 1987). On the other hand, it is important to consider specific aspects of the potential utility of exercise training programs in attenuating the insulin resistance and glucose intolerance associated with aging.

Of major importance is understanding of the rate at which the beneficial metabolic effects dissipate when a program of regular exercise is discontinued (Burstein et al., 1985; Heath et al., 1983). For example, Heath et al. (1983) studied physically trained men and women with normal glucose tolerance, measuring glucose and insulin responses to oral glucose the day following a usual bout of exercise and again after 10 d without any exercise. After 10 d of inactivity, the subjects had an increase in their average plasma glucose response to the glucose challenge and a doubling of their average insulin response compared to their responses the day following exercise. This was consistent with a marked diminution in their insulin sensitivity during the period of inactivity. As indicated by an unchanged average VO_2max, there was no decrease in fitness levels nor was there any change in percent body fat or body weight to account for the apparent decrease in insulin sensitivity. Because a single bout of exercise restored insulin and glucose responses almost to their values in the trained state, it was suggested that acute bouts of exercise are primarily responsible for the enhanced insulin sensitivity seen in physically trained individuals.

Although a single bout of exercise may be sufficient to improve glucose and insulin responses to oral glucose in trained athletes, more may be required in previously sedentary patients with impaired glucose tolerance and NIDDM. A study by Rogers et al. (1988) addressed the issue of the acute effects of exercise in 3 subjects with impaired glucose tolerance and in 8 subjects with mild NIDDM, all of whom were sedentary. A single bout of exercise in these subjects had no effect on glucose or insulin responses to the oral glucose. However, after 7 d of 60-min exercise sessions at 68% $\dot{V}O_2$max (an energy expenditure of 470 kcal per session), and with the oral glucose challenge 16 h after the last bout of exercise, subjects had an average 36% reduction in the glucose response and 32% reduction in the insulin response. The improved responses to oral glucose occurred despite the fact that there were no significant changes in body weight, percent body fat, or $\dot{V}O_2$max, i.e., with no detectable cardiovascular training effect. The difference between this study and that by Heath et al. (1983), in which a single bout of exercise in trained athletes resulted in a marked improvement of the insulin response to oral glucose, may be that the exercise stimulus for these sedentary patients with NIDDM was much milder than that for the trained athletes in the study by Heath's group. (The mean baseline $\dot{V}O_2$max was less than half that of the subjects in the study by Heath's group.) Nonetheless, a relatively brief, 1-wk period of training was responsible for significant improvements in oral glucose tolerance and insulin sensitivity in these subjects with impaired glucose tolerance or mild NIDDM.

Although the data discussed above demonstrate that exercise training can have beneficial effects on insulin sensitivity and glucose tolerance, they also indicate that the degree of apparent benefit depends on the duration and intensity of the exercise, and that the effect is markedly diminished within 10 d following the last exercise session. Therefore, it appears that the improvements in glucose tolerance and insulin sensitivity seen with exercise are largely the result of the individual exercise bouts, and not of the trained state *per se*. This means that exercise must be performed regularly in order to be of benefit to carbohydrate metabolism.

Because previously sedentary older individuals are less physically fit (Hollenbeck et al., 1985), long-term physical training may be required to improve their fitness levels so they can perform the duration and intensity of exercise necessary to produce improvements in insulin sensitivity or glucose tolerance. For example, Holloszy et al. (1986) estimated that for subjects with NIDDM who normalized their glucose responses to oral glucose, an exercise load of approximately 25–35 km of running per week at a speed that elicits 70–85% of $\dot{V}O_2$max was required. This level of training may be difficult or impossible to achieve in older patients who have been overweight and sedentary for years and who may have other medical problems such as arthritis or heart disease that limit their activities. Therefore, exercise should optimally be initiated at much younger ages and be continued throughout the life span. Data from the study of Frisch et al. (1986) support this contention and suggest that much less intense exercise than that achieved by the subjects in the study by Holloszy et al. (1986) can be beneficial if engaged in habitually.

FUTURE RESEARCH DIRECTIONS

Two general lines of research need to be undertaken. The first involves unanswered biological questions as to the effect of age on insulin secretion and insulin action and the second involves behavior modification issues. Perhaps the most fundamental impact of age on insulin function is the progressive and apparently inexorable decrease in insulin secretion per β-cell described in rats. In addition to providing an explanation for why β-cell function declines with age, understanding this phenomenon is likely to provide insight into the mechanism responsible for other examples of endocrine cell failure with age. Of potentially greater importance is the possibility that the knowledge gained by solving this unresolved issue may help explain why insulin secretory capacity fails in patients with NIDDM.

Although there are certainly other unanswered biological questions concerning the effect of age on insulin secretion and insulin action, none of them seems to be as important as our current inability to use the information available to prevent age-related changes in insulin secretion and insulin action. Specifically, it is research in the area of behavior modification that is most needed. At the simplest level, techniques must be found to make individuals aware of the unfortunate health-related implications of adiposity and a sedentary lifestyle. In addition, health care professionals must be made aware of the fact that a significant decline in glucose tolerance is not an inevitable consequence of getting older, and that the morbid events associated with this phenomenon can, at least to a considerable extent, be prevented by lifestyle modifications. Finally, clinically effective approaches to weight loss and exercise programs must be found to increase the likelihood that overweight individuals can lose weight, become more active, and maintain these practices as they age. Unfortunately, our ability to accomplish these goals is at an infinitely more rudimentary level than is our understanding of the effect of age on carbohydrate metabolism. The greatest hindrance to overcoming the medical consequences of the effect of age on glucose tolerance is not ignorance of the biology of this process, but understanding how to put into practice what is known. Consequently, it is the information that will come from thoughtful research in this area that is most needed.

SUMMARY

In this chapter emphasis has been placed on differentiating the inexorable effects of age on insulin secretion and insulin action from those secondary to age-related variables. The results of studies in both animals and human beings have been critically reviewed. Given the complexity of the issues that have been addressed, care must be exercised in order to avoid dangerous oversimplification in an attempt to summarize succinctly the information that has been presented. Perhaps the safest statement that can be made is that a progressive decline in glucose tolerance is not an inevitable consequence of aging. Whether or not age *per se* is responsible for a decrease in glucose tolerance in those older than 60 remains to be seen.

As a corollary, age-related changes must be held accountable for a good deal, it not all, of the glucose intolerance previously demonstrated to occur as human beings get older. In this context, an increase in degree of obesity and a decrease in level of habitual physical activity both play a major causal role in the glucose intolerance of aging. Of even greater pragmatic interest are the results showing that little, if any, loss of glucose tolerance can be shown in older individuals who are both nonobese and physically active.

The generalizations outlined above also hold true, in general, if more specific attention is focussed on the effect of age on the ultimate determinants of glucose tolerance, i.e., insulin secretion and insulin action. In the latter instance, there appears to be no evidence that the ability of insulin to stimulate glucose disposal decreases with age. This does not mean that age *per se* may not be associated with some decline in insulin action, and it is most difficult to rule out this possibility. On the other hand, it is quite clear that insulin-mediated glucose disposal does not decrease with age in healthy, nonobese, physically active individuals, up to the age of 60.

The relationship between age and insulin secretory function is more complicated. In the case of rats, there is substantial evidence that insulin secretory function per β-cell declines progressively with age. Fortunately, rats, at least, are able to compensate for this defect by making more β-cells. Whether or not the same inevitable loss of β-cell function with age occurs in human beings is not clear, nor do we understand the capacity for β-cell hyperplasia in nonrodent species. It is tempting to speculate that insulin secretory function also decreases progressively and inexorably with age in human beings, but that our ability to increase β-cell mass is limited. If this were the case, it provides a rational explanation for why the prevalence of NIDDM increases so dramatically with age, and it is totally consistent with comparisons of insulin secretory function in younger and older individuals. On the other hand, as tempting as this point of view may be, it is necessary to emphasize that it requires further experimental validation.

Although unresolved issues remain about the relationship among age, obesity, physical activity, and glucose tolerance, the health-related implications of what is already known are substantial. There is substantial evidence that resistance to insulin-mediated glucose disposal is the earliest discernible defect in patients with NIDDM and that the insulin resistance associated with aging can be largely prevented if individuals can remain non-obese and physically active as they grow older. Given this information, there is every reason to believe that the age-related increase in prevalence of NIDDM would be dramatically attenuated if individuals were able to remain non-obese and physically active.

Of even greater clinical relevance is the importance of insulin resistance and/or compensatory hyperinsulinemia in the genesis of CHD. These defects in insulin metabolism lead to a variety of abnormalities in lipid metabolism, blood pressure regulation, and fibrinolytic activity, all of which are changes that increase the risk of CHD. Again, the untoward results of insulin resistance and/or compensatory hyperinsulinemia are unlikely to be inevitable consequences of aging, but rather events that could be largely avoided if the weight gain and decreased physical activity that are too often associated with aging could be prevented.

The ultimate message is a simple one. Weight gain and physical inactivity are not inevitable consequences of growing older. Understanding this simple notion and having the ability to modulate behavior would reduce to a tremendous degree the changes in insulin action and the consequences of this defect that are now accepted as inevitable consequences of aging. What must be done is clear; ways to effectively accomplish this goal must be recognized as a major societal need. The consequences of not understanding these issues, and the inability to respond to them, must be ultimately rectified if the goal is to prevent the deleterious consequences of age-related changes in glucose, insulin, and lipoprotein metabolism.

BIBLIOGRAPHY

Anderson, E.A., and A.L. Mark (1993). The vasodilator action of insulin: Implications for the insulin hypothesis of hypertension. *Hypertension* 21:136–141.

Andres, R. (1971). Aging and diabetes. *Med. Clin. North Am.* 55:835–846.

Assmann, G., and H. Schulte (1992). Relation of high-density lipoprotein cholesterol and triglycerides to incidence of atherosclerotic coronary artery disease (the PROCAM experience). *Am. J. Cardiol.* 70:733–737.

Austin, M.A. (1991). Plasma triglyceride and coronary heart disease. *Arterioscler. Thromb.* 11:2–14.

Austin, M.A., J.L. Breslow, C.H. Hennekens, J.E. Buring, W.S. Willett, and R.M. Krauss (1988). Low-density lipoprotein subclass patterns and risk of myocardial infarction. *J. Am. Med. Assoc.* 260:1917–1921.

Boden, G., X. Chen, R.A. DeSantis, Z. Kendrick (1993). Effects of age and body fat on insulin resistance in healthy men. *Diabetes Care* 16:728–733.

Bogardus, C., S. Lillioja, D.M. Mott, C. Hollenbeck, and G. M. Reaven (1985). Relationship between degree of obesity and in vivo insulin action in man. *Am. J. Physiol.* 248 (Endocrinol. Metab. 11):E286–E291.

Borkan, G.A., D.E. Hults, S.G. Gerzof, A.H. Robbins, and C.K. Silbert (1983). Age changes in body composition revealed by computed tomography. *J. Gerontol.* 38:673–677.

Bouchard, C., J.-P. Despres, and P. Mauriege (1993). Genetic and nongenetic determinants of regional fat distribution. *Endocr. Rev.* 14:72–93.

Bracho-Romero, E., and G.M. Reaven (1977). Effect of age and weight on plasma glucose and insulin responses in the rat. *J. Am. Geriatr. Soc.* 25:299–302.

Brands, M.W., D.A. Hildebrandt, H.L. Mizelle, and J.E. Hall (1991). Sustained hyperinsulinemia increases arterial pressure in conscious rats. *Am. J. Physiol.* 260:R764–768.

Burstein, R., C. Polychronakos, C.J. Towes, J.D. McDougall, H.J. Guyda, and B.I. Posner (1985). Acute reversal of the enhanced insulin action in trained athletes. Association with insulin receptor changes. *Diabetes* 34:756–760.

Castelli, W.P., J.T. Doyle, T. Gordon, C.B. Hames, M.C. Hjortland, S.B. Hulley, A. Kagan, and W.J. Zukel (1977). HDL cholesterol and other lipids in coronary heart disease. *Circulation* 55:767–772.

Criqui, M.H., G. Heiss, R. Cohn, L.D. Cowan, C.M. Suchindran, S. Bangdiwala, S. Kritchevsky, D.P. Jacobs, H.K. O'Grady, and C.E. Davis (1993). Plasma triglyceride level and mortality from coronary heart disease. *N. Engl. J. Med.* 328:1220–1225.

Curry, D.L., G.M. Reaven, and E. Reaven (1984). Glucose-induced secretion by perfused pancreas of 2- and 12-mo-old Fischer 344 rats. *Am. J. Physiol.* 247 (Endocrinol. Metab. 10):E385–388.

Davidson, M.D. (1979). The effect of aging on carbohydrate metabolism. A review of the English literature and a practical approach to the diagnosis of diabetes mellitus in the elderly. *Metabolism* 28:688–705.

DeFronzo, R.A. (1979). Glucose intolerance and aging: Evidence for tissue insensitivity to insulin. *Diabetes* 28:1095–1101.

Donner, C.C., E. Fraze, Y.-D.I. Chen, C.B. Hollenbeck, J.E. Foley, and G.M. Reaven (1985). Presentation of a new method for specific measurement of in vivo insulin-stimulated glucose disposal in humans: Comparison of this approach with the insulin clamp and minimal model techniques. *J. Clin. Endocrinol. Metab.* 60:723–726.

Facchini, F., Y.-D.I. Chen, C. Clinkingbeard, J. Jeppesen, and G.M. Reaven (1992). Insulin resistance, hyperinsulinemia, and dyslipidemia in nonobese individuals with a family history of hypertension. *Am. J. Hypertension* 5:694–699.

Falkner, B., S. Hulman, and H. Kushner (1993). Insulin-stimulated glucose utilization and borderline hypertension in young adult blacks. *Hypertension* 22:18–25.

Falkner, B., S. Hulman, J. Tennenbaum, and H. Kushner (1990). Insulin resistance and blood pressure in young black men. *Hypertension* 16:706–711.

Farquhar, J.W., A. Frank, R.C. Gross, and G.M. Reaven (1966). Glucose, insulin, and triglyceride responses to high- and low-carbohydrate diets in man. *J. Clin. Invest.* 45:1648–1656.

Ferrannini, E., S.M. Haffner, B.D. Mitchell, and M.P. Stern (1991). Hyperinsulinaemia: the key feature of a cardiovascular and metabolic syndrome. *Diabetologia* 3:416–422.

Ferrari, P., P. Weidmann, S. Shaw, D. Giachino, W. Riesen, Y. Allemann, and G. Heynen (1991). Altered insulin sensitivity, hyperinsulinemia, and dyslipidemia in individuals with a hypertensive parent. *Am. J. Med.* 91:589–596.

Fink, R.I., O.G. Kolterman, J. Griffin, and J.M. Olefsky (1983). Mechanisms of insulin resistance in aging. *J. Clin. Invest.* 71:1523–1535.

Fink, R.I., P. Wallace, and J.M. Olefsky (1986). Effects of aging on glucose-mediated glucose disposal and glucose transport. *J. Clin. Invest.* 77:2034–2041.

Fraze, E., Y-A.M. Chiou, Y-D.I. Chen, and G.M. Reaven (1987). Age-related changes in postprandial plasma glucose, insulin, and free fatty acid concentrations in nondiabetic individuals. *J. Am. Geriatr. Soc.* 35:224–228.

Fraze, E., C.C. Donner, A.L.M. Swislocki, Y.-A.M. Chiou, Y.-D.I. Chen, and G.M. Reaven (1985). Ambient plasma free fatty acid concentrations in noninsulin-dependent diabetes mellitus: Evidence for insulin resistance. *J. Clin. Endocrinol. Metab.* 61:807–811.

Frisch, R.E., G. Wyshak, T.E. Albright, N.L. Albright, and J. Schiff (1986). Lower prevalence of diabetes in female former college athletes compared with nonathletes. *Diabetes* 35:1101–1105.

Garg, A., J.H. Helderman, M. Koffler, R. Ayuso, J. Rosenstock, and P. Raskin (1988). Relationship between lipoprotein levels and in vivo insulin action in normal young white men. *Metabolism* 37:982–987.

Ginsberg, H., G. Kimmerling, J.M. Olefsky, and G.M. Reaven (1975). Demonstration of insulin resistance in untreated adult onset diabetic subjects with fasting hyperglycemia. *J. Clin. Invest.* 55:454–461.

Golay, A., A.L.M. Swislocki, Y.-D.I. Chen, and G.M. Reaven (1987). Relationships between plasma free fatty acid concentration, endogenous glucose production, and fasting hyperglycemia in normal and non-insulin dependent diabetic individuals. *Metabolism* 36:692–696.

Goodman, M.N., S.M. Dluz, M.A. McElaney, E. Belur, and N.B. Ruderman (1983). Glucose uptake and insulin sensitivity in rat muscle: changes during 3-96 weeks of age. *Am. J. Physiol.* 244 (Endocrinol. Metab. 7):E93–E100.

Haffner, S.M., M.P. Stern, H.P. Hazuda, B.D. Mitchell, and J.K. Patterson (1990). Cardiovascular risk factors in confirmed prediabetic individuals: does the clock for coronary heart disease start ticking before the onset of clinical diabetes? *J. Amer. Med. Assoc.* 263:2893–2898.

Haffner, S.M., M.P. Stern, B.D. Mitchell, H.P. Hazuda, and J.K. Patterson (1990). Incidence of type II diabetes in Mexican Americans predicted by fasting insulin and glucose levels, obesity, and body-fat distribution. *Diabetes* 39:283–288.

Hall, J.E., M.W. Brands, S.D. Kivlighn, H.L. Mizelle, A. Hildebrandt, and C.A. Gaillard (1990). Chronic hyperinsulinemia and blood pressure. *Hypertension* 15:519–527.

Harris, M.I. (1985). Prevalence of non-insulin-dependent diabetes and impaired glucose tolerance. In: *National Diabetes Data Group. Diabetes in Americans:Diabetes Data Compiled 1984*, Publ. No. 85–1468, Bethesda, MD: National Institutes of Health.

Harris, M.I., W.C. Hadden, W.C. Knowler, and P.H. Bennet (1987). Prevalence of diabetes and impaired glucose tolerance and plasma glucose levels in US population aged 20-74 years. *Diabetes* 36:523–534.

Heath, G.W., J.R. Gavin, III, J.M. Hinderliter, J.M. Hagberg, S.D. Bloomfield, and J.O. Holloszy (1983). Effects of exercise and lack of exercise on glucose tolerance and insulin sensitivity. *J. Appl. Physiol.: Respir. Environ. Exerc. Physiol.* 55:512–517.

Helmrich, S.P., D.R. Ragland, R.W. Leung, and R.S. Paffenbarger, Jr. (1991). Physical activity and reduced occurrence of non-insulin-dependent diabetes mellitus. *N. Engl. J. Med.* 325:147–152.

Hollenbeck, C., W. Haskell, M. Rosenthal, and G. Reaven (1985). Effect of habitual physical activity on regulation of insulin-stimulated glucose disposal in older males. *J. Am. Geriatr. Soc.* 33:273–277.

Hollenbeck, C.B., and G.M. Reaven (1987). Variations in insulin-stimulated glucose uptake in healthy individuals with normal glucose tolerance. *J. Clin. Endocrinol. Metab.* 64:1169–1173.

Holloszy, J.O., J. Schultz, J. Kusnierkiewicz, J.M. Hagberg, and A.A. Ehsani (1986). Effects of exercise on glucose tolerance and insulin resistance: Brief review and some preliminary results. *Acta Med. Scand.* 711 (Suppl):55–65.

Hulley, S.B., R.H. Rosenman, R.D. Bawol, and R.J. Brand (1980). Epidemiology as a guide to clinical decisions. The association between triglyceride and coronary heart disease. *N. Engl. J. Med.* 302:1383–1389.

Huse, D.M., G. Oster, A.R. Killen, M.L. Lacoy, and G.D. Colditz (1989). The economic costs of non-insulin-dependent diabetes mellitus. *JAMA* 262:2708–2713.

Juhan-Vague, I., M.C. Alessi, and P. Vague (1991). Increased plasma plasminogen activator inhibitor 1 levels. A possible link between insulin resistance and atherothrombosis. *Diabetologia* 34:457–462.

Juhan-Vague, I., S.G. Thompson, and J. Jespersen, on Behalf of the ECAT Angina Pectoris Study Group (1993). Involvement of the hemostatic system in the insulin resistance syndrome: A study of 1500 patients with angina pectoris. *Arterioscler. Thromb.* 13:1865–1873.

Kane, R.L., D.H. Solomon, and J.C. Beck (1981). *Geriatrics in the United States: Manpower Projections and Training Considerations.* Lexington, MA: Heath.

Kaplan, N.M. (1989). The deadly quartet. Upper-body obesity, glucose intolerance, hypertriglyceridemia, and hypertension. *Arch. Intern. Med.* 149:1514–1520.

Klimas, J.E. (1968). Oral glucose tolerance during the life span of a colony of rats. *J. Gerontol.* 23:31–34.

Krotkiewski, M., K. Mandroukas, L. Sjostrom, L. Sullivan, H. Wetterqvist, and P. Bjornstorp (1979). Effects of long-term physical training on body fat, metabolism, and blood pressure in obesity. *Metabolism* 28:650–658.

Lampman, R.M., J.T. Santinga, P.J. Savage, D.R. Bassett, C.R. Hydrick, J.D. Flora, and W.D. Block (1985). Effect of exercise training on glucose tolerance, in vivo insulin sensitivity, lipid and lipoprotein concentrations in middle-aged men with mild hypertriglyceridemia. *Metab. Clin. Exp.* 34:205–211.

Landin, K., L. Tengvory, and U. Smith (1990). Elevated fibrinogen and plasminogen activator (PAI-1) in hypertension are related to metabolic risk factors for cardiovascular disease. *J. Intern. Med.* 227:273–278.

Laws, A., and G.M. Reaven (1992). Evidence for an independent relationship between insulin resistance and fasting plasma HDL-cholesterol, triglyceride and insuin concentrations. *J. Int. Med.* 231:25–30.

Laws, A., and G.M. Reaven (1993). Insulin resistance and risk factors for coronary heart disease. In: *E. Ferrannini (ed.) Clinical Endocrinology and Metabolism: Insulin Resistance and Disease.* London:Baillière Tindall, pp. 1063–1078

Maclean, N., and R.F. Ogilvie (1955). Quantitative estimation of the pancreatic islet tissue in diabetic subjects. *Diabetes* 4:367–376.

Maneatis, T., R. Condie, and G. Reaven (1982). Effect of age on plasma glucose and insulin responses to a mixed meal. *J. Am. Geriatr. Soc.* 30:178–182.

Manninen, V., L. Tenkanen, P. Koskinen, J.K. Huttenen, M. Manttari, O.P. Heinonen, and M.H. Frick (1992). Joint effects of serum triglyceride and LDL cholesterol and HDL cholesterol concentrations on coronary heart disease risk in the Helsinki heart study: Implications for treatment. *Circulation* 85:37–45.

Manson, J.E., D.M. Nathan, A.S. Krolewski, M.J. Stampfer, W.C. Willet, and C.H. Hennekens (1992). A prospective study of exercise and incidence of diabetes among US male physicians. *J. Am. Med. Assoc.* 268:63–67.

Manson, J.E., E.B. Rimm, M.J. Stampfer, G.A. Colditz, W.C. Willett, A.S. Krolewski, B. Rosner, C.H. Hennekens, F.E. Speizer (1991). Physical activity and incidence of non-insulin-dependent diabetes mellitus in women. *Lancet* 338:774–778.

Miller, G.J., and N.E. Miller (1975). Plasma-high-density-lipoprotein concentration and development of ischaemic heart-disease. *The Lancet* 1:16–19.

Modan, M., H. Halkin, S. Almog, A. Lusky, A. Eshkol, M. Shefi, Shitrit, A., and Fuchs, Z. (1985). Hyperinsulinemia:a link between hypertension, obesity and glucose intolerance. *J. Clin. Invest.* 75:809–817.

Moody, A.J., S.L. Jeffcoate, and A. Volund (1970). The effects of anti-insulin serum on the disposal of an oral load of (6¹⁴C) glucose by the tissues of the rat. *Horm. Metab. Res.* 4:193–199.

Narimiya, M., S. Azhar, C.B. Dolkas, C.E. Mondon, C. Sims, D.W. Wright, and G. Reaven (1984). Insulin resistance in older rats. *Am. J. Physiol.* 246 (Endocrinol Metab 9):E397–E404.

National Diabetes Data Group. (1979). Classification and diagnoses of diabetes mellitus and other categories of glucose intolerance. *Diabetes* 28:1039–1057.

Novak, L.P. (1972). Aging, total body potassium, fat-free mass, and cell mass in males and females between ages 18 and 85 years. *J. Gerontol.* 27:438–443.

Ohlson, L.-O., B. Larsson, K. Svardsudd, L. Welin, H. Erikkson, L. Wilhelmsen, P. Björntorp, and G. Tibblin (1985). The influence of body fat distribution on the incidence of diabetes mellitus. 13.5 Years of follow-up of the participants in the study of men born in 1913. *Diabetes* 34:1055–1058.

Olefsky, J.M., J.W. Farquhar, and G.M. Reaven (1974a). Reappraisal of the role of insulin in hypertriglyceridemia. *Am. J. Med.* 57:551–560.

Olefsky, J.M., G.M. Reaven, and J.W. Farquhar (1974b). Effects of weight reduction on obesity: Studies of carbohydrate and lipid metabolism. *J. Clin. Invest.* 53:64–76.

Pacini, G., A. Valerio, F. Beccaro, R. Nosadini, C. Cobelli, and G. Crepaldi (1988). Insulin sensitivity and beta-cell responsivity are not decreased in elderly subjects with normal OGTT. *J. Am. Geriatr. Soc.* 36:317–323.

Park, K.S., B.D. Rhee, K.U. Lee, S.Y. Kim, H.K. Lee, C.S. Koh, and H.K. Min (1991). Intra-abdominal fat is associated with decreased insulin sensitivity in healthy young men. *Metabolism* 40:600–603.

Patsch, J.R., G. Miesenböck, T. Hopferwieser, V. Mühlberger, E. Knapp, J.K. Dunn, A.M. Gotto, Jr., and W. Patsch (1992). Relation of triglyceride metabolism and coronary artery disease: Studies in the postprandial state. *Arterioscler. Thromb.* 12:1336–1345.

Potter van Loon, B.J., C. Kluft, J.K. Radder, M.A. Blankenstein, and A.E. Meinders (1993). The cardiovascular risk factor plasminogen activator inhibitor Type I is related to insulin resistance. *Metabolism* 42:945–949.

Rabinowitz, D., and K.L. Zierler (1962). Forearm metabolism in obesity and its response to intraarterial insulin. *J. Clin. Invest.* 41:2173–2181.

Randeree, H.A., M.A.K. Omar, A.A. Motala, M.A. Seedat (1992). Effect of insulin therapy on blood pressure in NIDDM patients with secondary failure. *Diabetes Care* 15:1258–1263.

Reaven, G.M. (1983). Insulin resistance in noninsulin-dependent diabetes mellitus: does it exist and can it be measured? *Am. J. Med.* 74 (Suppl 1A):3–17.

Reaven, G.M. (1988). Role of insulin resistance in human disease. *Diabetes* 37:1595–1607.

Reaven, G.M. (1991). Relationship between insulin resistance and hypertension. *Diabetes Care* 14:33–38.

Reaven, G.M. (1993). Are triglycerides important as a risk factor for coronary disease? *Heart Dis. Stroke* 2:44–48.

Reaven, G.M., and Y.-D.I. Chen (1988). Role of insulin in regulation of lipoprotein metabolism in diabetes. *Diabetes/Metab. Rev.* 4:639–652.

Reaven, G.M., N. Chen, C. Hollenbeck, and Y-D.I. Chen (1989a). Effect of age on glucose tolerance and glucose uptake in healthy individuals. *J. Am. Geriatr. Soc.* 37:735–740.

Reaven, G.M., Y.-D.I. Chen, J. Jeppesen, P. Maheux, and R.M. Krauss (1993). Insulin resistance and hyperinsulinemia in individuals with small, dense, low density lipoprotein particles. *J. Clin. Invest.* 92:141–146.

Reaven, E., D. Curry, J. Moore, and G.M. Reaven (1983a). Effect of age and environmental factors on insulin release from the perfused pancreas of the rat. *J. Clin. Invest.* 71:345–350.

Reaven, E.P., D.L. Curry, and G.M. Reaven (1987). Effect of age and sex on rat endocrine pancreas. *Diabetes* 36:1397–4000.

Reaven, E.P., G. Gold, and G.M. Reaven (1979). Effect of age on glucose-stimulated insulin release by the b-cell of the rat. *J. Clin. Invest.* 64:591–599.

Reaven, G.M., C.B. Hollenbeck, and Y.-D.I. Chen (1989b). Relationship between glucose tolerance, insulin secretion, and insulin action in non-obese individuals with varying degrees of glucose tolerance. *Diabetologia* 32:52–55.

Reaven, G.M., R.L. Lerner, M.P. Stern, and J.W. Farquhar (1967). Role of insulin in endogenous hypertriglyceridemia. *J. Clin. Invest.* 46:1756–1767.

Reaven, G.M., and R. Miller (1968). Study of the relationship between glucose and insulin responses to an oral glucose load in man. *Diabetes* 17:560–569.

Reaven, E.P., and G.M. Reaven (1981). Structure and function changes in the endocrine pancreas of aging rats with reference to the modulating effects of exercise and caloric restriction. *J. Clin. Invest.* 68:75–84.

Reaven, G.M., and E.P. Reaven (1985). Age, glucose intolerance, and non-insulin-dependent diabetes mellitus. *J. Am. Geriatr. Soc.* 33:286–290.

Reaven, G.M., and Staff, Palo Alto GRECC Aging Study Unit (1985). Beneficial effect of moderate weight loss in older patients with non-insulin-dependent diabetes mellitus poorly controlled with insulin. *J. Am. Geriatr. Soc.* 33:93–95.

Reaven, E., D. Wright, C.E. Mondon, R. Solomon, H. Ho, and G.M. Reaven (1983b). Effect of age and diet on insulin secretion and insulin action in the rat. *Diabetes* 32:175–180.

Reisin, E., R. Abel, M. Moden, D.S. Silverberg, H.E. Eliahou, and B. Modan (1978). Effect of weight loss without salt restriction on the reduction of blood pressure in overweight hypertensive patients. *N. Engl. J. Med.* 298:1–6.

Rodnick, K.J., W.L. Haskell, A.L.M. Swislocki, J.E. Foley, and G.M. Reaven (1987). Improved insulin action in muscle, liver, and adipose tissue in physically trained human subjects. *Am. J. Physiol.* 253 (Endocrinol. Metab. 16):E489–E495.

Rogers, M.A., M.S. Yamamoto, D.S. King, J.M. Hagberg, A.A. Ehsani, and J.O. Holloszy (1988). Improvement in glucose tolerance after 1 wk of exercise in patients with mild NIDDM. *Diabetes Care* 11:613–618.

Rosenthal, M., W.L. Haskell, R. Solomon, A. Widstrom, and G.M. Reaven (1983). Demonstration of a relationship between level of physical training and insulin-stimulated glucose utilization in normal humans. *Diabetes* 32:408–411.

Rowe, J.W., K.L. Minnaker, J.A. Pallotta, and J.S. Flier (1983). Characterization of the insulin resistance of aging. *J. Clin. Invest.* 71:1581–1587.

Saad, M., S. Lillioja, B.L. Myomba, C. Castillo, R. Ferraro, M. DeGregorio, E. Raussin, W.C. Knowles, P.H. Bennett, B.V. Howard, and C. Bogardus (1991). Racial differences in the relation between blood pressure and insulin resistance. *N. Engl. J. Med.* 324:733–739.

Saad, M.F., D.J. Pettitt, D.M. Mott, W.C. Knowler, R.G. Nelson, and P.H. Bennett (1989) Sequential changes in serum insulin concentration during development of non-insulin-dependent diabetes. *Lancet* 1:1356–1359.

Santos, R. F., S. Azhar, C. Mondon, and E. Reaven (1989). Prevention of insulin resistance by environmental manipulation as young rats mature. *Horm. Metab. Res.* 21:55–58.

Schwartz, R.S. (1987). The independent effects of dietary weight loss and aerobic training on high density lipoproteins and apolipoprotein A-I concentrations in obese men. *Metabolism* 36:165–171.

Seals, D.R., J.M. Hagberg, W.K. Allen, B.F. Hurley, G.P. Dalsky, A.A. Ehsani, and J.O. Holleszy (1984). Glucose tolerance in young and older athletes and sedentary men. *J. Appl. Physiol.* 56:1521–1525.

Shamiss, A., J. Carroll, and T. Rosenthal (1992). Insulin resistance in secondary hypertension. *Am. J. Hypertension* 5:26–28.

Shen, S-W., G.M. Reaven, and J.W. Farquhar (1970). Comparison of impedance to insulin mediated glucose uptake in normal and diabetic subjects. *J. Clin. Invest.* 49:2151–2160.

Sheu, W.H.-H., C.-Y. Jeng, S.-M. Shieh, M.M.-T. Fuh, D.D.-C. Shen, Y.-D.I. Chen, and G.M. Reaven (1992). Insulin resistance and abnormal electrocardiograms in patients with high blood pressure. *Am. J. Hypertension* 5:444–448.

Shimokata, H., D.C. Muller, J.L. Fleg, J. Sorkin, A.W. Ziemba, and R. Andres (1991). Age as independent determinant of glucose tolerance. *Diabetes* 40:44–51.

Sicree, R.A., P.Z. Zimmet, H.O.M. King, and J.S. Coventry (1987). Plasma insulin response among Nauruans: Prediction of deterioriation in glucose tolerance over 6 yr. *Diabetes* 36:179–186.

Swislocki, A.L.M., Y.-D.I. Chen, A. Golay, M.-O. Chang, and G.M. Reaven (1987). Insulin suppression of plasma-free fatty acid concentration in normal individuals and patients with type 2 (non-insulin-dependent) diabetes. *Diabetologia* 30:622–626.

Tedde, R., L.A. Sechi, A. Marigliano, A. Palo, and L. Scano (1989). Antihypertensive effect of insulin reduction in diabetic-hypertensive patients. *Am. J. Hypertension* 2:163–170.

Tobey, T.A., M. Greenfield, F. Kraemer, and G.M. Reaven (1981). Relationship between insulin resistance, insulin secretion, very low density lipoprotein kinetics and plasma triglyceride levels in normotriglyceridemic man. *Metabolism* 30:165–171.

U.S. Department of Health and Human Services (1986). *Current Estimates from the National Health Interview Survey: United States*. Publication No. (PHS)87-1592. Hyattsville, MD: National Center for Health Statistics.

Vaccaro, O., K.J. Ruth, and J. Stamler (1992). Relationship of postload plasma glucose to mortality with 19-yr follow-up. *Diabetes Care* 13:1328–1334.

Wang, J.T., L.T. Ho, K.T. Tang, L.M. Wang, Y.-D.I. Chen, and G. M. Reaven (1989). Effect of habitual physical activity on age-related glucose intolerance. *J. Am. Geriatr. Soc.* 37:203–209.

Warram, J.H., B.C. Martin, A.S. Krolewski, J.S. Soeldner, and C.R. Kahn (1990). Slow glucose removal rate and hyperinsulinemia precede the development of type II diabetes in the offspring of diabetic parents. *Ann. Intern. Med.* 113:909–915.

Yki-Järvinen, H., and V.A. Koivisto (1983). Effects of body composition on insulin sensitivity. *Diabetes* 32:965–969.

Zavaroni, I., L. Bonini, M. Fantuzzi, E. Dall'Aglio, M. Passeri, and G.M. Reaven (1994). Hyperinsulinaemia, obesity, and syndrome X. *J. Int. Med.* 235:51–56.

Zavaroni, I., E. Dall'Aglio, O. Alpi, F. Bruschi, E. Bonora, A. Pezzgrossa, and V. Ruttorini (1985). Evidence for an independent relationship between plasma insulin and concentration of high density lipoprotein cholesterol and triglyceride. *Atherosclerosis* 55:259–266.

Zavaroni, I., E. Dall'Aglio, F. Bruschi, E. Bonora, O. Alpi, A. Pezzavossa, and U. Butturini (1986). Effect of age and environmental factors on glucose tolerance and insulin secretion in a worker population. *J. Am. Geriatr. Soc.* 34:271–275.

Zimmet, P., S. Whitehouse, F. Alford, and D. Chisholm (1978). The relationship of insulin response to a glucose stimulus over a wide range of glucose tolerance. *Diabetologia* 15:23–27.

DISCUSSION

BOUCHARD: When people age, even when they do not gain weight, their body composition evolves in the direction of a greater fat content; in addition, men and some women develop a masculine pattern of fat distribution as they age, which means that they tend to store fat primarily in the abdominal area. Finally, with aging, even when people remain lean, there is an increase in abdominal visceral fat. This progressive accretion of adipose tissue in the abdominal area, especially in the visceral depot, has considerable implications for the lipid and lipoprotein profile, for glucose and insulin metabolism, and perhaps even for blood pressure. It may not have a direct relation to the ability of the pancreas to meet the demand for insulin, but indirectly, upper body fat and visceral fat eventually augment the risk of becoming insulin resistant. I believe this is a critically important concept.

REAVEN: We differ somewhat in the relative importance we place on the role of visceral versus generalized obesity. I certainly would not deny the importance of obesity; in fact, I believe that adiposity *per se* is a crucial issue. I think the major reason that plasma glucose concentration rises when insulin begins to fall in patients with Type II diabetes is because of the inability to control free-fatty acid levels, which are obviously linked to adiposity. Also, there are two reports showing that chronic elevation of free-fatty acids inhibits glucose-stimulated insulin secretion. If, as I believe, plasma glucose levels begin to increase as insulin levels begin to decline, the resulting hyperglycemia would further decrease the insulin response because of glucose toxicity to the β cells. Concentrations of circulating free-fatty acids would then rise even more. If fatty acids do, in fact, inhibit insulin secretion, this would be an example of a substrate-related loss of insulin secretory function.

EVANS: I think perhaps the tissue to focus on in aged humans is skeletal muscle because there are age-associated reductions in skeletal muscle mass, even if subjects are matched on fat-free mass. Visceral fat-free mass is preserved with aging, while skeletal muscle mass is reduced. Rubin Andres's paper on ideal body weight at age 60 suggests that there should be an average gain of about 9 kg relative to weight at age 20. In other words, he concludes that the body-mass index associated with the lowest all-cause mortality is significantly greater at age 60 than it is at age 20. My guess is that if we specifically measured muscle mass, the ideal muscle mass would not change with advancing age. I think the reason that increased body weight with advancing age appears beneficial is that when people gain weight as they age, they tend to preserve muscle mass that would otherwise be lost. What is your interpretation of Andres's data?

REAVEN: I agree that muscle mass is crucial. For example, if one compares insulin action in weightlifters versus runners, whole-body glucose uptake values are essentially the same in the individuals in these two groups. But if the data are normalized to muscle mass, weightlifters have the same glucose uptake per kg muscle as do untrained people, whereas runners have much higher values for glucose uptake. Also, if one compares whole-body, insulin-stimulated glucose uptake in women and men, women have less glucose uptake, but if the data are normalized for muscle mass, the sexes are comparable. I believe that neither laboratory animals nor human beings have a progressive and inexorable loss of insulin action on muscle with age; the loss seen in the oldest age group is likely to be due to loss of muscle mass. In response to your specific question about Andres's data, I must confess that interpreting them is too complicated for me.

BOUCHARD: I think we need to be very cautious on this particular issue. There are plenty of contradictory data. The paper by Reuben Andres published about 10 y ago is almost alone in claiming that an increase in body weight with age is associated with a decreased mortality rate.

BLOOMFIELD: John Holloszy has made the argument that these body composition changes, i.e., an increase in body fat and a decrease in lean muscle mass, are really epiphenomena as regards their contribution to insulin resistance with aging and that the primary causal factor is a lack of physical activity throughout the life span that causes both the body composition changes and the increased insulin resistance.

REAVEN: I agree with this in principle, but I wouldn't want to denigrate the effect of obesity. If a person's weight is modified, his or her insulin action will also be modified. With a weight gain, he or she becomes more insulin resistant; with a loss, less resistant. On the other hand, the impact of obesity is often overemphasized and that of physical activity is given short shrift. That became very clear to me when we first described the fact there was a direct relationship between insulin-mediated glucose uptake and physical activity level as estimated by either $\dot{V}O_2$max or activity questionnaire. At that time we tried to point out the importance of physical activity in modulating *in vivo* insulin action and that the association between obesity and insulin resistance was at least partly due to the fact that obese individuals are often also physically inactive. I still believe this to be true.

BOUCHARD: All the evidence you have reviewed suggests that physical activity is particularly useful in the prevention rather than in the treatment of NIDDM once the diabetic state has been established. Thus, regular physical activity may have little to do with the capacity of the pancreas to compensate and meet the demands for higher insulin levels. This raises the question of what factors determine the capacity of the β cells of the endocrine pancreas to adapt to increasing insulin needs. British investigators have suggested that a low adaptive capacity may result from a lower

β cell complement during fetal growth as a result of maternal nutritional deficiencies and detrimental maternal environmental conditions. What is your view on this "stunted-growth" hypothesis?

REAVEN: I believe the most important unanswered question in terms of glucose regulation is why one person can and one person cannot compensate for the insulin resistance. Is it genetic? So far there is no evidence to support this view. Is it something that happens early in nutrition? Could it be that having mumps destroys some β cells in certain individuals and not in others? One of the problems is that techniques to quantify insulin secretion in human beings have been not very sensitive.

EICHNER: Is Syndrome X principally restricted to Caucasians?

REAVEN: You are probably referring to publications suggesting that the link between insulin resistance and blood pressure is more prominent in European individuals as compared to Afro-Americans or Pima Indians. I think those conclusions are not entirely persuasive. For example, there is at least one report showing a lack of correlation between blood pressure and either plasma insulin levels or insulin resistance in Afro-Americans. However, there are two very nice papers from Bonnie Falkner, showing that if one compares hypertensive Afro-Americans with those who are normotensive, the hypertensive group is more insulin resistant and has higher insulin levels. You have to take your choice as which study you think is more convincing.

SUTTON: You reviewed a number of clinical studies. Would you comment on the degree of control the investigators had over such factors as time of the last exercise bout and the nature of the diet immediately preceding the various observations? I'm also interested in whether or not the subjects in these clinical studies had medical complications such as cerebral vascular disease.

REAVEN: The evidence linking plasma levels of lipoproteins, glucose, or insulin to cerebral vascular disease is weak. It is not clear if these poor correlations are real or if the studies have been inadequate. On the other hand, the link between these variables and hypertension is very clear and powerful. In the study by Shimokata, there was no control over most of the variables you mentioned, but there was a large number of individuals. In the other studies I reviewed, the subjects were hospitalized on a research ward and those variables were carefully controlled.

BALDWIN: At the City of Hope Hospital in Duarte, California, Tom Balon's group is studying the Zucker diabetic-prone strain of rat. They find that a 2% magnesium dietary supplement can normalize insulin levels, glucose tolerance, and other markers of diabetes. Is this a phenomenon unique to the Zucker rat model, or is it something that has implications in the human system as well?

REAVEN: It's a very good question and one I can't answer. We have tried very hard to avoid animals like the Zucker rat, the Ob/Ob mouse, etc., because it seems clear that the central nervous systems of these animals causes an initial over-secretion of insulin, and I believe this does not happen in Type II diabetes. I cannot say that these data are not relevant to humans, but I find most of the data that come from these genetic models difficult to evaluate. There are some other interesting models of insulin resistance that can be used to study the physiology of Type II diabetes. For example, rats with spontaneous hypertension (SHR) are insulin resistant and hyperinsulemic. If they are injected with a relatively low dose of streptozotocin, a β-cell toxin, they will respond with only minor decreases in insulin level, but they will become very hyperglycemic. If you inject the control WKY rat with the same dose of streptozotocin, nothing happens. The SHR rat may not be the perfect model for Type II diabetes, but it closely replicates the natural history of the disease.

TIPTON: I am also fond of the SHR model, but the WKY is probably not a good control model. Tomanek at Iowa conclusively demonstrated that the WKY rat will die sooner than the SHR. I have come to the conclusion that the WKY is probably the most non-physiological control animal model available in scientific research. Consequently, we must be cautious in the extrapolation of animal results to humans.

REAVEN: I agree. We have used over the years several rat models for Type II diabetes. A 4-month-old Sprague-Dawley rat is insulin resistant and hyperinsulinemic, like a prediabetic human. You give Sprague-Dawley rats a little streptozotocin, and they become diabetic. If you feed a normal, healthy Sprague-Dawley rat a fructose-enriched diet, they become insulin resistant, hyperinsulinemic, and hypertriglyceridemic. Again, a small dose of streptozotocin makes them very diabetic. So whether it's an SHR, a 4-month-old Sprague-Dawley, or a fructose-fed Sprague-Dawley, the metabolic effects of a small decrease in insulin secretion are essentially identical in insulin resistant rats. There is not a perfect rat model for Type II diabetes, but the three models I have described all mimic the pathophysiology of patients with Type II diabetes. The results of studies with all three of these models are quite consistent.

WHITE: When comparisons are made between 2 month-old rats and 9 or 12-month-old animals, it seems that it is maturation and not aging *per se* that is being studied. Do you have data from very old rats showing that there is a further decrease in insulin production per β cell, and that hyperplasia of β cells continues?

REAVEN: Yes! Furthermore, we tried everything we could do to make the β cell fail. For example, if we kept rats sedentary, and give them high-fructose diets, which make even a young animal very insulin resistant, we ended up over time with islets that looked terrible. Observing those islets though a microscope made us wonder how the rat was living, let alone secreting insulin. The rat has an incredible capacity to continue to compensate; the islets get progressively larger, the pancreas gets larger, and the rat eventually adapts! Experimentally, one can change the degree of hyperplasia enormously, depending upon whether the rats run or don't run. Whether they are females or male rats, the phenomenon is absolutely the same. The islets will look different as a function of degree of insulin resistance, but the progressive loss of insulin secretory response per β cell that occurs will age does not change.

WHITE: But if you contrast a 12-month-old animal to a 27-month-old animal, is it a continued change or simply a maintenance of the change seen during earlier maturation?

REAVEN: It is progressive change.

SEALS: Do you see a role for the increased activity of the sympathetic nervous system in older persons who display the insulin resistance syndrome?

REAVEN: I don't think that a primary increase in sympathetic activity is usually the cause of insulin resistance. Some of the abnormalities we see in triglyceride metabolism and blood pressure, etc., in insulin-resistant individuals could be related to the hyperinsulinemia that stems from this resistance and increases sympathetic nervous system activity, rather than vice versa. For example, insulin acts on the kidney to retain sodium. When insulin resistance reduces glucose uptake in muscles, the kidney still responds very nicely to insulin's action to promote sodium retention. Consequently, I believe increased activity of the sympathetic nervous system may play a role in some of the events secondary to insulin resistance, but that it is not the cause of the resistance.

TERJUNG: It's apparent that thyroid status sets the stage for sympathetic responsiveness. Do you see any role for thyroid influence?

REAVEN: No. Excess thyroid hormone will lead to insulin resistance. But early on we measured every hormone that we could think of measuring and could find no link to any change in hormone level in the normal population. There are more recent studies which suggest that changes in androgen level can alter insulin resistance in women, but not in men. It is not a clear story yet, but in terms of classic hormones, insulin antagonist hormones do not seem responsible for the insulin resistance in the world at large.

TIPTON: What about the central nervous system action of insulin in your model? Does it have a role?

REAVEN: There are certainly insulin receptors in the brain, and there has been a good deal of discussion of insulin's role in this tissue. It is not a field I follow closely, and I will only say that I am not overcome with the evidence that there is a regulatory role for insulin at that level. That comment should not be construed as an expert opinion.

LAKATTA: Please elaborate on how we might motivate the population to change its lifestyle?

REAVEN: I think it is unfortunate that we know more about the possible mechanisms of insulin resistance than we do about methods that will permit an insulin resistant individual to lose 10 kg and maintain that weight loss. We clearly need to know how to help individuals to make lifestyle changes before the untoward events associated with insulin resistance take place. I just don't know how to bring that about.

LAKATTA: My intuition tells me that it may be a hopeless cause to expect that our generation will modify its lifestyle substantially. I think the way to win is through educating children, i.e., making exercise a part of their ordinary daily lives and educating them about nutrition and ideal body weights and how their bodies will change later. In that sense, we need a marketing arm to translate what we sit here and discuss among ourselves into material useful in the elementary educational system. Maybe there are mechanisms in place that already do that. If it is not being done, it may be attributed to the fact that the data we present might not be in the right form. Also, we really need more hard data on the types of activities that lead to improvements in specific endpoints, i.e., we need more research that will lead to better, more refined prescriptions for lifestyle change.

REAVEN: I agree; I think early intervention is the only hope we have.

BAR-OR: I knew you were going to bring us to the crux of the problem—the child. I would like to provide just a hint of a possible behavioral approach. There are recent data comparing the efficacy of two behavior modification approaches for inducing longstanding beneficial effects of increased physical activity in obese adolescents. One approach was based on prescribing an exercise program, whereas the other focused on giving incentives for reducing participation in sedentary activities such as watching TV; this latter approach did not include any exercise prescription. The behavioral method of attempting to minimize sedentary activities yielded longer-lasting effects than did the actual exercise intervention. Whether the same applies for older populations is obviously a question.

BOUCHARD: If we are to prevent the advent of obesity in children and adolescents, I believe that any recommendation that dietary fat should contribute up to 40% of energy intake is counterproductive. Such a recommendation may have some validity in older people, but with children, young adults, and middle-aged adults, I think it is a breeding ground for obesity.

EVANS: Sue Roberts published a study of infants in which she found that in the first year of life, weight gain was not associated at all with milk consumption, but rather with the physical activity levels of the babies. According to the work of Ravussin, physical activity also seems to be a dominant factor in the weight gain of adults. Dietary energy intake plays a smaller role in causing obesity and differences in body fat than does activity. In untrained individuals—old and young—differences in activity explain almost 80% of the difference in body fat. So I think a real focus on activity rather than the appropriate amount of dietary fat is important.

REAVEN: I don't disagree. My recollection of the Ravussin paper is that they estimated energy expenditure very elegantly, but I don't think that energy intake was quantified as well as expenditure was; I could be wrong about that. We need to measure both really well to make general conclusions.

10

Immune Function

David C. Nieman, DrPH

INTRODUCTION

During the last century, dramatic improvements in life expectancy have been achieved in many countries worldwide. In the United States, for example, life expectancy has increased from 47 y to nearly 76 y during the 1900s and is expected to exceed 82 y by the year 2050 (Brody et al., 1987; NCHS, 1992; NCHS, 1993). In 1900 only 40% of Americans lived beyond age 65, whereas in 1990 this proportion had risen to 80%. The fastest growing minority in the United States is the "very old" (85 and older population), a group that is projected to increase from 3.1 million in 1990 to approximately 17.7 million by the year 2050.

The central issue raised by increasing longevity is that of net gain in active functional years versus total years of disability and dysfunction (Van Nostrand et al., 1993). The National Center for Health Statistics (1993) has estimated that 15% of the average American's life is spent in an unhealthy state (i.e., impaired by disabilities, injuries, and/or disease).

435

Among those reaching age 65, 5 of their remaining 17–18 y, on average, will be unhealthy ones as assessed by these criteria.

Immune senescence or age-associated immune deficiency appears to be partly responsible for some of the afflictions of old age (Ben-Yehuda & Weksler, 1992a, 1992b; Plewa, 1990). Elderly persons are more susceptible to many infections, autoimmune disorders, and cancers when compared with younger adults. Death rates from pneumonia and influenza, for example, are much higher among the very old (1361 deaths per 100,000 for those 85 y and over) as compared to adults of late middle age (17.8 per 100,000 for those 55–59 y of age) (Van Nostrand et al., 1993). Death rates for cancer also climb steeply with increasing age (NCHS, 1993). The elderly, while comprising only about 15% of the total American population, account for at least 50% of the hospitalizations and 75–85% of the deaths attributed to influenza. Additionally, there is increasing evidence that this can be linked to defects in T cell-mediated immune mechanisms, particularly cytotoxic T lymphocytes that are involved in viral clearance and host recovery (Mbawuike et al., 1993; Powers, 1993; Powers & Belshe, 1993). Ben-Yehuda and Weksler (1992b) have proposed that immune senescence contributes to the diseases of aging, which, in turn, further compromise immune competence.

Although aging is a very complex process that ultimately leads to irreversible biological changes, it appears to be influenced by genetic, environmental, and lifestyle factors. There is mounting evidence that health habits can have a sizable influence on life expectancy and quality of life, even in old age (Institute of Medicine, 1990).

A new and growing area of research interest is the relationship between certain lifestyle factors (in particular, physical activity and diet) and immune senescence (Meydani, 1993; Nieman & Henson, 1994). The purpose of this chapter is to summarize the available research in this area. Although the elderly as a group have lower immune function than do younger adults, there is considerable variation, and researchers have sought to determine if some of this variation is due to differences in nutrient intake and physical activity patterns. Before exploring this issue, a brief review of immune senescence will be provided.

IMMUNE SENESCENCE

The age-related decline of immune function has been well documented in humans and animals, although the onset, magnitude, and rate differ both between and within species (Ben-Yehuda & Weksler, 1992a, 1992b; Plewa, 1990; Solomon et al., 1988). The results of animal experiments have shown that mice exhibiting the greatest age-related declines in immune function have shorter life spans than those showing slower rates of decline (Hirokawa et al., 1992). In a prospective study of 199 elderly humans, Roberts-Thomson et al. (1974) reported that those with lower T cell immune function experienced greater mortality rates than did those within the normal range. These results are consistent with the finding that Japanese centenarians have immune systems that function at levels comparable to adults in their 40s (Sonoda et al., 1988).

The immune system comprises two functional divisions: the innate, which acts as a first line of defense against infectious agents, and the adaptive, which when activated produces a specific reaction and immunological memory to each infectious agent (Male & Roitt, 1989). Antigen presentation to the adaptive immune system results in a complex series of events leading to the development of memory B cell and T cell populations. Upon subsequent exposure to the antigen, these memory cells produce a more rapid and effective immune response (McElhaney et al., 1993).

The innate immune system comprises cells (natural killer cells and phagocytes, including neutrophils, eosinophils, basophils, monocytes, and macrophages) and soluble factors (acute phase proteins, complement, lysozyme, and interferons). The adaptive immune system also comprises cells (B- and T-lymphocytes) and soluble factors (immunoglobulins). Significant populations of cells found in these two systems are listed in Tables 10-1 and 10-2.

In general, the innate immune system acts nonspecifically on various microorganisms, begins to function early in life, and does not show ap-

TABLE 10.1. *Leukocyte subsets and normal proportions within the blood compartment. Data from Male & Roitt, 1989.*

Total leukocytes	$5-10 \times 10^9$/L of blood
Granulocytes	60–70%
Neutrophils	55–65%
Eosinophils	2–5%
Basophils	$< 1\%$
Monocytes	3–9%
Lymphocytes	25–33%

TABLE 10.2. *Characterization of major monoclonal antibodies to human lymphocyte subpopulations by cell surface structures. Data from Lydyard & Grossi, 1989.*

Cell Type	Antigen Cluster Designation	Antibody	% of Lymphocytes (Mean ± SD)
T cells	CD5	Anti-Leu-1	72 ± 7%
T cytotoxic/suppressor cells	CD8	Anti-Leu-2a	28 ± 8%
T helper/inducer cells	CD4	Anti-Leu-3a	45 ± 10%
B cells	CD19	Anti-Leu-12	10 ± 5%
Natural killer cells (NK)	CD16	Anti-Leu-11a	15 ± 7%
		Anti-Leu-11b	
		Anti-Leu-11c	
NK cells, cytotoxic T cells	CD56	Anti-Leu-19	15 ± 6%

preciable age-related decline (Hirokawa et al., 1992). In contrast, the acquired immune system, which specifically reacts with antigens, does not function well at the time of birth, shows gradual development until about the time of puberty, and then declines as age increases. The age-related decline is most apparent in T cell-dependent immune functions and appears to be directly related to thymus involution (Ben-Yehuda & Weksler, 1992b).

Circulating Concentrations of Immune Cells

Circulating concentrations of total leukocytes, granulocytes, monocytes, and total lymphocytes do not change appreciably with age, although decreased lymphocyte counts have been measured in extreme old age (Goto & Nishioka, 1989; Utsuyama et al., 1992). Of the various lymphocyte subsets, B cells decline slightly in old age, whereas natural killer (NK) cells often increase (Facchini et al., 1987; Krishnaraj & Blandford, 1988; Pagenelli et al., 1992; Vitale et al., 1992). T cell concentrations tend to decrease with age, the decline being greater among the T cytotoxic/suppressor subset (CD8$^+$) than the T helper/inducer subset (CD4$^+$), resulting in a small increase in the CD4:CD8 ratio. Other documented changes in the distribution of T cell subsets include a reduced number of circulating CD45RA$^+$ "naive" T cells and an increased number of CD45RO$^+$ "memory" T lymphocytes (McElhaney et al., 1993; Thoman & Weigle, 1989).

Natural Killer Cells, Cytotoxic Activity, and Other Nonspecific Defense Mechanisms

NK cells are unique in the immune domain because they express spontaneous cytolytic activity against a variety of tumor and virus-infected cells, and they play an important role in limiting the growth and spread of a variety of microbial infections. Laboratory measurement of natural killer cell cytotoxic activity (NKCA) involves separating mononuclear cells (lymphocytes and monocytes, i.e., effector cells) from whole blood samples and incubating them for 4 h with ^{51}Cr-labelled K562 cancer cells (targets) at several effector-to-target ratios (for example, 40:1, 20:1, 10:1, and 5:1). Killed targets are quantified by measuring the amount of ^{51}Cr released into the supernatant solution (Nieman, 1994b). The NK cells are the only mononuclear cell that exhibit cytotoxicity capabilities within 4 h of exposure to target cells. Unlike T lymphocytes, NK cells do not require the involvement of major histocompatibility (MHC) antigens to initiate cytotoxicity, and they can respond rapidly to foreign materials such as viruses and bacteria, exerting protective effects in advance of the antigen-specific immune system.

Data in humans are contradictory with respect to the function of NK cells, with NKCA reported to increase, decrease, or not change with age (Facchini et al., 1987; Fiatarone et al., 1989; Krishnaraj, 1992; Krishnaraj & Blandford, 1987; Ligthart et al., 1989; Vitale et al., 1992). The divergence of these findings can be attributed in part to the different techniques employed to evaluate the binding and killing activities of NK cells to tumor targets. Krishnaraj (1992), for example, has produced data consistent with the viewpoint that the NK cell system is highly preserved, if not slightly hyperactive, during healthy human aging. Krishnaraj and Svanborg (1992) have reported that with increase in age, there is a relative increase in circulating concentrations of "mature" NK cells ($CD16^+CD57^+$) versus "immature" NK cells ($CD56^+57^-$).

As the ratio of mature to immature NK cells increases, there is a corresponding enhancement of NKCA that may represent an immunobiological advantage to the elderly, who often experience impaired T cell immunity. In other words, the relative increase in mature NK cells that function in a MHC-unrestricted manner (nonspecific) may be a compensatory mechanism to overcome the age-associated decrease in activity of cytotoxic T cells, which operate in a MHC-restricted manner (specific). Mature NK cells can also synthesize and secrete gamma interferon (a cytokine with several immunoregulatory properties) (Krishnaraj, 1992). Thus, when T cells are functioning at suboptimal levels in the elderly, mature NK cells may assume a critical role in maintaining some of the homeostatic immune mechanisms.

In contrast, Vitale et al. (1992) have reported that although circulating concentrations of NK cells increase among the very old, when NKCA is analyzed at a single cell level, function is impaired, with the defect located at the postbinding level. These results are in agreement with morphological evidence that samples of natural killer cell ($CD16^+$) from old subjects contain significant numbers of large agranular lymphocytes that appear less efficient in target lysis than large granular lymphocytes. Nonetheless, overall NKCA appears to be unaffected because of the greater numbers of NK cells among the elderly. Further research is needed before these opposing viewpoints can be resolved.

Other nonspecific defense mechanisms such as granulocyte, monocyte, and macrophage function appear to be preserved in old age (Ben-Yehuda & Weksler, 1992a). In one study comparing 20 elderly (mean age 77 y) and 20 young adults (mean age 30 y), age did not seem to affect the capability of monocytes to express certain cytokines (interleukin-1, interleukin-6, and tumor necrosis factor), the cell adhesion molecules ICAM-1 and LFA-3, and the class II-MHC HLA-DR (Rich et al., 1993). Antigen-presenting cells from young and aged humans also appear to be comparable in their abilities to provide accessory functions for T cells (Gilhar et al., 1992; Schwab et al., 1992).

B Lymphocytes and Serum Immunoglobulins

Many of the cofactors necessary for B lymphocyte secretion of immunoglobulins are produced by T lymphocytes (Ben-Yehuda & Weksler, 1992b). For this reason, optimal antibody response of most antigens requires the cooperation of both B lymphocytes and T lymphocytes. Although the antibody response of B lymphocytes from elderly humans is often reduced (depending on the antigen), the "decline" in B cell function seems to be indirectly related to a decline in T cell function. B cell function itself appears to be largely preserved with age (Murasko et al., 1991). For example, when B cells are co-cultured with enriched autologous CD4[+] lymphocytes, pokeweed mitogen-induced immunoglobulin production is reduced among the elderly by about two-thirds when compared to younger adults, but that production can be partially restored by adding interleukin-2 and/or interleukin-5 (T cell cytokines) (Antonaci et al., 1992).

An age-related decline in the antibody response to tetanus toxoid, hepatitis B, and other vaccines has been reported (Ben-Yehuda & Weksler, 1992b; Denis et al., 1984; Powers, 1993). The seroconversion rate to hepatitis-B vaccine, for example, is only 45% among the elderly compared to 96% for younger adults (Denis et al., 1984). The literature is less than clear regarding the antibody response of the elderly to the influenza vaccine. In one analysis of 30 studies evaluating antibody induction by influenza vaccines, 10 studies showed a better response by young versus elderly subjects, 16 could not detect any significant difference, and 4 found better responses in the elderly (Beyer et al., 1989).

There is some speculation that elderly people, despite impaired immune responses, may be able to mount appropriate antibody responses to influenza vaccine antigens because they have been primed by more than one contact (either by natural infection or by vaccination) with several subtypes of influenza virus during their lifetimes (Glathe et al., 1993). In this situation, the infuenza vaccine acts as a booster and activates preexisting B-memory cells. However, as mentioned earlier in this chapter, the elderly still experience high levels of morbidity and mortality from the influenza virus because of reduced activity of certain lymphocytes, namely, influenza virus-specific, MHC class I-restricted, cytotoxic T lymphocytes; this lymphocytic activity is important in viral clearance following infection (Bender & Small, 1993; Mbawuike et al., 1993; Powers, 1993).

Serum levels of IgM appear unchanged or slightly diminished in the very old, whereas IgG and IgA levels may be increased compared to those of younger adults. Nonetheless, the observed increase in circulating concentrations of autoantibodies and monoclonal immunoglobulins is considered to be a more important reflection of the aging immune system (Hirokawa et al., 1992; Pagenelli et al., 1992). Although the immune system normally discerns between self and nonself, in autoimmune diseases abnormal antibodies against self molecules are produced, causing various organ disorders (Hirokawa et al., 1992). The age-related increase in production of autoantibodies and monoclonal immunoglobulins further demonstrates that B cells are poorly regulated in some elderly individuals (Crawford et al., 1989).

T Lymphocytes and Proliferative Response to Mitogens

T cells are indisputably the component of the immune system most sensitive to the aging process. The most significant decrements occur in cellular immunity, reducing resistance to tumor cells, viruses, and primary allograft rejection (Canonica et al., 1985; Gamble et al., 1990; Hessen et al., 1991; Matour et al., 1989; Murasko et al., 1986; Nagel et al., 1988, 1989).

Thymic involution, which begins soon after puberty and is virtually complete by midlife, precedes the age-related decline of T cell-dependent immune function. The result is that the microenvironment of the aging thymus is unable to promote T cell differentiation at the levels observed during youth (Hirokawa et al., 1992; Schwab et al., 1992). A concomitant decrease in thymic hormone production is such that by age 60 thymic hormones are undetectable (Plewa, 1990). As a result, the number of circulating immature T cells increases while that of functionally mature T cells decreases with age. These changes have been associated with depression of several T cell-dependent functions such as the delayed-type hypersensitivity skin test (DTH) and mixed lymphocyte culture reaction test (Canonica et al., 1985; Gilhar et al., 1992). One of the critical functions of the thymus gland is the positive selection of T cells that recognize antigens in association with self-MHC molecules, and this too has been shown to be impaired among the elderly (Schwab et al., 1992).

A team of researchers from Japan has confirmed in a series of elaborate experiments that the thymus plays a pivotal role in the age-related decline of immune functions (Hirokawa et al., 1992). They have attempted to counteract this through various means and have found that multiple, sequential grafting of thymuses taken from newborn mice is effective in preventing and delaying the onset of the murine age-related decline of immune function. A single grafted thymus involutes in 2–3 mo, and obviously, in humans, this makes the method impractical. As a result, this team of researchers is developing an *in vitro* culture system to promote the growth and maturation of T lymphocytes using various interleukins and a novel cofactor produced by thymic epithelial cells.

The ability of T cells to proliferate (or clone themselves) after coming in contact with specific antigens is an important component of the adaptive immune response. In comparison to the T lymphocytes from young persons, those from healthy old persons exhibit a decreased mitogen response to the plant lectins phytohemagglutinin (PHA) and concanavalin A (Con A). A common finding among researchers is that the elderly, when compared to young subjects, exhibit a 45%–65% decrease in the ability of T lymphocytes to proliferate in response to mitogens (Canonica et al., 1985; Hessen et al., 1991; Murasko et al., 1991; Nagel et al., 1989). However, although 60% of elderly subjects may experience a much lower T cell proliferative response, 40% may respond in a pattern similar to that of young adults (Hessen et al., 1991).

Interleukin-2 (IL-2) production following mitogen stimulation of T cells from old subjects is also decreased, which appears to be due to the failure of a large fraction of activated T cells to express IL-2 receptors (Candore et al., 1992; Hessen et al., 1991; Nagel et al., 1989; Orson et al., 1989). Additionally, the elderly are less able to express certain proto-oncogenes (e.g., c-*jun*) that play key roles in cell growth, differentiation, and development (Song et al., 1992).

The response of lymphocytes to mitogenic stimulation is very complex, and more than 70 molecules are specifically regulated during this response (Pieri et al., 1992). In principle, impairment of any step in the process could contribute to the age-related decline in the proliferative response, and a multitude of factors that vary from one individual to another may be responsible (Di Pietro et al., 1993). Nonetheless, it seems clear that lymphocytes from aged individuals display a number of defects that prevent normal T cell cycle entry and transit (Thoman & Weigle, 1989). The end result is that aging leads to an accumulation of T cells that do not respond well to activators.

Table 10-3 summarizes data comparing immune function of young versus elderly females (Nieman & Henson, 1994). Although circulating concentrations of immune cells and NKCA were found to be similar

TABLE 10-3. *Comparison of immune function tests between young and elderly women. Data from Nieman & Henson (1994) are used with permission.*

	Young Female College Students	Elderly Women
Number of subjects	13	30
Age (y)	21.5 ± 0.5	73.4 ± 0.8
Total leukocytes (10^9/L)	6.08 ± 0.54	6.28 ± 0.30
Lymphocytes (10^9/L)	2.42 ± 0.15	2.21 ± 0.12
T cells (CD3+) (10^9/L)	2.09 ± 0.13	1.91 ± 0.11
NK cells (CD3-CD16+CD56+) (10^9/L)	0.26 ± 0.04	0.35 ± 0.04
Lymphocyte proliferation		
Concanavalin A	46.2 ± 2.9	31.1 ± 2.4*
Phytohemagglutinin	55.8 ± 3.2	28.9 ± 2.6*
Mixed lymphocyte culture		
reaction test (cpm·10^{-3})	6.78 ± 1.01	2.08 ± 0.26*
NK cell cytotoxic activity (lytic units)	41.7 ± 4.2	50.4 ± 4.8

* = P<0.01

between groups, T cell function measured by two plant lectins (PHA and Con A) and the mixed lymphocyte culture reaction test was substantially lower in the elderly subjects (33%, 48%, and 69%, respectively). Figure 10-1 depicts the PHA data from this table in scatterplot form.

EXERCISE AND AGE-ASSOCIATED IMMUNE DEFICIENCY

National surveys have shown that older adults exercise less and have lower levels of cardiorespiratory fitness than do younger adults (Institute of Medicine, 1990). Both acute and chronic endurance exercise have a major influence on various measures of immune function in younger adults (Nieman 1994a, 1994b; Nieman & Nehlsen-Cannarella, 1992). Although research on the role of endurance exercise on the immune systems of elderly subjects is just beginning, data from the few available studies are intriguing and have potential for widespread public health influence.

Table 10-4 summarizes seven studies published in this area (Nieman & Henson, 1994). Only three of these studies involved human subjects, and all but two evaluated the effect of chronic exercise training on the resting immune response.

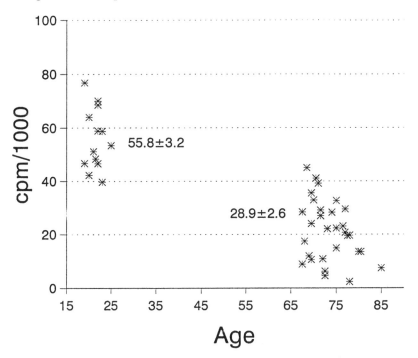

FIGURE 10-1. *A scatterplot of the lymphocyte proliferative response to PHA in young (N = 13, age = 21.5 ± 0.5 y) versus old (N = 30, age = 73.4 ± 0.8 y) female adults.* Data from Nieman et al. (1993a).

TABLE 10-4. *Summary of seven studies on the role of endurance exercise on immune senescence. Table from Nieman & Henson (1994) is used with permission.*

Investigator	Subjects	Research Design	Exercise Intervention	Immune Measures	Major Results
RATS & MICE					
Pahlavani et al., 1988	34 Fischer-344 male rats; 4 age groups: 7, 12, 18, 24 mo	Pair-matched and assigned to trained or untrained groups	60 min swimming, 2×/d, 5×/wk for 6 mo	Splenic lymphocyte response to Con A and LPS; IL-2 production (bioassay)	Age-related decline in Con A or LPS response and IL-2 production not prevented by training; decrease seen in rats 7 mo old
Barnes et al., 1991	30 Fischer-344 male rats; 6 and 24 mo old	10 young controls; 11 old controls; 9 old exercised	60 min treadmill run at 75% capacity, 5×/wk for 10 wk	Antigen KLH injected 3 wk before end, with serum anti-KLH-specific IgG measured	Age-related decline in antibody response to KLH not affected by exercise in old rats
Nasrullah Mazzeo 1992	48 Fischer-344 male rats; 3 age groups: 3, 12, 22 mo	Pair-matched and assigned to trained or untrained groups	60 min treadmill run at 75% capacity, 5×/wk for 15 wk	Splenic lymphocyte response to Con A; IL-2 production; NK cytotoxic activity	Age-related decline in Con A response and IL-2 production countered; suppressed in younger rats. No effect of training on NK cytotoxic activity.
de la Fuente, et al., 1992	60 BALB/c male mice; 2 age groups: 15 or 60 wk	Young & old mice, 3 groups of 10 each	Controls vs. swim to exhaustion (194 min) or 90 min/d for 20 d	PHA-induced response cells from axillary nodes, spleen, and thymus	Single swim bout decreased PHA response in all compartments, but after 20 d of exercise, 90 min swim led to increase in young and old.
HUMAN BEINGS					
Crist et al., 1989	14 elderly women, age 72 y	Assigned to trained or untrained groups	20-30 min aerobics, 3×/wk for 16 wk	NK cytotoxic activity (only at end of study)	NK cytotoxic activity 33% higher in trained vs. untrained elderly women
Fiatarone et al., 1989	8 young (30 y) and 9 old (71 y) active women	Acute response to maximal exercise; samples before/after	Maximal bike test	NK cytotoxic activity with and without IL-2; NK cell counts	All measures the same between young and old, both before and after maximal bike exercise
Nieman et al., 1993	30 sedentary old (73 y), 12 highly fit old (73 y), and 13 young (22 y) women	Cross-sectional comparisons among groups; sedentary were divided into exercise or control	High fit women trained 1.6 h/d for 11 y; exercise group walked 35 min/d, 5×/wk, for 12 wks at 60% capacity	PHA-induced response of blood lymphocytes; NK cell cytotoxic activity;	High fit vs. sedentary elderly women had higher NK cell activity and PHA response; 12 wk of walking had no effect on NK or T cell function.

Age and the Acute Immune Response to Exercise

The sudden, temporary changes in the immune system caused by one bout of exercise are called "acute" responses to exercise, and they usually disappear within 6 h after the exercise period is finished. Although a growing number of published reports on exercise immunology provides evidence that the immune system is profoundly affected by acute exercise, the clinical significance of these large but transient alterations is disputed (Nieman, 1994b).

Fiatarone et al. (1989) are the only researchers to have investigated the acute immune response to exercise in elderly humans, and more research is needed in this area because of its importance in helping to define potential differences between young and old. Mazzeo (1994) has emphasized that because the aging process is associated with a decline in a number of variables linked to the neuroendocrine system and because this system plays an important role in modulating immune function, research comparing the immune response to a single bout of exercise between young and old is essential.

Numerous studies have now established that high-intensity, cardio-respiratory exercise is associated with a unique biphasic perturbation of the circulating leukocyte count (Nieman & Nehlsen-Cannarella, 1992). Immediately after exercise, total leukocytes increase 50%–100%, represented evenly by lymphocytes and neutrophils with a small contribution from monocytes. Within 30 min of recovery from exercise, however, the lymphocyte count dips 30%–50% below preexercise levels, remaining low for 3–6 h. Meanwhile, a marked and prolonged neutrophilia can be measured. Moderate-intensity exercise induces a much smaller leukocytosis, lymphocytosis, neutrophilia, and lymphocytopenia.

Of the three major lymphocyte subpopulations (T, B, and NK cells), NK cells are by far most responsive to exercise (Nieman, 1994a, 1994b). It is typical for NK cells to increase 150–300% immediately following high-intensity exercise and to contribute substantially to the overall lymphocytosis before falling below pre-exercise levels for several hours. T cells (especially T cytotoxic/suppressor cells) also respond in a similar fashion, although the relative changes are smaller. The function of NK and T cells changes in a parallel fashion to the numerical changes. Study of the acute immune response to exercise is a useful model because it allows researchers to examine the immune system while it is under varying degrees of stress. Potentially, this research model could also better define how the immune system differs between young and old.

In the study by Fiatarone et al. (1989), the responsiveness of blood NK cells from eight young (mean age 30 y) and nine old (71 y) female subjects to a maximal bicycle ergometer test was measured. Females from both age groups had similar NK cell numbers and cytotoxic activity levels both at baseline and during 15 min of recovery from the maximal exercise bout. When NK cells were stimulated *in vitro* with IL-2, no difference in response was measured between age groups. Although this study is limited by small subject numbers, it confirms the growing consensus that NKCA is preserved in old age. It is unfortunate that T cell function was not measured in this study; it would have provided more useful information because it is more strongly influenced by the aging process than is NKCA.

de la Fuente et al. (1992) measured the acute PHA-induced response of lymphocytes taken from the axillary nodes, spleen, and thymus of young and old BALB/c mice. Sixty young and old mice were divided into 3 groups of 10 each. One group of mice was required to swim in individual glass baths until exhaustion (a mean of 194 min), a second swam 90 min/d for 20 d, and the third served as a sedentary control group. All animals were killed immediately after exercise. The PHA-induced response of spleen lymphocytes was significantly depressed in both young and old animals immediately after a single bout of exhaustive swimming, but the response was elevated immediately after the last 90 min bout of swimming. A similar pattern was seen for cells from the axillary nodes and thymus. All immune responses were much reduced in the older than in younger mice, however. The authors concluded that while exhaustive exercise is detrimental to the proliferative ability of lymphocytes, regular endurance exercise triggers an adaptation process reflecting an enhanced response in younger mice, and to a lesser extent, in older mice.

Age and Immune System Adaptations to Exercise Training

The persistent changes in the structure and function of the immune system following regular exercise training are called "chronic" adaptations to exercise. Several studies have made cross-sectional comparisons of the immune systems of athletes and non-athletes or have compared immune responses in both control subjects and in previously sedentary individuals who initiated exercise training programs (Nieman & Nehlsen-Cannarella, 1992; Nieman, 1994a, 1994b). Most of these studies have failed to demonstrate any important effects of regular exercise training on circulating concentrations of total leukocytes or lymphocytes or on their various subpopulations.

Several studies on animals and humans, however, have shown significant improvements in NKCA with exercise training (Nieman, 1994a, 1994b). In a randomized controlled study of 36 sedentary, young adult women, subjects in the exercise group walked 45 min per session, 5 times per wk for 15 continuous weeks and experienced a 57% increase in NKCA after 6 wk (Nieman et al., 1990). However, this contrast between groups was not maintained after 15 wk of training. In a randomized controlled study of mice, 9 wk of moderate-intensity training was associated with significantly higher NKCA (MacNeil & Hoffman-Goetz, 1993). Investigators from Denmark measured higher NKCA in elite cyclers relative to untrained subjects (Pedersen et al., 1989). The mechanism underlying the higher NKCA in trained individuals has not yet been established.

In contrast to NKCA, mitogen-stimulated lymphocyte proliferation does not appear to be altered substantially with exercise training in young adult human subjects, but it may be decreased in young rodents (Nieman, 1994a, 1994b). Pahlavani et al. (1988) studied the effects of heavy swim training (two 60-min bouts per day, 5 times per wk for 6 mo) on proliferation of spleen lymphocytes taken from 34 male rats ranging in age from 7 mo (young) to 24 mo (old). This lymphocyte proliferation was induced by Con A (cell-mediated immunity) and by lipopolysaccharide (LPS) (humoral-mediated immunity). IL-2 production was also determined after incubating lymphocytes with Con A and then measuring the ability of the supernatant liquid in the culture medium to support the growth of IL-2 dependent T cells. Animals were pair-matched, assigned to exercise training or sedentary control groups, and killed 24 h after the last exercise bout. The older sedentary control rats had a significantly lower Con A-induced proliferative response than did their sedentary counterparts, and exercise training had no effect on this relationship except to reduce the response in the two younger age groups. LPS-induced proliferation and IL-2 production followed a similar pattern. The authors concluded that intense swim exercise did not prevent the age-related decline in immune function. However, swim exercise is probably not a suitable modality for evaluating exercise effects on the immune system of rodents because of the stress swimming imposes on the animal.

A similar study design was employed by Nasrullah and Mazzeo (1992), but the exercise intervention was 60 min of treadmill exercise at 75% of maximal running capacity for 15 wk. Although exercise training led to a significant decrease in Con A-induced splenic lymphocyte proliferation in the youngest age group, an increase was also measured in the oldest animals, findings contrasting those of Pahlavani et al. (1988). The IL-2 production followed a pattern similar to that of Con A-induced proliferation, except that IL-2 levels among the trained older animals were comparable to those of the youngest sedentary age group (Mazzeo & Nasrullah, 1992). The ability of spleen cytotoxic cells to lyse YAC-1 target cells (a murine T cell lymphoma) declined with advancing age and was unaffected by endurance exercise training. The authors concluded that 15 wk of endurance training can suppress Con A-induced lymphocyte proliferation and IL-2 production in young animals and cause modest improvements in older animals.

Barnes et al. (1991) studied the effects of 10 wk of endurance training (60 min of treadmill running at 75% of maximal running capacity, 5 times a wk) on humoral immunity in old male rats. Three weeks prior to the end of the study, an antigen, keyhole limpet hemocyanin (KLH), was injected into the animals (including young and old controls). Seventeen days later, serum levels of anti-KLH specific IgG were measured and found to be significantly lower in the older rats; exercise training had no effect. The authors concluded that endurance training had no effect on the *in vivo* ability of male rats to mount an antibody response to KLH.

Only two human studies have considered the response of the aging immune system to exercise training. Crist et al. (1989) reported that moderately trained elderly women had NKCA levels 33% greater than those of untrained elderly women. Subjects trained moderately 3 times per wk for 16 wk. Baseline measurements were not taken, however, and it is difficult to determine if differences were present before the women were assigned to exercise or sedentary control groups.

The relationship between cardiorespiratory exercise, immune function, and upper respiratory tract infections in 30 sedentary elderly women (mean age, 73 y) was investigated using a 12-wk randomized, controlled, clinical design (Nieman et al., 1993a). Cross-sectional comparisons were made at baseline with a group of 12 highly conditioned elderly women (mean age, 73 y) who were active in state and national senior game and road race endurance events. The highly conditioned elderly women (average $\dot{V}O_2$max of 31 mL·kg^{-1}·min^{-1}) had been physically active for an average of 11 y and had trained an average of 1.6 h daily during the previous year. The intervention group walked 30–40 min, 5 d per wk, for 12 wk at an intensity equivalent to 60% of heart rate reserve. At baseline, the highly conditioned subjects exhibited superior NKCA and PHA-induced lymphocyte proliferation compared to the 30 sedentary elderly women (Figures 10-2, 10-3 and Table 10-5). The $\dot{V}O_2$max was positively correlated with PHA-induced lymphocyte proliferation, whereas NKCA correlated negatively with body fatness (as determined from the sum of four skinfolds).

Twelve weeks of moderate cardiorespiratory exercise training improved the $\dot{V}O_2$max of the previously sedentary elderly subjects 12.6% (from 19.0 ± 0.1 to 21.4 ± 0.2 mL·kg^{-1}·min^{-1}) but did not result in any improvement in NK or T cell function relative to the sedentary control group (Nieman et al., 1993a, 1993b, 1993c; Warren et al., 1993). (Figures 10-2, 10-3, 10-4 and Table 10-6). A variety of T cell function tests known to be negatively affected by aging were measured in the elderly women at baseline and after 5 and 12 wk of training. These tests included mitogen-induced lymphocyte proliferation with both PHA and Con A, the mixed lymphocyte culture reaction test, and the delayed-type hypersensitivity skin test (DTH).

Findings from this study demonstrate the importance of controlling for time and seasonal effects on immune function. As shown in Table 10-6 and Figures 10-2 and 10-3, for the 30 elderly female subjects, NKCA

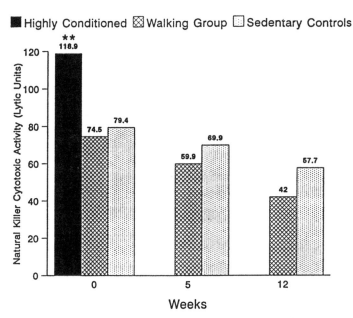

FIGURE 10-2. *At baseline, natural killer cytotoxic activity (NKCA) was significantly higher in 12 highly conditioned versus 30 sedentary elderly women. Twelve weeks of moderate exercise training had no significant effect on NKCA in the walking group relative to the sedentary control group.* Data from Nieman et al. (1993a). ** $P < 0.01$

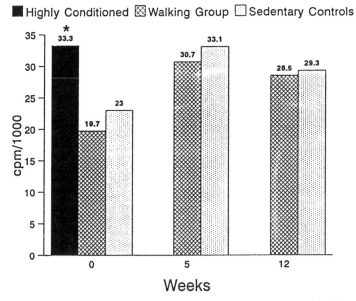

FIGURE 10-3. *At baseline, the lymphocyte proliferative response to PHA was significantly higher in the highly conditioned versus the sedentary elderly women. Twelve weeks of moderate exercise training had no significant effect on the PHA-induced proliferative response relative to the control group.* Data from Nieman et al. (1993a). * $P < 0.05$

TABLE 10-5. *Cross-sectional comparisons between highly conditioned and sedentary elderly females. Data from Nieman et al., 1993a.*

	Highly Conditioned Elderly Females (N=12)	Sedentary Elderly Females (N=30)
Age (years)	72.5 ± 1.8	73.4 ± 0.8
Height (cm)	161 ± 2	160 ± 1
Weight (kg)	55.6 ± 2.6	66.3 ± 2.1**
Sum of 4 skinfolds (mm)	49.2 ± 7.0	78.8 ±4.8**
$\dot{V}O_2$max (ml·kg^{-1}·min^{-1})	31.3 ± 0.9	18.7 ± 0.6**
Total leukocytes (10⁹/L)	5.73 ± 0.33	6.28 ± 0.30
Neutrophils (10⁹/L)	2.81 ± 0.23	3.44 ± 0.22
Lymphocytes (10⁹/L)	2.27 ± 0.15	2.21 ± 0.12
T cells (CD3⁺) (10⁹/L)	1.68 ± 0.12	1.62 ± 0.10
T helper/inducer (CD3⁺CD4⁺) (10⁹/L)	1.03 ± 0.09	1.04 ± 0.07
T cytotoxic/suppressor (CD3⁺CD8⁺) (10⁹/L)	0.66 ± 0.08	0.57 ± 0.06
Natural killer (CD3⁻CD16⁺CD56⁺) (10⁹/L)	0.33 ± 0.04	0.35 ± 0.04
B cells (CD20⁺) (10⁹/L)	0.20 ± 0.05	0.19 ± 0.02
Lymphocyte proliferative response (cpm·10⁻³)		
Concanavalin A	32.1 ± 3.8	26.0 ± 2.2
Phytohemagglutinin	33.3 ± 4.9	21.4 ± 2.1*
Mixed lymphocyte culture reaction test (cpm·10⁻³)	11.7 ± 3.0	6.9 ± 0.9*
Natural killer cell activity; Effector:target ratio, 40:1 (% lysis)	52.5 ± 3.5	40.1 ± 2.4**
Immunoglobulin G (g/L)	10.7 ± 0.7	11.4 ± 0.7

  * P<0.05; **P<0.01

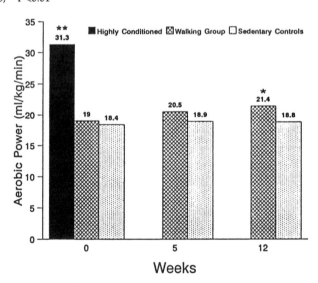

FIGURE 10-4. *At baseline, $\dot{V}O_2$max was significantly higher in the highly conditioned versus sedentary elderly women. Twelve weeks of moderate exercise training (5 sessions/wk, 35–40 min, at 60% of heart rate reserve) led to a significant 12.6% improvement in $\dot{V}O_2$max compared to the control group.* Data from Warren et al. (1993) and Nieman et al. (1993a). * P<0.05, change from baseline between groups.

TABLE 10.6 *Lymphocyte function test data at baseline, 5 wk, and 12 wk in exercise versus control groups of elderly women (mean age, 73 y). Subjects in the walking group walked 30–40 min/d, 5 d/wk for 12 wk. No significant effect of moderate exercise on any of the immune function tests was measured relative to the control group. Table from Nieman & Henson (1994); used with permission of Williams & Wilkins.*

Variable	Walking Group (N=14)			Control Group (N=16)			Effect, Group × Time P Value
	Baseline	5 wk	12 wk	Baseline	5 wk	12 wk	
$\dot{V}O_2$max (mL·kg^{-1}·min^{-1})	19.0+1.1	20.5+1.2	21.4+1.2*	18.4+0.7	18.9+0.6	18.8+0.7	0.005
Lymphocyte proliferation (cpm·10^{-3})							
Concanavalin A	24.0+3.0	27.0+3.6	32.2+3.8	27.7+3.1	27.4+3.2	30.1+3.1	0.263
Phytohemagglutinin	19.7±3.5	30.7±4.6	28.5±4.1	23.0±2.4	33.1±4.8	29.3±3.3	0.807
Mixed lymphocyte culture reaction test (cpm·10^{-3})	8.45±1.54	4.85±0.8	2.18±0.41	5.55±0.81	4.23±0.73	1.99±0.35	0.106
Delayed type hypersensitivity skin test (7 antigens, mm)	13.6+2.3		10.9+1.9	13.4+2.6		10.7+1.2	0.982
NK cell cytotoxic activity (lytic units)	74.5±10.7	59.9±9.1	42.0±5.8	79.4±11.4	69.9±10.0	57.7±7.0	0.694

*P<0.05, change from baseline different between groups

fell 35% during the 12-wk study (September through November), while the PHA lymphocyte proliferative response rose 35%. Other researchers have also reported strong seasonal variations in several types of NK and T cell function measures, with the change in NK activity being a mirror image of lymphocyte responsiveness to mitogens (Pati et al., 1987).

Log books for daily recording of health problems were provided to each highly conditioned and sedentary subject at baseline. Careful verbal and written instructions were given to the subjects to record health problems using symptom codes each day of the study. The rates of occurrence of upper respiratory tract infections (URTI) in the highly conditioned, walking, and calisthenic control groups were compared during the study (September through November). Half of the elderly women in the calisthenic group suffered an URTI during the study as compared with 3 of 14 subjects in the walking group and 1 of 12 subjects in the highly conditioned group (Chi-square = 6.36, P = 0.042). (Figure 10-5). These data suggest that elderly women not engaging in cardiorespiratory exer-

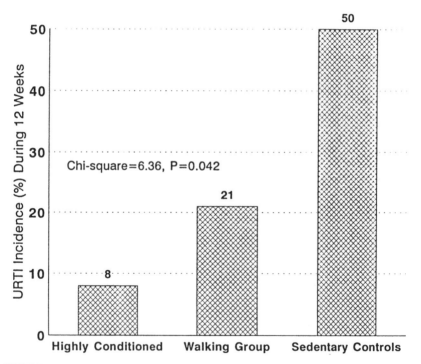

FIGURE 10-5. *During 12 wk of the fall season, elderly female subjects kept daily logs of health status and sickness symptoms. Increased endurance training (185 min per wk by the walking group, 600 min per wk by the highly conditioned group) was associated with a reduced incidence of upper respiratory tract infections.* Data from Nieman et al., 1993a.

cise are more likely than their exercising counterparts to experience an URTI during the fall season.

The authors concluded that highly active, highly conditioned, relatively lean, elderly women who regularly competed in endurance competitions had NKCA levels that were superior to those of sedentary elderly or even to levels measured in young adult women. T cell function, which is most affected by the aging process, was significantly greater in the highly conditioned than in the sedentary elderly women but remained below the levels of untrained, young adult women. In contrast, 12 wk of moderate cardiorespiratory training failed to alter immune function in the previously sedentary women. Although the incidence of URTI was lowest in the highly conditioned group, walkers were able to achieve a lower URTI incidence than that of the control group, despite no differences in chronic, resting immune function. The authors speculated that each walking bout may be associated with temporary but positive improvements in immunosurveillance that improve host protection, but this has yet to be measured in elderly subjects.

NUTRITION AND IMMUNE SENESCENCE

Many cells of the immune system depend on metabolic pathways that utilize various nutrients as critical cofactors (Chandra, 1988, 1991). Enzymes and various immune processes require the presence of zinc, iron, copper, selenium, vitamins C, A, E, and B-6, and other micronutrients, whereas deficiencies of these nutrients have been associated with negative immune changes in many studies (Bowman et al., 1990; Chandra, 1991; Dallman, 1987; Meydani et al., 1991; Prasad et al., 1993; Talbott et al., 1987). As a result, changes in immune function occur early in the course of nutritional deficiency. Chandra (1988, 1991) has provided extensive evidence linking protein-energy malnutrition (PEM) with lymphoid tissue atrophy and a corresponding decrease in most host defense mechanisms and an increase in infectious disease. For example, PEM has been associated with a marked reduction in DTH response, phagocytosis, cytokine and immunoglobulin production, and circulating concentrations of several types of lymphocytes. Although PEM and deficiencies of many vitamins and minerals have been found to impair various aspects of immune function, obesity, excess lipid intake, and excessive nutrient supplementation may also have negative effects (Chandra, 1988, 1991).

Several surveys have demonstrated the existence of specific nutritional deficiencies in a significant proportion of the elderly, especially those residing in nursing homes (Chandra, 1991; Kerstetter et al., 1992; Mowé et al., 1994). Reports of malnutrition in institutionalized older persons vary widely, from 10% to as high as 85%, depending on the study.

The causes include changes in nutrient requirements secondary to disease processes and drug regimens, the aging process itself, and social-psychological, physical, and economic barriers to adequate food intake (Kerstetter et al., 1992).

A vicious cycle can develop among malnutrition, impaired immunity, and infection. Studies conducted in Veterans Administration nursing homes indicate that patients acquire a new infection every three months and are hospitalized several times yearly, primarily because of infectious illnesses (Kerstetter et al., 1992). At any given time, 15%–20% of nursing home residents have an infection, in most cases associated with serious nutritional deficiencies.

Can improvements in nutrient intake lead to positive immune changes among the elderly? In a one-year, double-blind, placebo-controlled trial of 96 elderly subjects (mean age 75 y), supplementation with a modest physiological amount of micronutrients improved various measures of immunity and decreased the frequency of infection-related illness (Chandra, 1992). Dietary supplementation with vitamin E, vitamin B-6, zinc, selenium, and other nutrients has been shown to enhance immunity in elderly subjects (Meydani et al., 1990; Moriguchi et al., 1990; Peretz et al., 1991; Prasad et al., 1993; Talbott et al., 1987).

Potential Interaction Among Exercise, Diet, and Immune Function

In the study by Nieman et al. (1993a) of highly conditioned and sedentary elderly women, intake of energy and most vitamins and minerals (on a weight-adjusted basis) was found to be significantly higher in the fit subjects (Butterworth et al., 1993; Nieman et al., 1993c) (Table 10-7). When the nutrient intake was expressed by nutrient density (nutrient per 1000 kcal), however, no difference was found between the highly conditioned and sedentary groups. This suggests that high volumes of physical activity by elderly subjects lead to an improvement in the quantity but not the quality of food intake. Statistical tests for correlations between the immune function measures (T and NK cell function) and the nutritional measures were performed, but none of the resulting correlation coefficients was statistically significant, a common finding in other studies of healthy, ambulatory elderly subjects (Goodwin & Garry, 1988; Payette et al., 1990).

Nonetheless, it makes sense that a greater intake of minerals and vitamins per kilogram of body weight over many years by lean and highly active elderly subjects may prove to be an important factor contributing to their superior immune function (which probably cannot be detected using simple correlational statistics). In other words, when the elderly become more active, their intake of food may increase in parallel with

TABLE 10-7. *Selected nutrient intake comparisons between highly conditioned and sedentary elderly females.* Data adapted from Butterworth et al. (1993). kg = kilogram of body weight; * P<0.05

Nutrient	Highly Conditioned (N=12)	Sedentary (N=30)
energy Intake (kcal)	2027±61	1546±8*
energy Intake (kcal/kg)	37.1±.9	24.1±.2*
protein (g/kg)	1.47±.12	0.97±.05*
carbohydrate (g/kg)	5.19±.45	3.25±.20*
fat (g/kg)	1.26±.14	0.86±.06*
dietary fiber (g/kg)	0.48±.06	0.27±.02*
vitamin A (RE/kg)	32.9±.2	17.4±.9
vitamin C (mg/kg)	4.36±.23	1.79±.18
vitamin E, total (mg/kg)	0.26±.03	0.19±.02*
thiamin (mg/kg)	0.03±.01	0.02±.001*
vitamin B-6 (mg/kg)	0.04±.005	0.03±.002*
folate (μ/kg)	6.34±.92	3.92±.33*
calcium (mg/kg)	16.3±.1	9.89±.57*
iron (mg/kg)	0.28±.03	0.21±.02*
zinc (mg/kg)	0.19±.01	0.14±.01*
selenium (μ/kg)	1.96±.20	1.30±.07*
copper (mg/kg)	0.03±.003	0.02±.001*

activity, improving their overall nutritional status. This improved nutritional status, working in combination with increased physical activity, maintenance of desirable weight, and other factors, may enhance immune function over the long term. This hypothesis will need to be investigated using a long-term, longitudinal study, during which these variables can be manipulated and their influences on immunity measured.

DIRECTIONS FOR FUTURE RESEARCH

The aging process has a strong effect on decreasing many cell-mediated and humoral immune responses. While there are some indications that environmental and lifestyle factors may influence these responses, only a few researchers have attempted to measure the influence of exercise training, and their findings (Table 10-4) do not present a clear picture.

Further research is warranted to prospectively study the effect of exercise training on immune function in elderly subjects over long time periods. The cross-sectional study of Nieman et al. (1993a) has demonstrated that highly conditioned, lean, elderly women have improved T and NK cell function when compared to their sedentary counterparts. However, the relative importance of high volumes of physical activity (mean of 1.5 h/d) low body fat, and high nutrient intake (and many other confounders, including self-selection) is impossible to determine. Also, few elderly persons are likely to be motivated to attain the lifestyles adopted by the highly conditioned subjects. In the 12-wk, randomized and controlled phase of this study, five 35–40 min brisk walking sessions per wk (which is probably at the high end of what most elderly persons are willing to do) failed to have any effect on immune function, despite a modest improvement in aerobic fitness.

Together, these data suggest that exercise training may need to be conducted for perhaps one year or more and be of sufficient volume to induce changes in body weight and nutrient intake before any change in immunity can be expected. In other words, because the aging process is so dominant in old age, unusual amounts of physical activity and other lifestyle changes may be necessary before the immune system is positively affected. Research is needed to determine the exercise frequency, intensity, and duration thresholds necessary to evoke improvements in immune function among the elderly. If these thresholds appear to be too high, these recommendations will have limited public health usefulness.

More research is needed to compare the response of the immune system to acute exercise bouts. Whereas Fiatarone et al. (1989) compared the NKCA response of young and old adults to graded maximal exercise, a more useful approach would be to study the change in T cell function that occurs following a bout of brisk walking. In the study by Nieman et al. (1993a), even though no change was detected in the resting immune function of the walkers, the finding that regular moderate exercise was associated with a lower incidence of URTI suggests that changes in immune function during and for a short time after the walking bout may be important.

In many other exercise-health relationships (e.g., the effects of exercise on HDL-cholesterol or insulin sensitivity), the beneficial effects of exercise are related more to the accumulated acute responses rather than to a true chronic adaptation. Perhaps this is also true for the relationship between physical activity and immune function. In other words, even though physical activity may have limited effects on resting immune function, the acute immune response to each exercise bout may enhance host protection against disease by improving overall immunosurveillance.

SUMMARY

The immune system undergoes significant change and decline with advancing age. The increased incidence of malignancy, infectious disease, and autoimmune disorders with age is thought to be linked to this decline of immunocompetence. The immune system is not uniformly affected by the aging process. The most significant decrements occur in cellular immunity, affecting resistance to tumor cells, viruses, and primary allograft rejection. There is agreement that T cells are the component of the immune system most sensitive to the aging process. The involution of the thymus gland, which steadily progresses with age, may be a major factor responsible for the inevitable aging of the immune system. A common finding among researchers is that the elderly, when compared to young subjects, exhibit a 45%–65% decrease in the ability of T lymphocytes to proliferate in response to mitogens.

Several surveys have suggested that the elderly exercise less, are less fit, and have more nutritional deficiencies than do young adults. Each of these factors has negative effects on immunity. The complex relationships between these factors, the aging process, and the immune system make it unclear how much of the "age-related" change in immune function is unavoidable and irrevocable.

Data from a growing number of epidemiological and experimental studies on younger adults suggest that regular physical activity is associated with favorable changes in immune function and enhanced host protection from upper respiratory tract infections. Conversely, few researchers have investigated the acute or chronic effects of physical activity on the immune systems of elderly human subjects, and no one has determined if lifelong patterns of exercise retard or reverse the usual age-related decrements in immune function. Four exercise training studies using aged rats have produced conflicting findings on the value of 2–6 mo of vigorous cardiorespiratory exercise on the functions of B, T, or NK cells. These discordant results may stem from the inappropriate use of swim training in two of these studies.

In the only major exercise training study conducted with humans, highly active, highly conditioned, relatively lean, elderly women who regularly competed in endurance competitions had NK cell activity levels that were superior to those of sedentary elderly or young adult women. T cell function, which is most affected by the aging process, was greater in the highly conditioned than in the sedentary elderly women but was still inferior to that of untrained, young adult women. Twelve weeks of moderate cardiorespiratory training improved cardiorespiratory fitness but failed to alter body weight or immune function in the sedentary women. Incidence of upper respiratory tract infections (URTI) was lowest in the highly conditioned group and highest in the sedentary control group, with the walkers in an intermediate position. The walkers were able to achieve a lower URTI incidence than the control group, despite the absence of a training effect on chronic, resting immune function. This suggests that each walking bout may be associated with temporary improvements in immunosurveillance that enhance host protection. Research on the acute effects of walking on immune function in elderly subjects is certainly warranted to investigate this possibility more closely.

BIBLIOGRAPHY

Antonaci, S., A. Polignano, C. Tortorella, A.R. Garofalo, E. Jirillo, and L. Bonomo (1992). Role of interleukin 2, interleukin 4 and interleukin 5 in the T helper cell-driven B cell polyclonal differentiation in the elderly. *Cytobios* 70:77–85.

Barnes, C.A., M.J. Forster, M. Fleshner, E.N. Ahanotu, M.L. Laudenslager, R.S. Mazzeo, S.F. Maier, and H. Lal (1991). Exercise does not modify spatial memory, brain autoimmunity, or antibody response in aged F-344 rats. *Neurobiol. Aging* 12:47–53.

Bender, B.S., and P.A. Small (1993). Heterotypic immune mice lose protection against influenza virus infection with senescence. *J. Infect. Dis.* 168:873–880.

Ben-Yehuda, A., and M.E. Weksler (1992a). Immune senescence: mechanisms and clinical implications. *Cancer Invest.* 10:525–531.

Ben-Yehuda, A., and M.E. Weksler. (1992b). Host resistance and the immune system. *Clin. Geriatric Med.* 8:701–711.

Beyer, W.E.P., A.M. Palache, M. Baljet, and N. Masurel. (1989). Antibody inducation by influenza vaccines in the elderly: a review of the literature. *Vaccine* 7:385–394.

Bowman, T.A., I.M. Goonewardene, A.M.G. Pasatiempo, A.C. Ross, and C.E. Taylor (1990). Vitamin A deficiency decreases natural killer cell activity and interferon production in rats. *J. Nutr.* 120:1264–1273.

Brody, J.A., D.B. Brock, and T.F. Williams (1987). Trends in the health of the elderly population. *Ann. Rev. Public Health* 8:211–234.

Butterworth, D.E., D.C. Nieman, R. Perkins, B.J. Warren, and R.G. Dotson (1993). Exercise training and nutrient intake in elderly women. *J. Am Diet. Assoc.* 93:653–657.

Candore, G., G. Di Lorenzo, C. Caruso, M.A. Modica, A.T. Colucci, G. Crescimanno, A. Ingrassia, G.B. Sangiorgi, and A. Salerno (1992). The effect of age on mitogen responsive T cell precursors in human beings is completely restored by interleukin-2. *Mech. Ageing Dev.* 63:297–307.

Canonica, G.W., G. Ciprandi, M. Caria, W. Dirienzo, A. Shums, B. Norton-Koger, and H.H. Fudenberg (1985). Defect of autologous mixed lymphocyte reaction and interleukin-2 in aged individuals. *Mech. Ageing Dev.* 32:205–212.

Chandra, R.K. (1991). 1990 McCollum award lecture. Nutrition and immunity: lessons from the past and new insights into the future. *Am. J. Clin. Nutr.* 53:1087–1101.

Chandra, R.K. (1992). Effect of vitamin and trace-element supplementation on immune responses and infection in elderly subjects. *Lancet* 340:1124–1127.

Chandra, R.K. (1988). *Nutrition and Immunology.* New York: Alan R. Liss, Inc.

Crawford, J., S. Oates, L.A. Wolfe, and H.J. Cohen (1989). An in vitro analogue of immune dysfunction with altered immunoglobulin production in the aged. *J. Am. Geriatr. Soc.* 37:1140–1146.

Crist, D.M., L.T. Mackinnon, R.F. Thompson, H.A Atterbom, and P.A. Egan (1989). Physical exercise increases natural cellular-mediated tumor cytotoxicity in elderly women. *Gerontol.* 35:66–71.

Dallman, P.R. (1987). Iron deficiency and the immune response. *Am. J. Clin. Nutr.* 46:329–334.

de la Fuente, M., M.D. Ferrandez, J. Miquel, and A. Hernanz (1992). Changes with aging and physical exercise in ascorbic acid content and proliferative response of murine lymphocytes. *Mech. Ageing Dev.* 65:177–186.

Denis, F., M. Mounier, L. Hessel, J.P. Michel, N. Gualde, F. Dubois, F. Barin, and A. Goudeau (1984). Hepatitis-B-vaccination in the elderly. *J. Infect. Dis.* 149:1019–1023.

Di Pietro, R., R.A. Rana, A. Sciscio, S. Marmiroli, A.M. Billi, A. Cataldi, and L. Cocco (1993). Age-related events in human active T lymphocytes: changes in the phosphoinositidase C activity. *Biochem. Biophys. Res. Com.* 194:566–570.

Facchini, A., E. Mariani, A.R. Mariani, S. Papa, M. Vitale, and F.A. Manzoli (1987). Increased number of circulating Leu 11+ (CD16) large granular lymphocytes and decreased NK activity during human ageing. *Clin. Exp. Immunol.* 68:340–347.

Fiatarone, M.A., J.E. Morley, E.T. Bloom, D. Benton, G.F. Solomon, and T. Makinodan (1989). The effect of exercise on natural killer cell activity in young and old subjects. *J. Gerontol.* 44:M37–45.

Gamble, D.A., R. Schwab, M.E. Weksler, and P. Szabo (1990). Decreased steady state c-myc mRNA in activated T cell cultures from old humans is caused by a smaller proportion of T cells that transcribe the c-myc gene. *J. Immunol.* 144:3568–3573.

Gilhar, A., E. Aizen, T. Pillar, and S. Eidelman (1992). Response of aged versus young skin to intradermal administration of interferon gamma. *J. Am. Acad. Dermatol.* 27:710–716.

Glathe, H., S. Bigl, and A. Grosche (1993). Comparison of humoral immune responses to trivalent infuenza split vaccine in young, middle-aged and elderly people. *Vaccine* 11:702–705.

Goodwin, J.S., and P.J. Garry (1988). Lack of correlation between indices of nutritional status and immunologic function in elderly women. *J. Gerontol.* 43:M46–49.

Goto, M., and K. Nishioka (1989). Age- and sex-related changes of the lymphocyte subsets in healthy individuals: an analysis by two-dimensional flow cytometry. *J. Gerontol.* 44:M51–56.

Hessen, M.T., D. Kaye, and D.M. Murasko (1991). Heterogeneous effects of exogenous lymphokines on lymphoproliferation of elderly subjects. *Mech. Ageing Dev.* 58:61–73.

Hirokawa, K., M. Utsuyama, M. Kasai, and C. Kurashima (1992). Aging and immunity. *Acta. Pathol. Jpn.* 42:537–548.

Institute of Medicine. (1990). *The Second Fifty Years: Promoting Health and Preventing Disability.* Washington, D.C.: National Academy Press, pp. 202–223.

Kerstetter, J.E., B.A. Holthausen, and P.A. Fitz (1992). Malnutrition in the institutionalized older adult. *J. Am. Diet. Assoc.* 92:1109–1116.

Krishnaraj, R. (1992). Immunosenescence of human NK cells: effects on tumor target recognition, lethal hit and interferon sensitivity. *Immunol. Letters* 34:79–84.

Krishnaraj, R., and G. Blandford (1987). Age-associated alterations in human natural killer cells. 1. Increased activity as per conventional and kinetic analysis. *Clin. Immunol. Immunopathol.* 45:268–285.

Krishnaraj, R., and G. Blandford (1988). Age-associated alterations in human natural killer cells. 2. Increased frequency of selective NK subsets. *Cell. Immunol.* 114:137–148.

Krishnaraj, R., and A. Svanborg (1992). Preferential accumulation of mature NK cells during human immunosenescence. *J. Cell. Biochem.* 50:386–391.

Ligthart, G.J., H.R. Schuit, and W. Hijmans (1989). Natural killer cell function is not diminished in the healthy aged and is proportional to the number of NK cells in the peripheral blood. *Immunology* 68:396–402.

Lydyard, P., and C. Grossi (1989) Cells involved in the immune response. In: I.M. Roitt, J. Brostoff, and D.K. Male (eds.) *Immunology* (2nd edition). New York: Gower Medical Publishing, pp. 2.2–2.17.

MacNeil, B., and L. Hoffman-Goetz (1993). Chronic exercise enhances in vivo and in vitro cytotoxic mechanisms of natural immunity in mice. *J. Appl. Physiol.* 74:388–395.

Male, D., and I. Roitt (1989). Adaptive and innate immunity. In: I.M. Roitt, J. Brostoff, and D.K. Male (eds.) *Immunology* (2nd edition). New York: Gower Medical Publishing, pp. 1.1–1.10.

Matour, D., M. Melnicoff, D. Kaye, and D.M. Murasko (1989). The role of T cell phenotypes in decreased lymphoproliferation of the elderly. *Clin. Immunol. Immunopathol.* 50:82–99.

Mazzeo, R.S. (1994). The influence of exercise and aging on immune function. *Med. Sci. Sports Exerc.* 26:586–592.

Mazzeo, R.S., and M.S. Nasrullah (1992). Exercise and age-related decline in immune functions. In: M. Eisinger and R.W. Watson (eds.) *Exercise and Disease.* Boca Raton, FL: CRC Press, pp. 159–178.

Mbawuike, I.N., A.R. Lange, and R.B. Couch (1993). Diminished influenza A virus-specific MHC class I-restricted cytotoxic T lymphocyte activity among elderly persons. *Viral Immunol.* 6:55–64.

McElhaney, J.E., M.J. Pinkoski, and G.S. Meneilly (1993). Changes in CD45 isoform expression after influenza vaccination. *Mech. Ageing Dev.* 69:79–91.

Meydani, S.N. (1993). Vitamin/mineral supplementation, the aging immune response, and risk of infection. *Nutr. Rev.* 51:106–109.

Meydani, S.N., M.P. Barklund, S. Liu, M. Meydani, R.A. Miller, J.G. Cannon, F.D. Morrow, R. Rocklin, and J.B. Blumberg (1990). Vitamin E supplementation enhances cell-mediated immunity in healthy elderly subjects. *Am. J. Clin. Nutr.* 52:557–563.

Meydani, S.N., J.D. Ribaya-Mercado, R.M. Russell, N. Sahyoun, F.D. Morrow, and S.N. Gershoff (1991). Vitamin B-6 deficiency impairs interleukin 2 production and lymphocyte proliferation in elderly adults. *Am. J. Clin. Nutr.* 53:1275–1280.

Moriguchi, S., N. Kobayashi, and Y. Kishino (1990). High dietary intakes of vitamin E and cellular immune functions in rats. *J. Nutr.* 120:1096–1102.

Mowé, M., T. Bømer, and E. Kindt (1994). Reduced nutritional status in an elderly population (>70 y) is probable before disease and possibly contributes to the development of disease. *Am. J. Clin. Nutr.* 59:317–324.

Murasko, D.M., B.J. Nelson, D. Matour, I.M. Goonewardene, and D. Kaye. (1991). Heterogeneity of changes in lymphoproliferative ability with increasing age. *Exp. Gerontol.* 26:269–279.

Murasko, D.M., B.J. Nelson, R. Silver, D. Matour, and D. Kaye (1986). Immunologic response in an elderly population with a mean age of 85. *Am. J. Med.* 81:612–618.

Nagel, J.E., R.K. Chopra, F.J. Chrest, M.T. McCoy, E.L. Schneider, N.J. Holbrook, and W.H. Adler (1988). Decreased proliferation, interleukin 2 synthesis, and interleukin 2 receptor expression are accompanied by decreased mRNA expression in phytohemagglutinin-stimulated cells from elderly donors. *J. Clin. Invest.* 81:1096–1102.

Nagel, J.E., R.K. Chopra, D.C. Powers, and W.H. Adler (1989). Effect of age on the human high affinity interleukin 2 receptor of phytohaemagglutinin stimulated peripheral blood lymphocytes. *Clin. Exp. Immunol.* 75:286–291.

Nasrullah, I., and R.S. Mazzeo (1992). Age-related immunosenescence in Fischer 344 rats: influence of exercise training. *J. Appl. Physiol.* 73:1932–1938.

National Center for Health Statistics. (1993). *Health, United States, 1992.* Hyattsville, MD: Public Health Service.

National Center for Health Statistics. (1992). *Vital Statistics of the United States, 1989, Life Tables.* Hyattsville, MD: Public Health Service.

Nieman, D.C. (1994a). Physical activity, fitness and infection. In: C. Bouchard, R.J. Shephard, and T. Stephens (eds.) *Physical Activity, Fitness, and Health: International Proceedings and Consensus Statement.* Champaign, IL: Human Kinetics Books, pp. 796–813.

Nieman, D.C. (1994b). Exercise, upper respiratory tract infection, and the immune system. *Med. Sci. Sports Exerc.* 26:128–139.

Nieman, D.C., and D.A. Henson (1994). Role of endurance exercise in immune senescence. *Med. Sci. Sports Exerc.* 26:172–181.

Nieman, D.C., D.A. Henson, G. Gusewitch, B.J. Warren, R.C. Dotson, D.E. Butterworth, and S.L. Nehlsen-Cannarella (1993a). Physical activity and immune function in elderly women. *Med. Sci. Sports Exerc.* 25:823–831.

Nieman, D.C., and S.L. Nehlsen-Cannarella. (1992). Exercise and infection. In: M. Eisinger, and R.W. Watson (eds.) *Exercise and Disease.* Boca Raton, FL: CRC Press, pp. 121–148.

Nieman, D.C., S.L. Nehlsen-Cannarella, P.A. Markoff, A.J. Balk-Lamberton, H. Yang, D.B.W. Chritton, J.A. Lee, and K. Arabatzis (1990). The effects of moderate exercise training on natural killer cells and acute upper respiratory tract infections. *Int. J. Sports Med.* 11:467–473.

Nieman, D.C., B.J. Warren, R.G. Dotson, D.E. Butterworth, and D.A. Henson (1993b). Physical activity, psychological well-being, and mood state in elderly women. *J. Aging Phys. Act.* 1:22–33.

Nieman, D.C., B.J. Warren, K.A. O'Donnell, R.G. Dotson, D.E. Butterworth, and D.A. Henson (1993c). Physical activity and serum lipids and lipoproteins in elderly women. *J. Am Geriatr. Soc.* 41:1339–1344.

Orson, F.M., C.K. Saadeh, D.E. Lewis, and D.L. Nelson (1989). Interleukin 2 receptor expression by T cells in human aging. *Cell Immunol.* 124:278–291.

Pagenelli, R., I. Quinti, U. Fagiolo, A. Cossarizza, C. Ortolani, E. Guerra, P. Sansoni, L.P. Pucillo, E. Scala, E. Cozzi, L. Bertollo, D. Monti, and C. Franceschi (1992). Changes in circulating B cells and immuno-globulin classes and subclasses in a healthy aged population. *Clin. Exp. Immunol.* 90:351–354.

Pahlavani, M.A., T.H. Cheung, J.A. Chesky, and A. Richardson. (1988). Influence of exercise on the immune function of rats of various ages. *J. Appl. Physiol.* 64:1997–2001.

Pati, A.K., I. Florentin, V. Chung, M. De Sousa, F. Levi, and G. Mathe (1987). Circannual rhythm in natural killer activity and mitogen responsiveness of murine splenocytes. *Cell Immunol.* 108:227–234.

Payette, H., M. Rola-Pleszczynski, and P. Ghadirian (1990). Nutrition factors in relation to cellular and regulatory immune variables in a free-living elderly population. *Am. J. Clin. Nutr.* 52:927–932.

Pedersen, B.K., N. Tvede, L.D. Christensen, K. Klarlund, S. Kragbak, and J. Halkjr-Kristensen (1989). Natural killer cell activity in peripheral blood of highly trained and untrained persons. *Int. J. Sports Med.* 10:129–131.

Peretz, A., J. Nèe, J. Desmedt, J. Duchateau, M. Dramaix, and J.P. Famaey (1991). Lymphocyte response is enhanced by supplementation of elderly subjects with selenium-enriched yeast. *Am. J. Clin. Nutr.* 53:1323–1328.

Pieri, C., R. Recchioni, F. Moroni, F. Marcheselli, and S. Damjanovich (1992). The response of human lymphocytes to phytohemagglutinin is impaired at different levels during aging. *Ann. N.Y. Acad. Sci.* 673:110–118.

Plewa, M.C. (1990). Altered host response and special infections in the elderly. *Emer. Med. Clin. N. Amer.* 8:193–206.

Powers, D.C. (1993). Influenza A virus-specific cytotoxic T lymphocyte activity declines with advancing age. *J. Am. Geriatr. Soc.* 41:1–5.

Powers, D.C., and R.B. Belshe (1993). Effect of age on cytotoxic T lymphocyte memory as well as serum and local antibody responses elicited by inactivated influenza virus vaccine. *J. Infect. Dis.* 167:584–592.

Prasad, A.S., J.T. Fitzgerald, J.S. Hess, J. Kaplan, F. Pelen, and M. Dardenne (1993). Zinc deficiency in elderly patients. *Nutrition* 9:218–224.

Rich, E.A., M.A. Mincek, K.B. Armitage, E.G. Duffy, D.C. Owen, J.D. Fayen, D.L. Hom, and J.J. Ellner (1993). Accessory function and properties of monocytes from healthy elderly humans for T lympho-cyte responses to mitogen and antigen. *Gerontology* 39:93–108.

Roberts-Thomson, I.C., S. Whittingham, U. Youngchaiyud, and I.R. Mackay (1974). Ageing, immune response and mortality. *Lancet* 2:368–370.

Schwab, R., C. Russo, and M.E. Weksler (1992). Altered major histocompatibility complex-restricted antigen recognition by T cells from elderly humans. *Eur. J. Immunol.* 22:2989–2993.

Solomon, G.F., M.A. Fiatarone, D. Benton, J.E. Morley, E. Bloom, and T. Makinodan (1988). Psychoim-munologic and endorphin function in the aged. *Ann. N.Y. Acad. Sci.* 521:43–58.

Song, L., J.M. Stephens, S. Kittur, G.D. Collins, J.E. Nagel, P.H. Pekala, and W.H. Adler (1992). Expres-sion of c-*fos*, c-*jun* and *jun* B in peripheral blood lymphocytes from young and elderly adults. *Mech. Ageing Dev.* 65:149–156.

Sonoda, A., H. Takada, and S. Suzuki (1988). Immunological feature of centenarian (IV). *Proc. Jpn. Soc. Immunol.* 18:703–707.

Talbott, M.C., L.T. Miller, and N.I. Kerkvliet (1987). Pyridoxine supplementation: effect on lymphocyte responses in elderly persons. *Am. J. Clin. Nutr.* 46:659–664.

Thoman, M.L., and W.O. Weigle (1989). The cellular and subcellular bases of immunosenescence. *Adv. Immunol.* 46:221–261.

Utsuyama, M., K. Hirokawa, C. Kurashima, M. Fukayama, T. Inamatsu, K. Suzuki, W. Hashimoto, and K. Sato (1992). Differential age-changes in the numbers of CD4$^+$CD45RA$^+$ and CD4$^+$CD29$^+$ T cell subsets in human peripheral blood. *Mech. Ageing Dev.* 63:57–68.

Van Nostrand, J.F., S.E. Furner, and R. Suzman (1993). Health data on older Americans: United States, 1992. National Center for Health Statistics. *Vital Health Stat.* 3(27):103.

Vitale, M., L. Zamai, L.M. Neri, A. Galanzi, A. Facchini, R. Rana, A. Cataldi, and S. Papa (1992). The impairment of natural killer function in the healthy aged is due to a postbinding deficient mechanism. *Cell. Immunol.* 145:1–10.

Warren, B.J., D.C. Nieman, R.G. Dotson, C.H. Adkins, K.A. O'Donnell, B.L. Haddock, and D.E. Butterworth (1993). Cardiorespiratory responses to exercise training in septuagenarian Women. *Int. J. Sports Med.* 14:60–65.

DISCUSSION

NASH: You note that the progressive depression of host defense in humans is most associated with T cell dysfunction, primarily arising from thymic gland senescence. You also noted some of the other risk factors for immune suppression. This list is fairly long in the aging population. There are immunosuppressive drugs, chemicals, and biologicals that are commonly used by older persons. There are also immunosuppressive behavioral states and traits including stress, anxiety, and depression. Furthermore, musculoskeletal and neuropathic pain in the aged may exert psychic influences on the immune system and require the taking of aspirin and nonsteroidal inflammatory drugs, which are also immunosuppressive. Age-related changes in sleep patterns, life satisfaction, financial stability, and autonomic function, plus spousal bereavement, can also influence the immune system.

We can examine the effect of exercise on immune function in three ways. First, we can investigate the acute exercise-induced leucocytosis, but this is an acute transitory calamity at the mercy of the autonomic nervous system or cellular damage. Also, I would no more suggest that my immune system could be conditioned by an acute leucocytosis than propose that my cardiovascular morbidity might be reduced just because my heart rate goes up when I run. As well, many investigators use the term "heightened immune surveillance" in describing acute changes in NK cells, but we don't know what the association is between the transitory elevation of NK function and depressed illness or neoplastic susceptibility. Importantly, the immune system is so exquisitely counter-regulated that every yin seems to have a yang.

The second way to study exercise effects on immune function is to look at the effect of training on baseline mononuclear cells and their phenotypes, and their phenotypic distributions or functional characteristics, including NK function or mitogen challenge tests. There are very few of these studies, and they tend to be cross-sectional and therefore subject to the anticipated selection bias of their designs.

Third, we might investigate whether training attenuates the native, accepted, and inevitable aging-associated immune risk factors on host defense. At our center, Arthur LaPerrier's work in HIV-infected individuals is a model for this approach, as he has looked at the influence of exercise training on the blunting of psychic stress effects on immune responses. Because the immune system is subservient to neuroendocrine changes and cellular damage and because reversal of thymic senescence has yet to be established with exercise training, aren't we better off looking at the blunting of suppressive influences on host defense rather than whether more mononuclear cells enter the circulation after exercise?

NIEMAN: Immune senescence is powerfully correlated with age. Age is so dominant that all the other factors you mentioned are relatively minor. In our study, we had a long list of subject-selection criteria, including the absence of known diseases, psychic disorders, bone fractures, or medications that affected the immune system. Yet, despite the fact that we had a very healthy non-diseased group of sedentary women, their T cell function was still dramatically lower than that of the young subjects. We recruited the highly conditioned, lean, elderly women and found that the age-related decrease in T cell function was partially abrogated. The question is, Why? Was it a function of their leanness or their diet? Twelve weeks of walking was an inadequate stimulus to affect the immune system in the previously sedentary elderly. It may take years of conditioning, with substantial weight loss, for such an effect to be detected.

Regarding the acute immune response to exercise, there is only one study by Fiatarone et al. that compared NK activity between young and old and found no difference before and after a maximal exercise bout. I wish they had looked at T cell function to see if there may be favorable changes taking place during moderate activity that could explain the our infection results.

EICHNER: As Mark Nash stated, mental stresses such as school exams, divorce, bereavement, social isolation, and depression can impair immunity. In contrast, relaxation techniques, self-hypnosis, and even anonymous writing about personal traumas can rev up immunity. Perhaps whether exercise harms or helps immunity depends on whether the exercise regimen is a stress or a joy. Also, because most of the exercise-induced immune changes you reviewed were modest and brief, and ascertainment of upper respiratory tract infections was mainly by self-rated questionnaires, I wonder how certain you are that these were *bona fide* infections that were prevented by exercise.

NIEMAN: We were with the women every day, so we knew if they were sick or not.

EICHNER: I would cite Joseph Cannon's 1993 review in the *Journal of Applied Physiology.* He describes the limits of current research and cautions us on prematurely concluding whether exercise helps or harms immunity. He says, so what if salivary IgA dips briefly after an exercise bout, when one person in 500 is born without IgA, yet doesn't get infections; and so what if blood lymphocytes rise and fall briefly after exercise, when only one lymphocyte in 500 is in the bloodstream anyway, and most of our common infections occur at the body's interface with the environment, i.e. the mucosa and skin?

NIEMAN: First, all we have are the epidemiological results. For example, in our LA marathon study we showed that during the week after the race, the odds of getting sick were 5.9 times greater among the runners who ran the race versus those who didn't. We have run athletes for 2.5–3 h on the treadmill at race pace and have measured the immune response throughout an entire day. I am impressed that the large acute changes that take place for at least 6 h after such heavy exertion do seem to explain the epidemiological findings. I know Dr. Cannon is not convinced of that, but there are many other researchers who are. Dr. Bente Pedersen in Denmark and others feel that there is an open window of increased vulnerability when the immune system is down for several hours after heavy exertion.

In our randomized controlled study with elderly women, we found that a daily walk helped reduce the incidence of the common cold during the fall season. The question is, If there is no change in resting immune function, then what explains those results? Perhaps we need to look at the acute changes during the walk itself. We did a study with younger women who in random order would either sit in the lab or walk for 45 min at 60% $\dot{V}O_2$max. During that 45-min walk at 60% $\dot{V}O_2$max there was no elevation in cortisol or epinephrine and a mild increase in norepinephrine. I feel this hormonal milieu is favorable to immunosurveillance. We did find an acute increase in immunoglobulin concentrations that was not due to plasma volume changes. Also, there was an increased circulation of lymphocytes in the blood compartment.

EICHNER: I have two brief rejoinders. In the week after a marathon, everybody feels lousy—slight fever, sore muscles, scratchy throat. Many times it's just the acute-phase response, not an infection. So I urge that you document infections. Second, another way that walking outdoors can cut the incidence of upper respiratory infections is that it takes you away from the viruses. Rhinoviruses lurk in the noses of children; just getting out of the house for an hour will cut your incidence of respiratory tract infections.

NIEMAN: The only thing I say on that last point is that all 30 women, controls and walkers, met together in the same facility for a warm-up.

EICHNER: So the controls were spreading their colds in the room, and the walkers were getting away from them.

NIEMAN: No, they all met in the same facility together. I agree that being outdoors may help. In this situation, though, I don't think that was the reason. Regarding marathons and sickness, we ask runners to self-report sickness and how many days they have been sick. For example, last summer I did a study of the Grandfather Mountain Marathon with 300 runners. This is a very difficult marathon with a net altitude gain of 1200 feet. Only 3% of runners got sick during that summer marathon. In the winter (LA Marathon), 13% got sick. Of the 3% that got sick after the summer marathon, nearly every one of them was sick for 10 d or more. I don't think this can be explained by feeling lousy after the run. I do agree that the next step is to do studies with direct virus innoculation.

BLUMBERG: I would like to respond to your emphasis on the "moderate" nature of the formulation employed by Ranjit Chandra (1992) in his clinical trial examining the effect of daily nutrient supplementation on immune responses and infection in elderly subjects. While the amounts of most of the micronutrients were similar to the RDA, vitamin E was present at 44 mg and beta-carotene at 16 mg, a consumption level about 4 times the upper quartile of usual intakes, i.e., amounts very difficult to achieve through diet alone. Considering the remarkable efficacy of the supplement in enhancing immune responses and reducing infectious disease episodes, it is important to recognize that these results may reflect more than a simple correction of marginally inadequate intakes common to older adults and may rather suggest a rational role for supradietary intakes of antioxidants. When you performed the dietary assessment of your subjects, did you determine intakes from supplements as well as from foods?

NIEMAN: The subjects abstained from all supplements during the study. That was one of the requirements.

BLUMBERG: The data you presented do not indicate the magnitude of variability of the immune responses within and between subjects. There is a tremendous heterogeneity among older people with regard to many physiological functions, particularly immunity. Did you observe a small or a substantial degree of intra- and inter-subject variability, for example, with the CMI MultiTest used to assess cell-mediated immune responses to recall antigens? A large variability could mask real benefits.

NIEMAN: On many immune measures, although they are lower in the elderly, variability is really not much different than what you see in the young.

DAVIS: I would like to encourage you not to be too quick to dismiss the importance of monocytes and macrophages of the innate (non-specific) immune system with respect to exercise and aging.

NIEMAN: To the contrary, I think they are very important.

DAVIS: As you suggested, the literature on aging suggests that there are few, if any, deficiencies in the numbers of monocytes/macrophages and various functions of these cells with aging, whereas there are major decreases in T cell function. However, macrophages and monocytes play the most important role in the first line of defense against infection. With respect to susceptibility to infection, the possibility must be considered that even small reductions in alveolar macrophage function can play a major role in allowing viruses to take hold. This all occurs before the adaptive immune responses (T cells) even notice that anything is wrong. Secondly, macrophages and monocytes are antigen-presenting cells. T cells can't really fight infectious agents and other foreign products without the presentation of the processed antigen from macrophages. Therefore, I think it's a mistake to focus totally on T cell function. It's much too early in the development of the new field of exercise immunology to rule out any of the components of an integrated immune response to infection and cancer.

NIEMAN: Mark, in the papers I reviewed in which functions of neutrophils, macrophages, and monocytes were compared in the elderly versus young, no statistical difference was shown. Are you aware of data that have shown a difference?

DAVIS: No; unfortunately, there are few good papers. This leads me to my second point, which is to emphasize the importance of the animal literature in this area. It is very difficult to study tissue macrophage function in humans.

NIEMAN: I agree.

EVANS: It is clear from our research that following exercise there is an increase in complement that is not different between old and young. We do see, however, that the stimulation of complement to neutrophil activation is affected by aging. Plasma elastase activities were quite different between old and young in response to complement. Also, the neutrophilia following exercise, the macrophage level in skeletal muscle, and stimulation of monocytes to produce interleukin-1 are altered with age.

KENNEY: With respect to the seasonal changes in T cell function, are those changes predictable? Secondly, could you speculate on the primary stimulus for those changes? Specifically, are changes in T cell function related to the environment (e.g., temperature, sunlight periodicity, etc.) in humans?

NIEMAN: There are very interesting animal data indicating that over the course of one year there may be predictable changes in which T cell function will go up and then down and then up again, and in a mirror image pattern, natural killer cell activity will go down and then up and then down. With humans it is not quite as clear.

BALDWIN: I think it is interesting that about 10 y ago I was asked what I thought about the swimming rodent model. I said at the time that swimming was a poor model to study systemic physiology. I still believe that. Tipton has the best data to show that in the swimming animal, particularly in the swimming rat, hypoxic stress occurs. I don't think it is a joy for these animals to do this type of conditioning, which may have a negative impact on immune function.

On another issue, has gender been considered in the experiments you have focused on? We know that there are marked gender-related differences in the effects of training on the body composition of rats, which you pointed out is a critical issue. For example, when the male rat is conditioned on a treadmill over time, there is both the expenditure of calories and an appetite suppression effect occurring, such that at the end of the training program there is usually a reduction in the fat content of the animal. Running female rats, on the other hand increase their energy intake to compensate for the increased expenditure and don't change their body fat.

NIEMAN: Mark, do you know if Mazzeo used male rats?

DAVIS: As far as I know everybody has used males.

EVANS: Cannon has seen differences between men and women in their acute-phase responses to exercise, including differences in interleukin-1 antagonists.

NIEMAN: Of the variables we have measured, important gender differences have not been established.

BALDWIN: If the mouse appears to be suitable as an animal model for immune studies in comparison to the rat, the mouse is an excellent treadmill runner. In fact you can take a naive mouse, put it on a treadmill at the speed used to train a rat, i.e., 20–25 m/min, and the mouse will run for about 2.5 h without missing a beat.

NIEMAN: Unfortunately, none of these exercise studies with mice has looked at the aging issue.

EVANS: In Joe Cannon's review on exercise and immune function, he also pointed out that treadmill exercise is a stress for rats that may cause some immune changes that have been attributed to exercise. He recommends the use of running wheels, not treadmills, because voluntary running wheels are less stressful.

NEIMAN: Hoffman-Goetz at Waterloo University published a paper in which she had mice running in wheels versus a treadmill. She found that NK activity in these mice was improved, whether they were in the wheel or on the treadmill. At least in her hands, the stress of the exercise environment didn't abrogate the apparent effect of the exercise.

TIPTON: I would like to repeat the point made by Baldwin that swimming is a terrible exercise model. The results mislead the scientific community and cause erroneous conclusions because the rats are avoiding being drowned; they don't respond physiologically to swimming exercise in the same way the human does.

SEALS: We found in the early and mid-1980s, that training older (early to late 60s) sedentary men and women for as long as 6 mo at low exercise intensities caused very little change in body composition or changes in the traditional risk factors for cardiovascular disease, such as glucose tolerance and plasma lipids. But training for an additional 6 mo with exercise at moderate or even high intensities produced modest reductions in body fat and weight associated with favorable alterations in the metabolic risk factors for heart disease. Thus, your comment that 12 wk of training may not be enough, especially if the adaptation in immune function is somehow linked to body composition changes, may be an appropriate one.

NIEMAN: In the 12-wk study, we measured diet, body composition, and blood lipids. There was no change in either the quantity or quality of the diet or in body composition. Our experience with these women, average age 73, is that walking 40 min at 60% $\dot{V}O_2$max 5 d/wk was quite close to their limit. Two women dropped out of the study because of prior foot injuries that were exacerbated by the walking. All of the other women were able to finish. I question exercising women in their 70s at intensities greater than those we used. The highly conditioned women obviously exercised more intensely, but I think they were a special group that was willing and motivated to push much harder. If we can't demonstrate in 12 wk important changes in immune function with a walking program, I question the usefulness of telling women to exercise twice as hard.

DAVIS: I again suggest that you may have overlooked some important immune changes by testing only a specific part of the immune system (T cells).

TIPTON: What happens to the plasma complement with aging, and are there changes in the major histocompatibility complex (MHC) that have any relevance to your findings and conclusions?

NIEMAN: I don't know of any paper that has claimed an age-related effect on MHC.

SUTTON: Some of the studies on humans were not randomized and were poorly controlled. It is very important that we don't take home wrong messages from studies that are scientifically flawed.

NIEMAN: That's right.

Index

Activities of daily living (ADL), 26; effects of exercise, 27-29; effects of fitness components 29-36

Activity, increase longevity, 13-15

Acute exercise effects, arterial blood pressure, 246-247; cardiovascular regulation, 240-250; heart rate, 244-245; pulmonary system, 265-278; reflexes, 72; stroke volume/cardiac output, 245-246; systemic hemodynamic adjustment, 244-247

Acute immune response to exercise, 445-446

Adipose tissue, 366-367

Aerobic capacity, exercise effects, 19

Aerobic cardiovascular fitness, 29

Aerobic training, reflex chronic exercise effects, 72-73

Age, acute immune response to exercise, 445-446; immune system adaptations to exercise training, 446-453

Aging and exercise, limitations of existing data, 6-8; methodological issues, 6-8

Aging process, primary vs secondary effects, 7

Aging, and motor control, 53-114; demographics in United States, 2; physical inactivity, 5-6

Angina pectoris, physical activity/fitness, 15

Angiogenesis, 91

Assessment of disability, 26-27

Atherosclerotic cardiovascular diseases, 376-377

Athletes, skeletal muscle aging effects on performance, 116-117

B Lymphocytes, 440

Balance, effects of exercise, 23-25

Basic self care, 26

Blood glucose, diet-induced brain function fluctuations, 96-97

Blood pressure, exercise effects, 244-245

Body composition, adipose tissue, 366-367; aging effects on, 363-367; bone, 365-366; lean body mass, 363-365; peak bone mass, 365-366

Body fluid, 305-351; baseline temperature, 313-315; dehydration age response, 315-321; experimental approaches, 307-308; future research, 339-340; introduction, 306-308; renal fluid conservation, 315-318; spontaneous fluid ingestion, 314-315

Body mass, lean, 363-365

Body temperature regulation, baseline temperature, 313-315; cold environment response, 337-339; epidemiology, 308-313; experimental approaches, 307-308; future research, 339-340; heat exposure and exercise, 318-319; heat storage, 330-332; heat waves, 308-311; hypothermia, 311-312; introduction, 306-308; plasma volume control, 332-333; skin blood flow, 321-324; sweat gland function, 327-329; sweating responses, 329-330

Bones, 175-235; age-related alterations, 182-202; architecture, 177-179; architecture alterations, 187-191; biology, 177-181; calcium intake, 216-217; cell activity changes, 184-185; composition, 177-179; disuse adaptations, 196-202; disuse osteopenia, 198-199; endocrine interaction status, 217; endocrine regulator changes, 185-186; future research, 217-219; geometry alterations, 187-191; introduction, 176-181; mass decline with aging, 182-184; mass nutritional factors, 216-217; mechanical loading response, 202-210; medical/clinical concerns, 181-182; osteogenic response to exercise, 210-212; osteoporotic fracture, 181; peak mass, 365-366; quality decline with aging, 186-191; safety factors, 191-192; stiffness, 179-180; strength, 179-180; training adaptations, 202-216; ultrastructural changes, 186-187; Vitamin D intake, 216-217

Brain function, vitamin supplement effects, 97-98

Calcium, lifetime effects on bone mass, 216-217

Cancer, 376

Cardiac output, aging effects, 324-327

Cardiopulmonary functions, 237-304; acute exercise effects, 240-250; at rest, 239-240; introduction, 238

Cardiorespiratory exercise, immune system, 448

Cardiovascular function, human performance effects, 258-260

Cardiovascular mechanism, exercise effects on movement, 90-91

Cardiovascular regulation, acute exercise effects, 240-250; maximal oxygen consumption, 240-244

Cells, circling concentrations of immune, 438

Cellular aging, 4; facultative, 5-6

Cerebral blood flow, maintenance of, 90

Cerebrovascular mechanism, exercise effects on movement, 90-91

Chronic disease, societal costs, 2-4

Chronic exercise effects, body composition factors, 255-256; cardiovascular adaptations, 250-257; central circulatory factors, 254-255; coordinated movement, 89; locomotion, 83-84; motor unit, 67-70; movement, 86-89; neurosynergies, 76-77; peripheral oxidative factors, 255; pulmonary system, 278-281; reflexes, 72-73; static balance, 78-80; VO_2max, 250-256

Chronic health problems, 3

Circling concentrations of immune cells, 438

Clinical status, coronary heart disease, 15-16; hypertension, 16; NIDDM, 16-17; osteoporotic fractures, 17-18

Cold environments, aging response to, 337-339

Components of fitness, 26-27

Coordination, 88-89

Coronary Heart Disease (CHD), insulin resistance, 411-417; physical activity/fitness, 15-16

Costs, chronic disease, 2-4

Cytoxic activity, 438